Hearing Aid
Handbook
2011

Jeffrey J. DiGiovanni, Ph.D., CCC-A

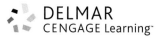

DELMAR
CENGAGE Learning

Australia • Brazil • Japan • Korea • Mexico • Singapore • Spain • United Kingdom • United States

DELMAR
CENGAGE Learning™

Hearing Aid Handbook, 2011

Jeffrey J. DiGiovanni, Ph.D., CCC-A

Vice President, Career and Professional Editorial: Dave Garza

Director of Learning Solutions: Matthew Kane

Senior Acquisitions Editor: Sherry Dickinson

Managing Editor: Marah Bellegarde

Product Manager: Laura J. Wood

Editorial Assistant: Anthony Souza

Vice President, Career and Professional Marketing: Jennifer Baker

Marketing Director: Wendy E. Mapstone

Senior Marketing Manager: Kristin McNary

Marketing Coordinator: Scott A. Chrysler

Production Director: Carolyn Miller

Senior Art Director: David Arsenault

For product information and technology assistance, contact us at **Cengage Learning Customer & Sales Support, 1-800-354-9706**

For permission to use material from this text or product, submit all requests online at **www.cengage.com/permissions**. Further permissions questions can be e-mailed to **permissionrequest@cengage.com**

Library of Congress Control Number: 2009939027

ISBN-13: 978-1-4354-8111-4

ISBN-10: 1-4354-8111-9

Delmar
5 Maxwell Drive
Clifton Park, NY 12065-2919
USA

Cengage Learning is a leading provider of customized learning solutions with office locations around the globe, including Singapore, the United Kingdom, Australia, Mexico, Brazil, and Japan. Locate your local office at: **international.cengage.com/region**

Cengage Learning products are represented in Canada by Nelson Education, Ltd.

To learn more about Delmar, visit **www.cengage.com/delmar**

Purchase any of our products at your local college store or at our preferred online store **www.CengageBrain.com**

Printed in the United States of America
1 2 3 4 5 6 7 12 11 10

To my nieces and nephews Frankie, Kathryn, Maddy, and Ryan
who are growing up much too quickly.

Table of Contents

Preface

If you are an audiologist, hearing aid dispenser, audiology student, or an employee of a hearing device company, then you are acutely aware of how complex the hearing device industry has become. For obvious reasons, dispensers (hearing aid dispensers or dispensing audiologists) generally dispense only a couple brands of hearing instruments. This fact points to the difficulty of keeping up with the industry. It's relatively easy to stay abreast of a couple companies. It is rather challenging to get the full story on all the other brands. If you are a student, it is likely your familiarity is derived from your clinical supervisors. Even then, you will probably only get a limited picture of the major players. But what about the other brands? What are their products, and what are their stories? The purpose of this book is to fill in the void between the entire industry and the hearing professional, whether the professional is a dispenser, a student, or in the industry.

Some time ago, it struck me that it is rather difficult to keep up with the technological advances, mergers, acquisitions, and branding changes in the hearing industry. The information seemed so diffuse. I concluded that a resource that provides a background on the various brands and their product offerings would be valuable to hearing professionals. With that, I made every attempt to be as objective as possible in reviewing the industry and each brand. To assist with this, I drew from published company analyses whenever possible.

Organization

The basic organization of the second edition is similar to that of the first, just expanded. This book begins with an overview of the hearing instrument industry. This includes a recent history of technology and business transactions. The current status of the marketplace is reviewed followed by a review of hearing instrument technology.

Following the first chapter are eleven more chapters, ten of which are dedicated to a particular hearing instrument brand. Brand history is detailed, complete with philanthropic activities and warranty information. After this, photos, features, and specifications are provided for the hearing instruments currently sold by each company. The final chapter is new in this edition and covers tinnitus as it relates to the hearing instrument industry. Tinnitus is a difficult problem to address, but there are effective devices and treatments for tinnitus, both of which have to be carefully implemented. This chapter provides a broad overview of the problem of tinnitus, available therapies that use sound therapy (with wearable devices), and a discussion of why more progress has not been made. Finally, as an added bonus, there are two appendixes. Contained in Appendix A is a series of philanthropic organizations related to hearing instruments. Generally, these organizations help get hearing aids to those without sufficient recourses to purchase them. This can be invaluable to compassionate dispensers who simply want to serve their patients. Contained in Appendix B is a list of acronyms and terms used in this book. This will assist the uninitiated in understanding the more discipline-specific terms.

It is important to note that the hearing instrument product information, including specifications, was provided by the manufacturers. In that regard, there is some variability in how the data was collected. For instance, in some cases, ANSI 1996 standards were used; in others, ANSI 2003 was used. Quite simply, the data reported by the manufacturers is reported here. However, there is also substantial variability in how the manufacturers *report* the data (e.g., format). To assist the reader, I have established a single presentation style across all companies.

While every attempt has been made to ensure accuracy and currency, neither the author nor the publisher are responsible for either errors in reporting or changes in the features and/or specifications.

New Online Companion Web Site Available

Log on to http://www.delmarlearning.com/companions to access the latest product information and updates from the hearing aid manufacturers profiled in this book.

About the Author

Jeffrey J. DiGiovanni is an associate professor and the coordinator of professional programs at Ohio University's School of Hearing, Speech, and Language Sciences. In his laboratory, the Auditory Psychophysics and Signal Processing Laboratory, he directs several doctoral students. He actively publishes in the areas of psychoacoustics and hearing-aid signal processing. He teaches various courses in the Au.D. program, including psychoacoustics, bioacoustics, balance, and, of course, hearing aids.

Jeff has worked with various hearing-related start-up companies, including a company that manufactures a surgically implantable hearing aid. He earned his bachelor's degree in electrical engineering, followed by his master's in audiology and Ph.D. in communication disorders with a focus on psychoacoustics and signal processing.

Acknowledgments

I am extremely grateful to Jessica Prewitt and Allison Mester, who, throughout this entire process, have kept detailed records of the hearing instrument companies' activities and product offerings. I am also grateful for the great level of interest and participation from the included hearing aid manufacturers.

Reviewers

Delmar Cengage Learning would like to thank the following reviewers for their time and valuable input throughout the development process:

Radhika Aravamudhan, Ph.D., CCC-A, FAAA
Assistant Professor, External Education Program Coordinator
George S. Osborne College of Audiology at Salus University
Elkins Park, Pennsylvania

Scott J. Bally, Ph.D., Professor
Gallaudet University
Department of Hearing, Speech, and Language Sciences
Washington, District of Columbia
Shanin L. Goodall, Au.D., CCC-A
Doctor of Audiology
Hear USA/HEARx
State Brandon, Florida

Myles Kessler, Au.D.
Adjunct Faculty
University of Connecticut
Storrs, Connecticut
Director of Audiology & Cochlear Implant Services
ENT Medical & Surgical Group, LLC
New Haven, Connecticut

Susan Ann T. Roberts, Au.D., CCC-A
Clinical Associate Professor
University at Buffalo
The State University of New York
Buffalo, New York

Christina Stocking, Au.D., CCC-A
Clinical Assistant Professor
University at Buffalo
The State University of New York
Buffalo, New York

CHAPTER ONE

The Hearing Instrument Industry

THE HEARING INSTRUMENT MARKETPLACE

Hearing instruments have evolved tremendously over the past 25 years. As of 1980, hearing instruments were fairly low-tech, with output compression the only available high-end feature. Certain technical innovations allowed for miniaturization to be the major research and development focus of the 1980s. In-the-canal (ITC) and then, in the early 1990s, completely-in-canal (CIC) hearing instruments were introduced and popularized to combat stigma issues (Mueller, 2006). The 2000s brought in the connectivity revolution by allowing small behind-the-ear (BTE) or open-fit hearing aids to be programmed wirelessly and connect to numerous peripheral devices. However, stigma still remains the largest reason for such poor market penetration.

Anyone who lived through the 1980s and 1990s knows how computers and related technologies developed at incredible rates. Computers went from novelty items without much utility to highly integrated, productive equipment for almost every sector. In the 1980s and 1990s, hearing instruments were still in the technological dark ages. Perhaps they were smaller, but they were still analog nonprogrammable devices at the turn of the decade, which makes the technological advances of the 1990s all the more significant. The early- to mid-1990s brought programmable hearing instruments to the forefront. Through a computer interface, though not required for all programmable hearing instruments, the hearing professional could program the hearing aid to the specific needs of the patient. Finally, in the mid-1990s, fully digital hearing instruments were introduced. Being in the field at that time, I remember all the exuberance surrounding this. Company representatives and audiologists at conferences swore up

1

and down how much clearer digital hearing instruments sounded. Companies touted these as better than the analog hearing instruments. Although the first generation of fully digital hearing instruments facilitated the fitting process, the performance of these devices was not quite up to the claims. In their defense, these first-generation instruments were simply digital implementations of analog devices. Or, more simply, they were doing more or less exactly what analog hearing instruments did, but digitally.

It is interesting to consider why hearing instrument technology lagged behind many other technologies. Digitally encoded music (i.e., the compact disc and players) has been widely available since the early 1980s. So why has that, and all other technologies, been late to be integrated into hearing instruments? The single, biggest reason for this is simple: Hearing instruments are small. Miniaturization follows innovation. Digital theory and application to sound may have been well developed in the 1980s, but it took another decade before the hardware was ready for hearing instrument applications. And even then, this generation did not provide more benefit to patients than their analog counterparts. But size encompasses more than just fitting the technology into a small package. Hearing instruments run on extremely low power, around 1 milliampere for all the components combined. To make this feasible, these digital systems had to be designed for low power to keep the battery small, thus keeping the overall package a reasonable size.

The transition from analog hearing instruments to their digital counterparts represented a critically important, one-time transition. This transition into the "digital domain" opened up endless signal-processing avenues to improve the speech signal for the hearing impaired, especially in noisy situations. While the first step into the digital world simply asked, "Can we do it?" the question now is, "What should we do with it?" This latter question involves determining and implementing signal-processing strategies that will improve the effective speech-to-noise ratio for hearing instrument users. Great strides have been made in this direction by different companies taking on different approaches to this challenge. Generally, companies aim to improve the signal-to-noise ratio or the effects of noise and reverberation, improve microphone directionality, process the speech signal to improve intelligibility, and reduce negative aspects of fittings (e.g., occlusion effect), all while streamlining the fitting process.

To better understand the hearing instrument industry, several aspects of it are analyzed in the following sections. First, a view of the market, or potential market, is described. Then, a broad view of the corporate standings, including market share, branding, and mergers and acquisitions, is provided. Finally, a profile of each company is provided at the beginning of each company's chapter to understand better how each company has its place in the industry.

The Market

As of 2008, there were approximately 36 million adults in the United States with some degree of hearing loss (NIDCD, 2009). This is expected to grow to over 50 million by 2030 and 80 million by 2040 (Kochkin, 2004, 2005). This is not surprising given the Baby Boomer population bubble, the first of which turned 60 in 2006. However, despite a large population of the hearing-impaired, U.S. market penetration remains a challenge at less than 25 percent, and as low as 20 percent (Kochkin, 2005, 2009; NIDCD, 2009). This has been attributed, at least in part, to the Baby Boomers' cultural fear of aging; they tend to remain in denial of hearing loss (Clemens & Sørensen, 2003). Aging populations represent a large proportion of the hearing-impaired, with 47 percent of Americans over 75, and 30 percent aged 65 to 74, having hearing loss (NIDCD, 2009). On a positive note, user satisfaction from hearing instruments has increased more than 10 percentage points since the MarkeTrak series was initiated in 1991. Satisfaction rates for new devices or devices between 1 and 4 years old are 77.5 percent and 73 percent, repectively, according to a survey of hearing instrument users (Kochkin, 2005). Other estimates show customer satisfaction rates closer to 70 percent (Stursberg, 2005). Although these numbers are encouraging, they do suggest that there is still room for improvement, especially in technology. In fact, market strategists are banking not only on technology, as it improves the performance of hearing instruments, but also on the belief that this will attract the more techno-friendly, active, communicative elderly (Phonak, 2006a). The hearing instrument industry is relying on open-fit hearing instruments to attract the traditionally resistant aging population as their main strategy to break the so-far impenetrable 20- to 25-percent market penetration (Clemens & Sørensen, 2003; Handelsbanken, 2006a; NIDCD, 2009). Unfortunately, because of the barriers to entry—and therefore to innovation—in this industry, some industry analysts remain doubtful of the industry's ability to increase penetration and reduce stigma (Clemens & Sørensen, 2003).

Hearing instruments are becoming more expensive despite a consistently low insurance reimbursement. The average cost of BTE, in-the-ear (ITE), and ITC hearing instruments has systematically increased from just over $600 per device in 1989 to just under $1,400 in 2005 (Kochkin, 2005). The average price paid for a digital hearing instrument is just over $2,000 (Clemens & Sørensen, 2003). Knowing that the latest high-end open-fit hearing instruments can exceed $3,500 each leads one to conclude that the market is bottom-heavy. That is, the majority of hearing instrument buyers purchase lower-end (i.e., lower-cost) hearing instruments, bringing the average price down. Despite the increasing prices of hearing instruments, third-party payments, which do not include purchases made by Veterans Affairs (VA), remain under 23 percent. As the average age of hearing instrument buyers is about 70, this puts an increasing financial burden on the aging population.

It is well-known that those eligible for VA and Medicare/Medicaid benefits typically receive some, if not total, hearing aid coverage. A recent benefit has been implemented as of January 1, 2009, for federal employees enrolled in the Federal Employees Health Benefits Plan. The coverage varies depending on the carrier, but ranges from a lifetime benefit of $500 to $1,000 per ear every 36 months (Healthy Hearing, 2009a). Another federal mandate in process is a $500 tax credit per hearing aid every 60 months for either all persons (as the Senate version dictates) or for persons under 18 years of age or over 55 (according to the House version) (Healthy Hearing 2009b). In addition, in the past few years, states have begun to mandate private insurance coverage. Most states with such mandates include age caps, usually 18 years of age. Rhode Island is the only state that has no age limit. A summary of coverage is as follows; note that some of these bills may still be pending (ASHA, 2009a,b; Audiology Online, 2008; Blue Cross Blue Shield, 2009; Hearing Loss Association of America, 2009; Hearing Loss Web, 2009; Hearing Review, 2008; LSHA, 2009; Rhode Island State House, 2006):

- California: $1,500 for children under 18 years; in process; refer to Senate Bill 1638
- Colorado: no cap, every 60 months for children under 18 years
- Connecticut: $1,000 coverage every 24 months for persons 12 years or younger
- Delaware: $1,000 per hearing aid every 36 months for children under 18 years
- Kentucky, Louisiana, and Maryland: $1,400 per hearing aid every 36 months for children under 18 years
- Illinois: $2,500 per hearing aid every 36 months; currently in Illinois State Legislature (State of Illinois, 2009)
- Louisiana: $1,400 per hearing aid every 36 months for children under 18 years
- Maine: $1,400 per hearing aid every 36 months for children up to 18
- Maryland: $1,400 per hearing aid every 36 months for minors who purchase, are fit and dispensed by a licensed audiologist
- Minnesota: no cap, one hearing aid per ear every 36 months for children under 18 years
- Missouri: varying coverage for screening, audiological assessment and hearing aids for newborns
- New Jersey: $1,000 per hearing aid every 24 months for children 15 years and younger
- New Mexico: $2,200 maximum coverage for up to two hearing aids every 36 months for children under 18 years, or up to 21 years if still attending high school (New Mexico State Legislature, 2007)
- Ohio: 50 percent coverage minus insurer-imposed co-payment; bill pending (HB No 110, 124th General Assembly)
- Oklahoma: no cap, every 48 months for children under 18 years
- Oregon: HB 3185 failed in committee; would have covered $1,200 per hearing aid every 48 months
- Rhode Island: $1,500 per hearing aid every 36 months for individuals under 19 years, and $700 per hearing aid every 36 months for individuals 19 years and older
- Virginia: HB 237 failed; would have covered $1,500 per hearing aid every 24 months for children under 18 years (State of Virginia, 2009)
- Wisconsin: uncapped cost of cochlear implants and hearing aids every 36 months for children 18 years and younger

The Marketplace: Consolidation and Market Share

The corporate scene has evolved dramatically in recent history. Most of this evolution is the natural maturing process of the hearing instrument industry, leading to fewer companies with greater market share. For example, in 1994, it took 20 manufacturers to hold 80 percent of the market share, whereas in 2003, the top 6 companies held 87 percent of the market share. In 2004, the "big six" held 94 percent (Parkhøi & Jessen, 2003; Stursberg, 2005). This process has occurred in part because of shorter product life cycles and thus increased cost of research and development (Parkhøi & Jessen, 2003). These reasons also create two sets of barriers: (a) barriers to entry, or new companies entering the industry, and (b) barriers to innovation. With this knowledge, it would be tempting to think that the industry and marketplace would be simplified. This is far from the case. Understanding the hearing instrument industry is still challenging because, despite mergers and acquisitions, separate brand names are often maintained. Table 1–1 shows the various brands under each manufacturer. A brand holds a certain value; brands are recognizable. Branding is so strong that most Americans still ask for a Kleenex® when really asking for a tissue. Nevertheless, consolidation in the hearing instrument industry brought greater market share to fewer players.

Ninety-five percent of the market share is held by the largest six hearing instrument companies (in order of worldwide market share from greatest to least): Siemens, William Demant Holding (hereafter William Demant), Sonova Holding AG (hereafter Sonova), Resound, Starkey Laboratories (hereafter Starkey), and Widex (Gretler et al., 2008; Phonak 2007; Gretler, 2004; Stursberg, 2005). Sonic Innovations has started to make its presence known with a notable 2 percent market share (Gretler et al., 2008). A breakdown of the market share holdings is shown in Figure 1–1. However, there are difficulties in making

Resound	Siemens	Sonova	Starkey	Widex	William Demant
Resound	Siemens Hearing	Phonak	Starkey	Widex	Oticon
Beltone	Rexton	Unitron Direct	Micro-Tech		Bernafon
Danavox	Electone	Lori Unitron	Audibel		Avada
Viennatone	A&M Hearing	Argosy	NU-EAR		
Philips Hearing					
Interton					

TABLE 1–1. Various brandings of the "big six" hearing instrument manufacturers, each with less than 5 percent market share. The top row is the manufacturer; below the manufacturer are their brands (Global Markets Direct, 2008a; Gretler et al., 2008; Kirkwood, 2006; Parkhøi & Jessen, 2003; Klemme, 2008a, 2008b).

Delmar/Cengage Learning

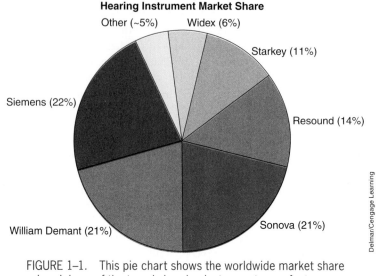

Hearing Instrument Market Share

Other (~5%)   Widex (6%)

Starkey (11%)

Siemens (22%)

Resound (14%)

William Demant (21%)

Sonova (21%)

Delmar/Cengage Learning

FIGURE 1–1.   This pie chart shows the worldwide market share breakdown of the top six hearing instrument manufacturers (Gretler et al., 2008; Phonak, 2007; Gretler, 2004; Stursberg, 2005).

a detailed analysis of the industry. One difficulty is that, despite consolidation, it is common for the acquiring company to maintain the branding of the subsidiary. Sonova purchased Unitron Direct (hereafter Unitron) in 2000, but Unitron maintains its own product line and branding (Parkhøi & Jessen, 2003, 2005). As far as any consumer is concerned, or dispenser for that matter, they are totally separate companies. However, the market share data are reported together. Therefore, it is difficult to discern what part of Sonova's overall market share can be attributed to its individual brands. The other challenge is that some of the major players in this industry are private companies, and therefore are not required to make detailed reports as are publicly traded companies. Starkey Laboratories and Widex are two such companies.

It is unlikely that the hearing instrument industry has completed its consolidation. The factors that have driven consolidation still continue, namely the shorter product cycle (2 to 3 years) and the increased cost to bring new products to market (i.e., research and development). The size of the hearing instrument market grows by about 4 to 6 percent per year, while the cost of research and development grows 10 to 15 percent per year (Parkhøi & Jessen, 2003, 2005). The Phonak Group officially changed its name to Sonova in August 2007. In doing so, they are maintaining the Phonak brand while providing a level playing field for their other brands (Phonak, 2007).

As far as further consolidation goes, both Starkey and Widex are desirable companies, but their owners have so far been unwilling to sell. Siemens is unlikely to sell, as its brand could not be part of the deal. Siemens Hearing represents about 0.5 percent of Siemens Global, which has enormous product offerings in numerous sectors. The name Siemens is highly recognized in each of these sectors. The drawback to this is that if Siemens desires to sell a particular division, the brand "Siemens" could not go along with it, thus reducing its desirability.

Return Rates

There are two types of return rates that get reported and that, on the surface, disagree. It is important to understand the actual and functional meaning of each. Both are useful pieces of information and should be reported together. As of 1999, the overall return rate for hearing instruments was about 18 percent, which is within 1 percent of what it was in 1995 (Northern & Beyer, 1999). As of 2006, return rates for all form factors combined dropped to 15.6 percent, the highest returns observed for BTEs (17.6 percent) and the lowest for ITEs (12.8 percent) (Strom, 2007). These numbers represent patients who buy hearing instruments and subsequently return them, but they do not track whether the patient purchased a different hearing instrument or simply walked away with nothing. In more than half of these cases, the patient ends up with a different hearing instrument. This number is often referred to as the "return for credit."

The second number that is reported as a "return rate" represents situations of actual lost sales, where the patient walks away with nothing, as does the hearing professional. Across all hearing instruments' form factors (e.g., BTE, ITE, etc.) and technology, 7 percent of hearing instrument purchasers return the device(s) without purchasing another one (Strom, 2001). This "lost sale" rate represents a true loss of revenue and service effort. The difference between the two rates, about 11 percent, represents the percentage of time the hearing professional will have to return a hearing instrument and purchase a different hearing instrument for the same patient. For specific form factors, CIC lost-sales rates are 6 percent, and those for digital hearing instruments are 9 percent (Strom, 2001). However, for this group of repurchasers, about half of them purchase a different brand in an attempt to get a better-functioning hearing instrument for the price (Kochkin, 2003). It has been suggested that the addition of aural rehabilitation can reduce the 7 percent lost-sale rate to 3 percent (Wayner, 2005).

Hearing Instruments: Technology Overview

The past few years have been good for hearing instruments. Finally, the promises of digital signal processing are paying off, and in some surprising ways. While direct processing of sound has certainly increased and improved, the most significant advancements have been largely due to applications of technology that are enabled by the hearing instrument's digital processor. What does that mean? As we discussed earlier, early digital hearing instruments had features similar to those of their analog counterparts. Once this technology was proven, research and development moved toward creating the signal processing to reduce noise and otherwise make speech more intelligible. This consisted largely of noise-reduction algorithms, processing for multiple microphones, and various forms of speech enhancement (e.g., spectral enhancement, speech-feature enhancements). As these algorithms became fairly well-established, a new algorithm came on the scene: feedback reduction. The successful application of acoustic cancellation to the feedback problem helped usher in the open-fit phenomenon. In the nonhearing technology sector, wireless technology had been advancing rapidly, so the time was right for the hearing industry to apply wireless technologies to hearing instruments. This new direction has already made a substantial, tangible difference to hearing instruments. The major recent advancements for hearing instruments have related to the application of wireless technology and the ability to make in situ measurements. The application of digital and related technologies has permanently changed the scene of hearing instruments, which has drastically improved both the speed and quality of the fitting process when performed by well-trained hearing professionals.

Signal Processing and Software

Once manufacturers established their digital platforms, the world became wide open to advancements in signal processing. Initially, efforts were put toward the processing of the sound stream to improve speech intelligibility. The payoffs of these strategies were mixed, but I think it is safe to say that there were not any home runs. Once it became clear that there weren't going to be quick returns in these early processing algorithms, the majority of "new" types of digital software were developed to support other technologies. Strictly speaking, the term "signal processing" becomes a misnomer as it indicates processing of a signal, presumably the incoming sound signal. However, software written and used within hearing instruments uses the same hardware resources as the true signal-processing software. This other software can be used to support other features of the hearing instrument, such as data logging, wireless connectivity, and the ability to make in situ measurements. A summary of signal processing specific to the incoming signal will be provided here, followed by some other applications of digital software.

The development and innovation of digital signal-processing strategies is complicated, as some came in and out of fashion while others have stayed and continually improved. So rather than expend considerable space on detailing this development and innovation of the strategies, they are discussed in broader, more categorical terms, including noise reduction, multiple microphones, and the like. Noise reduction represents one of the earlier efforts in digital sound processing. Noise, as opposed to the bulk of speech, is a random signal. Speech also has a syllabic rate that can be detected as amplitude modulation. These modulations allow for speech to be differentiated from the noise. These speech detectors, integrated into the hearing instrument, allow for the differentiation of speech and noise in various frequency bands. Finally, gain is decreased in the bands with the worst signal-to-noise ratios (SNR) to improve the overall SNR. The success of this type of algorithm was not terribly impressive when employed on a single-microphone instrument. A critical factor in allowing these noise reduction algorithms to work is separating the noise from the speech, or more generally, source separation. It turns out that separating the incoming signal into separate sources and categorizing them as "signal" or "noise" is an incredibly difficult task for hearing instruments. This undoubtedly will be a major emphasis for signal processing in the future. Research has well established the principles our brain uses to determine one "auditory object" from another, but employing these principles in a hearing instrument to work in real time will be a programming challenge. In the meantime, the current, most effective method of noise reduction is the use of multiple microphones. Multiple microphones allow for a sort of spatial filtering, reducing the relative intensity level of a signal based on location. Multimicrophone systems require processing to set the directional pattern of the array. Generally, it is assumed that zero degrees azimuth (i.e., straight ahead) is the preferred direction for listening. Various patterns have been developed, which may vary over time with added intelligence called *adaptive directionality*. The directionality of a microphone array can be altered via the processing associated with the microphone array, and if the software is well-designed, the directional pattern can automatically adjust to maximize the signal-to-noise ratio, even as these noise sources change location. While having more microphones requires more processing, it also provides greater flexibility. Theoretically, one fewer noise source than the number of microphones can be managed, meaning a *three*-microphone system can adequately amplify the signal in front of the listener while attenuating the input level of *two* noise sources. The system becomes less effective as the noise sources become more diffuse or occur in the presence of reverberation. Also, these microphones need to have fairly specific spacing, so there is a pretty tight limitation on the number of microphones a single device can handle. Generally, three microphones is the maximum for a larger BTE. Advances in binaural processing enabled by wireless technology offer encouraging improvements by allowing the microphones on both ears to work together, as is discussed in the next section.

Digital processing also implies that there must be some type of storage or memory. As with any digital system, software needs to be written to literally instruct the device how to function. This software is stored on the device. In recent years, added memory has been included in digital hearing instruments allowing for much greater storage than what is required for the core function of the instrument. Despite this greater storage, it is still quite limited when compared to your average personal music player (PMP). For example, the memory in a hearing instrument would only be able to hold a couple seconds of a single song, as opposed to a common PMP's capacity of thousands of songs. Nevertheless, this storage capacity has allowed for other data to be stored over time. This has led to a new feature in digital hearing instruments: data logging.

Data logging has evolved in two directions. First, with sufficient memory, the hearing instrument can store information about the user's environment and usage patterns over time. The hearing instrument can log in changes in volume, memory settings, usage duration, and the like. Similarly, a separate device can be worn. This second device has a microphone, some signal processing, and memory storage to store information about the listening environment. In both cases, the hearing professional can take these logged data from the appropriate device. These data can be analyzed to understand better the various listening situations to which the patient is exposed. Finally, these data can lead to a better prescription for the patient. Many current hearing instruments contain the intelligence to make adjustments for the user in real time. For instance, the hearing instrument may track volume position throughout the day and, eventually, make automatic adjustments, anticipating the user's needs. Similarly, the hearing instrument will be able to automatically enable the directional microphone system in appropriate situations, and even change frequency and compression profiles depending on the ambient noise level, spectrum, temporal properties, and signal-to-noise ratio. These are a sampling of various way manufacturers have implemented learning technologies into their products.

Despite multiple innovations in signal processing, the limitations in overcoming the distortion imposed by an impaired ear are even more challenging. When one considers the significant distortion created by inner hair cell or nerve loss (i.e., cochlear dead regions), audibility of the signal at appropriate frequencies may not lead to the best speech understanding. As a possible solution to this problem, manufacturers have resurrected an old processing idea and implemented in novel ways. Frequency transposition is when some or all of the frequency content of an input signal is remapped at the output. Originally introduced in the 1960s, frequency compression was a common way to employ this. Frequency compression is proportionally decreasing the frequencies. For example, a 5 percent compression would remap 100 Hz to 95 Hz and 1,000 Hz to 950 Hz. The goal of such a method is to improve audibility of higher frequency for those with a severe high-frequency loss. Unfortunately, some of the side effects, such as sound quality changes, of this classic method have made it non-preferred by hearing-aid users.

Over the past couple of years, manufacturers have released several new implementations of frequency transposition. One such method uses the frequency compression idea but limits it to a range of frequencies. By doing so, the goal is to improve the audibility of high-frequency sounds without changing the sound quality of low-frequency sounds. Another method that is offered uses a type of linear frequency transposition. In this case, a frequency range is moved to a different range. For example, for a precipitous loss with severe hearing loss at and above 2.0 kHz, either the more prominent aspects of the input signal above 2.0 kHz will be lowered or a fixed range of frequencies (e.g., 2.0–4.0 kHz) will be shifted and overlapped with a lower range of frequencies (e.g., 1.0–2.0 kHz). The sophistication in modern hardware allows for a great deal of customization in how transposition is implemented for particular patients. It is not known, however, how to predict which patients seeking hearing instruments will benefit from this technology. In sum, frequency transposition, being several decades old, may just have been an idea well before its time.

The technology in hearing instruments is limited largely by its physical size. Technology such as microphones, processors, memory chips, and wireless chips take up space and require power, both of which are precious commodities in hearing instruments. As memory size and power requirements decrease, it will be possible to integrate large memory chips into the devices to allow a multitude of capabilities. Think hearing instrument plus PMP. The current method that manufacturers employ to achieve broad functionality without sacrificing significant size or battery life is through a third device, often worn around the neck. This is discussed in detail below.

Throughout the short history of digital hearing instruments, a great deal of innovation has transpired. From the initial digital device that simply emulated the analog device to such advancements as multimicrophone arrays and adaptive directionality, the possibilities of the digital platform have yet to be maximized.

Feedback, Form Factors, and Fittings

Historically, hearing instruments have rarely exceeded a 4000-Hz frequency response. While this response is only a portion of the frequency response of the normal ear, it made great strides toward amplifying frequencies important for speech understanding. It has long been known that ~3000 Hz is the minimum frequency bandwidth for speech communication, which is how telephony specifications were determined. However, this bandwidth was determined using sentences. Since sentences are rich in context and only represent a portion of our listening experience, this bandwidth should only serve as an absolute minimum for communication and not the ideal. This is why we still have to say things like, "*Esss*, as in *Sam*" or "*Efff*, as in *Frank*," as they sound nearly identical with this reduced frequency response. At the very least, a broader frequency response will improve the listening experience and can perhaps improve speech perception, especially in the presence of competing sounds.

Poor frequency response historically has been limited by technology. Hearing instrument dispensers constantly try to strike a balance between minimizing the occlusion effect while prescribing appropriate gain at high frequencies. With the close proximity of the microphone and receiver, the entire amplification system is prone to feedback. Until recently, the preferred method of reducing feedback has been to reduce the size of the vent or eliminate it altogether. In addition, the occlusion effect often became problematic, especially in situations where the patient has decent low-frequency thresholds. When CICs were introduced in the 1980s, the proposed solution was to have a deep fit evidenced by going past the second bend of the external auditory meatus (EAM). Once it was assured that the ear mold or shell did this, it became reasonable to expect that the end of the ear mold or shell was in the bony region of the EAM. Much of the occlusion effect is a result of sounds being conducted into the EAM through the cartilaginous region. So, if the medial end of the ear mold or shell goes beyond this region, the occlusion effect can be dramatically reduced. Eventually, this method was employed in all form factors, including BTE ear molds. The success of this remedy was limited by active ears, less-than-ideal fits, and other complications. If a person is said to have "active ears," his or her jaw movement causes changes in ear canal morphology such that it interferes with the quality of the fit of the hearing instrument during such movements. Other ideas have been developed, such as adaptive notch filters, but the real winner in this arena has been the integration of acoustic-cancellation technology to reduce the occurrence of feedback.

Acoustic cancellation is a technique that can be applied to reduce the energy of a known signal. Perhaps the easiest way to explain this technology is through a common application: noise-reducing headphones. Noise-reducing headphones look and sound similar to any other headphone but have the added feature of acoustic-cancellation technology. For instance, if one wears these headphones on an airplane, there is significant background noise that can interfere with the listening experience. The headphones, however, have a feature where they can sample the noise via a microphone on the outside and estimate what time, level, and spectral changes there will be at the output of the headphone. The circuitry in the headphone performs these operations and then inverts the phase. If the headphones do their job, the ambient sounds entering the EAM will be exactly the same as the processed ambient sounds reproduced by the headphone, except that the phase is inverted. In this manner, the two otherwise identical sounds are added together like a positive number and its negative equivalent, and the noise is eliminated. Of course, this is an idealized scenario. In the real world, these headphones have more modest reduction of ambient noise and work best for low-level, constant, low-frequency sounds.

For hearing instruments, acoustic cancellation represents a dramatic improvement in the reduction of feedback. To do this, a more sophisticated processing algorithm had to be developed. For this technology to work with hearing instruments, the device first needs to detect the occurrence of feedback. Once feedback is detected, the parameters, including frequency and level, are assessed. Following this, the device creates an identical signal, phase-inverted at the sound output. To maximize efficiency, the phase is adjusted to maintain maximal feedback reduction. In a well-designed system, the occurrence, detection, and elimination of the feedback signal is almost transparent to the user. This type of transparency of technology to the end user is critical for the success of hearing instruments.

This application of acoustic-cancellation technology enabled the hearing industry to add a form factor, the "open fit." On the face of it, one could argue that a BTE with a skeletal mold is an open fit. However, this new form factor represents a more substantial departure from the traditional BTE. First, being true to its name, it departs from the standard requirement of a custom ear mold. Of course, these are digital instruments. Open-fit hearing instruments have some other characteristics, including a typically small body for the "BTE" case, thin tubing with a noncustom ear bud, and some form of feedback management system, usually using a specialized application of acoustic cancellation. Because of the standard ear buds, patients can have a hearing evaluation and a hearing instrument fitting, and can take their new instruments with them, all on the same day.

As an alternative to the open fit just described, most manufacturers offer the option of placing the receiver in the ear canal, thus the so-called receiver-in-the-ear (RITE) or receiver-in-the-canal (RIC). This slight change in receiver placement allows the body of the instrument to be smaller (by removing the receiver), and manufacturers have argued that a greater amount of gain can be attained. This certainly facilitates greater high-frequency response without the high-frequency energy-sucking thin tubing. Also, the physical setup of an unoccluded ear has limited the amount of low- and mid-frequency gain that has been available. Over the past couple of years, however, receiver manufacturers have made significant progress toward improving receiver technology such that greater (or actual) gains may be provided at mid- and mid-low frequencies for both RITE and open-fit instruments. Limitations in high-frequency gain are generally due to feedback rather than driver technology (Rickets et al., 2007). Nevertheless, many manufacturers have devices with frequency responses beyond 10.0 kHz. So while this technology offers promising returns, some of these promises are being realized now, and further progress is certainly to come.

So if open-fit instruments can be dispensed in the same day, what about those times when an open fit is inappropriate (e.g., excessive high-frequency loss, any audible low-frequency loss)? Does the patient *still* have to wait a week or two to get the new hearing instruments? Well, the simple answer is no, but there is still a wait. Multiple manufacturers (e.g., Siemens iScan, Widex CAMISHA) offer electronic scanning of impressions. These devices, while embodying incredible technology, are simple to use. Essentially, once the hearing professional makes the impressions, they are placed in the scanner, which makes a three-dimensional rendering of the impressions. These "e-impressions" can be directly uploaded to the manufacturer. Until this technology became available, the physical impression was the only part of the order that prevented an electronic submission of the order. Now, with e-impressions, the entire order can be submitted electronically (Lesiecki, 2006). This process, combined with advances in ear mold and shell manufacturing, saves many days between the prescription and fit of the custom hearing instrument.

Finally, digital technology has facilitated the fitting process through in situ measurements. This application allows various measurements to be made while the hearing instrument is worn by the patient as fit by the hearing professional. In situ measurements require the generation of stimuli and/or the measurement of sound levels. Sound generation and/or analysis is not difficult with a digital platform. Currently, multiple manufacturers offer technology that can measure in situ audiograms and/or make real-ear measurements with the hearing instrument. Unfortunately, only a small proportion of hearing professionals actually make real-ear measurements. It is difficult to say if this is due to lack of training or awareness of the importance of real-ear measurements, an unwillingness to spend the money on appropriate hardware, or the resistance to spending the extra few minutes to know—truly know—how much gain the patient is receiving from his or her hearing instruments. The technology allowing for the hearing instrument to make real-ear measurements eliminates one of those reasons as a factor.

Wireless Applications

As stated, the application of various technologies to hearing instruments seems to come after many other applications of technology. Whether it is digital technology, directional microphones, or even wireless technology, they have all existed in a fairly mature form before they became popular in hearing instruments. Hearing instruments have a market that will only entertain the products within certain physical dimensions. This has worked against hearing instruments in two ways: (a) the physical size of the technology (e.g., digital microchip), and (b) increased power consumption that often requires a larger battery to provide an acceptable interval between battery changes. Despite great improvements in these areas, this one-two punch is still the limiting factor in the development of wireless technologies in hearing instruments.

The Hearing Aid Compatibility Act of 1988 and the Federal Communication Commission's (FCC's) subsequent modification now require compatibility between digital wireless phones and hearing instruments (Myers, 2005). Part of the hearing industry's response to this includes the introduction of Bluetooth™ technology that can "plug into" hearing instruments. The first thing this allows is cell phone compatibility. Unfortunately, the power required for Bluetooth means that the Bluetooth technology cannot be integrated into the hearing instrument. One current solution consists of a large Bluetooth appendage to the instrument. Alternatively, more devices are required. In the latter case, a third device with a bigger, rechargeable battery houses the Bluetooth technology to interface with a cell phone. This third remote device communicates with the hearing instrument through a much lower power and proprietary wireless protocol that the hearing instrument can house (Yanz, 2006). So, to make this work, this remote device acts as an intermediary between the cell phone and the hearing instrument. If this sounds clunky, it is. But this still represents an important step in the integration of common wireless protocols into hearing instruments. Eventually, power sources for hearing instruments will improve, while wireless systems will become smaller and more efficient, allowing the more consumer-friendly wireless protocol to be housed within the hearing instrument. Eventually, it is likely that a large proportion of hearing instruments will convert their power sources to rechargeable batteries; only a few models currently have this feature. Even though rechargeable batteries have a lower power density, meaning they will have less charge for the physical size of the battery, they only have to run for 1 or 2 days before recharging. This is in contrast to disposable batteries that consumers demand run for at least 5 to 7 days. At about a dollar apiece, this could represent a savings of $100 per year for hearing instrument users. This can also result in an overall increase in available power as the reduction in time required to run on a charge is less than the reduced power density of rechargeable batteries relative to disposable batteries. Up until 2008, rechargeable lithium-ion and lithium-polymer batteries were limited to about 300 charges or so before the charge capacity significantly decreased. However, new innovations have increased that to beyond 1,000, or even 1,400, charges (Lane, 2009; Nickish, 2008).

This means that, with careful integration into the hearing instruments, new rechargeable batteries in hearing aids should last at least 3 years, and up to 6 years with charging every 2 days. With these battery advancements in longevity and available power, the transition into rechargeable batteries will facilitate the integration of new technologies into hearing instruments.

As wireless technologies improve, especially in the areas of size and power consumption, hearing instruments will benefit more from them. Eventually, it can be expected that commonly used wireless protocols will be housed inside hearing instruments, an event that will be made possible as rechargeable hearing instruments become a standard, at least for high-end instruments. Furthermore, I believe that the improved integration of wireless technologies will allow greater compatibility with many devices in addition to cell phones for improved listening experiences. Some examples of this include personal music listening, computer interfacing, and even public performance situations like churches, live shows, movie theaters, and the like. Hearing professionals will be greatly relieved when wireless protocols are standardized with a universal, wireless programming system. This application alone will save the hearing professional time and inconvenience in connecting and programming hearing instruments. It is plausible, even, that hearing instruments may be programmable virtually through a secure Internet connection to the hearing professional's office.

Only recent releases of hearing instruments have been able to wirelessly communicate at a high data rate. Several brands offer hearing instruments that can "talk" to each other to maintain the same memory mode or volume level, or otherwise react similarly and simultaneously to ambient conditions. This basic communication requires a very low-speed data transfer and allows the instrument on each ear to remain synchronized. As advances are made, the communication rates have increased greatly and allowing for the signal received in each ear to be processed by both devices. This will almost certainly not only improve the directionality of microphone systems, but also enable better calculation of source locations for sounds and provide better localization cues to the user. Eventually, hearing instruments will take into account elevation of sound sources, rather than only incorporating the assumption that sound sources are all in the horizontal plane. In addition, digital binaural processing will improve the CROS (contralateral routing of signals) and BiCROS (bilateral-CROS) applications. There are already wireless devices that can transmit the audio signal from one device to the other, but this is generally an analog signal without much sophisticated processing. The application of a digital, wireless system will improve the efficiency, connectivity, and effectiveness of these devices.

The application of wireless technologies to hearing systems has started to blur the line between the medically prescribed hearing instrument and consumer electronics. It has even been suggested that a hearing instrument dispensing office may serve both hearing-impaired and normal-hearing populations (Yanz, 2006). In fact, I have heard from hearing professionals that normal-hearing individuals are purchasing hearing instruments to obtain the connectivity these devices offer. The future of hearing instruments is indeed bright, and the devices are in a rapid advancement phase. These innovations are absolutely welcomed by users and hearing professionals. It is critical, however, that these highly touted technologies are developed responsibly, using rigorous test methods to ensure that they actually benefit the user in real-world listening situations. With the advancements in technology and improved manufacturing techniques, I continue to be hopeful that the prices of hearing instruments will level off or, even better, come down. A streamlined fitting process, higher success rates, and off-site programming requiring fewer office visits almost demand this.

CHAPTER TWO

Bernafon

BERNAFON: SWISS ENGINEERING WITH LATIN NAMING

International Headquarters
Bernafon AG
International Headquarters
Morgenstrasse 131
CH-3018 Bern
Switzerland
Web site: http://www.bernafon.com

U.S. Headquarters
Bernafon, LLC
200 Cottontail Lane, Bldg. B
Somerset, NJ 08873
USA
Phone: 1 (888) 941-4203
Web site: http://www.bernafon-us.com

The year 2006 represented an important milestone for Bernafon as it celebrated its sixtieth anniversary of manufacturing hearing instruments. The story, however, began 22 years prior to 1946, when it introduced its first hearing instrument. Founded in 1924, Gfeller AG in Flamatt, France, developed and manufactured electromechanical devices. The founder, Hans Gfeller, suffered from a severe hearing loss, which led the company to develop its first hearing instrument in 1946.

Bernafon's mission is specific: "to help people hear and communicate better by providing Innovative Hearing Solutions" (Bernafon, 2007a). The company has stated its strengths to be in the devices themselves, including electroacoustic systems, design and manufacture of hearing instrument hardware, and software design (Bernafon, 2006a). This stated focus on innovation seems to play out in its corporate structure. Of the 110 employees at its headquarters, 70 are directly involved in the various aspects of product development. The company has a total of 500 employees worldwide on four continents (Bernafon, 2006b). From all appearances, despite being a wholly owned subsidiary of William Demant Holding, it is run as a relatively independent entity.

Some of Bernafon's milestones are as follows (from Bernafon, 2009, 2007a, unless otherwise stated):

1924: founded as Gfeller AG in Flamatt, France
1946: introduced its first hearing instrument, called the A1 2-pack, a body-worn hearing instrument
1951: introduced a body-worn hearing instrument with an integrated battery (C TG)
1955: innovated the hearing instrument by adding three controls (F400)
1963: introduced its first BTE (H70)
1972: reworked the BTE to use a size 13 battery (S4)
1986: acquired Maico Hearing Instrument in Minneapolis, MN
Ascom group integrated Gfeller AG and Autophon and became Ascom Audiosys AG
1986: introduced the Charisma, its first ITC
1988: introduced first digitally programmable BTE (PHOX) as well as the programming console (PX 8)
1992: acquired Robert Bosch GmbH
1992: introduced a remote control with digitally programmable hearing instruments
1995: acquired by William Demant Holding A/S and the division was renamed to Bernafon; Bernafon's new headquarters were established in Bern, Switzerland
1997: introduced its first two-channel wide dynamic range compression (WDRC) hearing instrument (Dualine and Dualine Digital)
1999: introduced a family of fully digital hearing instruments with multiple programs and directional microphones (SMILE)
2000: acquired Dahlberg Inc., a Canadian hearing instrument company
2001: opened up sales to Poland
2003: moved its U.S. hearing division from Minneapolis, MN, to Franklin Township, NJ—2 miles from Oticon, Inc. (also owned by William Demant Holding) (*HJ Report*, 2003)
2004: opened up sales to the Netherlands
2005: introduced its first mini-BTE for open fittings (SwissEar™)
2006: sixtieth anniversary of hearing-related product activities
2006: introduced data logging with software to interpret the data and program the device to the user's typical listening experience (ICOS)
2006: introduced receiver-in-the-ear hearing instrument which won the "red dot" design award (Brite)
2009: binaural communication between hearing instruments was included in new device line, also allowing Bluetooth connectivity (Vérité)

Warranty

Bernafon's hearing instruments generally include a standard 2-year warranty and a 1-year loss and damage warranty. Loss and damage extensions for an additional year or two can be purchased (Bernafon, 2007b).

PRODUCT INFORMATION

PRODUCT 1: VÉRITÉ

Product Application

VÉRITÉ 505 M-speaker
VÉRITÉ 505 P-speaker

Features of VÉRITÉ M-speaker and VÉRITÉ P-speaker

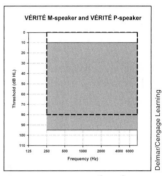

Fitting range for VÉRITÉ 505 M-speaker (outlined region) and VÉRITÉ 505 P-speaker (shaded region)

- Bernafon ChannelFree™ DSP
- Wireless binaural coordination between left and right instrument
- Multi-environment program with spectral enhancement
- Adaptive directionality
- Adaptive noise reduction – reduces gain when signal is suspected to be noise
- Soft Noise Management™ – reduces level of soft environmental noise
- Fast transient signal compression system
- Data logging and learning
- 2 receiver power options
- Automatic telephone detection
- Personalization by lifestyle profile and data learning
- 4 freely assignable program memories
- Multi-environment
- Dedicated programs for specific situations

Options of VÉRITÉ M-speaker and VÉRITÉ P-speaker

- Optional RC-P remote control
- Optional SoundGate for Bluetooth wireless technology or aired DAI reception
- Telephone, GPS and TV reception microphone with Bluetooth wireless technology

Typical Specifications		VÉRITÉ M-speaker	VÉRITÉ P-speaker
Standard ANSI S3.22-2003			
Output sound pressure level	Max OSPL 90 (dB SPL)	109	120
	HF-Average OSPL 90 (dB SPL)	104	117
Full-on gain	Peak gain (dB)	47	59
	HF-Average-Full-on gain (dB)	41	58
Total harmonic distortion	500 Hz	<0.5%	<1.5%
	800 Hz	<0.5%	<1.5%
	1600 Hz	<1%	<1%
Equivalent input noise (dB SPL)		17	15
Telecoil sensitivity	HFA-SPLITS (dB SPL)	n/a	n/a
Battery	Operating current (mA)	1.2	1.3
	Battery type	312	312

Delmar/Cengage Learning

PRODUCT 2: MOVE

Product Application

MOVE 106 BTE DM
MOVE 105 BTE DM VC
MOVE 112 BTE VC
MOVE 315 ITC DM VC
MOVE 305 ITC DM
MOVE 400 CIC

Features of MOVE 106 BTE DM

- 7-channel advanced signal processing
- Automatic program with 9 modes
- Adaptive 4-band directionality
- Adaptive noise reduction in 8 bands – reduces gain when signal is suspected to be noise
- Soft Noise Management – reduces level of soft environmental noise
- Adaptive feedback canceller – uses acoustic cancellation to reduce feedback
- Feedback manager – a component of the fitting software that allows the practitioner to minimize the likelihood of feedback
- Tracker data logging with fine-tuning suggestions
- Music, telephone, and auditorium programs
- Individually adjustable programs for direct audio input and telecoil
- Program copy function
- Multi-program assistant
- Adaptive directional microphone system

- Push-button control of hearing instrument functions
- Remote-control reception coil
- Best for mild to moderately severe hearing loss

Options of MOVE 106 BTE DM

- Earhook/SPIRA^{flex} option
- Optional remote control
- 10 color options

Features of MOVE 105 BTE DM VC

- 7-channel advanced signal processing
- Automatic program with 9 modes
- Adaptive 4-band directionality
- Adaptive noise reduction in 8 bands – reduces gain when signal is suspected to be noise
- Soft Noise Management – reduces level of soft environmental noise
- Adaptive feedback canceller – uses acoustic cancellation to reduce feedback
- Feedback manager – a component of the fitting software that allows the practitioner to minimize the likelihood of feedback
- Tracker data logging with fine-tuning suggestions
- Music, telephone, and auditorium programs
- Individually adjustable programs for direct audio input/FM and telecoil
- Program copy function
- Multi-program assistant
- Adaptive directional microphone system
- Push-button control of hearing instrument functions
- Volume control
- Remote-control reception coil
- Best for mild to severe hearing loss

Options of MOVE 105 BTE DM VC

- Earhook/SPIRA^{flex} option
- Optional remote control
- 6 color options

Features of MOVE 112 BTE VC

- 7-channel advanced signal processing
- Automatic program with 9 modes
- Adaptive noise reduction in 8 bands – reduces gain when signal is suspected to be noise
- Soft Noise Management – reduces level of soft environmental noise
- Adaptive feedback canceller – uses acoustic cancellation to reduce feedback
- Feedback manager – a component of the fitting software that allows the practitioner to minimize the likelihood of feedback

- Tracker data logging with fine-tuning suggestions
- Music, telephone, and auditorium programs
- Individually adjustable programs for direct audio input/FM and telecoil
- Program copy function
- Multi-program assistant
- Omnidirectional response
- Push-button control of hearing instrument functions
- Volume control
- Remote-control reception coil
- Best for mild to severe/profound hearing loss

Options of MOVE 112 BTE VC

- Earhook/SPIRA^{flex} Option
- Optional remote control
- 6 color options

Features of MOVE 315 ITC DM VC

- 7-channel advanced signal processing
- Automatic program with 9 modes
- Adaptive 4-band directionality
- Adaptive noise reduction in 8 bands – reduces gain when signal is suspected to be noise
- Soft Noise Management – reduces level of soft environmental noise
- Adaptive feedback canceller – uses acoustic cancellation to reduce feedback
- Feedback manager – a component of the fitting software that allows the practitioner to minimize the likelihood of feedback
- Tracker data logging with fine-tuning suggestions
- Music, telephone, and auditorium programs
- Program copy function
- Multi-program assistant
- Adaptive directional half-shell and canal instrument
- Push-button control of hearing instrument functions
- Volume control
- Omnidirectional response
- Best for mild to moderately severe hearing loss

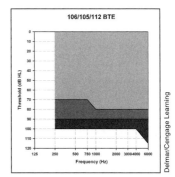

Fitting range for MOVE 106 BTE DM SPIRA^{flex} (light gray only), MOVE 105/106 BTE DM VC Earhook (medium and light gray), and MOVE 112 BTE VC (all shaded regions)

Options of MOVE 315 ITC DM VC

- Optional telecoil
- Optional remote-control reception coil
- Optional remote control

- Optional auto telephone
- Optional without volume control
- 4 color options

Features of MOVE 305 ITC DM

- 7-channel advanced signal processing
- Automatic program with 9 modes
- Adaptive 4-band directionality
- Adaptive noise reduction in 8 bands – reduces gain when signal is suspected to be noise
- Soft Noise Management – reduces level of soft environmental noise
- Adaptive feedback canceller – uses acoustic cancellation to reduce feedback
- Feedback manager – a component of the fitting software that allows the practitioner to minimize the likelihood of feedback
- Tracker data logging with fine-tuning suggestions
- Music, telephone, and auditorium program
- Program copy function
- Multi-program assistant
- Adaptive directional canal instrument
- Push-button control of hearing instrument functions
- Best for mild to moderately severe hearing loss

Options of MOVE 305 ITC DM

- Optional telecoil
- Optional remote-control reception coil
- Optional remote control
- Optional auto telephone
- 4 color options

Features of MOVE 400 CIC

- 7-channel advanced signal processing
- Automatic program with 9 modes
- Adaptive noise reduction in 8 bands – reduces gain when signal is suspected to be noise
- Soft Noise Management – reduces level of soft environmental noise
- Adaptive feedback canceller – uses acoustic cancellation to reduce feedback
- Feedback manager – a component of the fitting software that allows the practitioner to minimize the likelihood of feedback
- Tracker data logging with fine-tuning suggestions

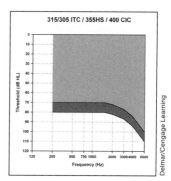

315/305 ITC / 355HS / 400 CIC

Fitting range for MOVE 400 CIC (light gray only) and MOVE 305 ITC DM, MOVE 315 ITC DM VC, and MOVE 355 HS DM VC (all shaded regions)

- Music, telephone, and auditorium programs
- Program copy function
- Multi-program assistant
- Best for mild to moderate hearing loss

Options of MOVE 400 CIC

- Optional remote-control reception coil
- Optional remote control
- 4 color options

Typical Specifications		MOVE 400 CIC	MOVE 305	MOVE 315
Standard ANSI S3.22-2003				
Output sound pressure level	Max OSPL 90 (dB SPL)	104	110	112
	HF-Average OSPL 90 (dB SPL)	98	104	107
Full-on gain	Peak gain (dB)	34	41	43
	HF-Average Full-on gain (dB)	31	34	38
Total harmonic distortion	500 Hz	<1%	<1%	<1%
	800 Hz	<1%	<1%	<1%
	1600 Hz	<1%	<1%	<1%
Equivalent input noise (dB SPL)		17	15	15
Telecoil sensitivity	HFA-SPLITS (dB SPL)	n/a	84	85
Battery	Operating current (mA)	0.8	1.2	1.2
	Battery type	10	312	312

Delmar/Cengage Learning

Typical Specifications		MOVE 106 BTE Earhook	MOVE 105 BTE Earhook	MOVE 112 BTE Earhook
Standard ANSI S3.22-2003				
Output sound pressure level	Max OSPL 90 (dB SPL)	124	123	133
	HF-Average OSPL 90 (dB SPL)	117	113	126
Full-on gain	Peak gain (dB)	57	60	71
	HF-Average Full-on gain (dB)	50	53	65
Total harmonic distortion	500 Hz	<2%	<1%	<2%
	800 Hz	<2%	<1%	<1%
	1600 Hz	<1%	<1%	<1%
Equivalent input noise (dB SPL)		13	13	12
Telecoil sensitivity	HFA-SPLITS (dB SPL)	101	96	109
Battery	Operating current (mA)	1.3	1.2	1.4
	Battery type	312	13	13

Delmar/Cengage Learning

PRODUCT 3: BRITE

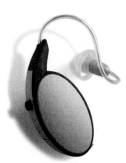

Brite BTE
Courtesy of Bernafon

Product Application

Brite 502 RITE DM
Brite 503 RITE DM

Features of Brite 502 RITE DM and Brite 503 RITE DM

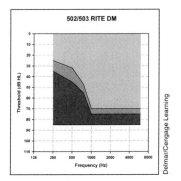

Fitting range for Brite 502 RITE DM and Brite 503 RITE DM for a micro mold (all shaded regions), tulip dome (medium and light gray), and open dome (light gray only)

- Receiver-in-the-ear technology
- Enhanced cosmetics due to small size
- Lifestyle-driven technology allows fittings to be individually customized
- Adaptive directional microphones
- Adaptive noise reduction system – reduces gain when signal is suspected to be noise
- Manual programs
  - Brite 502 RITE DM – audio navigation and 1 manual program
  - Brite 503 RITE DM – performance priority and 2 manual programs
- Audio Navigation Program™ – automatically changes settings appropriate for current listening environment (Brite 503 RITE DM only)
- Performance priority in the automatic program (Brite 502 RITE DM only)
- Remote control compatibility
- Compatible with open domes, tulip domes, and custom micro molds
- Programmable via OASIS plus 8.5

Options of Brite 502 RITE DM and Brite 503 RITE DM

- Colors: anthracite, mocha brown, birch beige, dune beige, stone, Sahara gold, olive green, copper, cranberry red, and pinot blue

Typical Specifications		Brite 503 RITE DM	Brite 502 RITE DM
Standard ANSI S3.22-2003			
Output sound pressure level	Max OSPL 90 (dB SPL)	109	109
	HFA OSPL 90 (dB SPL)	103	103
Full-on gain	Peak gain (dB)	50	50
	HFA (dB)	43	43
Total harmonic distortion	500 Hz	<1%	<1%
	800 Hz	<1%	<1%
	1600 Hz	<2%	<2%
Equivalent input noise (dB SPL)*		18	18
Telecoil sensitivity	HFA SPLITS (dB SPL)	n/a	n/a
Battery	Operating current (mA)	1.3	1.3
	Battery type	312	312

*Technical data measured with expansion, corresponding to Soft Noise Management level 3.

Delmar/Cengage Learning

PRODUCT 4: ICOS

Product Application

ICOS 106 BTE DM
ICOS 105 BTE DM
ICOS 105 BTE DM VC
ICOS 205 ITE DM VC
ICOS 315 ITC DM VC
ICOS 355 HS DM VC
ICOS 305 ITC DM
ICOS 415 MC DM
ICOS 410 MC/ICOS 400 CIC

Features of ICOS 106 BTE DM

- Micro-size BTE housing
- Lifestyle-driven technology
- Audio Navigation Program – automatically changes settings appropriate for current listening environment
- 7 channels
- Multidimensional directionality in 4 bands
- Adaptive noise reduction in 8 bands – reduces gain when signal is suspected to be noise
- Soft Noise Management – reduces level of soft environmental noise
- Adaptive feedback cancellation
- OpenFit™
- Adaptive signal unification
- 3 configurable listening programs (choice of 11 different programs)

- ICOS tracker data logging system
- Compatible with open dome, tulip dome, custom tip, and canal molds
- Suitable for mild to moderate hearing loss

Options of ICOS 106 BTE DM

- Colors: titan, platinum, gold, anthracite, black, gray, gray-brown, beige, brown, and graphite
- Compatible with SPIRA^{flex} sound tube system
- Remote control
- DAI compatibility
- Mute function

Features of ICOS 105 BTE DM and ICOS 105 BTE DM VC

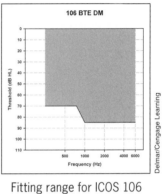

- Audio Navigation Program – automatically changes settings appropriate for current listening environment
- 3 configurable listening programs
- Dedicated DAI/FM listening program
- Multidimensional directionality – adaptive directional microphone system and automatic mode selection
- Adaptive noise reduction in 8 bands – reduces gain in the band(s) in which signal is suspected to be noise

Fitting range for ICOS 106 BTE DM

- Audio Recognition™ with 4 different monitors to detect presence of speech, noise, or wind
- Soft Noise Management – reduces level of soft environmental noise
- Adaptive feedback cancellation – uses acoustic cancellation to reduce feedback
- OpenFit with low-frequency compensation
- 7-channel digital signal processing
- ICOS tracker (data logging) with fine-tune proposals
- Sound Check™ within OASIS fitting software helps verify first fit
- 7-channel TriQualizer™ within OASIS fitting software allows for 3 different input levels (50, 60, and 85 dB) within each channel
- Clinical and lifestyle profile – audiometric data customized to the listening situations of the patient
- Remote control reception
- Ear hooks
- Programmable telecoil
- Push-button control of hearing instrument functions
- Volume control (ICOS 105 BTE DM VC only)
- Recommended for mild to severe hearing loss
- Programmed with OASIS plus, version 6.0 or later

Options of ICOS 105 BTE DM and ICOS 105 BTE DM VC

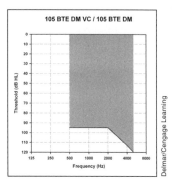

Fitting range for ICOS 105 BTE DM VC/105 BTE DM

- FMA3 adaptor for FM communication systems only
- DAI2 adaptor for connection to Hi-Fi, TV set, PC, etc.
- Optional ear hooks and children's ear hooks available
- SPIRA thin sound tube 0.9
- Colors: blue, platinum, gold, anthracite, black, white, green, yellow, rose, blue, gray, gray-brown, beige, brown, and graphite

Features of ICOS 205 ITE DM VC, ICOS 315 ITC DM VC, ICOS 355 HS DM VC, ICOS 305 ITC DM, ICOS 415 MC DM, and ICOS 410 MC/ICOS 400 CIC

- Audio Navigation Program – automatically changes settings appropriate for current listening environment
- 3 configurable listening programs
- Additional auto telephone program
- Multidimensional directionality – adaptive directional microphone system and automatic mode selection
- Adaptive noise reduction in 8 bands – reduces gain in the band(s) in which signal is suspected to be noise
- Audio Recognition with 4 different monitors to detect presence of speech, noise, or wind
- Soft Noise Management – reduces level of soft environmental noise
- Adaptive feedback cancellation – uses acoustic cancellation to reduce feedback
- OpenFit with low-frequency compensation
- 7-channel digital signal processing
- Clinical and lifestyle profile – audiometric data customized to the listening situations of the patient
- Push-button control of hearing instrument functions (ICOS 205 ITE DM VC, ICOS 315 ITC DM VC, ICOS 355 HS DM VC, and ICOS 306 ITC DM only)
- Volume control (ICOS 205 ITE DM VC, ICOS 315 ITC DM VC, and ICOS 355 HS DM VC only)
- ICOS tracker (data logging) with fine-tune proposals
- Sound Check within OASIS fitting software helps verify first fit
- 7-Channel TriQualizer within OASIS fitting software allows for 3 different input levels (50, 60, and 85 dB) within each channel
- ICOS 205 ITE DM VC, ICOS 315 ITC DM VC, ICOS 355 HS DM VC, and ICOS 305 ITC DM are recommended for mild to moderately severe hearing loss

- ICOS 415 MC DM, ICOS 410 MC, and ICOS 400 CIC are recommended for mild to moderate hearing loss
- Programmable via OASIS plus, version 6.0 or later

Options of ICOS 205 ITE DM VC, ICOS 315 ITC DM VC, ICOS 355 HS DM VC, ICOS 305 ITC DM, ICOS 415 MC DM, and ICOS 410 MC/ICOS 400 CIC

- Remote-control reception coil
- Programmable telecoil (ICOS 205 ITE DM VC, ICOS 315 ITC DM VC, ICOS 355 HS DM VC, and ICOS 305 ITC DM only)
  - Auto telephone – automatically switches to telecoil with detection of telephone (ICOS 205 ITE DM VC, ICOS 315 ITC DM VC, ICOS 355 HS DM VC, and ICOS 305 ITC DM only)
- Colors: beige, pink, brown, and dark brown

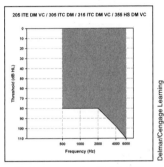

Fitting range for ICOS 305 ITC DM/315 ITC DM/205 ITE DM/VC

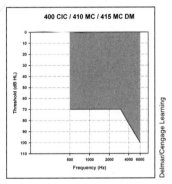

Fitting range for ICOS 400 CIC/410 MC/415 MC DM

Typical Specifications		ICOS 106 BTE DM SPIRA^{flex} Tube 0.9	ICOS 106 BTE DM SPIRA^{flex} Tube 1.3	ICOS 105 BTE DM VC	ICOS 105 BTE DM
Standard ANSI S3.22-2003					
Output sound pressure level	Max OSPL 90* (dB SPL)	117	121	123	123
	HFA OSPL 90 (dB SPL)	108	113	113	113
Full-on gain	Peak gain* (dB)	47	50	60	60
	HFA (dB)	41	46	53	53
Total harmonic distortion	500 Hz	<1%	<1%	<1%	<1%
	800 Hz	<1%	<1%	<1%	<1%
	1600 Hz	<1%	<1%	<1%	<1%
Equivalent input noise (dB SPL)		16	12	13	13

continues

continued

Typical Specifications		ICOS 106 BTE DM SPIRA^{flex} Tube 0.9	ICOS 106 BTE DM SPIRA^{flex} Tube 1.3	ICOS 105 BTE DM VC	ICOS 105 BTE DM
Telecoil sensitivity	HFA-SPLITS (dB SPL)	n/a	n/a	96	96
Battery	Operating current (mA)	1.3	1.3	1.2	1.2
	Battery type	312	312	13	13

*Measurements made according to IEC 60118-7 (2cc).

Delmar/Cengage Learning

Typical Specifications		ICOS 205 ITE DM VC	ICOS 315 ITC DM VC/ICOS 255 HS DM VC	ICOS 305 ITC DM	ICOS 415 MC DM	ICOS 410 MC/ ICOS 400 CIC
Standard ANSI S3.22-2003						
Output sound pressure level	Max OSPL 90* (dB SPL)	112	112	110	104	104
	HFA OSPL 90 (dB SPL)	107	107	104	98	98
Full-on gain	Peak gain* (dB)	46	43	41	34	34
	HFA (dB)	41	38	34	30	31
Total harmonic distortion	500 Hz	<1%	<1%	<1%	<1%	<1%
	800 Hz	<1%	<1%	<1%	<1%	<1%
	1600 Hz	<1%	<1%	<1%	<1%	<1%
Equivalent input noise (dB SPL)		14	15	15	14	17
Telecoil sensitivity	HFA-SPLITS (dB SPL)	85	85	84	n/a	n/a
Battery	Operating current (mA)	1.2	1.2	1.2	1.1	0.8
	Battery type	13	312	312	10	10

*Measurements made according to IEC 60118-7 (2cc).

Delmar/Cengage Learning

PRODUCT 5: SYMBIO^{XT}

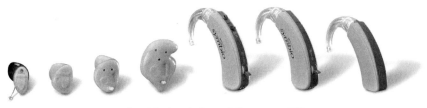

Symbio family from CIC though BTE
Courtesy of Bernafon

Product Application

Symbio XT 100 BTE
Symbio XT 110 BTE
Symbio XT 115 BTE DM
Symbio XT 200 ITE
Symbio XT 205 ITE DM
Symbio XT 320 ITC
Symbio XT 325 ITC DM
Symbio XT 410 MC
Symbio XT 400 CIC

Features of Symbio XT 100 BTE, Symbio XT 110 BTE, and Symbio XT 115 BTE DM

- OpenFit to avoid occlusion
- ChannelFree™ – frequency-based gain without filtering signal into separate bands
- Adaptive feedback canceller – uses acoustic cancellation to reduce feedback
- Battery end-of-life signal
- High cellular phone immunity
- Developed for FM communication (Symbio XT 110 BTE and Symbio XT 115 BTE DM only)
- DAI (Symbio XT 110 BTE and Symbio XT 115 BTE DM only)
- Dual microphones for directionality (Symbio XT 115 BTE DM only)
- Mini-BTE (Symbio XT 100 BTE only)
- Compact power BTE (Symbio XT 110 BTE and Symbio XT 115 BTE DM only)
- Switches to change programs (excludes Symbio XT 100 BTE)
- Programmable telecoil (Symbio XT 110 BTE and Symbio XT 115 BTE DM only)
- Symbio XT 100 BTE recommended for mild to moderately severe hearing loss
- Symbio XT 110 BTE and Symbio XT 115 BTE DM recommended for moderate to severe hearing loss
- Programmed via OASIS plus fitting software

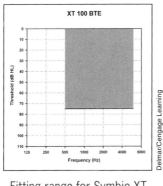

Fitting range for Symbio XT
100 BTE

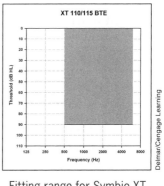

Fitting range for Symbio XT
110 BTE/115 BTE

Options of Symbio XT 100 BTE, Symbio XT 110 BTE, and Symbio XT 115 BTE DM

- FMA2 adaptor used for FM communication, CROS 2 (accessory), and connection to Hi-Fi, TV set, PC, etc. (Symbio XT 100 BTE, Symbio XT 110 BTE, and Symbio XT 115 BTE DM only)
- Colors: beige, brown, gray, black, and dark gray
- Optional ear hooks and children's ear hooks available

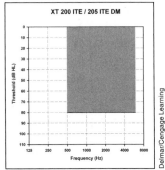

Fitting range for Symbio XT 200 ITE/205 ITE DM

Features of Symbio XT 200 ITE, Symbio XT 205 ITE DM, Symbio XT 320 ITC, Symbio XT 325 ITC DM, Symbio XT 410 MC, and Symbio XT 400 CIC

- OpenFit to avoid occlusion
- ChannelFree – frequency-based gain without filtering signal into separate bands
- Adaptive feedback canceller – uses acoustic cancellation to reduce feedback
- Battery end-of-life signal
- High cellular phone immunity
- Dual microphones for directionality (Symbio XT 205 ITE DM and Symbio XT 325 ITC DM only)
- Symbio XT 200 ITE and Symbio XT 205 ITE DM recommended for moderate to severe hearing loss
- Symbio XT 320 ITC, Symbio XT 325 ITC, Symbio XT 410 MC, and Symbio XT 400 CIC recommended for mild to moderately severe hearing loss
- M/DM switch (Symbio XT 205 ITE DM and Symbio XT 325 ITC DM only)
- Programmed via OASIS plus fitting software

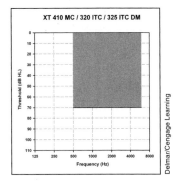
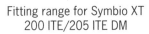

Fitting range for Symbio XT 400 MC/320 ITC/325 ITC DM

Options of Symbio XT 200 ITE, Symbio XT 205 ITE DM, Symbio XT 320 ITC, Symbio XT 326 ITC DM, Symbio XT 410 MC, and Symbio XT 400 CIC

- Programmable or automatic T-coil (Symbio XT 200 ITE, Symbio XT 205 ITE DM, Symbio XT 320 ITC, and Symbio XT 325 ITC DM only)

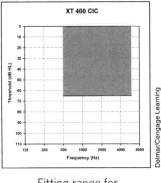

Fitting range for Symbio XT 400 CIC

- M/T switch (Symbio XT 200 ITE, Symbio XT 205 ITE DM, Symbio XT 320 ITC, and Symbio XT 325 ITC DM only)
- ON/OFF switch (Symbio XT 200 ITE, Symbio XT 205 ITE DM, Symbio XT 320 ITC, and Symbio XT 325 ITC DM only)
- Colors: beige, pink, brown, dark brown (Symbio XP 200 ITE, Symbio XP 320 ITC, Symbio XP ITE DM, and Symbio XP 325 ITC DM)

Typical Specifications		Symbio XT 100 BTE	Symbio XT 110 BTE	Symbio XT 115 BTE DM
Standard ANSI S3.22-1996				
Output sound pressure level	Max OSPL 90* (dB SPL)	127	131	131
	HFA OSPL 90 (dB SPL)	119	125	125
Full-on gain	Peak gain* (dB)	52	62	62
	HFA (dB)	45	56	56
Total harmonic distortion	500* Hz	0.5%	1.4%	2%
	800* Hz	0.5%	0.4%	0.5%
	1600* Hz	0.4%	0.2%	0.3%
Equivalent input noise (dB SPL)		22	23	23
Telecoil sensitivity	HFA-SPLITS (dB SPL)	n/a	104	104
Battery	Operating current (mA)	1.0	1.1	1.1
	Battery type	13	13	13

*Measurements made according to IEC 60118-7 (2cc).
Delmar/Cengage Learning

Typical Specifications		Symbio XT 200 ITE	Symbio XT 320 ITC	Symbio XT 410 MC	Symbio XT 400 CIC
Standard ANSI S3.22-1996					
Output sound pressure level	Max OSPL 90* (dB SPL)	120	110	110	106
	HFA SSPL 90 (dB SPL)	116	105	105	102
Full-on gain	Peak gain* (dB)	55	45	38	34
	HFA (dB)	50	39	32	30
Total harmonic distortion	500 Hz	0.8%	0.6%	0.8%	1.1%
	800 Hz	0.5%	0.6%	0.9%	1.0%
	1600 Hz	0.4%	0.6%	1.2%	1.8%
Equivalent input noise (dB SPL)		22	22	25	24
Telecoil sensitivity	10 mA/m 1000 Hz (dB SPL)	100	90	n/a	n/a
Battery	Operating current (mA)	1.0	1.0	1.0	1.0
	Battery type	13	312	10	10

*Measurements made according to IEC 60118-7 (2cc).
Delmar/Cengage Learning

Typical Specifications		Symbio XT 205 ITE DM	Symbio XT 325 ITC DM
Standard ANSI S3.22-1996			
Output sound pressure level	Max OSPL 90* (dB SPL)	120	110
	HFA SSPL 90 (dB SPL)	116	106
Full-on gain	Peak gain* (dB)	55	45
	HFA (dB)	49	40
Total harmonic distortion	500 Hz	0.4%	0.5%
	800 Hz	0.5%	0.5%
	1600 Hz	0.3%	0.5%
Equivalent input noise (dB SPL)		23	22
Telecoil sensitivity	10 mA/m 1000 Hz (dB SPL)	91	90
Battery	Operating current (mA)	1.1	1.1
	Battery type	13	312

*Measurements made according to IEC 60118-7 (2cc).

Delmar/Cengage Learning

PRODUCT 6: SWISSEAR

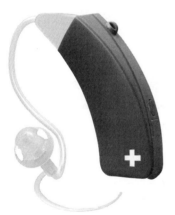

SwissEar BTE with earhook
Courtesy of Bernafon

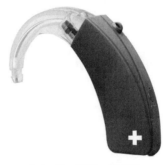

SwissEar BTE with Thin
Sound Tube
Courtesy of Bernafon

Product Application

SwissEar 106 BTE D

Features of SwissEar 106 BTE D

- Directional microphone
- Phonemic compression using fast time constants

- Soft Noise Management – reduces level of soft environmental noise
- ChannelFree Signal Unification – frequency-based gain without filtering signal into separate bands
- Adaptive feedback canceller – uses acoustic cancellation to reduce feedback
- No occlusion allows for comfortable fitting
- Fully automatic
- ON/OFF function via battery drawer
- Switches easily between thin tube to ear hook
- 3-step conversion function to full gain BTE
- SoundMaster™ for client-oriented fitting
- In situ audiometry for more precise fit
- SwissEar 106 BTE D with thin sound tube is a mini-BTE for mild to moderately severe ski-slope hearing loss
- Programmed via OASIS plus fitting software

Fitting range for Swiss Ear 106 BTE D with Thin Sound Tube

Options of SwissEar 106 BTE D

- Ear hook
- Wide range of colors: black/silver, gray/silver, beige, and pearl white

Typical Specifications		SwissEar 106 BTE D Thin Sound Tube	SwissEar 106 BTE D Earhook
Standard ANSI S3.22-2003			
Output sound pressure level	Max OSPL 90* (dB SPL)	115	126
	HFA OSPL 90 (dB SPL)	105	119
Full-on gain	Peak gain* (dB)	38	61
	HFA (dB)	36	50
Total harmonic distortion	500* Hz	n/a	n/a
	800* Hz	0.3%	1.5%
	1600* Hz	0.3%	0.5%
Equivalent input noise* (dB SPL)		24	23
Telecoil sensitivity	HFA-SPLITS (dB SPL)	n/a	n/a
Battery	Operating current (mA)	1.2	1.2
	Battery type	13	13

*Measurements made according to IEC 60118-7 (2cc).

Delmar/Cengage Learning

PRODUCT 7: SMILE PLUS

Product Application

Smile Plus 100/110/120 BTE
Smile Plus 115 BTE DM
Smile Plus 200 ITE
Smile Plus 310/320/321 ITC
Smile Plus 410 MC
Smile Plus 401 CIC
Smile Plus 205 ITE DM
Smile Plus 315 ITC DM
Smile Plus 325 ITE DM

Features of Smile Plus 100/110/120 BTE and Smile Plus 115 BTE DM

- Dual microphone technology accessed via a local switch or an optional remote control (excludes Smile Plus 100/110/120 BTE)
- Programmable via Oticon plus fitting software
- Three-dimensional fitting system
- High fitting success rate thanks to multi-channel technology
- 2 listening programs to meet individual client needs
- Feedback management – a notch filter centered ~3000 Hz
- Individualized fitting solutions with the Smile Plus concept for user controls (local controls/fully automatic/optional remote control)
- User-operated rotated digital loudness control (DLC)
- Optimized speech intelligibility with the NAL-NL1 fitting
- Other common fitting algorithms are available
- High immunity from mobile telephone interference
- Programmable indicator for startup and low battery warning
- FM compatibility
- Digital technology for advanced sound quality and comfort
- Smile Plus 100 BTE recommended for mild to moderate hearing loss

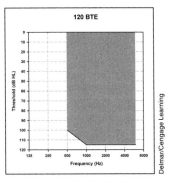

Fitting range for Smile Plus
120 BTE

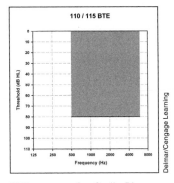

Fitting range for Smile Plus
110/115 BTE

- Smile Plus 110 and 115 BTE recommended for moderate to severe hearing loss
- Smile Plus 120 BTE recommended for moderate to profound hearing loss
- Telecoil
- Switches to change between programs or settings (excludes Smile Plus 100 BTE)

Options of Smile Plus 100/110/120 BTE and Smile Plus 115 BTE DM

- Optional ear hooks and children's ear hooks available
- Remote control
- Audio shoe/FM shoe (excludes Smile Plus 100 BTE)

Fitting range for Smile Plus 100 BTE

Features of Smile Plus 200 ITE, Smile Plus 205 ITE DM, Smile Plus 310/320/321 ITC, Smile Plus 410 MC, Smile Plus 401 CIC, Smile Plus 315 ITC DM, and Smile Plus 325 ITE DM

- Dual microphone technology assessed with a local switch or an optional remote control
- Programmable via OASIS plus fitting software
- Three-dimensional fitting system
- High fitting success rate thanks to multichannel technology
- 2 listening programs to meet individual client needs
- Feedback management – a notch filter centered ~3000 Hz
- Individualized fitting solutions with the Smile Plus concept for user controls (local controls/fully automatic/optional remote control)
- User-operated, rotary DLC
- Optimized speech intelligibility with the NAL-NL1 fitting algorithm
- Other common fitting algorithms available
- High immunity from mobile telephone interference
- Programmable indicator for startup and low battery warning
- Digital technology for advanced sound quality and comfort
- Efficient wax protection systems
- In situ audiometry
- Smile Plus 200 ITE, Smile Plus 205 ITE DM recommended for moderate to severe hearing loss
- Smile Plus 321 ITC, Smile Plus 325 ITE DM, Smile Plus 310 ITC DM, Smile Plus 321 ITC DM, Smile Plus 315 ITC DM, and Smile Plus 320 ITC recommended for mild to moderately severe hearing loss
- Smile Plus 410 MC and Smile Plus 401 CIC recommended for mild to moderate hearing loss

Options of Smile Plus 200 ITE, Smile Plus 205 ITE DM, Smile Plus 310/320/321 ITC, Smile Plus 410 MC, Smile Plus 401 CIC, Smile Plus 315 ITC DM, and Smile Plus 325 ITE DM

- Colors: beige, pink, and brown (brown only available with Smile Plus 410 MC and Smile Plus 410 CIC)
- Telecoil (excludes Smile Plus 315 ITC DM, Smile Plus 310 ITC DM, Smile Plus 410 MC, and Smile Plus 401 CIC)
- Automatic telecoil – automatically switches to telecoil with detection of telephone (excludes Smile Plus 315 ITC DM, Smile Plus 310 ITC DM, Smile Plus 410 MC, and Smile Plus 401 CIC)
- M/T switch or P1/P2 switch (excludes Smile Plus 310 ITC, Smile Plus 410 MC, and Smile Plus 401 CIC)
- Remote control

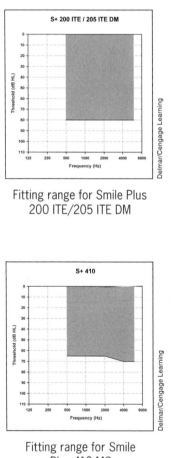

Fitting range for Smile Plus
200 ITE/205 ITE DM

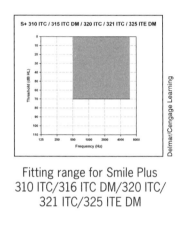

Fitting range for Smile Plus
310 ITC/316 ITC DM/320 ITC/
321 ITC/325 ITE DM

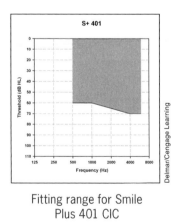

Fitting range for Smile
Plus 410 MC

Fitting range for Smile
Plus 401 CIC

BERNAFON

Typical Specifications		Smile Plus 100 BTE	Smile Plus 110 BTE	Smile Plus 115 BTE DM	Smile Plus 120 BTE
Standard ANSI S3.22-1996					
Output sound pressure level	Max OSPL 90* (dB SPL)	128	131	131	136
	HFA SSPL 90 (dB SPL)	120	124	124	130
Full-on gain	Peak gain* (dB)	54	67	64	74
	HFA (dB)	47	61	58	68
Total harmonic distortion	500 Hz	≤2%	≤2%	≤2%	≤4%
	800 Hz	≤2%	≤2%	≤2%	≤4%
	1600 Hz	≤2%	≤2%	≤2%	≤4%
Equivalent input noise (dB SPL)		26	26	26	26
Telecoil sensitivity	HFA-SPLITS (dB SPL)	100	109	108	127
Battery	Operating current (mA)	1.4	1.7	1.7	1.8
	Battery type	13	13	13	675

*Measurements made according to IEC 60118-7 (2cc).
Delmar/Cengage Learning

Typical Specifications		Smile Plus 200 ITE	Smile Plus 205 ITE DM	Smile Plus 315 ITC DM	Smile Plus 325 ITE DM
Standard ANSI S3.22-1996					
Output sound pressure level	Max OSPL 90* (dB SPL)	123	123	112	116
	HFA SSPL 90 (dB SPL)	117	117	107	110
Full-on gain	Peak gain* (dB)	55	55	40	48
	HFA (dB)	48	47	35	39
Total harmonic distortion	500 Hz	1%	1%	1%	1%
	800 Hz	1%	1%	1%	1%
	1600 Hz	1%	1%	1%	1%
Equivalent input noise (dB SPL)		26	26	28	27
Telecoil sensitivity	HFA-SPLITS (dB SPL)	96	96	n/a	89
Battery	Operating current (mA)	1.2	1.4	1.3	1.4
	Battery type	13	13	312	312

*Measurements made according to IEC 60118-7 (2cc).
Delmar/Cengage Learning

Typical Specifications		Smile Plus 320/321 ITC	Smile Plus 310 ITC	Smile Plus 410 MC	Smile Plus 401 CIC
Standard ANSI S3.22-1996					
Output sound pressure level	Max OSPL 90* (dB SPL)	116	113	109	107
	HFA SSPL 90 (dB SPL)	110	108	104	102
Full-on gain	Peak gain* (dB)	48	43	38	34
	HFA (dB)	39	39	33	27
Total harmonic distortion	500 Hz	1%	1%	1%	1%
	800 Hz	1%	1%	1%	1%
	1600 Hz	1%	1%	1%	1%
Equivalent input noise (dB SPL)		26	26	25	27
Telecoil sensitivity	HFA-SPLITS (dB SPL)	89	n/a	n/a	n/a
Battery	Operating current (mA)	1.2	1.2	1.1	1.1
	Battery type	312	312	10	10

*Measurements made according to IEC 60118-7 (2cc).

Delmar/Cengage Learning

PRODUCT 8: XTREME

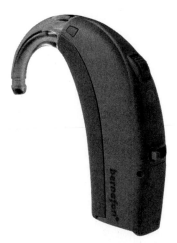

Xtreme 120 BTE
Courtesy of Bernafon

Product Application

Xtreme 120 BTE

Features of Xtreme 120 BTE

- 5-channel digital signal processing
- Adaptive feedback canceller
- Adaptive noise reduction
- Soft Noise Management – reduces level of soft environmental noise
- Independent MPO (maximum power output) shaping – 1 dB steps
- Variable time constants
- Fully programmable telecoil
- Fully programmable DAI
- Volume control with rotary function and OFF-function
- Status light
- 3 program switch
- Compatible with external inputs (FM, DAI, etc.)
- Xtreme 120 BTE suitable for severe to profound hearing loss

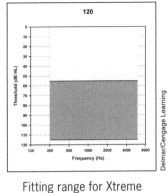

Fitting range for Xtreme 120 BTE

Options of Xtreme 120 BTE

- DAI
- Bone conductor
- CROS/BiCROS

Typical Specifications		Xtreme 120 BT
Standard ANSI S3.22-1996		
Output sound pressure level	Max OSPL 90 (dB SPL)	140
	HFA OSPL 90 (dB SPL)	132
Full-on gain	Peak gain (dB)	82
	HFA (dB)	73
Total harmonic distortion	500 Hz	2%
	800 Hz	2%
	1600 Hz	1%
Equivalent input noise (dB SPL)		27
Telecoil sensitivity	HFA SPLITS (dB SPL)	114
Battery	Operating current (mA)	2.6
	Battery type	675

Delmar/Cengage Learning

PRODUCT 9: PRIO

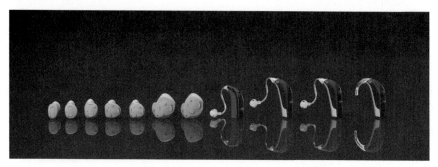

PRIO family from CIC though BTE
Courtesy of Bernafon

Product Application

Prio 112 BTE VC
Prio 105 BTE DM VC
Prio 105 BTE DM
Prio 202 ITE VC
Prio 205 ITE DM VC
Prio 322 ITC VC
Prio 315 ITC DM VC
Prio 305 ITC DM
Prio 415 MC DM
Prio 400 CIC

Features of Prio 112 BTE VC, Prio 105 BTE DM VC, and Prio 105 BTE DM

- Signal processing in 7 frequency channels
- Fully automatic program with 5 performance priorities
- Music, telephone, and auditorium programs
- Adaptive dual-band directionality (Prio 105 BTE DM VC and Prio 105 BTE DM only)
- Adaptive noise reduction – reduces gain when signal is suspected to be noise
- Soft Noise Management – reduces level of soft environmental noise
- Adaptive feedback manager – uses acoustic cancellation to reduce feedback
- Adaptive Signal Unification™ for optimal sound quality
- OpenFit with low-frequency compensation
- Tracker (data logging) with fitting recommendations
- Client profile with client lifestyle priorities – first fit based on audiometric data and lifestyle parameters

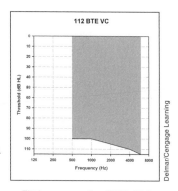

Fitting range for PRIO 112 BTE VC

Delmar/Cengage Learning

- Programmable telecoil
- Push-button control of hearing instrument functions
- FM communication
- DAI
- Volume control (excludes Prio 105 BTE DM)
- Ear hooks
- Performance priorities in the automatic program
- Individually adjustable programs for DAI/FM and telecoil
- Choice of cosmetic open fittings with SPIRA^{flex}
- Prio 112 BTE VC recommended for mild to severe/profound hearing loss
- Prio 105 BTE DM VC and Prio 105 BTE DM recommended for mild to severe hearing loss
- Programmable via OASIS plus fitting software

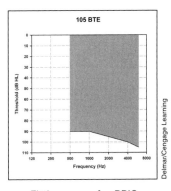

Fitting range for PRIO 105 BTE

Options of Prio 112 BTE VC, Prio 105 BTE DM VC, and Prio 105 BTE DM

- Colors: beige, gray-brown, anthracite, and black
- Optional remote control
- Optional ear hooks and children's ear hooks available
- SPIRA^{flex} sound tube 0.9/1.3 available

Features of Prio 202 ITE VC, Prio 205 ITE DM VC, Prio 322 ITC VC, Prio 315 ITC DM VC, Prio 305 ITC DM, Prio 415 MC DM, and Prio 400 CIC

- Signal processing in 7 frequency channels
- Fully automatic program with 5 performance priorities
- Music, telephone, and auditorium programs
- Adaptive dual-band directionality (Prio 205 ITE DM VC, Prio 315 ITC DM, Prio 305 ITC DM, and Prio 415 MC DM only)
- Adaptive noise reduction – reduces gain when signal is suspected to be noise
- Soft Noise Management – reduces level of soft environmental noise
- Adaptive feedback manager – uses acoustic cancellation to reduce feedback
- Adaptive Signal Unification reduces level of soft environmental noise
- OpenFit with collection vents
- Tracker (data logging) with fitting recommendations
- Client profile with client lifestyle priorities – first fit based on audiometric data and lifestyle parameters
- Performance priorities in the automatic program
- Adjustable programs for telecoil
- Automatic telephone program (Prio 415 MC DC and Prio 400 CIC only)
- Push-button control of hearing instrument functions (optional features of Prio 415 MC DM and Prio 400 CIC)

- Volume control (excludes Prio 305 ITC DM, Prio 415 MC DM, and Prio 400 CIC)
- Prio 202 ITE VC and Prio 400 CIC recommended for mild to moderate hearing loss
- Prio 205 ITE DM VC, Prio 322 ITC VC, Prio 315 ITC DM VC, Prio 305 ITC DM, and Prio 405 MC DM recommended for mild to moderate hearing loss
- Programmable via OASIS plus fitting software

Options of Prio 202 ITE VC, Prio 205 ITE DM VC, Prio 322 ITC VC, Prio 315 ITC DM VC, Prio 305 ITC DM, Prio 415 MC DM, and Prio 400 CIC

- Optional remote-control reception coil
- Programmable telecoil (excludes Prio 415 MC DM and Prio 400 CIC)
- Auto telephone – automatically switches to telecoil with detection of telephone (excludes Prio 415 MC DM and Prio 400 CIC)
- Colors: beige, pink, brown, and dark brown

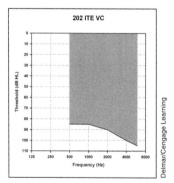

Fitting range for PRIO 202 ITE VC

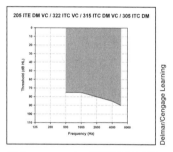

Fitting range for PRIO 205 ITE DM VC/322 ITC VC/315 ITC DM/305 ITC DM

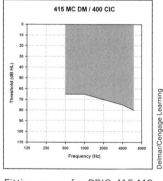

Fitting range for PRIO 415 MC DM/400 CIC

Typical Specifications		Prio 112 BTE VC	Prio 105 BTE DM VC	Prio 105 BTE DM
Standard ANSI S3.22-2003				
Output sound pressure level	Max OSPL 90* (dB SPL)	133	123	123
	HFA OSPL 90 (dB SPL)	126	113	113
Full-on gain	Peak gain* (dB)	71	60	60
	HFA (dB)	65	53	53
Total harmonic distortion	500 Hz	<2%	<1%	<1%
	800 Hz	<1%	<1%	<1%
	1600 Hz	<1%	<1%	<1%
Equivalent input noise (dB SPL)		12	13	13
Telecoil sensitivity	HFA-SPLITS (dB SPL)	109	96	96
Battery	Operating current (mA)	1.4	1.2	1.2
	Battery type	13	13	13

*Measurements made according to IEC 60118-7 (2cc).
Delmar/Cengage Learning

Typical Specifications		Prio 202 ITE VC	Prio 205 ITE DM VC	Prio 322 ITC VC	Prio 315 ITC DM VC	Prio 305 ITC DM
Standard ANSI S3.22-2003						
Output sound pressure level	Max OSPL 90* (dB SPL)	120	112	115	112	110
	HFA OSPL 90 (dB SPL)	115	107	107	107	104
Full-on gain	Peak gain* (dB)	55	46	44	43	41
	HFA (dB)	47	41	37	38	34
Total harmonic distortion	500 Hz	<1%	<1%	<1%	<1%	<1%
	800 Hz	<1%	<1%	<1%	<1%	<1%
	1600 Hz	<1%	<1%	<1%	<1%	<1%
Equivalent input noise (dB SPL)		15	14	16	15	15
Telecoil sensitivity	HFA-SPLITS (dB SPL)	94	85	83	85	84
Battery	Operating current (mA)	1.3	1.2	1.2	1.2	1.2
	Battery type	13	13	312	312	312

*Measurements made according to IEC 60118-7 (2cc).
Delmar/Cengage Learning

Typical Specifications		Prio 415 MC DM	Prio 400 CIC
Standard ANSI S3.22-2003			
Output sound pressure level	Max OSPL 90* (dB SPL)	104	104
	HFA OSPL 90 (dB SPL)	98	98
Full-on gain	Peak gain* (dB)	34	34
	HFA (dB)	30	31
Total harmonic distortion	500 Hz	<1%	<1%
	800 Hz	<1%	<1%
	1600 Hz	<1%	<1%
Equivalent input noise (dB SPL)		14	17
Telecoil sensitivity	HFA-SPLITS (dB SPL)	n/a	n/a
Battery	Operating current (mA)	1.1	0.8
	Battery type	10	10

*Measurements made according to IEC 60118-7 (2cc).

Delmar/Cengage Learning

PRODUCT 10: NEO

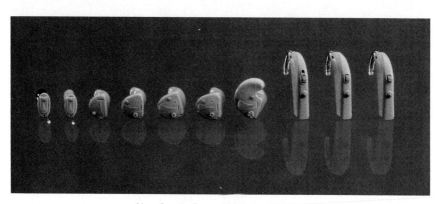

Neo family from CIC through BTE
Courtesy of Bernafon

Product Application

Neo 102 BTE
Neo 112 BTE
Neo 105 BTE DM
Neo 202 TE
Neo 322 ITC
Neo 301 ITC

Neo 302 ITC
Neo 401 CIC
Neo 411 MC
Neo 315 ITC DM

Features of Neo 102 BTE, Neo 112 BTE, and Neo 105 BTE DM

- 5 channels
- OpenFit
- Adaptive feedback cancellation – uses acoustic cancellation to reduce feedback
- Adaptive noise reduction in 8 frequency bands – reduces gain in band(s) in which the signal is suspected to be noise
- Directional microphone system with active microphone matching (Neo 105 BTE DM only)
- Multiple listening programs
- Soft Noise Management – reduces level of soft environmental noise
- Programmable beep indicators
- Telecoil boost
- Push-button control of hearing instrument functions
- Rotary volume control
- ON/OFF function on battery drawer
- FM communication
- DAI
- Programmable via OASIS plus fitting software
- Neo 102 BTE and Neo 105 BTE DM recommended for mild to severe hearing loss
- Neo 112 BTE recommended for mild to severe/profound hearing loss

Options of Neo 102 BTE, Neo 112 BTE, and Neo 105 BTE DM

- Colors: beige, gray-brown, gray, and brown
- Optional ear hooks and children's ear hooks available
- SPIRA^flex thin sound tube 0.9

Features of Neo 202 ITE, Neo 322 ITC, Neo 301 ITC, Neo 302 ITC, Neo 401 CIC, Neo 411 MC, and Neo 315 ITC DM

- 5 channels
- OpenFit
- Adaptive feedback cancellation – uses acoustic cancellation to reduce feedback
- Adaptive noise reduction in 8 frequency bands – reduces gain in the band(s) in which signal is suspected to be noise

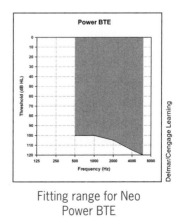

Fitting range for Neo Power BTE

- Directional microphone system with active microphone matching (Neo 315 ITC DM only)
- Multiple listening programs
- Soft Noise Management – reduces level of soft environmental noise
- Programmable beep indicators
- Push-button control of hearing instrument functions (optional feature of Neo 401 CIC and Neo 411 MC (P1, P2))
- Volume control (excludes Neo 310 ITC, Neo 401 CIC, and Neo 411 MC)
- Programmable via OASIS plus fitting software
- Neo 202 ITE recommended for moderate to severe hearing loss
- Neo 322 ITC, Neo 315 ITC DM, and Neo 302 ITC recommended for mild to moderately severe hearing loss
- Neo 301 ITC, Neo 411 MC, and Neo 401 CIC recommended for mild to moderate hearing loss

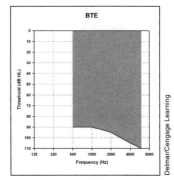

Fitting range for Neo BTE

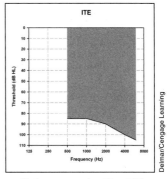

Fitting range for Neo ITE

Options of Neo 202 ITE, Neo 322 ITC, Neo 301 ITC, Neo 302 ITC, Neo 401 CIC, Neo 411 MC, and Neo 315 ITC DM

- Colors: beige, pink, brown, and dark brown
- Automatic telecoil – automatically switches to telecoil with detection of telephone (excludes Neo 401 CIC and Neo 411 MC)
- Telecoil boost (excludes Neo 401 CIC and Neo 411 MC)
- Programmable telecoil (excludes Neo 401 CIC and Neo 411 MC)

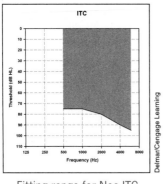

Fitting range for Neo ITC

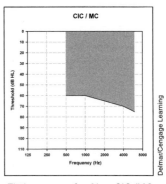

Fitting range for Neo CIC/MC

Typical Specifications		Neo 102 BTE	Neo 112 BTE	Neo 105 BTE DM
Standard ANSI S3.22-1996				
Output sound pressure level	Max OSPL 90 (dB SPL)	123	132	123
	HFA OSPL 90 (dB SPL)	118	126	113
Full-on gain	Peak gain* (dB)	60	71	60
	HFA (dB)	55	65	50
Total harmonic distortion	500 Hz	<1%	<1%	<1%
	800 Hz	<1%	<1%	<1%
	1600 Hz	<1%	<1%	<1%
Equivalent input noise (dB SPL)		14	15	19
Telecoil sensitivity	HFA-SPLITS (dB SPL)	103	111	95
Battery	Operating current (mA)	1.0	1.2	1.0
	Battery type	13	13	13

*Measurements made according to IEC 60118-7 (2cc).
Delmar/Cengage Learning

Typical Specifications		Neo 202 ITE	Neo 322 ITC	Neo 302 ITC
Standard ANSI S3.22-1996				
Output sound pressure level	Max OSPL 90* (dB SPL)	120	114	110
	HFA OSPL 90 (dB SPL)	114	106	104
Full-on gain	Peak gain* (dB)	53	44	40
	HFA (dB)	45	34	32
Total harmonic distortion	500 Hz	<1%	<1%	<1%
	800 Hz	<1%	<1%	<1%
	1600 Hz	<1%	<1%	<1%
Equivalent input noise (dB SPL)		18	20	20
Telecoil sensitivity	HFA-SPLITS (dB SPL)	97	90	83
Battery	Operating current (mA)	1.1	1.0	1.0
	Battery type	13	312	312

*Measurements made according to IEC 60118-7 (2cc).
Delmar/Cengage Learning

Typical Specifications		Neo 315 ITC DM	Neo 301 ITC	Neo 411 MC/ Neo 401 CIC
Standard ANSI S3.22-1996				
Output sound pressure level	Max OSPL 90 (dB SPL)	113	110	104
	HFA OSPL 90 (dB SPL)	106	104	98
Full-on gain	Peak gain* (dB)	43	40	34
	HFA (dB)	36	32	27

continues

continued

Typical Specifications		Neo 315 ITC DM	Neo 301 ITC	Neo 411 MC/ Neo 401 CIC
Total harmonic distortion	500 Hz	<2%	<1%	<1%
	800 Hz	<1%	<1%	<1%
	1600 Hz	<1%	<1%	<1%
Equivalent input noise (dB SPL)		22	20	21
Telecoil sensitivity	HFA SPLITS (dB SPL)	89	83	n/a
Battery	Operating current (mA)	1.0	1.0	0.9
	Battery type	312	312	10

*Measurements made according to IEC 60118-7 (2cc).

Delmar/Cengage Learning

PRODUCT 11: FLAIR

Product Application

Flair 100/110/112 BTE
Flair 115 BTE DM
Flair 200 ITE
Flair 310/320/321 ITC
Flair 321 ITC VC-A
Flair 410 MC
Flair 401 CIC
Flair 315 ITC DM

Features of Flair 100/110/112 BTE and Flair 115 BTE DM

- Programmable via OASIS plus fitting software
- Feedback management – a notch filter centered ~3000 Hz
- Upper-operated, rotary DLC or absolute analog loudness control
- Optimized speech intelligibility with the NAL-NL1 fitting algorithm
- Other common fitting algorithms available
- FM compatibility
- High immunity from mobile telephone interference
- Programmable battery indicator for startup and low battery warning
- Digital technology for enhanced sound quality and comfort
- Dual microphones for directionality (Flair 115 BTE DM only)
- Push-button control of hearing instrument modes
- Telecoil (excludes Flair 100 BTE)
- DAI (excludes Flair 100 BTE)
- Flair 100 BTE recommended for mild to moderately severe hearing loss
- Flair 110 BTE, Flair 112 BTE, and Flair 115 BTE DM recommended for moderate to severe hearing loss

BERNAFON

Options of Flair 100/110/112 BTE and Flair 115 BTE DM

- Colors: beige, brown, and gray
- Optional ear hooks and children's ear hooks available
- FM communication available (excludes Flair 100 BTE)

Features of Flair 200 ITE, Flair 310/320/321 ITC, Flair 321 ITC VC-A, Flair 410 MC, Flair 401 CIC, and Flair 315 ITC DM

- Programmable via OASIS plus fitting software
- High fitting success rate thanks to 2-channel technology
- Feedback management – a notch filter centered ~3000 Hz
- User-operated, rotary DLC or absolute analog volume control (VC-A)
- Optimized speech intelligibility with the NAL-NL1 fitting algorithm
- Other common fitting algorithms available
- High immunity from mobile telephone interference
- Programmable battery indicator for startup and low battery warning
- Efficient wax protection systems
- Digital technology for enhanced sound quality and comfort
- Push-button control of hearing instrument modes
- Dual microphones for directionality (Flair 315 ITC DM only)
- Flair 200 ITE recommended for mild to severe hearing loss
- Flair 320 ITC, Flair 320 ITC, Flair 321 ITC VC-A recommended for mild to moderately severe hearing loss
- Flair 310 ITC, Flair 315 ITC DM, Flair 410 MC, and Flair 401 CIC recommended for mild to moderate hearing loss

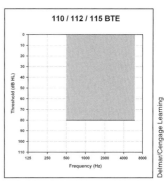

Fitting range for Flair 110/112/115 BTE

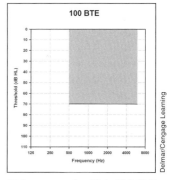

Fitting range for Flair 100 BTE

Options of Flair 200 ITE, Flair 310/320/321 ITC, Flair 321 ITC VC-A, Flair 410 MC, Flair 401 CIC, and Flair 315 ITC DM

- Colors: beige and pink (Flair 200 ITE, Flair 320/321 ITC, Flair 321 ITC VC-A, Flair 315 ITC DM, and Flair 310 ITC only)
- Colors: pink and brown (Flair 410 MC and Flair 401 CIC only)
- Telecoil (Flair 200 ITE, Flair 320/321 ITC, and Flair 321 ITC VC-A only)
- Automatic telecoil (Flair 200 ITE, Flair 320/321 ITC, and Flair 321 ITC VC-A only)

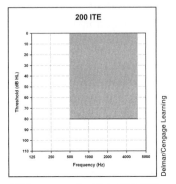

Fitting range for Flair 200 ITE

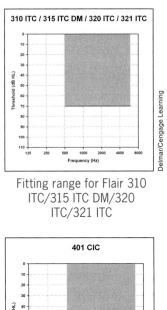

Fitting range for Flair 310 ITC/315 ITC DM/320 ITC/321 ITC

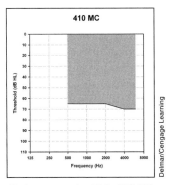

Fitting range for Flair 410 MC

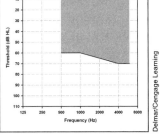

Fitting range for Flair 401 CIC

Typical Specifications		Flair 100 BTE	Flair 110 BTE, Flair 112 BTE	Flair 115 BTE DM
Standard ANSI S3.22-1996				
Output sound pressure level	Max OSPL 90 (dB SPL)	128	131	131
	HFA SSPL 90 (dB SPL)	120	124	124
Full-on gain	Peak gain* (dB)	54	67	64
	HFA (dB)	47	61	58
Total harmonic distortion	500 Hz	≤2%	≤2%	≤2%
	800 Hz	<2%	<2%	<2%
	1600 Hz	<2%	<2%	<2%
Equivalent input noise (dB SPL)		26	26	26
Telecoil sensitivity	HFA-SPLITS (dB SPL)	n/a	109	108
Battery	Operating current (mA)	1.3	1.6	1.7
	Battery type	13	13	13

*Measurements made according to IEC 60118-7 (2cc).

Delmar/Cengage Learning

Typical Specifications		Flair 200 ITE	Flair 320 ITC, Flair 321 ITC	Flair 321 ITC VC-A	Flair 315 ITC DM
Standard ANSI S3.22-1996					
Output sound pressure level	Max OSPL 90 (dB SPL)	123	116	116	112
	HFA OSPL 90 (dB SPL)	117	110	110	107
Full-on gain	Peak gain* (dB)	55	48	48	40
	HFA (dB)	48	39	39	35
Total harmonic distortion	500 Hz	1%	1%	1%	1%
	800 Hz	1%	1%	1%	1%
	1600 Hz	1%	1%	1%	1%
Equivalent input noise (dB SPL)		26	26	26	28
Telecoil sensitivity	HFA-SPLITS (dB SPL)	96	89	89	n/a
Battery	Operating current (mA)	1.1	1.1	1.1	1.2
	Battery type	13	312	312	312

*Measurements made according to IEC 60118-7 (2cc).

Delmar/Cengage Learning

Typical Specifications		Flair 310 ITC	Flair 410 MC	Flair 401 CIC
Standard ANSI S3.22-1996				
Output sound pressure level	Max OSPL 90* (dB SPL)	113	109	107
	HFA OSPL 90 (dB SPL)	108	104	102
Full-on gain	Peak gain* (dB)	43	38	34
	HFA (dB)	39	33	27
Total harmonic distortion	500 Hz	1%	1%	1%
	800 Hz	1%	1%	1%
	1600 Hz	1%	1%	1%
Equivalent input noise (dB SPL)		26	25	27
Telecoil sensitivity	HFA-SPLITS (dB SPL)	n/a	n/a	n/a
Battery	Operating current (mA)	1.1	1.0	1.0
	Battery type	312	10	10

*Measurements made according to IEC 60118-7 (2cc).

Delmar/Cengage Learning

PRODUCT 12: WIN

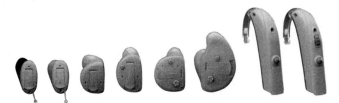

Win family from CIC through BTE
Courtesy of Bernafon

Product Application

Win 102 BTE
Win 112 BTE
Win 105 BTE DM
Win 202 ITE
Win 322 ITC
Win 301 ITC
Win 302 ITC
Win 401 CIC
Win 411 MC
Win 315 ITC DM

Features of Win 102 BTE, Win 112 BTE, and Win 105 BTE DM

- 3 channels
- Adaptive noise reduction – reduces gain when signal is suspected to be noise
- Directional microphone system with active microphone matching (Win 105 BTE DM only)
- Soft Noise Management – reduces level of soft environmental noise
- Feedback management – a notch filter centered ~3000 Hz
- Programmable beep indicators
- Telecoil boost
- Push-button control of hearing instrument modes
- FM compatibility
- DAI
- Volume control
- ON/OFF function on battery drawer
- Programmable via OASIS plus fitting software
- Win 102 BTE and Win 105 BTE DM recommended for mild to severe hearing loss
- Win 112 BTE recommended for mild to severe/profound hearing loss

Options of Win 102 BTE, Win 112 BTE, and Win 105 BTE DM

- Colors: beige
- Optional ear hooks and children's ear hooks available

Features of Win 202 ITE, Win 322 ITC, Win 301 ITC, Win 302 ITC, Win 401 CIC, Win 411 MC, and Win 315 ITC DM

- 3 channels
- Adaptive noise reduction – reduces gain when signal is suspected to be noise
- Directional microphone system with active microphone matching (Win 315 ITC DM only)
- Soft Noise Management – reduces level of soft environmental noise
- Feedback management – a notch filter centered ~3000 Hz
- Programmable beep indicators
- Push-button control of hearing instrument modes
- Volume control
- Programmable via Oasis plus fitting software
- Win 202 ITE recommended for moderate to severe hearing loss
- Win 322 ITC, Win 315 ITC DM, Win 302 ITC recommended for mild to moderately severe hearing loss
- Win 301 ITC, Win 411 MC, and Win 401 CIC recommended for mild to moderate hearing loss

Options of Win 202 ITE, Win 322 ITC, Win 301 ITC, Win 302 ITC, Win 401 CIC, Win 411 MC, and Win 315 ITC DM

- Colors: beige, pink, brown, and dark brown
- Automatic telecoil – automatically switches to Telecoil with detection of telephone (excludes Win 401 CIC and Win 411 MC)
- Telecoil boost (excludes Win 401 CIC and Win 411 MC)

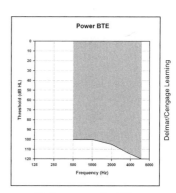

Fitting range for Win Power BTE

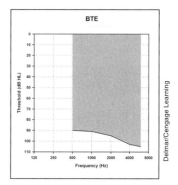

Fitting range for Win BTE

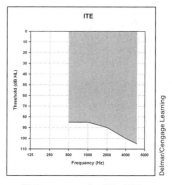

Fitting range for Win ITE

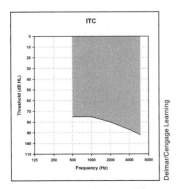

Fitting range for Win ITC

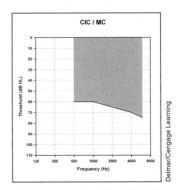

Fitting range for Win CIC/MC

Typical Specifications		Win 102 BTE	Win 112 BTE	Win 105 BTE DM
Standard ANSI S3.22-1996				
Output sound pressure level	Max OSPL 90* (dB SPL)	123	132	123
	HFA OSPL 90* (dB SPL)	118	126	113
Full-on gain	Peak gain (dB)	60	71	60
	HFA (dB)	55	65	50
Total harmonic distortion	500 Hz	<1%	<1%	<1%
	800 Hz	<1%	<1%	<1%
	1600 Hz	<1%	<1%	<1%
Equivalent input noise (dB SPL)		14	15	19
Telecoil sensitivity	HFA-SPLITS (dB SPL)	103	111	95
Battery	Operating current (mA)	1.0	1.2	1.0
	Battery type	13	13	13

*Measurements made according to IEC 60118-7 (2cc).

Delmar/Cengage Learning

Typical Specifications		Win 202 ITE	Win 322 ITC	Win 302 ITC
Standard ANSI S3.22-1996				
Output sound pressure level	Max OSPL 90* (dB SPL)	120	114	110
	HFA OSPL 90 (dB SPL)	114	106	104
Full-on gain	Peak gain (dB)	53	44	40
	HFA (dB)	45	34	32
Total harmonic distortion	500 Hz	<1%	<1%	<1%
	800 Hz	<1%	<1%	<1%
	1600 Hz	<1%	<1%	<1%

continues

continued

Typical Specifications		Win 202 ITE	Win 322 ITC	Win 302 ITC
Equivalent input noise (dB SPL)		18	20	20
Telecoil sensitivity	HFA-SPLITS (dB SPL)	97	90	83
Battery	Operating current (mA)	1.1	1.0	1.0
	Battery type	13	312	312

*Measurements made according to IEC 60118-7 (2cc).

Delmar/Cengage Learning

Typical Specifications		Win 315 ITC DM	Win 301 ITC	Win 411 MC, Win 401 CIC
Standard ANSI S3.22-1996				
Output sound pressure level	Max OSPL 90* (dB SPL)	113	110	104
	HFA OSPL 90 (dB SPL)	106	104	98
Full-on gain	Peak gain* (dB)	43	40	34
	HFA (dB)	36	32	27
Total harmonic distortion	500 Hz	<2%	<1%	<1%
	800 Hz	<1%	<1%	<1%
	1600 Hz	<1%	<1%	<1%
Equivalent input noise (dB SPL)		22	20	21
Telecoil sensitivity	HFA-SPLITS (dB SPL)	89	83	n/a
Battery	Operating current (mA)	1.0	1.0	0.8
	Battery type	312	312	10

*Measurements made according to IEC 60118-7 (2cc).

Delmar/Cengage Learning

CHAPTER THREE

General Hearing Instruments

GENERAL HEARING INSTRUMENTS (GHI): THE UNDERDOG WITH BIG PLANS

International Headquarters
175 Brookhollow
Harahan, LA 70123
Phone: 1 (800) 824-3021
E-mail: customerservice@generalhearing.com
Web site: http://www.generalhearing.com

General Hearing Instruments (GHI), currently located in Harahan, Louisiana, is a relatively recent player and, not unlike many companies, was started by a general dissatisfaction with the current (read: mid-1980s) state of the industry. Roger Juneau cofounded GHI in 1984 in Roanoke, Virginia, and, wasting no time, went into production in the spring of 1985. The driving force behind this new venture was, in Juneau's view, the limitations of available hearing devices at that time. He was particularly perturbed by the poor fidelity and bandwidth of hearing instruments. Apparently, being an avid portable music listener, he believed that the sound quality of available hearing instruments paled in comparison to the Sony Walkman™ (Krcmar, 2006). The reason for the discrepancy between these two devices is not a mystery. As discussed in Chapter 1, hearing instruments had—and to some extent still have—a pretty narrow frequency response, much of which was because of limitations in technology. Current components have the capability for a high-end frequency response of 12,000 or even 14,000 Hz. With the application of acoustic feedback cancellation, hearing instruments have been able to improve not only the quality of fit in terms of an improved gain to target match and reduced occlusion effect, but also an increase in frequency response without negating proper gain or reintroducing the occlusion effect.

In my view, what makes GHI distinctive is what they are despite being a speck on the industry's market-share and revenue radar. Admittedly, market data is difficult to obtain, as GHI is a privately held company. However, given the stiff competition in a quickly maturing industry, GHI has developed into a company with a passion for innovation to truly improve hearing instruments and related products where much of the industry has not exerted tangible effort. Because of their innovation and sincere efforts to improve the state of the industry, I have included them in this book.

In my opinion, there are three areas in which GHI has invested significant efforts to make their mark in the industry. First, they have reapplied existing centrifuge technology to the problem of cerumen in hearing instruments. While this may not be the most profound problem facing the hearing-impaired, it is a very real, annoying, inconvenient, expensive, and time-consuming problem. This ingenious little device is designed to clear the soft materials in hearing instruments of cerumen at minimal risk to the hearing instrument. As a bonus, this Spindoctor is available to consumers, reducing—probably significantly— the number of office visits. Perhaps its greatest claim is sub-60s cleaning time.

Second, they are expending significant energy in soft hearing devices. The current product offering in this category includes a series of silicon-based, soft-shell, in-the-ear hearing aids. This soft-shell feature relates to two product lines, Simply Soft and SmartWear™, an in-the-ear, noncustom hearing instrument, which looks like an ITC or CIC form factor. Think of the disposable SongBird without the annoying aspect of throwing them out every month, but the devices look like traditional ITCs or CICs. An important application of their soft-shell hearing instruments is for pediatric patients. Their Kustom for Kids line embodies similar features just described, but is customized for children. Some of the claims include a secure fit for active children, broad frequency response, and reduced number of remakes (GHI, 2009). GHI is working to improve further this technology for infant applications. They are working to be able to make the soft "shell" self-forming, which will allow some ability to grow with the child, further reducing the number of remakes (Krcmar, 2006). Of course, this technology promises to create a better seal, thus reducing feedback.

Third, GHI seems to be one of the few companies in the world that truly cares about the tinnitus patient. In my experience, tinnitus patients feel alienated by hearing device companies that produce a token tinnitus device to complete their product line. Moreover, with over 12 million tinnitus sufferers who seek medical attention, 2 million of whom are debilitated by it, tinnitus remains a seriously underserved medical problem. Any hearing professionals can tell you there is no cure, but at the same time, highly effective treatments exist. GHI's tinnitus devices integrate their soft-shell technology as well as other traditional tinnitus sound therapy, namely noise generation, for the purpose of habituation or "masking." Their line of tinnitus devices includes a so-called combination device where amplification is combined with complex sound generation as well as simple sound-generating devices in both custom and noncustom form factors. GHI's strong belief in helping the tinnitus patient is backed by their production of informational materials, including a tinnitus documentary, to educate people on tinnitus (GHI, 2009).

Philanthropy

Along with some high-quality tinnitus devices, GHI is dedicated to broadly disseminating information about tinnitus. They have rallied some of the top researchers and clinicians in tinnitus to be included in a documentary intended to educate the public about tinnitus (GHI, 2009). GHI has developed an accompanying information packet that includes a DVD copy of the documentary and associated sundries such as brochures, displays, and premade ads (GHI, 2009).

Warranty

GHI offers a 1-year manufacturer's warranty, including loss and damage, on their custom devices. There is a processing fee for loss and damage claims, which varies with device. GHI's Simply Soft noncustom devices are covered with a 6-month manufacturer's warranty, which does not include loss and damage coverage. Additional coverage for these devices can be purchased (GHI, 2007).

PRODUCT INFORMATION

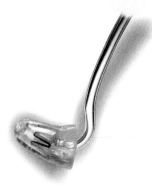

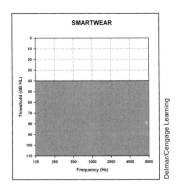

SmartWear SFE: Soft, silicone noncustom ear mold featuring temperature-sensitive, self-forming technology. Stent allows device to conform to any ear canal and eliminate feedback.
Courtesy of GHI

Fitting range for SmartWear SFE

PRODUCT 1: MUSICIANS' LISTENING DEVICE

Product Application

Musicians' Listening Device

Features of Musicians' Listening Device Micro OTE

- Micro case design
- 4 Channel
- 4 Memory
- Soft, free field dome
- Different size domes available
- Micro-poly tube
- No ear impressions
- Same-day fitting
- Adaptive feedback cancellation
- Layered noise reduction
- 12 Band gain adjustment
- 16 kHz Bandwidth
- Electronic damping – allows for better elimination of unwanted response peaks from the outgoing signal
- Programmable tone generator
- Low battery warning
- Memory button plays audible beeps to indicate the memory selected
- Programmable power-on delay
- Expanded headroom
- High coherence
- Designed for high fidelity music listening

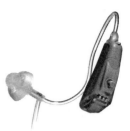

Musicians' Listening Device
Courtesy of GHI

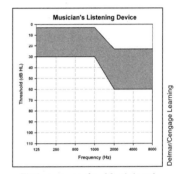

Fitting range for Musicians' Listening Device

Typical Specifications		Musicians' Listening Device Micro OTE
Standard ANSI S3.22-1996		
Saturation sound pressure level	Max OSPL 90 (dB SPL)	
	HFA AVG (dB SPL)	
Reference test gain	Target (dB)	
	Measured (dB)	
Equivalent input noise (dB SPL)		
Battery	Operating current (mA)	
	Battery type	10

Delmar/Cengage Learning

PRODUCT 2: SIMPLICITY

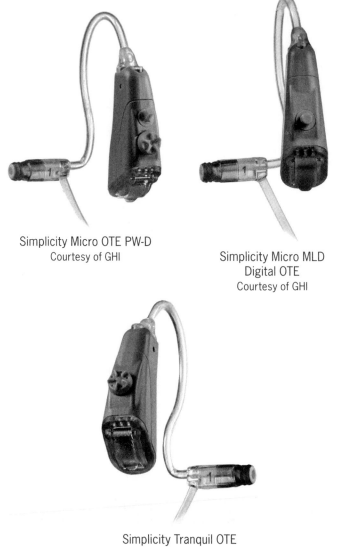

Simplicity Micro OTE PW-D
Courtesy of GHI

Simplicity Micro MLD
Digital OTE
Courtesy of GHI

Simplicity Tranquil OTE
Courtesy of GHI

Product Application

Simplicity Micro OTE PW-D
Simplicity Micro Digital OTE
Simplicity Tranquil OTE

Features of Simplicity Micro OTE PW-D

- Micro case design
- Same-day fitting
- Micro-poly tube
- No ear impressions
- Speech-in-noise switch
- Economically priced
- Recommended for mild to moderate high-frequency hearing loss

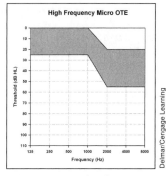

Fitting ranges for Simplicity Micro OTE PW-D

Features of Simplicity Micro Digital OTE

- Music Lover's Design™ (MLD) feature
- Micro case design
- Same-day fitting
- Micro-poly tube
- No ear impressions
- 4 memories
- Economically priced
- Recommended for mild to moderate high-frequency hearing loss

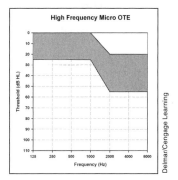

Fitting ranges for Simplicity Micro OTE PW-D and Micro OTE

Features of Simplicity Tranquil OTE

- Broadband noise generator
- Micro case design
- Same-day fitting
- Micro-poly tube
- No ear impressions
- Volume control wheel
- Speech-in-noise switch
- Economically priced

Typical Specifications		Simplicity Micro OTE PW-D
Standard ANSI S3.22-1996		
Saturation sound pressure level	Max OSPL 90 (dB SPL)	119.3
	HFA AVG (dB SPL)	109.7
Reference test gain	Target (dB)	32.7
	Measured (dB)	22.9
Equivalent input noise (dB SPL)		29.4
Battery	Operating current (mA)	0.21
	Battery type	10

Delmar/Cengage Learning

Typical Specifications	Simplicity Micro OTE Digital – Memory 1	Simplicity Micro OTE Digital – Memory 2	Simplicity Micro OTE Digital – Memory 3	Simplicity Micro OTE Digital – Memory 4
Standard ANSI S3.22-1996				
Source (dB)	40	40	40	40
Peak (dB)	15.1	16.8	22	25.6
Peak frequency (Hz)	2.900	3.300	3.100	3.100
RMS out (dB)	47.1	49.2	53.5	57.7
Noise reduction (dB)	16	16	16	16

Note: Each program has progressively louder gain and output. Memories and settings can be modified via General Hearing's Evolution digital software.

Delmar/Cengage Learning

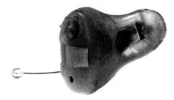

Typical Specifications	Simplicity Tranquil
Standard ANSI S3.22-1996	
Source (dB)	0
Peak (dB)	62.7
Peak frequency (Hz)	2,800
RMS out (dB)	74.1
Noise reduction (dB)	16
Operating current (mA)	0

Delmar/Cengage Learning

PRODUCT 3: SIMPLY SOFT

Simply Soft: noncustom, soft silicone mild amplification device
Courtesy of GHI

Product Application

Simply Soft

Features of Simply Soft

- Small, in-the-ear design
- Soft, medical-grade silicone body
- Stacked manual volume control
- High-fidelity, Class-D circuitry
- Color-coded red/blue tips
- Dynamic wax system
- Slipstream pressure venting

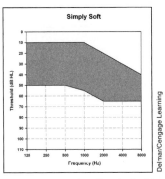

Fitting range for Simply Soft

Delmar/Cengage Learning

Typical Specifications		Simply Soft
Standard ANSI S3.22-1996		
Saturation sound pressure level	Max SSPL 90 (dB SPL)	111
	HFA SSPL 90 (dB SPL)	110
Full-on gain	Peak gain (dB)	23
	HFA (dB)	20
Total harmonic distortion		<3.5%
Equivalent input noise (dB SPL)		<34
Battery	Operating current (mA)	0.23
	Battery type	10

Delmar/Cengage Learning

PRODUCT 4: CANAL OPEN EAR

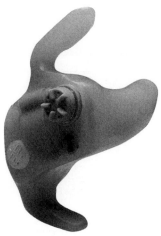

Canal Open Ear: free-field,
open-ear device for patients
with a high-frequency
hearing loss
Courtesy of GHI

Product Application

Canal Open Ear

Features of Canal Open Ear

- Small canal size
- Perfect for active patients
- 12-month warranty plus coverage
- Recommended for patients having normal hearing in the low frequencies, but a mild to moderate high-frequency hearing loss

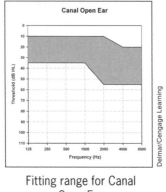

Fitting range for Canal
Open Ear

Options of Canal Open Ear

• Choice of circuitry – Class A (recommended)

Typical Specifications		Canal Open Ear
Standard ANSI S3.22-1996		
Saturation sound pressure level	Max SSPL 90 (dB SPL)	105
	HFA SSPL 90 (dB SPL)	100
Full-on gain	Peak gain (dB)	30
	HFA (dB)	30
Total harmonic distortion		<4.5%
Equivalent input noise (dB SPL)		<34
Battery	Operating current (mA)	0.35
	Battery type	10

Delmar/Cengage Learning

PRODUCT 5: TRANQUIL BTE

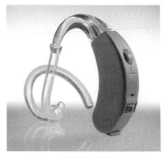

Tranquil BTE: BTE-style
device featuring Tranquil
noise-generating circuitry
Courtesy of GHI

Product Application

Tranquil BTE

Features of Tranquil BTE

- Slim-line case
- ON/OFF switch
- Manual linear VC
- Adjustable output trimmer
- Broadband noise generator
- Noncustom ear mold included

Typical Specifications	Tranquil BTE Trimmer at Full-On Setting	Tranquil BTE Trimmer at Midpoint Setting
Standard ANSI S3.22-1996		
Source (dB)	0.0	0.0
Peak (dB)	73	64
Peak frequency (Hz)	2200	5900
RMS out (dB)	82	66
Noise reduction (dB)	16	16
Operating current (mA)	0.65	0.65
Battery type	13	13

Delmar/Cengage Learning

PRODUCT 6: TRANQUIL®

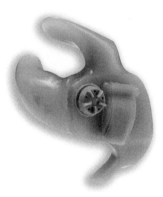

Tranquil: open-ear style device
for tinnitus treatment
Courtesy of GHI

Product Application

Tranquil Open Ear

Features of Tranquil Open Ear

- In-the-ear, open design
- Small, cosmetically appealing
- Manual, linear volume control
- Broadband noise
- High-fidelity, Class-D circuitry
- Wide, smooth frequency response
- 0 dB (HL) VC floor
- 3 output levels
- Low-frequency or high-frequency emphasis

Typical Specifications	Tranquil "NM" Circuit Style (Normal to Mild)	Tranquil "MM" Circuit Style (Mild to Moderate)	Tranquil "MS" Circuit Style (Moderate to Severe)
Standard ANSI S3.22-1996			
RMS out (dB SPL)	63	77	94
Peak output (Hz)	2800 and 6000	3000	3000
Operating current (mA)	0.4	0.4	0.5
Battery type	10	10	10

Delmar/Cengage Learning

PRODUCT 7: SIMPLY TRANQUIL

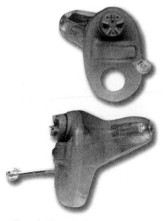

Simply Tranquil: noncustom,
soft silicone tinnitus
treatment device
Courtesy of GHI

Product Application

Simply Tranquil ITE

Features of Simply Tranquil ITE

- Open design
- Small, cosmetically appealing
- Soft, medical-grade silicone
- Color-coded red/blue tips
- Manual linear VC
- 0 dB (HL) VC floor
- High-fidelity, Class-D circuitry
- Wide, smooth frequency response
- Broadband noise generator with high-frequency emphasis

Typical Specifications	Simply Tranquil ITE
Standard ANSI S3.22-1996	
RMS out (dB SPL)	66
Peak output (Hz)	3600
Operating current (mA)	0.4
Battery type	5

Delmar/Cengage Learning

PRODUCT 8: TRANQUIL COMBO

Amplification/Sound Generator

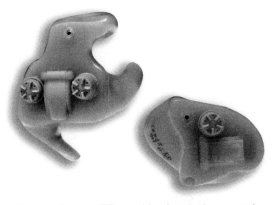

Tranquil Combo ITE: combination tinnitus sound
generator and hearing amplification circuit
Courtesy of GHI

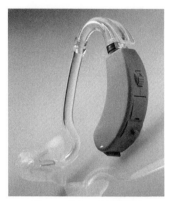

Tranquil Combo BTE:
combination tinnitus sound
generator and hearing
amplification circuit
Courtesy of GHI

Product Application

Tranquil Combo BTE
Tranquil Combo ITE

Features of Tranquil Combo BTE

- Slim-line case
- SmartWear SFE ear mold – combines the convenience of a noncustom ear mold with the security and comfort of a custom fit by continuously adapting to the ear canal shape
- Wide-band digital amplification
- 4 memories
- Telecoil
- NOAH 3 compatible
- Low battery warning
- Sound generator consists of broadband frequency spectrum and manual linear volume control
- Recommended for patients experiencing tinnitus and/or hyperacusis in addition to hearing loss

Features of Tranquil Combo ITE

- Cosmetic appeal
- Manual sound generator VC
- Low battery drain
- Broadband noise generator

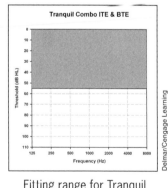

Fitting range for Tranquil
Combo BTE and ITE

- Independent or simultaneous operation of controls
- Recommended for patients experiencing tinnitus and/or hyperacusis in addition to hearing loss

Options of Tranquil Combo ITE

- Open shell
- Canal model available (size 10 A battery)

Typical Specifications	Tranquil Combo BTE	Tranquil Combo ITE-Analog	Tranquil Combo ITE-Digital
Standard ANSI S3.22-1996			
Source (dB)	0.0	0.0	0.0
Peak (dB)	62	73	54
Peak frequency (Hz)	2200	2200	3700
RMS out (dB)	73	82	89
Noise reduction (dB)	16	16	16
Operating current (mA)	1.22	0.65	1.20
Battery type	13	312	312

Delmar/Cengage Learning

CHAPTER FOUR

Micro-Tech

MICRO-TECH: MAINTAINING INDEPENDENCE

Recognizable "Minneapolis" Address
Micro-Tech Hearing Instruments
P.O. Box 59124
Minneapolis, MN 55459
USA
Phone: 1 (800) 745-4327
URL: http://www.mthearing.com

Corporate Headquarters
Micro-Tech Hearing Instruments
6425 Flying Cloud Drive
Eden Prairie, MN 55344
USA
Phone: 1 (952) 995-8800
Web site: http://www.mthearing.com

> *To be the preferred supplier of hearing instruments through quality, innovation, and caring.*
> — Micro-Tech vision statement

Despite being a new hearing instrument company founded in 1986, Micro-Tech had ability for innovation. A couple of trendsetting examples include a fully titanium and water-resistant (i.e., submersible) BTE shell (no longer offered) and the Touchless Telecoil® that automatically turns on the telecoil when a strong electromagnetic field is detected (Micro-Tech, 2006a).

In 1999, Micro-Tech was acquired by Starkey Laboratories. This allowed for a greater parts-sharing between companies to help Starkey catch up in their lagging technology. Since both companies are located in the suburbs of Minneapolis, Minnesota, the close geographic proximity assisted in this.

Philanthropy

Micro-Tech has been providing hearing instruments to the needy in other countries since 1992. Micro-Tech continues to send its team of audiologists outside the U.S. annually for these philanthropic hearing instrument fits. They even allow a few of their patients to attend these trips. The company is so passionate about its work that three-quarters of its employees donate money to the So The World May Hear Foundation, which has a similar focus to their own company missions (Micro-Tech, 2006b).

Warranty

Micro-Tech offers a standard 1-year warranty to its products. This includes loss and damage protection, which is good for one instance. During this time, remakes are free. Extensions can be purchased in 1-year increments for up to 3 years (Micro-Tech, 2003).

PRODUCT INFORMATION

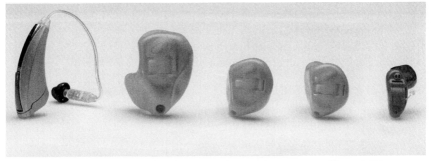

Micro-Tech's family product line consisting of BTE, ITE, ITC, and CIC
Courtesy of Micro-Tech

PRODUCT 1: AXIO™

Product Application

Axio iM32 RIC
Axio iM32 RIC Power
Axio iM32 ITE
Axio iM32 HS
Axio iM32 ITC
Axio iM32 CIC

Features of Axio iM32 RIC

- Sound imaging – high resolution sounds imaging with frequency shaping in all 16 channels and 16 bands
- Strategic feedback control – a feedback program that uses intelligent artifact elimination to give improve feedback cancellation
- Premium adaptive environmental sequencing – a system for managing noise and preserving speech intelligibility

- Full acoustic landscape – adapts to any listening environment by adjusting to the patients preferred settings
- Comfort control – allows hearing aids to be programmed to what is most comfortable to the patient
- Dynamic directional detection – automatically filters out background noise to improve speech understanding in noisy environments
- Live real ear measurement – providing the more precise information
- T^2 (Touch-tone) – allows patients to control their hearing aids using any cell or touch phone
- Automatic telephone solutions – automatically detects telephone use and adjusts the frequency response
- Auto path – an automatic fitting routine to help provide an accurate first fit
- 3D live speech mapping – verifies how hearing aid processes acoustic input, such as speech, in real time while including the patient and family in the fitting process
- Live speech mapping – verifies how hearing aid processes acoustic input, such as speech

Options of Axio iM32 RIC

- Self-check – allows a diagnostic check of the microphone, circuit, and receiver
- Appointment reminders – to remind patients of follow-up appointments and maintenance checks
- Leisure listening memories – for better processing music and television
- Voice indicators – alerts patient on status of battery, memory, and telephone modes
- Tonal indicators – different tones for memory, low battery, etc.
- Verify comfort
- In-situ audiometry
- Data logging

Features of Axio iM32 RIC mPower

- Sound imaging – high resolution sounds imaging with frequency shaping in all 16 channels and 16 bands
- Strategic feedback control – a feedback program that uses intelligent artifact elimination to give improved feedback cancellation
- Premium adaptive environmental sequencing – a system for managing noise and preserving speech intelligibility

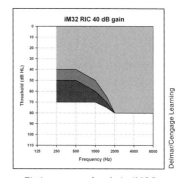

Fitting range for Axio iM32 RIC 40 dB of gain: Open earbud (light gray), occluded earbud (medium gray), custom occluded earmold (dark gray)

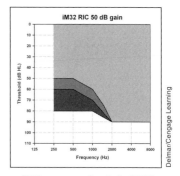

Fitting range for Axio iM32 RIC 50 dB of gain: Open earbud (light gray), occluded earbud (medium gray), custom occluded earmold (dark gray)

- Full acoustic landscape – adapts to any listening environment by adjusting to the patients preferred settings
- Comfort control – allows hearing aids to be programmed to what is most comfortable to the patient
- Dynamic directional detection – automatically filters out background noise to improve speech understanding in noisy environments
- T^2 (Touch-tone) – allows patients to control their hearing aids using any cell or touch phone
- Automatic telephone solutions – automatically detects telephone use and adjusts the frequency response
- Auto path – an automatic fitting routine to help provide an accurate first fit
- 3D Live speech mapping – verifies how hearing aid processes acoustic input, such as speech, in real time while including the patient and family in the fitting process
- Live speech mapping – verifies how hearing aid processes acoustic input, such as speech

Options of Axio iM32 RIC mPower

- Self-check – allows a diagnostic check of the microphone, circuit, and receiver
- Appointment reminders – to remind patients of follow-up appointments and maintenance checks
- Leisure listening memories – for better processing music and television
- Voice indicators – alerts patient on status of battery, memory, and telephone modes
- Tonal indicators – different tones for memory, low battery, etc.
- Verify comfort
- In-situ audiometry
- Data logging

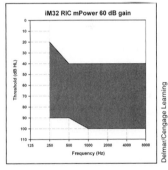

Fitting range for Axio iM32 Power RIC 60 dB of gain with custom occluded earmold

Features of Axio iM32 ITE, Axio iM32 HS, Axio iM32 ITC, and Axio iM32 CIC

- Sound imaging – high resolution sounds imaging with frequency shaping in all 16 channels and 16 bands
- Strategic feedback control – a feedback program that uses intelligent artifact elimination to give improved feedback cancellation
- Premium adaptive environmental sequencing – a system for managing noise and preserving speech intelligibility

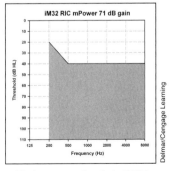

Fitting range for Axio iM32 Power RIC 71 dB of gain with custom occluded earmold

- Full acoustic landscape – adapts to any listening environment by adjusting to the patients preferred settings
- Comfort control – allows hearing aids to be programmed to what is most comfortable to the patient
- Dynamic directional detection – automatically filters out background noise to improve speech understanding in noisy environments
- Live real ear measurement – providing the more precise information
- T^2 (Touch-tone) – allows patients to control their hearing aids using any cell or touch phone
- Automatic telephone solutions – automatically detects telephone use and adjusts the frequency response
- Auto path – an automatic fitting routine to help provide an accurate first fit
- 3D Live speech mapping – verifies how hearing aid processes acoustic input, such as speech, in real time while including the patient and family in the fitting process
- Live speech mapping – verifies how hearing aid processes acoustic input, such as speech

Options of Axio iM32 ITE, Axio iM32 HS, Axio iM32 ITC, and Axio iM32 CIC

- Self-check – allows a diagnostic check of the microphone, circuit, and receiver
- Appointment reminders – to remind patients of follow-up appointments and maintenance checks
- Leisure listening memories – for better processing music and television
- Voice indicators – alerts patient on status of battery, memory, and telephone modes
- Tonal indicators – different tones for memory, low battery, etc.
- Verify comfort
- In-situ audiometry
- Data logging

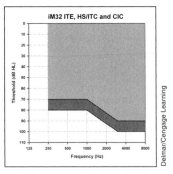

Fitting range for Axio iM32
ITC, HS, ITC, and CIC: ITE
(light gray), and HS/ITC, CIC
(dark gray)

Typical Specifications		Axio™iM32 RIC (40 gain)	Axio™iM32 RIC (50 gain)	Axio™iM32 RIC Power (60 gain)	Axio™iM32 RIC Power (71 gain)
Standard ANSI S3.22-1996					
Output sound pressure level	Max OSPL 90 (dB SPL)	110	115	123	131
	HF-average OSPL 90 (dB SPL)	102	108	115	125
Full-on gain	Peak gain (dB)	40	50	60	71
	HF-average-full-on gain (dB)	31	44	52	64
Total harmonic distortion	500 Hz	1.0%	1.0%	1.0%	1.0%
	800 Hz	1.6%	1.6%	1.6%	1.6%
	1600 Hz	2.5%	2.5%	2.5%	2.5%
Equivalent input noise (dB SPL)		<25	<25	<25	<25
Telecoil sensitivity	HFA-SPLITS (dB SPL)	n/a	n/a	n/a	n/a
Battery	Operating current (mA)	1.2	1.3	1.2	1.6
	Battery type	312	312	312	312
Compression characteristics – channel AGC	Attack (ms)	20	20	20	20
	Release 0.1s (ms)	5-150	5-150	5-150	5-150
	Release 2.0s (ms)	5-150	5-150	5-150	5-150

Delmar/Cengage Learning

Typical Specifications		Axio™iM32 ITE	Axio™iM32 HS/ITC	Axio™iM32 CIC
Standard ANSI S3.22-1996				
Output sound pressure level	Max OSPL 90 (dB SPL)	115-131	110-131	110-131
	HF-average OSPL 90 (dB SPL)	111-126	106-126	106-126
Full-on gain	Peak gain (dB)	45-71	40-71	35-71
	HF-average-full-on gain (dB)	41-65	36-65	35-65
Total harmonic distortion	500 Hz	1.0%	1.0%	1.0%
	800 Hz	1.6%	1.6%	1.6%
	1600 Hz	2.5%	2.5%	2.5%
Equivalent input noise (dB SPL)		<25	<25	<25

continues

continued

Typical Specifications		Axio™iM32 ITE	Axio™iM32 HS/ITC	Axio™iM32 CIC
Telecoil sensitivity	HFA-SPLITS (dB SPL)	n/a	n/a	n/a
Battery	Operating current (mA)	1.1-1.7	1.1-1.7	1.1-1.7
	Battery type	312 or 13	312, 13, or 10	312, 13, or 10
Compression characteristics – channel AGC	Attack (ms)	20	20	20
	Release 0.1s (ms)	5-150	5-150	5-150
	Release 2.0s (ms)	5-150	5-150	5-150

Delmar/Cengage Learning

PRODUCT 2: VECTOR

Product Application

Vector iM24 RIC
Vector iM24 ITE
Vector iM24 HS
Vector iM24 ITC
Vector iM24 CIC
Vector iM16 RIC
Vector iM16 ITE
Vector iM16 HS
Vector iM16 ITC
Vector iM16 CIC
Vector iM12 RIC
Vector iM12 ITE
Vector iM12 HS
Vector iM12 ITC
Vector iM12 CIC

Features of Vector iM24 RIC

• Sound imaging – high resolution sounds imaging with frequency shaping in all 12 channels and 12 bands
• Strategic feedback control – a feedback program that uses intelligent artifact elimination to give improved feedback cancellation
• Adaptive environmental sequencing – a system for managing noise and preserving speech intelligibility
• Acoustic landscape – adapts to any listening environment by adjusting to the patients preferred settings
• Dynamic directional detection – automatically filters out background noise to improve speech understanding in noisy environments
• Live real ear measurement – providing the more precise information

- T^2 (Touch-tone) – allows patients to control their hearing aids using any cell or touch phone
- Automatic telephone solutions – automatically detects telephone use and adjusts the frequency response
- Auto path – an automatic fitting routine to help provide an accurate first fit
- Live speech mapping – verifies how hearing aid processes acoustic input, such as speech

Options of Vector iM24 RIC

- Leisure listening memories – for better processing music and television
- Tonal indicators – different tones for memory, low battery, etc.
- Verify comfort
- In-situ audiometry
- Data logging

Features of Vector iM24 ITE, Vector iM24 HS, Vector iM24 ITE, and Vector iM24 CIC

- Sound imaging – high resolution sounds imaging with frequency shaping in all 12 channels and 12 bands
- Strategic feedback control – a feedback program that uses intelligent artifact elimination to give improved feedback cancellation
- Adaptive environmental sequencing – a system for managing noise and preserving speech intelligibility
- Acoustic landscape – adapts to any listening environment by adjusting to the patients preferred settings
- Dynamic directional detection – automatically filters out background noise to improve speech understanding in noisy environments
- Live real ear measurement – providing the more precise information
- T^2 (Touch-tone) – allows patients to control their hearing aids using any cell or touch phone
- Automatic telephone solutions – automatically detects telephone use and adjusts the frequency response
- Auto path – an automatic fitting routine to help provide an accurate first fit
- Live speech mapping – verifies how hearing aid processes acoustic input, such as speech

Options of Vector iM24 ITE, Vector iM24 HS, Vector iM24 ITE, and Vector iM24 CIC

- Leisure listening memories – for better processing music and television
- Voice indicators – alerts patient on status of battery, memory, and telephone modes
- Tonal indicators – different tones for memory, low battery, etc.
- Verify comfort
- In-situ audiometry
- Data logging

Features of Vector iM16 RIC

- Sound imaging – high resolution sounds imaging with frequency shaping in all 8 channels and 8 bands
- Strategic feedback control – a feedback program that uses intelligent artifact elimination to give improved feedback cancellation
- Adaptive Environmental Sequencing – a system for managing noise and preserving speech intelligibility
- Acoustic Landscape – adapts to any listening environment by adjusting to the patients preferred settings
- Dynamic directional detection – automatically filters out background noise to improve speech understanding in noisy environments
- Live real ear measurement – providing the more precise information
- T^2 (Touch-tone) – allows patients to control their hearing aids using any cell or touch phone
- Automatic telephone solutions – automatically detects telephone use and adjusts the frequency response
- Auto path – an automatic fitting routine to help provide an accurate first fit
- Live speech mapping – verifies how hearing aid processes acoustic input, such as speech

Options of Vector iM16 RIC

- Leisure listening memories – for better processing music and television
- Tonal indicators – different tones for memory, low battery, etc.
- Verify comfort
- In-situ audiometry
- Data logging

Features of Vector iM16 ITE, Vector iM16 HS, Vector iM16 ITE, and Vector iM16 CIC

- Sound imaging – high resolution sounds imaging with frequency shaping in all 8 channels and 8 bands
- Strategic feedback control – a feedback program that uses intelligent artifact elimination to give improved feedback cancellation
- Adaptive environmental sequencing – a system for managing noise and preserving speech intelligibility
- Acoustic landscape – adapts to any listening environment by adjusting to the patients preferred settings
- Dynamic directional detection – automatically filters out background noise to improve speech understanding in noisy environments
- Live real ear measurement – providing the more precise information
- T^2 (Touch-tone) – allows patients to control their hearing aids using any cell or touch phone

- Automatic telephone solutions – automatically detects telephone use and adjusts the frequency response
- Auto path – an automatic fitting routine to help provide an accurate first fit
- Live speech mapping – verifies how hearing aid processes acoustic input, such as speech

Options of Vector iM16 ITE, Vector iM16 HS, Vector iM16 ITE, and Vector iM16 CIC

- Leisure listening memories – for better processing music and television
- Voice indicators – alerts patient on status of battery, memory and telephone modes
- Tonal indicators – different tones for memory, low battery, etc.
- Verify comfort
- In-situ audiometry
- Data logging

Features of Vector iM12 RIC

- Sound imaging – high resolution sounds imaging with frequency shaping in all 6 channels and 6 bands
- Strategic feedback control – a feedback program that uses intelligent artifact elimination to give improved feedback cancellation
- Adaptive environmental sequencing – a system for managing noise and preserving speech intelligibility
- Acoustic landscape – adapts to any listening environment by adjusting to the patients preferred settings
- Dynamic directional detection – automatically filters out background noise to improve speech understanding in noisy environments
- Live real ear measurement – providing the more precise information
- T² (Touch-tone) – allows patients to control their hearing aids using any cell or touch phone
- Automatic telephone solutions – automatically detects telephone use and adjusts the frequency response
- Auto path – an automatic fitting routine to help provide an accurate first fit
- Live speech mapping – verifies how hearing aid processes acoustic input, such as speech

Options of Vector iM12 RIC

- Leisure listening memories – for better processing music and television
- Tonal indicators – different tones for memory, low battery, etc.
- Verify comfort
- In-situ audiometry
- Data logging

Features of Vector iM12 ITE, Vector iM12 HS, Vector iM12 ITE, and Vector iM12 CIC

- Sound imaging – high resolution sounds imaging with frequency shaping in all 6 channels and 6 bands
- Strategic feedback control – a feedback program that uses intelligent artifact elimination to give improved feedback cancellation
- Adaptive environmental sequencing – a system for managing noise and preserving speech intelligibility
- Acoustic landscape – adapts to any listening environment by adjusting to the patients preferred settings
- Dynamic directional detection – automatically filters out background noise to improve speech understanding in noisy environments
- Live real ear measurement – providing the more precise information
- T^2 (Touch-tone) – allows patients to control their hearing aids using any cell or touch phone
- Automatic telephone solutions – automatically detects telephone use and adjusts the frequency response
- Auto path – an automatic fitting routine to help provide an accurate first fit
- Live speech mapping - verifies how hearing aid processes acoustic input, such as speech

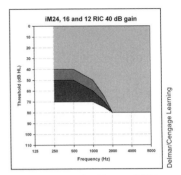

Fitting range for Vector iM24, iM16, and iM12 RIC 40 dB of gain: Open earbud (light gray), occluded earbud (medium gray), custom occluded earmold (dark gray)

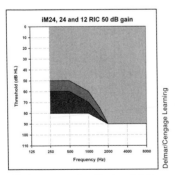

Fitting range for Vector iM24, iM16, and iM12 RIC 50 dB of gain: Open earbud (light gray), occluded earbud (medium gray), custom occluded earmold (dark gray)

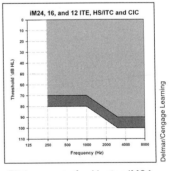

Fitting range for Vector iM24, iM16, and iM12 ITC, HS, ITC, and CIC: ITE (light gray), and HS/ITC, CIC (dark gray)

Options of Vector iM12 ITE, Vector iM12 HS, Vector iM12 ITE, and Vector iM12 CIC

- Leisure listening memories – for better processing music and television
- Voice indicators – alerts patient on status of battery, memory, and telephone modes
- Tonal indicators – different tones for memory, low battery, etc.
- Verify comfort
- In-Situ audiometry
- Data logging

Typical Specifications		Vector™iM24, iM16, and iM12 RIC (40 gain)	Vector™iM24, iM16, and iM12 RIC (50 gain)
Standard ANSI S3.22-1996			
Output sound pressure level	Max OSPL 90 (dB SPL)	110	115
	HF-average OSPL 90 (dB SPL)	102	108
Full-on gain	Peak gain (dB)	40	50
	HF-average-full-on gain (dB)	31	44
Total harmonic distortion	500 Hz	1.0%	1.0%
	800 Hz	1.6%	1.6%
	1600 Hz	2.5%	2.5%
Equivalent input noise (dB SPL)		<25	<25
Telecoil sensitivity	HFA-SPLITS (dB SPL)	n/a	n/a
Battery	Operating current (mA)	1.2	1.3
	Battery type	312	312
Compression characteristics – channel AGC	Attack (ms)	20	20
	Release 0.1s (ms)	5-150	5-150
	Release 2.0s (ms)	5-150	5-150

Delmar/Cengage Learning

Typical Specifications		Vector™iM24, iM16, and iM12 ITE	Vector™iM24, iM16, and iM12 HS/ITC	Vector™iM24, iM16, and iM12 CIC
Standard ANSI S3.22-1996				
Output sound pressure level	Max OSPL 90 (dB SPL)	115-131	110-131	110-131
	HF-average OSPL 90 (dB SPL)	111-126	106-126	106-126

continues

continued

Typical Specifications		Vector™iM24, iM16, and iM12 ITE	Vector™iM24, iM16, and iM12 HS/ITC	Vector™iM24, iM16, and iM12 CIC
Full-on gain	Peak gain (dB)	45-71	40-71	35-71
	HF-average-full-on gain (dB)	41-65	36-65	35-65
Total harmonic distortion	500 Hz	1.0%	1.0%	1.0%
	800 Hz	1.6%	1.6%	1.6%
	1600 Hz	2.5%	2.5%	2.5%
Equivalent input noise (dB SPL)		<28	<28	<28
Telecoil sensitivity	HFA-SPLITS (dB SPL)	n/a	n/a	n/a
Battery	Operating current (mA)	1.1-1.7	1.1-1.7	1.1-1.7
	Battery type	312 or 13	312, 13, or 10	312, 13, or 10
Compression characteristics – channel AGC	Attack (ms)	20	20	20
	Release 0.1s (ms)	5-150	5-150	5-150
	Release 2.0s (ms)	5-150	5-150	5-150

Delmar/Cengage Learning

PRODUCT 3: CURVE

Product Application

Curve m7 RIC
Curve m5 RIC
Curve m3 RIC

Features of Curve m7 RIC

- Integrated real ear measurement (IREM) – performs real-ear measurement and incorporates data immediately through Inspire® OS 3.0
- Auto-path fitting – initial fitting protocol designed to significantly shorten the fitting process
- Voice indicators – use speech to alert wearers of hearing aid status
- Patient reminders – reminds patient to schedule follow-up visits
- Self-check – a diagnostic check of the microphone, circuit, and receiver
- Acoustic signatures – type of environmental management that helps programs switch seamlessly
- Intelligent environmental adaptation – adjusts to different environments instantly
- Enhanced environmental adaptation – provides superior identification and detection of quiet and other sounds

- Environmental adaptation – transitions easily from one acoustic environment to the next
- Advanced data log with acoustic signature link – records use information, evaluates potential features, and makes recommendations for fitting adjustments
- Data log – records wide variety of data about the daily use of the hearing aid
- Precise fine-tuning – 8 channels and 12 bands
- Enhanced fine-tuning – 8 channels and 10 bands
- Fine-tuning – 4 channels and 8 bands
- Adaptive feedback intercept – eliminates feedback as well as the audible artifacts
- Adaptive indicator tones – indicator tones change intensity based on ambient noise levels
- Directional speech detector (DSD)
- Automatic telephone response – automatically switches to telephone mode
- 4-memory push-and-hold functionality

Options of Curve m7 RIC

- Open ear bud
- Occluded ear bud
- Custom occluded ear bud
- Colors: sterling, champagne, slate, pearl, bronze, and onyx

Features of Curve m5 RIC

- Auto-path fitting – initial fitting protocol designed to significantly shorten the fitting process
- Enhanced environmental adaptation – provides superior identification and detection of quiet and other sounds
- Environmental adaptation – transitions easily from one acoustic environment to the next
- Advanced data log with acoustic signature link – records use information, evaluates potential features, and makes recommendations for fitting adjustments
- Data log – records wide variety of data about the daily use of the hearing aid
- Precise fine-tuning – 8 channels and 12 bands
- Enhanced fine-tuning – 8 channels and 10 bands
- Fine-tuning – 4 channels and 8 bands
- Adaptive feedback intercept – eliminates feedback as well as the audible artifacts
- Adaptive indicator tones – indicator tones change intensity based on ambient noise levels
- Directional speech detector
- Automatic telephone response – automatically switches to telephone mode
- 4-memory push-and-hold functionality

Options of Curve m5 RIC

- Open ear bud
- Occluded ear bud
- Custom occluded ear bud
- Colors: sterling, champagne, slate, pearl, bronze, and onyx

Features of Curve m3 RIC

- Auto-path fitting – initial fitting protocol designed to significantly shorten the fitting process
- Environmental adaptation – transitions easily from one acoustic environment to the next
- Data log – records wide variety of data about the daily use of the hearing aid
- Fine-tuning – 4 channels and 8 bands
- Adaptive feedback intercept – eliminates feedback as well as the audible artifacts
- Adaptive indicator tones – indicator tones change intensity based on ambient noise levels
- Directional speech detector
- Automatic telephone response – automatically switches to telephone mode
- 4-memory push-and-hold functionality

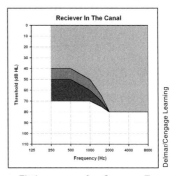

Options of Curve m3 RIC

- Open ear bud
- Occluded ear bud
- Custom occluded ear bud
- Colors: sterling, champagne, slate, pearl, bronze, and onyx

Fitting range for Curve m7 RIC, Curve m5 RIC, and Curve m3 RIC for a custom occluded ear bud (all shaded regions), occluded ear bud (medium and light gray), and open ear bud (light gray only)

Typical Specifications		Curve m7 RIC	Curve m5 RIC	Curve m3 RIC
Standard ANSI S3.22-1996				
Output sound Pressure level	Max OSPL 90 (dB SPL)	110	110	110
	HF-Average OSPL 90 (dB SPL)	105	105	105
Full-on gain	Peak gain (dB)	40	40	40
	HF-Average Full-on gain (dB)	36	36	36
Total harmonic distortion	500 Hz	1%	1%	1%
	800 Hz	1%	1%	1%
	1600 Hz	1%	1%	1%

continues

continued

Typical Specifications		Curve m7 RIC	Curve m5 RIC	Curve m3 RIC
Equivalent input noise (dB SPL)		25	25	25
Telecoil sensitivity	HFA-SPLITS (dB SPL)	n/a	n/a	n/a
Battery	Operating current (mA)	1.27-1.42	1.27-1.42	1.27-1.42
	Battery type	312	312	312
Compression characteristics – channel AGC	Attack (ms)	25	25	25
	Release 0.1s (ms)	57	57	57
	Release 2.0s (ms)	57	57	57

Delmar/Cengage Learning

PRODUCT 4: RADIUS

Product Application

Radius 16 Power BTE
Radius mini BTE
Radius 16 ITE
Radius 16 ITC
Radius 16 CIC

Features of Radius 16 Power BTE and Radius 16 mini BTE

- 8 channels
- 12 bands
- 4 program memories
- Active feedback intercept (off, adaptive (default), static) – uses acoustic cancellation to reduce feedback
- Environmental detection – detects acoustic signature (quiet, other sounds, mechanical sounds, wind)
- Directional speech detector – dynamic directional based on KEMAR (Knowles Electronic Manikin for Acoustic Research)
- Data log – records hearing aid use and makes recommendations for fitting changes in Inspire OS software
- Integrated real-ear measurement – performs real-ear measurements through hearing instrument and Inspire OS software
- Self-check – allows both patient and hearing care professional to perform a system diagnostic that checks the performance of the microphone, receiver, and circuit
- Audiometer
- Verify comfort
- Programmable reminder – alerts patients to schedule a follow-up appointment

- Voice indicators for self-check, reminder, battery, memory, and shutdown
- Indicator tones for memory selection, standby, volume control, low battery, telephone mode, and shutdown
- Automatic telephone response and induction coil
- Power-on delay
- Direct audio input (FM and Bluetooth)
- Tamper-resistant battery door

Options of Radius 16 Power BTE and Radius 16 mini BTE

- Colors: bisque, brushed platinum, brushed platinum duo, burnished iron, café, Cape Cod, Cape Cod duo, chestnut, chestnut duo, fairway, frost gold, latte, pebble, truffle, and tuxedo

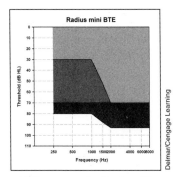

Fitting range for Radius 16, 12, 8, and 4 mini BTE thin tube open (light gray), thin tube occluded (light gray and medium gray), and standard earhook (all shaded regions)

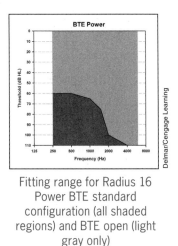

Fitting range for Radius 16 Power BTE standard configuration (all shaded regions) and BTE open (light gray only)

Features of Radius 16 ITE, Radius 16 ITC, and Radius 16 CIC

- 8 channels
- 12 bands
- 2 program memories
- Active feedback intercept (off, adaptive (default), static) – uses acoustic cancellation to reduce feedback
- Environment detection – detects acoustic signature (quiet, other sounds, mechanical sounds, wind)
- Directional speech detector – dynamic directional based on KEMAR
- Data log – records hearing aid use and makes recommendations for fitting changes in Inspire OS software
- Integrated real-ear measurement – performs real-ear measurements through hearing instrument and Inspire OS software

- Self-check – allows both patient and hearing care professional to perform a system diagnostic that checks the performance of the microphone, receiver, and circuit
- Audiometer
- Verify comfort
- Programmable reminder – alerts patients to schedule a follow-up appointment
- Voice indicators for self-check, reminder, battery, memory, and shutdown
- Indicator tones for memory selection, standby, volume control, low battery, telephone mode, and shutdown
- Automatic telephone response
- Volume control – up to 40 dB range

Options of Radius 16 ITE, Radius 16 ITC, and Radius 16 CIC

- 4 programmable memories
- Autocoil
- Colors: pink faceplate and shell, light-brown faceplate and shell, and medium-brown faceplate and shell (Radius 16 ITE and Radius 16 ITC)
- Colors: pink faceplate and pink shell, light-brown faceplate and clear shell, medium-brown faceplate and blue or red shell, and dark-brown faceplate and blue or red shell (Radius 16 CIC)

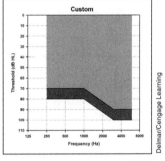

Fitting range for Radius 16 ITE (all shaded regions) and ITC/CIC (light gray only)

Product Application

Radius 12 Power BTE	Radius 12 BTE
Radius 12 Power Plus BTE	Radius 12 ITE
Radius 12 mini BTE	Radius 12 ITC
Radius 12 OTE	Radius 12 CIC
Radius 12 OTE DSD	

Features of Radius 12 Power BTE, Radius 12 Power Plus BTE, Radius 12 OTE, Radius 12 OTE DSD, and Radius 12 BTE, and Radius mini BTE

- 8 channels
- 12 bands
- Up to 4 memories*
- Active feedback intercept (off, adaptive (default), static) – uses acoustic cancellation to reduce feedback
- Environmental detection – detects acoustic signature (quiet, other sounds, mechanical sounds, wind)

- Directional speech detector – dynamic directional based on KEMAR (excludes Radius 12 OTE DSD)
- Directional speech detector – fixed directional (Radius 12 OTE DSD only)
- Data log* – records hearing aid use and makes recommendations for fitting changes in Inspire OS software
- Audiometer*
- Verify comfort*
- Tone indicators for memory selection, standby, volume control, low battery, telephone mode, and shutdown
- Automatic telephone response and induction coil (excludes Radius 12 OTE and Radius 12 OTE DSD)
  - Power-on delay
  - Direct audio input (DAI)* FM and Bluetooth
  - Tamper-resistant battery door
  - Programmed via Inspire OS software

*varies by product

Options of Radius 12 Power BTE, Radius 12 Power Plus BTE, Radius 12 OTE, Radius 12 OTE DSD, Radius 12 BTE, and Radius mini BTE

- Colors: ice, ice purple, light gray, brown, black, and beige (Radius 12 Power Plus BTE)
- Colors: beige, dark brown/beige, beige/dark brown, dark brown, light gray, light gray/dark gray, dark gray, black/dark gray, dark gray/black, black, ice, ice purple, and silver/blue (Radius 12 Power BTE and Radius 12 BTE)
- Colors: beige, smoke, light gray, dark gray, black, and brown (Radius 12 OTE)
- Colors: beige/brown, light gray/brown, and dark brown/brown (Radius 12 OTE DSD)

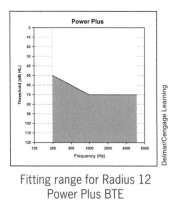

Fitting range for Radius 12
Power Plus BTE

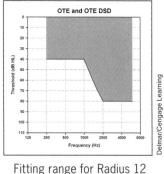

Fitting range for Radius 12
OTE and Radius 12 OTE DSD

Features of Radius 12 ITE, Radius 12 ITC, and Radius 12 CIC

- 8 channels
- 12 bands
- 2 program memories
- Active feedback intercept (off, adaptive (default), static) – uses acoustic cancellation to reduce feedback
- Environment detection: detects acoustic signature (quiet, other sounds, mechanical sounds, wind)
- Directional speech detector – dynamic directional based on KEMAR
- Data log – records hearing aid use and makes recommendations for fitting changes in Inspire OS software
- Audiometer
- Verify comfort
- Indicator tones – memory, low battery, volume control, battery shutdown, telephone
- Automatic telephone response
- Power-on delay
- Volume control (can disable in software) – up to 40 dB range

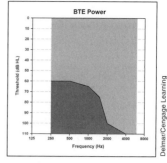

Fitting range for Radius 12 Power BTE standard configuration (all shaded regions) and open configuration (light gray only)

Options of Radius 12 ITE, Radius 12 ITC, and Radius 12 CIC

- 4 programmable memories
- Autocoil
- Colors: pink faceplate and shell, light-brown faceplate and shell, and medium-brown faceplate and shell (Radius 12 ITE and Radius 12 ITC)
- Colors: pink faceplate and pink shell, light-brown faceplate and clear shell, medium-brown faceplate and red or blue shell, and dark-brown faceplate and red or blue shell (Radius 12 CIC)

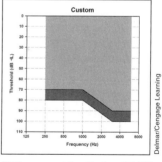

Fitting range for Radius 12 ITE (all shaded regions) and ITC/CIC (light gray only)

Product Application

Radius 8 Power BTE	Radius 8 ITC
Radius 8 mini BTE	Radius 8 CIC
Radius 8 ITE	

Features of Radius 8 Power BTE and Radius 8 mini BTE

- 8 channels
- 10 bands

- 4 program memories
- Active feedback intercept (off, adaptive (default), static) – uses acoustic cancellation to reduce feedback
- Environmental detection – detects acoustic signature (quiet, other sounds, mechanical sounds, wind)
- Directional speech detector – directional microphone system
- Data log – records hearing aid use and makes recommendations for fitting changes in Inspire OS software
- Audiometer*
- Verify comfort*
- Indicator tones – memory, low battery, volume control, battery shutdown, telephone
- Automatic telephone response and induction coil
- Power-on delay
- Direct audio input* – FM and Bluetooth
- Tamper-resistant battery door

*varies by product

Options of Radius 8 Power BTE and Radius 8 mini BTE

- Colors: beige, dark brown/beige, beige/dark brown, dark brown, light gray, light gray/dark gray, dark gray, black/dark gray, dark gray/black, black, ice, ice purple, and silver/blue

Features of Radius 8 ITE, Radius 8 ITC, and Radius 8 CIC

- 8 channels for sound adaptation
- 10 bands for fine-tuning
- 2 program memories
- Active feedback intercept (off, adaptive (default), static) – uses acoustic cancellation to reduce feedback
- Environmental detection – detects acoustic signature (quiet, other sounds, mechanical sounds, wind)
- Directional speech detector – dynamic directional based on KEMAR
- Data log – records hearing aid use and makes recommendations for fitting changes in Inspire OS software
- Audiometer
- Verify comfort
- Indicator tones – memory, low battery, volume control, battery shutdown, telephone
- Automatic telephone response

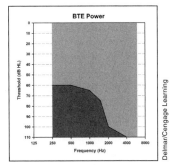

Fitting range for Radius 8 Power BTE standard configuration (all shaded regions) and open configuration (light gray only)

- Power-on delay
- Volume control – up to 40 dB range

Options of Radius 8 ITE, Radius 8 ITC, and Radius 8 CIC

- 4 programmable memories
- Autocoil
- Colors: pink faceplate and shell, light-brown faceplate and shell, and medium-brown faceplate and shell (Radius 8 ITE and Radius 8 ITC)
- Colors: pink faceplate and pink shell, light-brown faceplate and clear shell, medium-brown faceplate and red or blue shell, and dark-brown faceplate and red or blue shell (Radius 8 CIC)

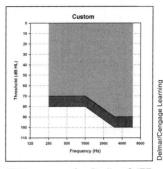

Fitting range for Radius 8 ITE (all shaded regions) and ITC/CIC (light gray only)

Product Application

Radius 4 Power BTE
Radius 4 mini BTE
Radius 4 ITE
Radius 4 ITC
Radius 4 CIC

Features of Radius 4 Power BTE and Radius 4 mini BTE

- 4 channels
- 8 bands
- 4 program memories*
- Active feedback intercept (off, adaptive (default), static) – uses acoustic cancellation to reduce feedback
- Environmental detection – detects acoustic signature (quiet, other sounds, mechanical sounds, wind)
- Directional speech detector – dynamic directional based on KEMAR
- Data log – records hearing aid use and makes recommendations for fitting changes in Inspire OS software
- Audiometer
- Verify comfort*
- Indicator tones – memory, low battery, volume control, battery shutdown, telephone
- Automatic telephone response
- Induction coil
- Power-on delay
- Direct audio input* – FM and Bluetooth
- Tamper-resistant battery door

*varies by product

Options of Radius 4 Power BTE and Radius 4 mini BTE

- Colors: beige, dark brown/beige, beige/dark brown, dark brown, light gray, light gray/dark gray, dark gray, black/dark gray, dark gray/ black, black, ice, ice purple, and silver/blue

Features of Radius 4 ITE, Radius 4 ITC, and Radius 4 CIC

- 4 channels
- 8 bands
- 2 program memories
- Active feedback intercept (off, adaptive (default), static) – uses acoustic cancellation to reduce feedback
- Environmental detection – detects acoustic signature (quiet, other sounds, mechanical sounds, wind)
- Directional speech detector – dynamic directional based on KEMAR
- Data log – records hearing aid use and makes recommendations for fitting changes in Inspire OS software
- Audiometer
- Verify comfort
- Indicator tones – memory, low battery, volume control, battery shutdown, telephone
- Automatic telephone response
- Power-on delay
- Volume control – up to 40 dB range

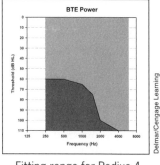

Fitting range for Radius 4 Power BTE standard configuration (all shaded regions) and open configuration (light gray only)

Options of Radius 4 ITE, Radius 4 ITC, and Radius 4 CIC

- 4 programmable memories
- Autocoil
- Colors: pink faceplate and shell, light-brown faceplate and shell, and medium-brown faceplate and shell (Radius 4 ITE and Radius 4 ITC)
- Colors: pink faceplate and pink shell, light-brown faceplate and clear shell, medium-brown faceplate and red or blue shell, and dark-brown faceplate and red or blue shell (Radius 4 CIC)

Product Application

Radius 2 Power BTE
Radius 2 BTE

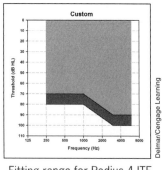

Fitting range for Radius 4 ITE (all shaded regions) and ITC/ CIC (light gray only)

Radius 2 ITE
Radius 2 ITC
Radius 2 CIC

Features of Radius 2 Power BTE and Radius 2 BTE

- 2 channels
- 8 bands
- 4 programmable memories*
- Active feedback intercept (off, adaptive (default), static) – uses acoustic cancellation to reduce feedback
- Environmental detection – detects acoustic signature (quiet, other sounds, mechanical sounds, wind)
- Indicator tones – memory, low battery, volume control, battery shutdown, telephone
- Programmable telecoil
- Power-on delay
- Tamper-resistant battery door

*varies by product

Options of Radius 2 Power BTE and Radius 2 BTE

- Colors: beige, dark brown/beige, beige/dark brown, dark brown, light gray, light gray/dark gray, dark gray, black/dark gray, dark gray/black, black, ice, ice purple, and silver/blue

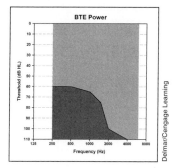

Fitting range for Radius 2 Power BTE standard configuration (all shaded regions) and open configuration (light gray only)

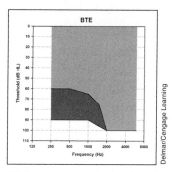

Fitting range for Radius 2 BTE standard (all shaded regions) and open configuration (light gray only)

Features of Radius 2 ITE, Radius 2 ITC, and Radius 2 CIC

- 2 channels
- 8 bands
- 1 programmable memory
- Active feedback intercept (off, adaptive (default), static) – uses acoustic cancellation to reduce feedback

- Environmental detection – detects acoustic signature (quiet, other sounds, mechanical sounds, wind)
- Indicator tones – memory, low battery, volume control, battery shutdown, telephone
- Power-on delay
- Volume control – up to 40 dB range

Options of Radius 12 ITE, Radius 2 ITC, and Radius 2 CIC

- 4 programmable memories
- Programmable Telecoil
- Colors: pink faceplate and shell, light-brown faceplate and shell, and medium-brown faceplate and shell (Radius 2 ITE and Radius 2 ITC)
- Colors: pink faceplate and pink shell, light-brown faceplate and clear shell, medium-brown faceplate and red or blue shell, and dark-brown faceplate and red or blue shell (Radius 2 CIC)

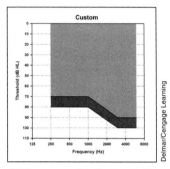

Fitting range for Radius 2 ITE (all shaded regions) and ITE/CIC (light gray only)

Typical Specifications		Radius 16, Radius 12, Radius 8, Radius 4 BTE	Radius 2 BTE	Radius 12 Open Ear BTE	Radius 12 Open Ear DSD	Radius 12 Power Plus BTE
Standard ANSI S3.22-1996						
Output sound Pressure level	Max OSPL (dB SPL)	135	128	115	115	140
	HF-Average OSPL 90 (dB SPL)	128	120	108	108	134
Full-on gain	Peak gain (dB)	70	60	40	40	80
	HF-Average Full-on gain (dB)	64	54	38	36	72
Total harmonic distortion	500 Hz	3%	2%	n/a	3%	<5%
	800 Hz	1%	1%	1%	3%	<2%
	1600 Hz	1%	1%	1%	3%	<1%
Equivalent input noise (dB SPL)		24	23	22	25	30
Telecoil sensitivity	HFA-SPLITS (dB SPL)	111	99	n/a	n/a	114
Battery	Operating current (mA)	1.6	1.4	1.3	1.32	2.8
	Battery type	13	13	312	10	675
Compression characteristics	Attack (ms)	5	10	5	5	5
	Release 0.1s (ms)	25	30	35	40	20
	Release 2.0s (ms)	25	30	35	40	20

Typical Specifications		Radius 16, Radius 12, Radius 8, Radius 4 mini BTE	Radius 16, Radius 12, Radius 8, Radius 4, Radius 2 ITE	Radius 12, Radius 16, Radius 12, Radius 8, Radius 4, Radius 2 ITC	Radius 12, Radius 16, Radius 12, Radius 8, Radius 4, Radius 2 CIC
Standard ANSI S3.22-1996					
Output sound Pressure level	Max OSPL (dB SPL)	123	113–120	110–115	110–113
	HF-Average OSPL 90 (dB SPL)	117	104–110	101–108	101–105
Full-on gain	Peak gain (dB)	55	30–55	30–50	30–50
	HF-Average Full-on gain (dB)	49	24–48	22–45	22–42
Total harmonic distortion (Hz)	500	6%	<3%	<3%	<3%
	800	3%	<3%	<3%	<3%
	1600	3%	<3%	<3%	<3%
Equivalent input noise (dB SPL)		28	<28	<28	<28
Telecoil sensitivity	HFA-SPLITS (dB SPL)	n/a	90–99	89–98	n/a
Battery	Operating current (mA)	1.25-1.6	1.1–1.5	1.1–1.5	1.1–1.5
	Battery type	312	13, 312	312, 10	10
Compression characteristics	Attack (ms)	25	5	5	5
	Release 0.1s (ms)	55	5–150	5–150	5–150
	Release 2.0s (ms)	55	5–150	5–150	5–150

Delmar/Cengage Learning

CHAPTER FIVE

Oticon

FOCUSING ON PEOPLE AND PRODUCTS

International Headquarters
Oticon A/S
Kongebakken 9
2765 Smørum
Denmark
Phone: +45 39 17 71 00
Fax: +45 39 27 79 00
E-mail: contact-us@oticon.com
Web site: http://www.oticon.com

U.S. Headquarters
Oticon, Inc.
29 Schoolhouse Road
Somerset, NJ 08873
Phone: 1-800-526-3921
Fax: 1-732-560-0029
E-mail: webmaster@oticonus.com
Web site: http://www.oticonus.com

> *To help people live the life they want with the hearing they have.*
> — Oticon vision (Oticon, 2007)

Founded in 1904, Oticon is one of the oldest names in the hearing industry. The company was originally founded as Oticon by Hans Demant, but the name was eventually changed to William Demant Holding to reflect the name of Hans's son and successor, William Demant, who took the helm in 1910. Hans Demant's main motivation was that his wife was hearing-impaired; he strongly desired to help his wife and others with hearing loss (Oticon, 2007a). It was at this time that Oticon moved to Copenhagen, Denmark. Oticon saw significant growth in the 1960s as it expanded into the United States, Switzerland, and Germany. In the 1980s, Oticon realized that not all technological solutions actually benefit the hearing instrument user and changed its focus likewise. Eriksholm, Oticon's independent research facility, looks for ways to improve hearing aids by considering the latest research in hearing science and hearing loss. Some of Oticon's other milestones are as follows (taken from Oticon, 2009, 2008a, 2008b, 2007c):

- 1930: Oticon's product lineup included hearing instruments for personal and church use, and hospital systems
- 1940: Employed 16 people and established its own production facility in Copenhagen due to the German trade block
- 1946: Introduced its first "all Oticon" hearing instrument (Oticon TA)
- 1957: The Oticon Foundation (originally the William Demant & Ida Emilie Foundation) was established through stock donations from William Demant and his wife
- 1977: Established its independent hearing research (read: *not* technology) facility, Eriksholm
- 1991: Introduced the first hearing instrument with automatic gain control, thus eliminating the volume control (MultiFocus)
- 1995: William Demant Holding (at the time Oticon Holding) went public on the Copenhagen Stock Exchange
- 2001: Introduced an advanced digital hearing instrument (Adapto)
- 2004: Included a level of intelligence in their hearing instruments (Syncro)
- 2006: Broadened the design elements of hearing instruments with their new device, which won the European Information Society Technology first grand prize (Delta)
- 2007: Introduced their first binaural communication-enabled device (Epoq)
- 2008: Expanded their premium product with value pricing line (Vigo and Vigo Pro)
- 2008: Released full-featured hearing instruments in a 2-cm package (Dual)
- 2009: Released latest high-end hearing instrument line (Hit Pro and Hit)

Philanthropy

Oticon sponsors a program, OtiKids (see http://otikids.com), which provides information resources to children with hearing loss and their parents; these resources include information on how to better cope with hearing loss. Ultimately, the goal of the program is to improve children's communication and performance in everyday situations (Oticon, 2007b).

Oticon has always espoused putting people first. Consistent with the Demant vision, and therefore Oticon's, the William Demant & Ida Emilie Foundation was established in 1957 (Oticon, 2007d). Eventually, this was renamed the Oticon Foundation. The Oticon Foundation seeks to "support the needs of hearing-impaired individuals as well as organizations" (Oticon, 2007d). Oticon also supports students with hearing loss through Sertoma International, a longtime U.S.-based civic service club. Through various fundraisers, Oticon recently donated $50,000 to the American Academy of Audiology Foundation (Hearing Review, 2009a).

Warranty

Oticon includes 2-year repair and 1-year loss-and-damage coverage for the Syncro, Delta, Safran, Tego, Tego Pro, and Sumo DM. The remainder of its hearing instruments is covered by a 1-year repair and loss-and-damage warranty (e.g., Sumo E and Sumo XP).

PRODUCT INFORMATION

PRODUCT 1: HIT PRO

Product Application

> Hit Pro RITE
> Hit Pro BTE 312
> Hit Pro BTE 13
> Hit Pro BTE Power
> Hit Pro HS/LP
> Hit Pro ITC
> Hit Pro CIC/MIC

Features of Hit Pro RITE

- Bandwidth 8000 Hz
- Single-band adaptive directionality – attenuates noise sources from the sides and behind
- Dual-mode automatic directionality
- Noise management (modulation) – uses speech detection to reduce the effects of noise without notably affecting important speech cues
- Automatic adaptation manager – gradually increases gain to the prescribed level to facilitate acclimatization
- Dynamic Feedback Cancellation 2 (DFC2) – eliminates feedback in most situations
- Front Focus – a directional system designed to aid in front/back sound source determination
- OpenEar Acoustics™
- Wind noise protection – an integrated filter designed to reduce the noise levels that occur when wind hits the microphone
- NAL – NL$_1$ and DSL v5.0 a m[i/o]
- Activity analyzer – a data-logging feature that suggests adjustments to the hearing professional
- Direct audio input (DAI) and FM
- Low-battery warning
- Sound indicators for program shifts
- Onset delay and "jingle" sound indicator
- Mute/Standby mode

- nEARcom cordless – enabled
- 6 fitting bands
- 4 user programs

Options of Hit Pro RITE

- 1 to 4 programs
- Cordless fitting (nEARcom)
- Telecoil
- AutoPhone™ – automatic shift to 1 of 2 dedicated phone programs, acoustic phone (AP): microphone or phone T (PT): telecoil
- Configurable volume control
- FM-compatible
- Speaker unit available in 4 lengths
- Ear grip
- NoWax speaker unit
- WaxStop in Micro Mold
- Tamper-resistant battery drawer
- AP_{900} DAI adapter
- R_{12} FM receiver
- FM_9 adapter

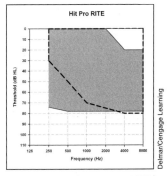

Fitting range for Hit Pro RITE: Dome (area within dotted line), micro mould (light gray)

Features of Hit Pro BTE 312

- Bandwidth 8000 Hz
- Single-band adaptive directionality – attenuates noise sources from the sides and behind
- Dual-mode automatic directionality
- Noise management (modulation) – attenuates interfering noise without notably affecting important speech cues
- Automatic adaptation manager – gradually increases gain to the prescribed level to facilitate acclimatization
- Dynamic Feedback Cancellation 2 – eliminates feedback in most situations
- Front Focus – a directional system designed to aid in front/back sound source determination
- OpenEar Acoustics
- Wind noise protection – an integrated filter designed to reduce the noise levels that occur when wind hits the microphone
- NAL – NL_1 and DSL v5.0 a m[i/o]
- Activity analyzer – a data-logging feature that suggests adjustments to the hearing professional
- DAI and FM
- Low-battery warning
- Sound indicators for program shifts
- Onset delay and "jingle" sound indicator
- Mute/Standby mode

- nEARcom cordless – enabled
- 6 fitting bands
- 4 user programs

Options of Hit Pro BTE 312

- 1 to 4 programs
- Cordless fitting (nEARcom)
- Telecoil
- AutoPhone – automatic shift to 1 of 2 dedicated phone programs, acoustic phone (AP): microphone or phone T (PT): telecoil
- Configurable volume control
- FM-compatible
- Tamper-resistant battery drawer
- Interchangeable standard and pediatric sound hooks
- Damper – damping element for replacement
- Corda^2 thin-tube fitting
- AP$_{900}$ DAI adapter
- R$_{12}$ FM receiver
- FM$_9$ adapter

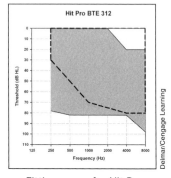

Fitting range for Hit Pro BTE 312: Corda^2 (area within dotted line), earmold (light gray)

Features of Hit Pro BTE 13

- Bandwidth 8000 Hz
- Single-band adaptive directionality – attenuates noise sources from the sides and behind
- Dual-mode automatic directionality
- Noise management (modulation) – uses speech detection to reduce the effects of noise without notably affecting important speech cues
- Automatic adaptation manager – gradually increases gain to the prescribed level to facilitate acclimatization
- Dynamic Feedback Cancellation 2 – eliminates feedback in most situations
- Front Focus – a directional system designed to aid in front/back sound source determination
- OpenEar Acoustics
- Wind noise protection – an integrated filter designed to reduce the noise levels that occur when wind hits the microphone
- NAL – NL$_1$ and DSL v5.0 a m[i/o]
- Activity analyzer – a data-logging feature that suggests adjustments to the hearing professional
- DAI and FM
- Low-battery warning
- Sound indicators for program shifts
- Onset delay and "jingle" sound indicator

- Mute/Standby mode
- nEARcom cordless – enabled
- 6 fitting bands
- 4 user programs

Options of Hit Pro BTE 13

- 1 to 4 programs
- Cordless fitting (nEARcom)
- Telecoil
- AutoPhone – automatic shift to 1 of 2 dedicated phone programs,
- acoustic phone (AP): microphone or phone T (PT): telecoil
- Configurable volume control
- FM-compatible
- Tamper-resistant battery drawer
- Interchangeable standard and pediatric sound hooks
- Damper – damping element for replacement
- Corda^2 thin-tube fitting
- AP$_{900}$ DAI adapter
- R$_{12}$ FM receiver
- FM$_9$ adapter

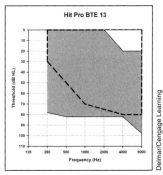

Fitting range for Hit Pro 13: Corda^2 (area within dotted line), earmold (light gray)

Features of Hit Pro BTE Power

- Bandwidth 8000 Hz
- Single-band adaptive directionality – attenuates noise sources from the sides and behind
- Dual-mode automatic directionality
- Noise management (modulation) – uses speech detection to reduce the effects of noise without notably affecting important speech cues
- Automatic adaptation manager – gradually increases gain to the prescribed level to facilitate acclimatization
- Dynamic Feedback Cancellation 2 – eliminates feedback in most situations
- Front Focus – a directional system designed to aid in front/back sound source determination
- OpenEar Acoustics
- Wind noise protection – an integrated filter designed to reduce the noise levels that occur when wind hits the microphone
- NAL – NL$_1$ and DSL v5.0 a m[i/o]
- Activity analyzer – a data-logging feature that suggests adjustments to the hearing professional
- DAI and FM
- Low-battery warning
- Sound indicators for program shifts

- Onset delay and "jingle" sound indicator
- Mute/Standby mode
- nEARcom cordless – enabled
- 6 fitting bands
- 4 user programs

Options of Hit Pro BTE Power

- 1 to 4 programs
- Cordless fitting (nEARcom)
- Telecoil
- AutoPhone – automatic shift to 1 of 2 dedicated phone programs, acoustic phone (AP): microphone or phone T (PT): telecoil
- Configurable volume control
- FM-compatible
- Tamper-resistant battery drawer
- Interchangeable standard and pediatric sound hooks
- Damper – damping element for replacement
- AP_{900} DAI adapter
- R_{12} FM receiver
- FM_9 adapter

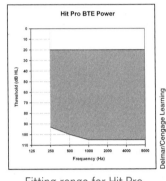

Fitting range for Hit Pro BTE Power

Features of Hit Pro HS/LP

- Bandwidth 8000 Hz
- Single-band adaptive directionality – attenuates noise sources from the sides and behind
- Dual-mode automatic directionality
- Noise management (modulation) – uses speech detection to reduce the effects of noise without notably affecting important speech cues
- Automatic adaptation manager – gradually increases gain to the prescribed level to facilitate acclimatization
- Dynamic Feedback Cancellation 2 – eliminates feedback in most situations
- Front Focus – a directional system designed to aid in front/back sound source determination
- OpenEar Acoustics
- Wind noise protection – an integrated filter designed to reduce the noise levels that occur when wind hits the microphone
- NAL – NL_1 and DSL v5.0 a m[i/o]
- Activity analyzer – a data-logging feature that suggests adjustments to the hearing professional
- DAI and FM

- Low-battery warning
- Sound indicators for program shifts
- Onset delay and "jingle" sound indicator
- Mute/Standby mode
- 6 fitting bands
- 4 user programs

Options of Hit Pro HS/LP

- 1 to 4 programs
- Optional telecoil
- Optional AutoPhone
- Optional volume control

Features of Hit Pro ITC

- Bandwidth 8000 Hz
- Single-band adaptive directionality – attenuates noise sources from the sides and behind
- Dual-mode automatic directionality
- Noise management (modulation) – uses speech detection to reduce the effects of noise without notably affecting important speech cues
- Automatic adaptation manager – gradually increases gain to the prescribed level to facilitate acclimatization
- Dynamic Feedback Cancellation 2 – eliminates feedback in most situations
- Front Focus – a directional system designed to aid in front/back sound source determination
- OpenEar Acoustics
- Wind noise protection – an integrated filter designed to reduce the noise levels that occur when wind hits the microphone
- NAL – NL$_1$ and DSL v5.0 a m[i/o]
- Activity analyzer – a data-logging feature that suggests adjustments to the hearing professional
- DAI and FM
- Low-battery warning
- Sound indicators for program shifts
- Onset delay and "jingle" sound indicator
- Mute/Standby mode
- 6 fitting bands
- 4 user programs

Options of Hit Pro ITC

- 1 to 4 programs
- Optional AutoPhone

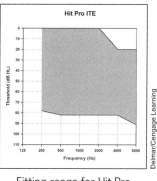

Fitting range for Hit Pro ITE, HS/LP

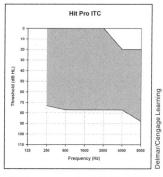

Fitting range for Hit Pro ITC

Features of Hit Pro CIC/MIC

- Bandwidth 8000 Hz
- Noise management (modulation) – uses speech detection to reduce the effects of noise without notably affecting important speech cues
- Automatic adaptation manager – gradually increases gain to the prescribed level to facilitate acclimatization
- Dynamic Feedback Cancellation 2 – eliminates feedback in most situations
- Front Focus – a directional system designed to aid in front/back sound source determination
- OpenEar Acoustics
- Wind noise protection – an integrated filter designed to reduce the noise levels that occur when wind hits the microphone
- NAL – NL$_1$ and DSL v5.0 a m[i/o]
- Activity analyzer – a data-logging feature that suggests adjustments to the hearing professional
- DAI and FM
- Low-battery warning
- Sound indicators for program shifts
- Onset delay and "jingle" sound indicator
- Mute/Standby mode
- 6 fitting bands
- 4 user programs

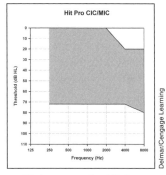

Fitting range for Hit Pro CIC/MIC

Options of Hit Pro CIC/MIC

- 1 program

Typical Specifications		Hit Pro RITE	Hit Pro BTE 312	Hit Pro BTE 13	Hit Pro Power
Standard ANSI S3.22-2003 and S3.7 (1995)					
Output sound pressure level	Max OSPL 90 (dB SPL)	108	115 (108*)	118 (117*)	127
	Avg OSPL 90 (dB SPL)	104	105 (94*)	114 (104*)	120
Full-on gain (50 dB SPL input)	Peak gain (dB)	46	51 (49*)	51 (49*)	61
	Avg (dB)	37	45 (34*)	45 (34*)	55
Total harmonic distortion (Hz)	500	0.1%	0.7%	0.2%	1.0%
	800	0.3%	0.9%	0.4%	0.5%
	1600	0.4%	0.1%	0.2%	0.3%
Equivalent input noise (dB SPL)	Omni	19	17	18	15
	Dir	25	26	27	26
Telecoil sensitivity	SPLITS (dB SPL) L/R	87/89	88/88	95/95	99/99
Battery	Operating current (mA)	1.3	1.1	1.2	1.2
	Battery type	312	312	13	13

*Devices fit with Corda[2] fitting system

Typical Specifications		Hit Pro CIC/MIC	Hit Pro ITC	Hit Pro HS/LP
Standard ANSI S3.22-2003 and S3.7 (1995)				
Output sound pressure level	Max OSPL 90 (dB SPL)	109	113	113
	Avg OSPL 90 (dB SPL)	104	107	102
Full-on gain (50 dB SPL input)	Peak gain (dB)	37	41	46
	Avg (dB)	33	37	41
Total harmonic distortion (Hz)	500	0.3%	0.6%	0.5%
	800	0.4%	0.6%	0.4%
	1600	0.9%	0.6%	0.4%
Equivalent input noise (dB SPL)	Omni	18	17	17
	Dir	n/a	n/q	25
Telecoil sensitivity	SPLITS (dB SPL) L/R	n/a	n/a	87/87
Battery	Operating current (mA)	0.8	1.2 (1.0*)	1.3 (1.1*)
	Battery type	10	312	312

*Devices fit with Corda^2 fitting system

Delmar/Cengage Learning

PRODUCT 2: HIT

Product Application

Hit RITE
Hit BTE 312
Hit BTE 13
Hit BTE Power
Hit HS/LP
Hit ITC
Hit CIC/MIC

Features of Hit RITE

- Bandwidth 8000 Hz
- Dual-mode automatic directionality
- Noise management (modulation) – uses speech detection to reduce the effects of noise without notably affecting important speech cues
- Dynamic Feedback Cancellation 2 – eliminates feedback in most situations
- Front Focus – a directional system designed to aid in front/back sound source determination
- OpenEar Acoustics
- Wind noise protection – an integrated filter designed to reduce the noise levels that occur when wind hits the microphone
- NAL – NL$_1$ and DSL v5.0 a m[i/o]
- Activity analyzer – a data-logging feature that suggests adjustments to the hearing professional

- DAI and FM
- Low-battery warning
- Sound indicators for program shifts
- Onset delay and "jingle" sound indicator
- Mute/Standby mode
- nEARcom cordless – enabled
- 4 fitting bands
- 4 user programs

Options of Hit RITE

- 1 to 4 programs
- Cordless fitting (nEARcom)
- Telecoil
- AutoPhone – automatic shift to 1 of 2 dedicated phone programs, acoustic phone (AP): microphone or phone T (PT): telecoil
- Configurable volume control
- FM-compatible
- Speaker unit available in 4 lengths
- Ear grip
- NoWax speaker unit
- WaxStop in Micro Mold
- Tamper-resistant battery drawer
- AP_{900} DAI adapter
- R_{12} FM receiver
- FM_9 adapter

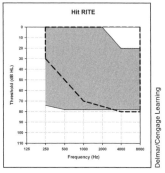

Fitting range for Hit RITE: Dome (area within dotted line), micro mould (light gray)

Features of Hit BTE 312

- Bandwidth 8000 Hz
- Dual-mode automatic directionality
- Noise management (modulation) – uses speech detection to reduce the effects of noise without notably affecting important speech cues
- Dynamic Feedback Cancellation 2 – eliminates feedback in most situations
- Front Focus – a directional system designed to aid in front/back sound source determination
- OpenEar Acoustics
- Wind noise protection – an integrated filter designed to reduce the noise levels that occur when wind hits the microphone
- NAL – NL_1 and DSL v5.0 a m[i/o]
- Activity analyzer – a data-logging feature that suggests adjustments to the hearing professional
- DAI and FM
- Low-battery warning

- Sound indicators for program shifts
- Onset delay and "jingle" sound indicator
- Mute/Standby mode
- nEARcom cordless – enabled
- 4 fitting bands
- 4 user programs

Options of Hit BTE 312

- 1 to 4 programs
- Cordless fitting (nEARcom)
- Telecoil
- AutoPhone – automatic shift to 1 of 2 dedicated phone programs, acoustic phone (AP): microphone or phone T (PT): telecoil
- Configurable volume control
- FM-compatible
- Tamper-resistant battery drawer
- Interchangeable standard and pediatric sound hooks
- Damper – damping element for replacement
- Corda^2 thin-tube fitting
- AP$_{900}$ DAI adapter
- R$_{12}$ FM receiver
- FM$_9$ adapter

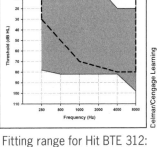

Fitting range for Hit BTE 312: Corda^2 (area within dotted line), earmold (light gray)

Features of Hit BTE 13

- Bandwidth 8000 Hz
- Dual-mode automatic directionality
- Noise management (modulation) – uses speech detection to reduce the effects of noise without notably affecting important speech cues
- Dynamic Feedback Cancellation 2 – eliminates feedback in most situations
- Front Focus – a directional system designed to aid in front/back sound source determination
- OpenEar Acoustics
- Wind noise protection – an integrated filter designed to reduce the noise levels that occur when wind hits the microphone
- NAL – NL$_1$ and DSL v5.0 a m[i/o]
- Activity analyzer – a data-logging feature that suggests adjustments to the hearing professional
- DAI and FM
- Low-battery warning
- Sound indicators for program shifts
- Onset delay and "jingle" sound indicator

- Mute/Standby mode
- nEARcom cordless – enabled
- 4 fitting bands
- 4 user programs

Options of Hit BTE 13

- 1 to 4 programs
- Cordless fitting (nEARcom)
- Telecoil
- AutoPhone – automatic shift to 1 of 2 dedicated phone programs, acoustic phone (AP): microphone or phone T (PT): telecoil
- Configurable volume control
- FM-compatible
- Tamper-resistant battery drawer
- Interchangeable standard and pediatric sound hooks
- Damper – damping element for replacement
- Corda^2 thin-tube fitting
- AP$_{900}$ DAI adapter
- R$_{12}$ FM receiver
- FM$_9$ adapter

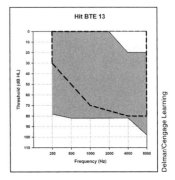

Fitting range for Hit BTE 312: Corda^2 (area within dotted line), earmold (light gray)

Features of Hit BTE Power

- Bandwidth 8000 Hz
- Dual-mode automatic directionality
- Noise management (modulation) – uses speech detection to reduce the effects of noise without notably affecting important speech cues
- Dynamic Feedback Cancellation 2 – eliminates feedback in most situations
- Front Focus – a directional system designed to aid in front/back sound source determination
- OpenEar Acoustics
- Wind noise protection – an integrated filter designed to reduce the noise levels that occur when wind hits the microphone
- NAL – NL$_1$ and DSL v5.0 a m[i/o]
- Activity analyzer – a data-logging feature that suggests adjustments to the hearing professional
- DAI and FM
- Low-battery warning
- Sound indicators for program shifts
- Onset delay and "jingle" sound indicator
- Mute/Standby mode
- nEARcom cordless – enabled
- 4 fitting bands
- 4 user programs

Options of Hit BTE Power

- 1 to 4 programs
- Cordless fitting (nEARcom)
- Telecoil
- AutoPhone – automatic shift to 1 of 2 dedicated phone programs, acoustic phone (AP): microphone or phone T (PT): telecoil
- Configurable volume control
- FM-compatible
- Tamper-resistant battery drawer
- Interchangeable standard and pediatric sound hooks
- Damper – damping element for replacement
- AP_{900} DAI adapter
- R_{12} FM receiver
- FM_9 adapter

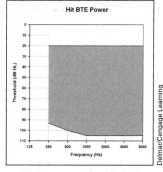

Fitting range for Hit BTE Power

Features of Hit HS/LP

- Bandwidth 8000 Hz
- Dual-mode automatic directionality
- Noise management (modulation) – uses speech detection to reduce the effects of noise without notably affecting important speech cues
- Dynamic Feedback Cancellation 2 – eliminates feedback in most situations
- Front Focus – a directional system designed to aid in front/back sound source determination
- OpenEar Acoustics
- Wind noise protection – an integrated filter designed to reduce the noise levels that occur when wind hits the microphone
- NAL – NL_1 and DSL v5.0 a m[i/o]
- Activity analyzer – a data-logging feature that suggests adjustments to the hearing professional
- DAI and FM
- Low-battery warning
- Sound indicators for program shifts
- Onset delay and "jingle" sound indicator
- Mute/Standby mode
- 4 fitting bands
- 4 user programs

Options of Hit HS/LP

- 1 to 4 programs
- Optional telecoil
- Optional AutoPhone
- Optional volume control

Features of Hit ITC

- Bandwidth 8000 Hz
- Dual-mode automatic directionality
- Noise management (modulation) – uses speech detection to reduce the effects of noise without notably affecting important speech cues
- Dynamic Feedback Cancellation 2 – eliminates feedback in most situations
- Front Focus – a directional system designed to aid in front/back sound source determination
- OpenEar Acoustics
- Wind noise protection – an integrated filter designed to reduce the noise levels that occur when wind hits the microphone
- NAL – NL$_1$ and DSL v5.0 a m[i/o]
- Activity analyzer – a data-logging feature that suggests adjustments to the hearing professional
- DAI and FM
- Low-battery warning
- Sound indicators for program shifts
- Onset delay and "jingle" sound indicator
- Mute/Standby mode
- 4 fitting bands
- 4 user programs

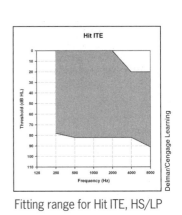

Fitting range for Hit ITE, HS/LP

Options of Hit ITC

- 1 to 4 programs
- Optional AutoPhone

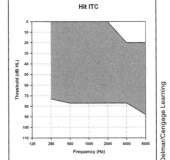

Fitting range for Hit ITC

Features of Hit CIC/MIC

- Bandwidth 8000 Hz
- Noise management (modulation) – uses speech detection to reduce the effects of noise without notably affecting important speech cues
- Dynamic Feedback Cancellation 2 – eliminates feedback in most situations
- Front Focus – a directional system designed to aid in front/back sound source determination
- OpenEar Acoustics
- Wind noise protection – an integrated filter designed to reduce the noise levels that occur when wind hits the microphone
- NAL – NL$_1$ and DSL v5.0 a m[i/o]
- Activity analyzer – a data-logging feature that suggests adjustments to the hearing professional

- DAI and FM
- Low-battery warning
- Sound indicators for program shifts
- Onset delay and "jingle" sound indicator
- Mute/Standby mode
- 4 fitting bands
- 4 user programs

Options of Hit CIC/MIC

- 1 program

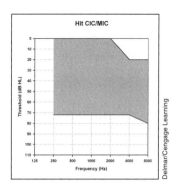

Fitting range for Hit CIC/MIC

Typical Specifications		Hit RITE	Hit BTE 312	Hit BTE 13	Hit BTE Power
Standard ANSI S3.22-2003 and S3.7 (1995)					
Output sound pressure level	Max OSPL 90 (dB SPL)	108	115 (108*)	118 (117*)	127
	Avg OSPL 90 (dB SPL)	104	105 (94*)	114 (104*)	120
Full-on gain (50 dB SPL input)	Peak gain (dB)	46	51 (49*)	51 (49*)	61
	Avg (dB)	37	45 (34*)	45 (34*)	55
Total harmonic distortion (Hz)	500	0.1%	0.7%	0.2%	1.0%
	800	0.3%	0.9%	0.4%	0.5%
	1600	0.4%	0.1%	0.2%	0.3%
Equivalent input noise (dB SPL)	Omni	19	17	18	15
	Dir	25	26	27	26
Telecoil sensitivity	SPLITS (dB SPL) L/R	87/89	88/88	95/95	99/99
Battery	Operating current (mA)	1.3	1.1	1.2	1.2
	Battery type	312	312	13	13

*for instruments fitted with Corda[2]

Delmar/Cengage Learning

Typical Specifications		Hit CIC/MIC	Hit ITC	Hit HS/LP
Standard ANSI S3.22-2003 and S3.7 (1995)				
Output sound pressure level	Max OSPL 90 (dB SPL)	109	113	113
	Avg OSPL 90 (dB SPL)	104	107	102
Full-on gain (50 dB SPL input)	Peak gain (dB)	37	41	46
	Avg (dB)	33	37	41

continues

continued

Typical Specifications		Hit CIC/MIC	Hit ITC	Hit HS/LP
Total harmonic distortion (Hz)	500	0.3%	0.6%	0.5%
	800	0.4%	0.6%	0.4%
	1600	0.9%	0.6%	0.4%
Equivalent input noise (dB SPL)	Omni	18	17	17
	Dir	n/a	n/q	25
Telecoil sensitivity	SPLITS (dB SPL) L/R	n/a	n/a	87/87
Battery	Operating current (mA)	0.8	1.2 (1.0*)	1.3 (1.1*)
	Battery type	10	312	312

*for non-wireless instruments

PRODUCT 3: DUAL

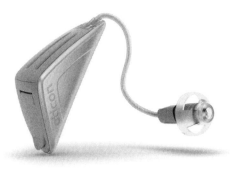

Dual Mini
Photos granted by Oticon, Inc.

Product Application

Dual XW RITE
Dual W RITE
Dual V RITE
Dual PRO RITE
Dual Mini m9 RITE
Dual Mini m7 RITE
Dual Mini m5 RITE

Features of Dual XW RITE

- Receiver-in-the-ear (RITE) hearing aid – receiver is placed in the ear canal and amplifier is placed behind the ear
- Advanced binaural processing
- Binaural synchronization
- Binaural coordination

- Binaural DFC
- MyVoice
- 10 kHz bandwidth
- 10 fitting bands
- Multiband adaptive directionality – adaptive directional microphone system utilizing four frequency bands
- Front Focus – a directional system designed to aid in front/back sound source determination
- TriState noise management – uses modulations in speech to determine speech and noise content in eight bands to improve the overall speech-to-noise ratio
- VAC/Clarity$_2$ rationales
- Dynamic Feedback Cancellation
- Memory/data-logging
- Phonecoil
- AutoPhone – automatic shift to 1 of 2 dedicated phone programs, acoustic phone (AP): microphone or phone T (PT): telecoil
- nEARcom provides a wireless link between NOAHlink and 1 or 2 hearing aids

Options of Dual XW RITE

- Speaker unit available in 4 lengths: short, medium, long, and extra-long
- 4 different earpieces available:
  - Open dome – available in 3 sizes: 6 mm, 8 mm, and 10 mm
  - Plus dome – available in only 1 size
  - Power dome – available in 3 sizes: 8 mm, 10 mm, and 12 mm
  - Micro Mold – requires taking an impression
- Ear grip – ensures a secure and comfortable grip: one version to fit the right ear and another version to fit the left ear
- Streamer optional
- 5 programs

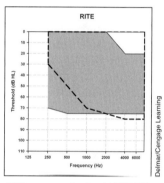

Fitting range for Dual XW RITE, Dual W RITE, Dual V RITE, and Dual PRO RITE. Micro Mold with power dome (gray), open dome and plus dome (dotted line)

Features of Dual W RITE

- Receiver-in-the-ear (RITE) hearing aid – receiver is placed in the ear canal and amplifier is placed behind the ear
- Binaural synchronization
- Binaural coordination
- Binaural DFC
- 8 kHz bandwidth
- 8 fitting bands
- Multiband adaptive directionality – adaptive directional microphone system utilizing four frequency bands

- Front Focus – a directional system designed to aid in front/back sound source determination
- TriState noise management – uses modulations in speech to determine speech and noise content in eight bands to improve the overall speech-to-noise ratio
- VAC/Clarity$_2$ rationales
- Dynamic Feedback Cancellation
- Memory/data-logging
- Phonecoil
- AutoPhone – automatic shift to 1 of 2 dedicated phone programs, acoustic phone (AP): microphone or phone T (PT): telecoil
- nEARcom provides a wireless link between NOAHlink and 1 or 2 hearing aids

Options of Dual W RITE

- Speaker unit available in 4 lengths: short, medium, long, and extra-long
- 4 different earpieces available:
  - Open dome – available in 3 sizes: 6 mm, 8 mm, and 10 mm
  - Plus dome – available in only 1 size
  - Power dome – available in 3 sizes: 8 mm, 10 mm, and 12 mm
  - Micro Mold – requires taking an impression
- Ear grip – ensures a secure and comfortable grip: one version to fit the right ear and another version to fit the left ear
- Streamer optional
- 5 programs

Features of Dual V RITE

- RITE hearing aid – receiver is placed in the ear canal and amplifier is placed behind the ear
- Binaural coordination
- Binaural DFC
- 8 kHz bandwidth
- 6 fitting bands
- Single-band adaptive directionality
- Front Focus – a directional system designed to aid in front/back sound source determination
- Two-state noise management
- VAC/Clarity$_2$ rationales
- Dynamic Feedback Cancellation
- Memory/data-logging
- Phonecoil
- AutoPhone – automatic shift to 1 of 2 dedicated phone programs, acoustic phone (AP): microphone or phone T (PT): telecoil
- nEARcom provides a wireless link between NOAHlink and 1 or 2 hearing aids

Options of Dual V RITE

- Speaker unit available in 4 lengths: short, medium, long, and extra-long
- 4 different earpieces available:
  - Open dome – available in 3 sizes: 6 mm, 8 mm, and 10 mm
  - Plus dome – available in only 1 size
  - Power dome – available in 3 sizes: 8 mm, 10 mm, and 12 mm
  - Micro Mold – requires taking an impression
- Ear grip – ensures a secure and comfortable grip: one version to fit the right ear and another version to fit the left ear
- Streamer optional
- 3 programs

Features of Dual PRO RITE

- RITE hearing aid – receiver is placed in the ear canal and amplifier is placed behind the ear
- 8 kHz bandwidth
- 6 fitting bands
- Single-band adaptive directionality
- Front Focus – a directional system designed to aid in front/back sound source determination
- Two-state noise management
- VAC/Clarity$_2$ rationales
- Dynamic Feedback Cancellation
- Memory/data-logging
- Phonecoil
- AutoPhone – automatic shift to 1 of 2 dedicated phone programs, acoustic phone (AP): microphone or phone T (PT): telecoil
- nEARcom provides a wireless link between NOAHlink and 1 or 2 hearing aids

Options of Dual PRO RITE

- Speaker unit available in 4 lengths: short, medium, long, and extra-long
- 4 different earpieces available:
  - Open dome – available in 3 sizes: 6 mm, 8 mm, and 10 mm
  - Plus dome – available in only 1 size
  - Power dome – available in 3 sizes: 8 mm, 10 mm, and 12 mm
  - Micro Mold – requires taking an impression
- Ear grip – ensures a secure and comfortable grip: one version to fit the right ear and another version to fit the left ear
- 3 programs

Features of Dual Mini m9 RITE

- RITE hearing aid – receiver is placed in the ear canal and amplifier is placed behind the ear
- 10 kHz bandwidth

- 10 fitting bands
- Multiband adaptive directionality – adaptive directional microphone system utilizing four frequency bands
- Front Focus – a directional system designed to aid in front/back sound source determination
- TriState noise management – uses modulations in speech to determine speech and noise content in eight bands to improve the overall speech-to-noise ratio
- VAC/Clarity$_2$ rationales
- Dynamic Feedback Cancellation
- Memory/data-logging
- Phonecoil
- AutoPhone – automatic shift to 1 of 2 dedicated phone programs, acoustic phone (AP): microphone or phone T (PT): telecoil

Options of Dual Mini m9 RITE

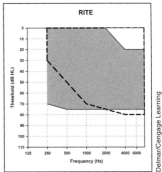

- Speaker unit available in 4 lengths: short, medium, long, and extra-long
- 4 different earpieces available:
  - Open dome – available in 3 sizes: 6 mm, 8 mm, and 10 mm
  - Plus dome – available in only 1 size
  - Power dome – available in 3 sizes: 8 mm, 10 mm, and 12 mm
  - Micro Mold – requires taking an impression
- Ear grip – ensures a secure and comfortable grip: one version to fit the right ear and another version to fit the left ear
- 5 programs

Fitting range for Dual Mini m9 RITE, Dual Mini m7 RITE, and Dual Mini m5 RITE for the Micro Mold with power dome (gray) and the open dome and plus dome (dotted line)

Features of Dual Mini m7 RITE

- RITE hearing aid – receiver is placed in the ear canal and amplifier is placed behind the ear
- 8 kHz bandwidth
- 8 fitting bands
- Multiband adaptive directionality – adaptive directional microphone system utilizing four frequency bands
- Front Focus – a directional system designed to aid in front/back sound source determination
- TriState noise management – uses modulations in speech to determine speech and noise content in eight bands to improve the overall speech-to-noise ratio
- VAC/Clarity$_2$ rationales
- Dynamic Feedback Cancellation

- Memory/data-logging
- Phonecoil
- AutoPhone – automatic shift to 1 of 2 dedicated phone programs, acoustic phone (AP): microphone or phone T (PT): telecoil

Options of Dual Mini m7 RITE

- Speaker unit available in 4 lengths: short, medium, long, and extra-long
- 4 different earpieces available:
  - Open dome – available in 3 sizes: 6 mm, 8 mm, and 10 mm
  - Plus dome – available in only 1 size
  - Power dome – available in 3 sizes: 8 mm, 10 mm, and 12 mm
  - Micro Mold – requires taking an impression
- Ear grip – ensures a secure and comfortable grip: one version to fit the right ear and another version to fit the left ear
- 5 programs

Features of Dual Mini m5 RITE

- RITE hearing aid – receiver is placed in the ear canal and amplifier is placed behind the ear
- 8 kHz bandwidth
- 6 fitting bands
- Single-band adaptive directionality
- Front Focus – a directional system designed to aid in front/back sound source determination
- TriState noise management – uses modulations in speech to determine speech and noise content in eight bands to improve the overall speech-to-noise ratio
- VAC/Clarity$_2$ rationales
- Dynamic Feedback Cancellation
- Memory/data-logging
- Phonecoil
- AutoPhone – automatic shift to 1 of 2 dedicated phone programs, acoustic phone (AP): microphone or phone T (PT): telecoil

Options of Dual Mini m5 RITE

- Speaker unit available in 4 lengths: short, medium, long, and extra-long
- 4 different earpieces available:
  - Open dome – available in 3 sizes: 6 mm, 8 mm, and 10 mm
  - Plus dome – available in only 1 size
  - Power dome – available in 3 sizes: 8 mm, 10 mm, and 12 mm
  - Micro Mold – requires taking an impression
- Ear grip – ensures a secure and comfortable grip: one version to fit the right ear and another version to fit the left ear
- 3 programs

OTICON

Typical Specifications		Dual W RITE	Dual XW RITE, Dual V RITE, Dual PRO RITE	Dual Mini m9 RITE	Dual Mini m7 RITE, Dual Mini m5 RITE
Standard ANSI S3.22-2003 and S3.7 (1995)					
Output sound pressure level	Max OSPL 90 (dB SPL)	108	108	108	108
	Avg OSPL 90 (dB SPL)	102	102	102	102
Full-on gain (50 dB SPL input)	Peak gain (dB)	47	47	47	47
	Avg (dB)	38	28	38	38
Total harmonic distortion (Hz)	500	0.4%	0.4%	0.4%	0.4%
	800	0.5%	0.5%	0.5%	0.5%
	1600	0.8%	0.8%	0.8%	0.8%
Equivalent input noise (dB SPL)	Omni	18	18	18	18
	Dir	29	29	29	29
Telecoil sensitivity	SPLITS (dB SPL) L/R	89/89	89/89	89/89	89/89
Battery	Operating current (mA)	1.1	1.1	0.9	0.9
	Battery type	312	312	10	10

Delmar/Cengage Learning

PRODUCT 4: VIGO PRO

Product Application

Vigo Pro RITE
Vigo Pro RITE Power
Vigo Pro BTE
Vigo Pro ITE
Vigo Pro ITC
Vigo Pro CIC/MIC

Features of Vigo Pro RITE and Vigo Pro RITE Power

- RITE hearing aid – receiver is placed in the ear canal and amplifier is placed behind the ear
- Best for mild to severe hearing losses
- DecisionMaker2™
- Bandwidth 8 kHz
- Multiband adaptive directionality – adaptive directional microphone system utilizing four frequency bands
- TriState noise management – uses modulations in speech to determine speech and noise content in eight bands to improve the overall speech-to-noise ratio
- VC learning – automatically adjusts the volume in specific sound environments in accordance with the user's behavioral pattern

- Automatic adaptation manager – gradually increases gain to the prescribed level to facilitate acclimatization
- Dynamic Feedback Cancellation 2
- Front Focus – a directional system designed to aid in front/back sound source determination
- OpenEar Acoustics
- Corda^2 thin-tube solution
- Wind noise protection – an integrated filter designed to reduce the noise levels that occur when wind hits the microphone
- NAL – NL$_1$ and DSL v5.0 m[i/o]
- Memory
- 4 customizable programs
- DAI and FM
- Telecoil
- AutoPhone program – automatic shift to 1 of 2 dedicated phone programs, acoustic phone (AP): microphone or phone T (PT): telecoil
- Low-battery warning
- Sound indicators for program shifts
- Onset delay and "jingle" sound indicator
- Mute/Standby mode
- nEARcom wireless – enabled

Options of Vigo Pro RITE and Vigo Pro RITE Power

- 1 to 4 programs
- Wireless fitting (nEARcom)
- Multiband adaptive directionality – adaptive directional microphone system utilizing four frequency bands
- Telecoil
- AutoPhone – automatic shift to 1 of 2 dedicated phone programs, acoustic phone (AP): microphone or phone T (PT): telecoil
- Configurable volume control

Features of Vigo Pro BTE

- Best for mild to severe hearing losses
- DecisionMaker2
- Bandwidth 8 kHz
- Multiband adaptive directionality – adaptive directional microphone system utilizing four frequency bands

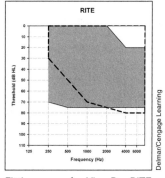

Fitting range for Vigo Pro RITE. Micro Mold with power dome (gray), open dome and plus dome (dotted line)

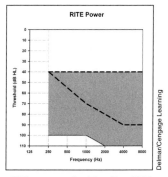

Fitting range for Vigo Pro RITE Power. Micro Mold with power dome (gray), open dome and plus dome (dotted line)

- TriState noise management – uses modulations in speech to determine speech and noise content in eight bands to improve the overall speech-to-noise ratio
- VC learning – automatically adjusts the volume in specific sound environments in accordance with the user's behavioral pattern
- Automatic adaptation manager – gradually increases gain to the prescribed level to facilitate acclimatization
- Dynamic Feedback Cancellation 2
- Front Focus – a directional system designed to aid in front/back sound source determination
- OpenEar Acoustics
- Corda^2 thin-tube solution
- Mind noise protection
- NAL – NL$_1$ and DSL v5.0 m[i/o]
- Memory
- 4 customizable programs
- DAI and FM
- Telecoil
- AutoPhone program – automatic shift to 1 of 2 dedicated phone programs, acoustic phone (AP): microphone or phone T (PT): telecoil
- Low-battery warning
- Sound indicators for program shifts
- Onset delay and "jingle" sound indicator
- Mute/Standby mode
- nEARcom wireless – enabled

Options of Vigo Pro BTE

- 1 to 4 programs
- Wireless fitting (nEARcom)
- Multiband adaptive directionality – adaptive directional microphone system utilizing four frequency bands
- Telecoil
- AutoPhone – automatic shift to 1 of 2 dedicated phone programs, acoustic phone (AP): microphone or phone T (PT): telecoil
- Configurable volume control

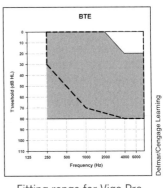

Fitting range for Vigo Pro BTE. Ear mold (gray), Corda^2 (white)

Features of Vigo Pro ITE

- Best for mild to severe hearing losses
- DecisionMaker2
- Bandwidth 8 kHz
- Multiband adaptive directionality – adaptive directional microphone system utilizing four frequency bands

- TriState noise management – uses modulations in speech to determine speech and noise content in eight bands to improve the overall speech-to-noise ratio
- VC learning – automatically adjusts the volume in specific sound environments in accordance with the user's behavioral pattern
- Automatic adaptation manager – gradually increases gain to the prescribed level to facilitate acclimatization
- Dynamic Feedback Cancellation 2
- Front Focus – a directional system designed to aid in front/back sound source determination
- OpenEar Acoustics
- Corda^2 thin-tube solution
- Mind noise protection
- NAL – NL_1 and DSL v5.0 m[i/o]
- Memory
- 4 customizable programs
- DAI and FM
- Telecoil
- AutoPhone program – automatic shift to 1 of 2 dedicated phone programs, acoustic phone (AP): microphone or phone T (PT): telecoil
- Low-battery warning
- Sound indicators for program shifts
- Onset delay and "jingle" sound indicator
- Mute/Standby mode
- nEARcom wireless – enabled

Options of Vigo Pro ITE

- 1 to 4 programs
- Optional wireless fitting (nEARcom)
- Multiband adaptive directionality – adaptive directional microphone system utilizing four frequency bands
- Optional telecoil
- Optional AutoPhone
- Optional volume control

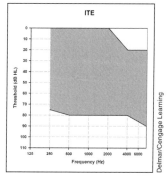

Fitting range for Vigo Pro ITE

Features of Vigo Pro ITC

- Best for mild to severe hearing losses
- DecisionMaker2
- Bandwidth 8 kHz
- Multiband adaptive directionality – adaptive directional microphone system utilizing four frequency bands
- TriState noise management – uses modulations in speech to determine speech and noise content in eight bands to improve the overall speech-to-noise ratio
- VC learning – automatically adjusts the volume in specific sound environments in accordance with the user's behavioral pattern

- Automatic adaptation manager – gradually increases gain to the prescribed level to facilitate acclimatization
- Dynamic Feedback Cancellation 2
- Front Focus – a directional system designed to aid in front/back sound source determination
- OpenEar Acoustics
- Corda[2] thin-tube solution
- Mind noise protection
- NAL – NL_1 and DSL v5.0 m[i/o]
- Memory
- 4 customizable programs
- DAI and FM
- Telecoil
- AutoPhone program – automatic shift to 1 of 2 dedicated phone programs, acoustic phone (AP): microphone or phone T (PT): telecoil
- Low-battery warning
- Sound indicators for program shifts
- Onset delay and "jingle" sound indicator
- Mute/Standby mode
- nEARcom wireless – enabled

Options of Vigo Pro ITC

- 1 to 4 programs
- Optional wireless fitting (nEARcom)
- Multiband adaptive directionality – adaptive directional microphone system utilizing four frequency bands
- Optional telecoil
- Optional AutoPhone

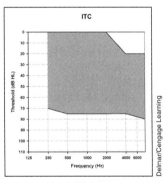

Fitting range for Vigo Pro ITC

Features of Vigo Pro CIC/MIC

- Best for mild to severe hearing losses
- DecisionMaker2
- Bandwidth 8 kHz
- Multiband adaptive directionality – adaptive directional microphone system utilizing four frequency bands
- TriState noise management – uses modulations in speech to determine speech and noise content in eight bands to improve the overall speech-to-noise ratio
- VC learning – automatically adjusts the volume in specific sound environments in accordance with the user's behavioral pattern
- Automatic adaptation manager – gradually increases gain to the prescribed level to facilitate acclimatization
- Dynamic Feedback Cancellation 2

- Front Focus – a directional system designed to aid in front/back sound source determination
- OpenEar Acoustics
- Corda[2] thin-tube solution
- Wind noise protection – an integrated filter designed to reduce the noise levels that occur when wind hits the microphone
- NAL – NL_1 and DSL v5.0 m[i/o]
- Memory
- 4 customizable programs
- DAI and FM
- Telecoil
- AutoPhone program – automatic shift to 1 of 2 dedicated phone programs, acoustic phone (AP): microphone or phone T (PT): telecoil
- Low-battery warning
- Sound indicators for program shifts
- Onset delay and "jingle" sound indicator
- Mute/Standby mode
- nEARcom wireless – enabled

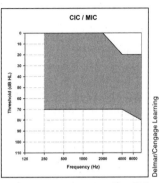

Options of Vigo Pro CIC/MIC

- 1 program

Fitting range for Vigo Pro CIC and Vigo Pro MIC

Typical Specifications		Vigo Pro RITE	Vigo Pro Power RITE	Vigo Pro BTE	Vigo Pro ITE	Vigo Pro ITC	Vigo Pro CIC/MIC
Standard ANSI S3.22-2003 and S3.7 (1995)							
Output sound pressure level	Max OSPL 90 (dB SPL)	108	124	115	113	113	109
	Avg OSPL 90 (dB SPL)	104	119	105	107	107	104
Full-on gain (50 dB SPL input)	Peak gain (dB)	46	55	51	46	41	37
	Avg (dB)	37	52	45	41	37	33
Total harmonic distortion (Hz)	500	0.1%	1.0%	0.7%	0.5%	0.6%	0.3%
	800	0.3%	0.5%	0.9%	0.4%	0.6%	0.4%
	1600	0.4%	0.5%	0.1%	0.4%	0.6%	0.9%
Equivalent input noise (dB SPL)	Omni	19	16	17	17	17	18
	Dir	25	30	26	25	26	n/a
Telecoil sensitivity	SPLITS (dB SPL) L/R	87/89	–	88/88	87/87	87/87	n/a
Battery	Operating current (mA)	1.3	1.3	1.2	1.3	1.2	0.9
	Battery type	312	312	312	312	312	10

PRODUCT 5: VIGO

Product Application

Vigo RITE
Vigo RITE Power
Vigo BTE
Vigo ITE
Vigo ITC
Vigo CIC/MIC

Features of Vigo RITE and Vigo RITE Power

- RITE hearing aid – receiver is placed in the ear canal and amplifier is placed behind the ear
- Best for mild to severe hearing losses
- DecisionMaker2
- Bandwidth 8 kHz
- Adaptive directionality – increases precision when attenuating noise in challenging situations by suppressing moving and stationary noise sources from the sides and behind
- Noise management – a modulation-based noise management system; uses a speech-weighted approach to ensure that interfering noise is attenuated without affecting important speech cues
- Automatic adaptation manager – gradually increases gain to the prescribed level to facilitate acclimatization
- Dynamic Feedback Cancellation 2
- Front Focus – a directional system designed to aid in front/back sound source determination
- OpenEar Acoustics
- Corda^2 thin-tube solution
- NAL – NL$_1$ and DSL v5.0 m[i/o]
- Memory
- 4 customizable programs
- DAI and FM
- Telecoil
- AutoPhone program – automatic shift to 1 of 2 dedicated phone programs, acoustic phone (AP): microphone or phone T (PT): telecoil
- Low-battery warning
- Sound indicators for program shifts
- Onset delay and "jingle" sound indicator
- Mute/Standby mode
- nEARcom wireless – enabled

Options of Vigo RITE and Vigo RITE Power

- 1 to 4 programs
- Wireless fitting (nEARcom)

- Adaptive directionality
- Telecoil
- AutoPhone
- Configurable volume control

Features of Vigo BTE

- Best for mild to severe hearing losses
- DecisionMaker2
- Bandwidth 8 kHz
- Adaptive directionality – increases precision when attenuating noise in challenging situations by suppressing moving and stationary noise sources from the sides and behind
- Noise management – a modulation-based noise management system; uses a speech-weighted approach to ensure that interfering noise is attenuated without affecting important speech cues
- Automatic adaptation manager – gradually increases gain to the prescribed level to facilitate acclimatization
- Dynamic Feedback Cancellation 2
- Front Focus – a directional system designed to aid in front/back sound source determination
- OpenEar Acoustics
- Corda^2 thin-tube solution
- NAL – NL$_1$ and DSL v5.0 m[i/o]
- Memory
- 4 customizable programs
- DAI and FM
- Telecoil
- AutoPhone program – automatic shift to 1 of 2 dedicated phone programs, acoustic phone (AP): microphone or phone T (PT): telecoil
- Low-battery warning
- Sound indicators for program shifts
- Onset delay and "jingle" sound indicator
- Mute/Standby mode
- nEARcom wireless – enabled

Options of Vigo BTE

- 1 to 4 programs
- Wireless fitting (nEARcom)

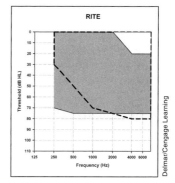

Fitting range for Vigo RITE. Micro Mold with power dome (gray), open dome and plus dome (dotted line)

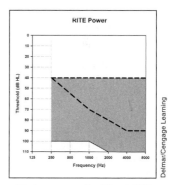

Fitting range for Vigo RITE Power. Micro Mold with power dome (gray), open dome and plus dome (dotted line)

OTICON

- Adaptive directionality
- Telecoil
- AutoPhone
- Configurable volume control
- FM-compatible

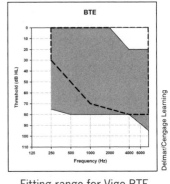

Fitting range for Vigo BTE RITE. Ear mold (gray), Corda² (white)

Features of Vigo ITE

- Best for mild to severe hearing losses
- DecisionMaker2
- Bandwidth 8 kHz
- Adaptive directionality – increases precision when attenuating noise in challenging situations by suppressing moving and stationary noise sources from the sides and behind
- Noise management – a modulation-based noise management system; uses a speech-weighted approach to ensure that interfering noise is attenuated without affecting important speech cues
- Automatic adaptation manager – gradually increases gain to the prescribed level to facilitate acclimatization
- Dynamic Feedback Cancellation 2
- Front Focus – a directional system designed to aid in front/back sound source determination
- OpenEar Acoustics
- Corda² thin-tube solution
- NAL – NL$_1$ and DSL v5.0 m[i/o]
- Memory
- 4 customizable programs
- DAI and FM
- Telecoil
- AutoPhone program – automatic shift to 1 of 2 dedicated phone programs, acoustic phone (AP): microphone or phone T (PT): telecoil
- Low-battery warning
- Sound indicators for program shifts
- Onset delay and "jingle" sound indicator
- Mute/Standby mode
- nEARcom wireless – enabled

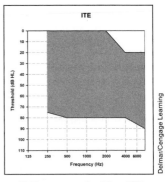

Fitting range for Vigo ITE

Options of Vigo ITE

- 1 to 4 programs
- Optional wireless fitting (nEARcom)
- Adaptive directionality
- Optional telecoil

- Optional AutoPhone
- Optional volume control

Features of Vigo ITC

- Best for mild to severe hearing losses
- DecisionMaker2
- Bandwidth 8 kHz
- Adaptive directionality – increases precision when attenuating noise in challenging situations by suppressing moving and stationary noise sources from the sides and behind
- Noise management – a modulation-based noise management system; uses a speech-weighted approach to ensure that interfering noise is attenuated without affecting important speech cues
- Automatic adaptation manager – gradually increases gain to the prescribed level to facilitate acclimatization
- Dynamic Feedback Cancellation 2
- Front Focus – a directional system designed to aid in front/back sound source determination
- OpenEar Acoustics
- Corda[2] thin-tube solution
- NAL – NL_1 and DSL v5.0 m[i/o]
- Memory
- 4 customizable programs
- DAI and FM
- Telecoil
- AutoPhone program – automatic shift to 1 of 2 dedicated phone programs, acoustic phone (AP): microphone or phone T (PT): telecoil
- Low-battery warning
- Sound indicators for program shifts
- Onset delay and "jingle" sound indicator
- Mute/Standby mode
- nEARcom wireless – enabled

Options of Vigo ITC

- 1 to 4 programs
- Optional wireless fitting (nEARcom)
- Adaptive directionality
- Optional telecoil
- Optional AutoPhone

Features of Vigo CIC/MIC

- Best for mild to severe hearing losses
- DecisionMaker2
- Bandwidth 8 kHz

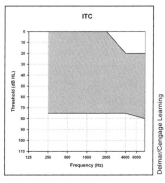

Fitting range for Vigo ITC

- Adaptive directionality – increases precision when attenuating noise in challenging situations by suppressing moving and stationary noise sources from the sides and behind
- Noise management – a modulation-based noise management system; uses a speech-weighted approach to ensure that interfering noise is attenuated without affecting important speech cues
- Automatic adaptation manager – gradually increases gain to the prescribed level to facilitate acclimatization
- Dynamic Feedback Cancellation 2
- Front Focus – a directional system designed to aid in front/back sound source determination
- OpenEar Acoustics
- Corda^2 thin-tube solution
- NAL – NL$_1$ and DSL v5.0 m[i/o]
- Memory
- 4 customizable programs
- DAI and FM
- Telecoil
- AutoPhone program – automatic shift to 1 of 2 dedicated phone programs, acoustic phone (AP): microphone or phone T (PT): telecoil
- Low-battery warning
- Sound indicators for program shifts
- Onset delay and "jingle" sound indicator
- Mute/Standby mode
- nEARcom wireless – enabled

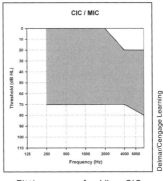

Fitting range for Vigo CIC and Vigo MIC

Options of Vigo CIC/MIC

- 1 program

Typical Specifications		Vigo RITE	Vigo Power RITE	Vigo BTE	Vigo ITE	Vigo ITC	Vigo CIC/ MIC
Standard ANSI S3.22-2003 and S3.7 (1995)							
Output sound pressure level	Max OSPL 90 (dB SPL)	108	124	115	113	113	109
	Avg OSPL 90 (dB SPL)	104	119	105	107	107	104
Full-on gain (50 dB SPL input)	Peak gain (dB)	46	55	51	46	41	37
	Avg (dB)	37	52	45	40	37	33
Total harmonic distortion (Hz)	500	0.1%	1.0%	0.7%	0.5%	0.6%	0.3%
	800	0.3%	0.5%	0.9%	0.4%	0.6%	0.4%
	1600	0.4%	0.5%	0.1%	0.4%	0.6%	0.9%

continues

continued

Typical Specifications		Vigo RITE	Vigo Power RITE	Vigo BTE	Vigo ITE	Vigo ITC	Vigo CIC/ MIC
Equivalent input noise (dB SPL)	Omni	19	16	17	17	17	18
	Dir	25	30	26	25	26	n/a
Telecoil sensitivity	SPLITS (dB SPL) L/R	87/89	–	88/88	87/87	87/87	n/a
Battery	Operating current (mA)	1.3	1.3	1.2	1.3	1.2	0.9
	Battery type	312	312	312	312	312	10

Delmar/Cengage Learning

PRODUCT 6: EPOQ

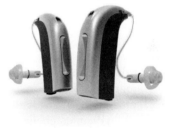

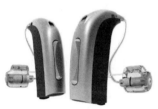

Epoq RITE
Photos granted by Oticon, Inc.

Epoq RITE Open Dome
Photos granted by Oticon, Inc.

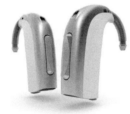

Epoq BTE
Photos granted by Oticon, Inc.

Product Application

Epoq W/XW RITE
Epoq W/XW RITE Power
Epoq W/XW BTE
Epoq W/XW ITE
Epoq W/XW ITC
Epoq W/XW CIC/MIC

Epoq V RITE
Epoq V RITE Power
Epoq V BTE
Epoq V ITE
Epoq V ITC
Epoq V CIC/MIC

Features of Epoq W/XW RITE and Epoq W/XW RITE Power

- RITE hearing aid – receiver is placed in the ear canal and amplifier is placed behind the ear
- True dynamics – a mixture of 2 parallel compression systems: a slow 15-channel and a fast 4-channel system
- **10 kHz bandwidth
- Front Focus – a directional system designed to aid in front/back sound source determination
- Life Learning – auto adjustments of volume control based on user habits
- *Spatial Sound – 2 binaurally fitted Epoqs work as 1 central processing unit
- *Binaural Dynamic Feedback Cancellation – cancels feedback using a binaural algorithm
- *MyVoice – makes adjustments depending on speech content
- Binaural broadband – high-speed binaural processing
- 4 memory programs
- AutoPhone program – automatic shift to 1 of 2 dedicated phone programs, acoustic phone (AP): microphone or phone T (PT): telecoil
- Activity analyzer – a data-logging feature that suggests adjustments to the hearing professional
- Epoq Memory – proprietary data-logging feature
- Sound indicators for phone call, program shifts
- Low-battery warning
- Onset delay and "jingle" sound indicator
- Wind noise protection – an integrated filter designed to reduce the noise levels that occur when wind hits the microphone
- TriState noise reduction – uses modulations in speech to determine speech and noise content in eight bands to improve the overall speech-to-noise ratio
- Multiband adaptive directionality – adaptive directional microphone system utilizing four frequency bands
- Voice-aligned compression (VAC) – a proprietary compression system designed to make speech more intelligible and comfortable
- DAI
- Telecoil
  - nEARcom-ready
  - Dynamic Feedback Cancellation 2
    - *Epoq XW only
    - **Excluding Epoq W/XW RITE Power

Options of Epoq W/XW RITE and Epoq W/XW RITE Power

- Streamer – companion device that connects the hearing instruments to different audio sources for communication, entertainment, or information purposes, such as mobile phones, MP3 players, PCs, etc.
- Push button for program options
- Volume control
- Telecoil
- AutoPhone program – automatic shift to 1 of 2 dedicated phone programs, acoustic phone (AP): microphone or phone T (PT): telecoil
- 4 different lengths of speaker unit: short, medium, long, and extra-long
- 3 earpiece options for RITE:
  - Open dome – available in 3 sizes: 6 mm, 8 mm, and 10 mm
  - Plus dome – available in 1 size
  - Micro Mold – requires taking an impression
- 3 earpiece options for RITE Power:
  - Plus dome – available in 1 size
  - Power dome – available in 3 sizes: 8 mm, 10 mm, and 12 mm
  - Power Mold – requires taking an impression
- Ear grip ensures a secure and comfortable grip
- Wax protection – NoWax/WaxStop
- 4 different black base colors: chroma beige, espresso, steel gray, and white-silver
- 4 different white base colors: ice blue, orchid, silver-gray, and gold dust
- 3 different neutral base colors: beige-silver, silver-beige, and steel silver
- Tamper-resistant battery drawer available in black, white, silver-gray, and beige

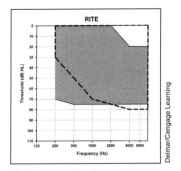

Fitting range for Epoq XW RITE, Epoq W RITE, and Epoq V RITE. Micro Mold with power dome (gray), open dome and plus dome (dotted line)

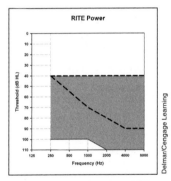

Fitting range for Epoq XW RITE Power, Epoq W RITE Power, and Epoq V RITE. Micro Mold with power dome (gray), open dome and plus dome (dotted line)

Features of Epoq W/XW BTE

- True dynamics – a mixture of 2 parallel compression systems: a slow 15-channel and a fast 4-channel system
- 10 kHz bandwidth
- Front Focus – a directional system designed to aid in front/back sound source determination

- Life Learning – auto adjustments of volume control based on user habits
  - *Spatial Sound – 2 binaurally fitted Epoqs work as 1 central processing unit
  - *Binaural Dynamic Feedback Cancellation – cancels feedback using a binaural algorithm
  - *MyVoice – makes adjustments depending on speech content
- Binaural broadband – high-speed binaural processing (excludes CIC/MIC)
- 4 memory programs
- AutoPhone program – automatic shift to 1 of 2 dedicated phone programs, acoustic phone (AP): microphone or phone T (PT): telecoil
- Activity analyzer – a data-logging feature that suggests adjustments to the hearing professional
- Epoq Memory – proprietary data-logging feature
- Sound indicators for phone call, program shifts
- Low-battery warning
- Onset delay and "jingle" sound indicator
- Wind noise protection – an integrated filter designed to reduce the noise levels that occur when wind hits the microphone
- 15-channel TriState noise reduction – uses modulations in speech to determine speech and noise content to improve the overall speech-to-noise ratio
- Multiband adaptive directionality – adaptive directional microphone system utilizing four frequency bands
- Voice-aligned compression – a proprietary compression system designed to make speech more intelligible and comfortable
- DAI
- Telecoil
  - *Epoq XW only

Options of Epoq W/XW BTE

- Streamer – companion device that connects the hearing instruments to different audio sources for communication, entertainment or information purposes, such as mobile phones, MP3 players, PCs, and the like
- Push button for program options
- Volume control
- Telecoil
- AutoPhone program – automatic shift to 1 of 2 dedicated phone programs, acoustic phone (AP): microphone or phone T (PT): telecoil
- 4 different black base colors: chroma beige, espresso, steel gray, and white-silver
- 4 different white base colors: ice blue, orchid, silver-gray, and gold dust

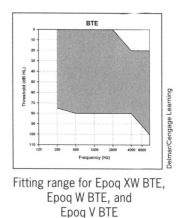

Fitting range for Epoq XW BTE, Epoq W BTE, and Epoq V BTE

- 3 different neutral base colors: beige-silver, silver-beige, and steel silver
- Tamper-resistant battery drawer available in black, white, silver-gray, and beige

Features of Epoq W/XW ITE and Epoq W/XW ITC

- True dynamics – a mixture of 2 parallel compression systems: a slow 15-channel and a fast 4-channel system
- 10 kHz bandwidth
- Front Focus – a directional system designed to aid in front/back sound source determination
- Life Learning – auto adjustments of volume control based on user habits
- *Spatial Sound – 2 binaurally fitted Epoqs work as 1 central processing unit
- *Binaural Dynamic Feedback Cancellation – cancels feedback using a binaural algorithm
- *MyVoice – makes adjustments depending on speech content
- Binaural broadband – high-speed binaural processing
- 4 memory programs
- AutoPhone program – automatic shift to 1 of 2 dedicated phone programs, acoustic phone (AP): microphone or phone T (PT): telecoil
- Activity analyzer – a data-logging feature that suggests adjustments to the hearing professional
- Epoq Memory – proprietary data-logging feature
- Sound indicators for phone call, program shifts
- Low-battery warning
- Onset delay and "jingle" sound indicator
- Wind noise protection – an integrated filter designed to reduce the noise levels that occur when wind hits the microphone
- 15-channel TriState noise reduction – uses modulations in speech to determine speech and noise content to improve the overall speech-to-noise ratio
- Multiband adaptive directionality – adaptive directional microphone system utilizing four frequency bands
- Voice-aligned compression – a proprietary compression system designed to make speech more intelligible and comfortable
- DAI
- Telecoil
- * Epoq XW only

Options of Epoq W/XW ITE and Epoq W/XW ITC

- Streamer – companion device that connects the hearing instruments to different audio sources for communication, entertainment or information purposes, such as mobile phones, MP3 players, PCs, etc.
- Push button for program options
- Volume control (excludes ITC)
- Telecoil (excludes ITC)

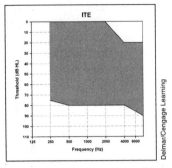

Fitting range for Epoq XW ITE, Epoq W ITE, and Epoq V BTE

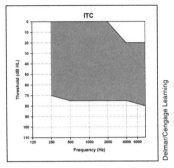

Fitting range for Epoq XW ITC, Epoq W ITE, and Epoq V BTE

- AutoPhone program – automatic shift to 1 of 2 dedicated phone programs, acoustic phone (AP): microphone or phone T (PT): telecoil
- 4 different skin colors available: pink, light brown, medium brown, and dark brown
- Wax protection – NoWax, MicroWaxBuster, and WaxBuster

Features of Epoq W/XW CIC/MIC

- True dynamics – a mixture of 2 parallel compression systems: a slow 15-channel and a fast 4-channel system
- 10 kHz bandwidth
- Front Focus – a directional system designed to aid in front/back sound source determination
- Life Learning – auto adjustments of volume control based on user habits
- 4 memory programs
- Activity analyzer – a data-logging feature that suggests adjustments to the hearing professional
- Epoq Memory – proprietary data-logging feature
- Sound indicators for phone call, program shifts
- Low-battery warning
- Onset delay and "jingle" sound indicator
- Wind noise protection – an integrated filter designed to reduce the noise levels that occur when wind hits the microphone
- 15-channel TriState noise reduction – uses modulations in speech to determine speech and noise content in eight bands to improve the overall speech-to-noise ratio
- Multiband adaptive directionality – adaptive directional microphone system utilizing four frequency bands
- Voice-aligned compression – a proprietary compression system designed to make speech more intelligible and comfortable
- DAI
- Telecoil

Options of Epoq W/XW CIC/MIC

- 4 different skin colors available: pink, light brown, medium brown, and dark brown
- Wax protection – NoWax, MicroWax-Buster, and WaxBuster

Features of Epoq V RITE and Epoq V RITE Power

- RITE hearing aid – receiver is placed in the ear canal and amplifier is placed behind the ear
- True dynamics – a mixture of 2 parallel compression systems: a slow 15-channel and a fast 4-channel system
- 8 kHz bandwidth
- Front Focus – a directional system designed to aid in front/back sound source determination
- Life Learning – auto adjustments of volume control based on user habits (VC only)
- 4 memory programs
- AutoPhone program – automatic shift to 1 of 2 dedicated phone programs, acoustic phone (AP): microphone or phone T (PT): telecoil
- Activity analyzer – a data-logging feature that suggests adjustments to the hearing professional
- Epoq Memory – proprietary data-logging feature
- Sound indicators for phone call, program shifts
- Low-battery warning
- Onset delay and "jingle" sound indicator
- Wind noise protection – an integrated filter designed to reduce the noise levels that occur when wind hits the microphone
- TriState noise reduction – uses modulations in speech to determine speech and noise content in eight bands to improve the overall speech-to-noise ratio
- Multiband adaptive directionality – adaptive directional microphone system utilizing four frequency bands
- Voice-aligned compression – a proprietary compression system designed to make speech more intelligible and comfortable
- DAI
- Telecoil
  - nEARcom-ready
  - Dynamic Feedback Cancellation 2

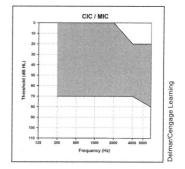

Fitting range for Epoq XW CIC, Epoq W CIC, Epoq V CIC, Epoq XW MIC, Epoq W MIC, and Epoq V MIC

Options of Epoq V RITE and Epoq V RITE Power

- Streamer – companion device that connects the hearing instruments to different audio sources for communication, entertainment, or information purposes, such as mobile phones, MP3 players, PCs, etc.

- Push button for program options
- Volume control
- Telecoil
- AutoPhone program – automatic shift to 1 of 2 dedicated phone programs, acoustic phone (AP): microphone or phone T (PT): telecoil
- 4 different lengths of speaker unit: short, medium, long, and extra-long
- 3 earpiece options for RITE:
  - Open dome – available in 3 sizes: 6 mm, 8 mm, and 10 mm
  - Plus dome – available in 1 size
  - Micro Mold – requires taking an impression
- 3 earpiece options for RITE Power:
  - Plus dome – available in 1 size
  - Power dome – available in 3 sizes: 8 mm, 10 mm, and 12 mm
  - Power Mold – requires taking an impression
- Ear grip ensures a secure and comfortable grip
- Wax protection – NoWax/WaxStop
- 4 different black base colors: chroma beige, espresso, steel gray, and white-silver
- 4 different white base colors: ice blue, orchid, silver-gray, and gold dust
- 3 different neutral base colors: beige-silver, silver-beige, and steel silver
- Tamper-resistant battery drawer available in black, white, silver-gray, and beige

Features of Epoq V BTE

- True dynamics – a mixture of 2 parallel compression systems: a slow 15-channel and a fast 4-channel system
- 8 kHz bandwidth
- Front Focus – a directional system designed to aid in front/back sound source determination
- Life Learning – auto adjustments of volume control based on user habits
- Binaural broadband – high-speed binaural processing (excludes CIC/MIC)
- 4 memory programs
- AutoPhone program – automatic shift to 1 of 2 dedicated phone programs, acoustic phone (AP): microphone or phone T (PT): telecoil
- Activity analyzer – a data-logging feature that suggests adjustments to the hearing professional
- Epoq Memory – proprietary data-logging feature
- Sound indicators for phone call, program shifts
- Low-battery warning
- Onset delay and "jingle" sound indicator
- Wind noise protection – an integrated filter designed to reduce the noise levels that occur when wind hits the microphone
- 15-channel TriState noise reduction – uses modulations in speech to determine speech and noise content to improve the overall speech-to-noise ratio
- Multiband adaptive directionality – adaptive directional microphone system utilizing four frequency bands

- Voice-aligned compression – a proprietary compression system designed to make speech more intelligible and comfortable
- DAI
- Telecoil

Options of Epoq V BTE

- Streamer – companion device that connects the hearing instruments to different audio sources for communication, entertainment or information purposes, such as mobile phones, MP3 players, PCs, and the like
- Push button for program options
- Volume control
- Telecoil
- AutoPhone program – automatic shift to 1 of 2 dedicated phone programs, acoustic phone (AP): microphone or phone T (PT): telecoil
- 4 different black base colors: chroma beige, espresso, steel gray, and white-silver
- 4 different white base colors: ice blue, orchid, silver-gray, and gold dust
- 3 different neutral base colors: beige-silver, silver-beige, and steel silver
- Tamper-resistant battery drawer available in black, white, silver-gray, and beige

Features of Epoq V ITE and Epoq V ITC

- True dynamics – a mixture of 2 parallel compression systems: a slow 15-channel and a fast 4-channel system
- 8 kHz bandwidth
- Front Focus – a directional system designed to aid in front/back sound source determination
- Life Learning – auto adjustments of volume control based on user habits
- Binaural broadband – high-speed binaural processing
- 4 memory programs
- AutoPhone program – automatic shift to 1 of 2 dedicated phone programs, acoustic phone (AP): microphone or phone T (PT): telecoil
- Activity analyzer – a data-logging feature that suggests adjustments to the hearing professional
- Epoq Memory – proprietary data-logging feature
- Sound indicators for phone call, program shifts
- Low-battery warning
- Onset delay and "jingle" sound indicator
- Wind noise protection – an integrated filter designed to reduce the noise levels that occur when wind hits the microphone
- 15-channel TriState noise reduction – uses modulations in speech to determine speech and noise content to improve the overall speech-to-noise ratio
- Multiband adaptive directionality – adaptive directional microphone system utilizing four frequency bands
- Voice-aligned compression – a proprietary compression system designed to make speech more intelligible and comfortable

- DAI
- Telecoil

Options of Epoq V ITE and Epoq V ITC

- Streamer – companion device that connects the hearing instruments to different audio sources for communication, entertainment or information purposes, such as mobile phones, MP3 players, PCs, etc.
- Push button for program options
- Volume control (excludes ITC)
- Telecoil (excludes ITC)
- AutoPhone program – automatic shift to 1 of 2 dedicated phone programs, acoustic phone (AP): microphone or phone T (PT): telecoil
- 4 different skin colors available: pink, light brown, medium brown, and dark brown
- Wax protection – NoWax, MicroWaxBuster, and WaxBuster

Features of Epoq V CIC/MIC

- True dynamics – a mixture of 2 parallel compression systems: a slow 15-channel and a fast 4-channel system
- 8 kHz bandwidth
- Front Focus – a directional system designed to aid in front/back sound source determination
- Life Learning – auto adjustments of volume control based on user habits
- 4 memory programs
- Activity analyzer – a data-logging feature that suggests adjustments to the hearing professional
- Epoq Memory – proprietary data-logging feature
- Sound indicators for phone call, program shifts
- Low-battery warning
- Onset delay and "jingle" sound indicator
- Wind noise protection – an integrated filter designed to reduce the noise levels that occur when wind hits the microphone
- 15-channel TriState noise reduction – uses modulations in speech to determine speech and noise content to improve the overall speech-to-noise ratio
- Multiband adaptive directionality – adaptive directional microphone system utilizing four frequency bands
- Voice-aligned compression – a proprietary compression system designed to make speech more intelligible and comfortable
- DAI
- Telecoil

Options of Epoq V CIC/MIC

- 4 different skin colors available: pink, light brown, medium brown, and dark brown
- Wax protection – NoWax, MicroWaxBuster, and WaxBuster

Typical Specifications		Epoq W/XW RITE	Epoq W/XW RITE Power	Epoq W/XW BTE	Epoq W/XW ITE	Epoq W/XW ITC	Epoq W/XW CIC/MIC
Standard ANSI S3.22-2003 and S3.7 (1995)							
Output sound pressure level	Max OSPL 90 (dB SPL)	109	124	115	113	113	109
	Avg OSPL 90 (dB SPL)	104	119	105	107	107	104
Full-on gain (50 dB SPL input)	Peak gain (dB)	46	55	50	46	41	37
	Avg (dB)	37	52	44	41	37	33
Total harmonic distortion (Hz)	500	0.1%	1.0%	0.7%	0.5%	0.6%	0.3%
	800	0.3%	0.5%	0.5%	0.4%	0.6%	0.4%
	1600	0.4%	0.5%	0.1%	0.4%	0.6%	0.9%
Equivalent input noise (dB SPL)	Omni	19	16	19	17	17	18
	Dir	25	30	25	25	26	n/a
Telecoil sensitivity	SPLITS (dB SPL) L/R	87/89	101/101	88/90	87/87	87	n/a
Battery	Operating current (mA)	1.3	1.4	1.2	1.3	1.2	0.9
	Battery type	312	312	312	312	312	10

Delmar/Cengage Learning

Typical Specifications		Epoq V RITE	Epoq V RITE Power	Epoq V BTE	Epoq V ITE	Epoq V ITC	Epoq V CIC/MIC
Standard ANSI S3.22-2003 and S3.7 (1995)							
Output sound pressure level	Max OSPL 90 (dB SPL)	108	124	115	113	113	109
	Avg OSPL 90 (dB SPL)	104	119	104	107	107	104
Full-on gain (50 dB SPL input)	Peak gain (dB)	46	55	50	46	41	37
	Avg (dB)	37	52	44	41	37	33
Total harmonic distortion (Hz)	500	0.1%	1.0%	0.7%	0.5%	0.6%	0.3%
	800	0.3%	0.5%	0.9%	0.4%	0.6%	0.4%
	1600	0.4%	0.5%	0.1%	0.4%	0.6%	0.9%
Equivalent input noise (dB SPL)	Omni	19	16	19	17	17	18
	Dir	25	30	25	25	26	n/a
Telecoil sensitivity	SPLITS (dB SPL) L/R	87/89	101/101	88/88	87/87	87/87	n/a
Battery	Operating current (mA)	1.3	1.4	1.2	1.3	1.2	0.9
	Battery type	312	312	312	312	312	10

Delmar/Cengage Learning

PRODUCT 7: SYNCRO 2

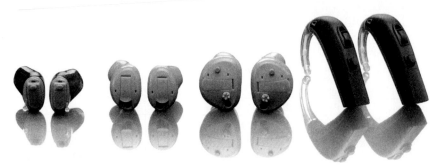

Syncro 2 family product line ranging from BTE through CIC
Photos granted by Oticon, Inc.

Product Application

Syncro 2 BTE
Syncro 2 BTE P
Syncro 2 HS/LP/FS
Syncro 2 ITC
Syncro 2 MIC
Syncro 2 CIC

Features of All Syncro 2 Products

- Multiband adaptive directionality – adaptive directional microphone system utilizing four frequency bands
- TriState noise management – uses modulations in speech to determine speech and noise content in eight bands to improve the overall speech-to-noise ratio
- Voice-aligned compression – a proprietary compression system designed to make speech more intelligible and comfortable; provides improved speech understanding, especially at high input levels
- Syncro activity analyzer – a data-logging feature that suggests adjustments to the hearing professional
- Up to 4 customizable programs
- Automatic adaptation manager – gradually increases gain to the prescribed level to facilitate acclimatization
- Automatic microphone matching – matches microphone response to minimize loss in directionality
- OpenEar Acoustics – a combination of an open fit with feedback cancellation, low-frequency emphasis, and a low processing delay
- Dynamic Feedback Cancellation – proprietary feedback cancellation algorithm
- Program sound indicators (beeps)

- Standby function
- Onset delay
- Right and left identification marking
- Recommended for all types of hearing losses, from mild to severe to profound
- Programmable via the Oticon Genie software 6.0 or higher

Features of Syncro 2 BTE and Syncro 2 BTE P

- DAI
- Fully programmable telecoil
- FM-compatible
- Adjustable sound hook

Options of Syncro 2 BTE and Syncro 2 BTE P

- Volume control with audible indication
- 9 dB, 5 dB, and undamped sound hooks
- Pediatric sound hooks
- Thin-tube fitting (Oticon Corda)
- Tamper-resistant battery door
- DAI and FM shoes
- Eyeglasses adapter
- Hair-tone colors: beige, light brown, dark brown, light gray, and dark gray
- Cool colors: black, transparent, yellow, orange, pink, purple, blue, and green

Features of Syncro 2 HS/LP/FS, Syncro 2 ITC, Syncro 2 MIC, and Syncro 2 CIC

- Design optimized for size and cosmetics
- Selection of 3 wax-protection systems – NoWax, MicroWaxBuster, and WaxBuster

Options of Syncro 2 HS/LP/FS, Syncro 2 ITC, Syncro 2 MIC, and Syncro 2 CIC

- AutoPhone program – automatic shift to 1 of 2 dedicated phone programs, acoustic phone (AP): microphone or phone T (PT): telecoil
  - Fully programmable telecoil and/or automatic telecoil
  - Volume control with audible indication

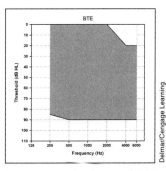

Fitting range for Syncro 2 BTE

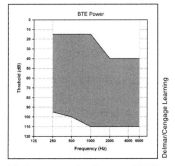

Fitting range for Syncro 2 BTE Power

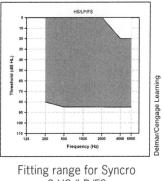

Fitting range for Syncro 2 HS/LP/FS

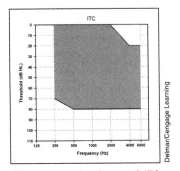

Fitting range for Syncro 2 ITC

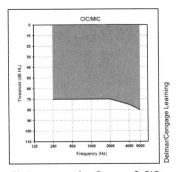

Fitting range for Syncro 2 CIC and Syncro 2 MIC

Typical Specifications		Syncro 2 BTE	Syncro 2 BTE Power
Standard ANSI S3.22-2003 and S3.7 (1995)			
Output sound pressure level	Max OSPL 90 (dB SPL)	112	126
	HFA OSPL 90 (dB SPL)	111	121
Full-on gain (50 dB SPL input)	Peak gain (dB)	54	62
	HFA (dB)	51	54
Total harmonic distortion (Hz)	500	0.5%	1.5%
	800	0.5%	1.0%
	1600	0.5%	0.5%
Equivalent input noise (dB SPL)	Typical/maximum, Omni	12/16	16/20
	Typical/maximum, Dir	20/24	26/30
Telecoil sensitivity	SPLITS (dB SPL)	93.5	99.5
Battery	Operating current (mA)	1.1	1.4
	Battery type	13	13

Delmar/Cengage Learning

Typical Specifications		Syncro 2 Full-Shell	Syncro 2 Half-Shell/Low-Profile	Syncro 2 ITC (312)	Syncro 2 ITC (10)	Syncro 2 CIC/MIC
Standard ANSI S3.22-2003 and S3.7 (1995)						
Output sound Pressure level	Max OSPL 90 (dB SPL)	113	112	110	104	103
	HFA OSPL 90 (dB SPL)	107	106	105	99	98
Full-on gain (50 dB SPL input)	Peak gain (dB)	52	47	41	37	37
	HFA (dB)	46	43	37	33	32
Total harmonic distortion (Hz)	500	1.5%	1.5%	0.5%	0.5%	1.0%
	800	1.0%	1.0%	0.5%	0.5%	0.5%
	1600	1.5%	1.0%	0.5%	0.5%	1.0%

continues

continued

Typical Specifications		Syncro 2 Full-Shell	Syncro 2 Half-Shell/Low-Profile	Syncro 2 ITC (312)	Syncro 2 ITC (10)	Syncro 2 CIC/MIC
Equivalent input noise (dB SPL)	Typical/maximum, Omni	17/21	19/23	20/24	18/22	20/24
	Typical/maximum, Dir	33/37	31/35	29/33	33/37	n/a
Telecoil sensitivity	SPLITS (dB SPL)	91	87	n/a	n/a	n/a
Battery	Operating current (mA)	1.2	1.2	1.2	1.1	0.7
	Battery type	13	312	312	10	10

Delmar/Cengage Learning

PRODUCT 8: DELTA SERIES 8000, 6000, AND 4000

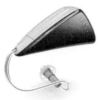

Delta 8000, 6000, and 4000 Receiver in the RITE hearing aids
Photos granted by Oticon, Inc.

Product Application

Delta 8000 BTE
Delta 6000 BTE
Delta 4000 BTE

Features of Delta 8000 BTE

- RITE – receiver is placed in the ear canal and amplifier is placed behind the ear
- Recommended for mid- to high-frequency hearing losses
- Frequency range – up to 8000 Hz
- Automatic multiband adaptive directionality – adaptive directional microphone system utilizing four frequency bands
- Activity analyzer – a data-logging feature that suggests adjustments to the hearing professional
- TriState noise management – uses modulations in speech to determine speech and noise content in eight bands to improve the overall speech-to-noise ratio
- Automatic adaptation manager – gradually increases gain to the prescribed level to facilitate acclimatization
- 6 channels with open dome

- 7 channels with plus dome
- Artificial intelligence (AI)
- Right and left identification marker rings (red/blue)
- Programmable via the Oticon Genie software

Options of Delta 8000 BTE

- Amplifier available in 17 different shell colors: champagne beige, chocolate brown, high-tech silver, charcoal gray, mother of pearl, diamond black, cabernet red, racing green, deep purple, shy violet, Samoa blue, midnight blue, sunset orange, green chameleon, check, Wall Street, wildlife
- 3 different back colors: beige, light gray, and dark gray
- 3 different lengths of speaker unit: short (#1), medium (#2), and long (#3)
- 2 dome versions:
  - Open dome – available in 3 sizes: 6 mm, 8 mm, and 10 mm)
  - Plus dome – closed

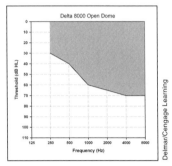

Fitting range for Delta 8000 BTE Open Dome

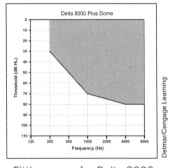

Fitting range for Delta 8000 BTE Plus Dome

Features of Delta 6000 BTE

- RITE hearing aid – receiver is placed in the ear canal and amplifier is placed behind the ear
- Recommended for mid- to high-frequency hearing losses
- Frequency range – up to 6000 Hz
- Automatic directionality – helps improve speech understating in noisy environments
- Noise management (speech-weighted) – reduces noise levels while enhancing speech
- Adaptation manager – gradually increases gain to the prescribed level to facilitate acclimatization
- 5 channels with open dome
- 6 channels with plus dome
- AI
- Programmable via the Oticon Genie software

Options of Delta 6000 BTE

- Amplifier available in 17 different shell colors: champagne beige, chocolate brown, high-tech silver, charcoal gray, mother of pearl, diamond black, cabernet red, racing green, deep purple, shy violet, Samoa blue, midnight blue, sunset orange, green chameleon, check, Wall Street, wildlife

- 3 different back colors: beige, light gray, and dark gray
- 3 different lengths of speaker unit: short (#1), medium (#2), and long (#3)
- 2 dome versions:
  - Open dome – available in 3 sizes: 6 mm, 8 mm, and 10 mm
  - Plus dome – closed

Features of Delta 4000 BTE

- RITE hearing aid – receiver is placed in the ear canal and amplifier is placed behind the ear
- Recommended for any configuration of hearing loss up to 80 dB flat
- Automatic fixed directionality
- Noise management (modulation) – uses speech detection to reduce the effects of noise without notably affecting important speech cues
- Frequency range up to 6000 Hz
- 3 to 5 channels depending on earpiece and amplification strategy
- Programmable via the Oticon Genie software

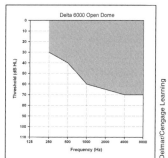

Fitting range for Delta 6000 BTE Open Dome

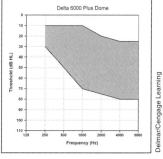

Fitting range for Delta 6000 BTE Plus Dome

Options of Delta 4000 BTE

- Choice of 2 amplification strategies: clarity (for mid- to high frequency hearing losses) and voice-aligned compression, a proprietary compression system designed to make speech more intelligible and comfortable (for broadband hearing losses)
- 3 types of earpieces:
  - Open dome – available in 3 sizes: 6 mm, 8 mm, and 10 mm
  - Plus dome – available in only 1 size
  - Micro Mold – requires taking an impression
- Amplifier available in 3 spine colors and a choice of 17 different shell colors
- 4 different lengths of receiver unit:
  - short (no. 1)
  - medium (no. 2)
  - long (no. 3)
  - extra long (no. 4)

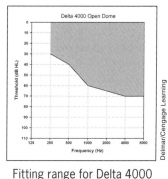

Fitting range for Delta 4000 BTE Open Dome

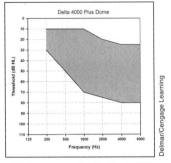

Fitting range for Delta 4000
BTE Plus Dome

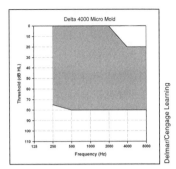

Fitting range for Delta 4000
Micro Mold

Typical Specifications		Delta 8000 BTE	Delta 6000 BTE	Delta 4000 BTE
Standard ANSI S3.22-2003 and S3.7 (1995)				
Output sound Pressure level	Max OSPL 90 (dB SPL)	105	105	105
	OSPL 90 1600 Hz (dB SPL)	97	97	97
Full-on gain (50 dB SPL input)	Peak gain (dB)	44	44	44
	1600 Hz (dB)	37	37	36
Total harmonic distortion (Hz)	500	n/a	n/a	n/a
	800	0.5%	0.5%	0.5%
	1600	0.5%	0.5%	0.5%
Equivalent input noise (dB SPL)		17	17	17
Telecoil sensitivity	SPLITS (dB SPL)	n/a	n/a	n/a
Battery	Operating current (mA)	1.2	1.2	1.2
	Battery type	10	10	10

Delmar/Cengage Learning

PRODUCT 9: ADAPTO

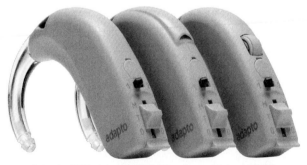

Adapto BTE, Adapto BTE Direct, and Adapto BTE
Power hearing aids
Photos granted by Oticon, Inc.

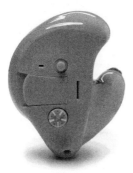
Adapto Full-Shell (FS)
Photos granted by Oticon, Inc.

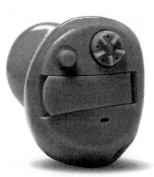
Adapto Half-Shell (HS)
Photos granted by Oticon, Inc.

Product Application

Adapto BTE
Adapto BTE D
Adapto BTE Power
Adapto Full-Shell Power (T)
Adapto Full-Shell Power P1/P2 (T)
Adapto Half-Shell/Low-Profile (T, VC)
Adapto Half-Shell/Low-Profile P1/P2 (T, VC)
Adapto Half-Shell/Low-Profile D (T)
Adapto ITC
Adapto MIC
Adapto CIC

Features of All Adapto Products

- VoiceFinder
- OpenEar Acoustics – a combination of an open fit with feedback cancellation, low-frequency emphasis, and a low processing delay; allows for open-ear fittings
- Dynamic Feedback Cancellation – proprietary feedback cancellation algorithm
- Advanced chip design
- Low power consumption
- Fully automatic operation
- Audible status indicator
- Designed for reduced interference with cell phones
- Recommended for all types of hearing losses, ranging from mild to severe
- 4 audiological rationales that consider different processing strategies based on different hearing losses:
  - FAST for sloping hearing losses
  - SLOW for adults over 70 with sloping hearing losses
  - SKI for ski-slope losses
  - LINEAR for flat hearing losses
- Programmable via the Oticon Genie software

Features of Adapto BTE, Adapto BTE D, and Adapto BTE Power

- Programs for dedicated listening situations
- Fully configurable function switches
- DAI
- Telecoil
- FM-compatible
- Adjustable sound hook

Options of Adapto BTE, Adapto BTE D, and Adapto BTE Power

- 9 dB and undamped sound hooks
- Pediatric sound hook
- Tamper-resistant battery drawer
- DAI and WTC (wireless transfer communication) shoes
- Eyeglasses adapter
- Hair-tone colors: beige, light brown, dark brown, light gray, and dark gray
- Cool colors: transparent, yellow, orange, pink, purple, blue, and green

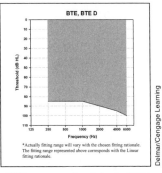

Fitting range for Adapto BTE and Adapto BTE D

Features of Adapto Full-Shell Power (T), Adapto Full-Shell Power P1/P2 (T), Adapto Half-Shell/Low-Profile (T, VC), Adapto Half-Shell/Low-Profile P1/P2 (T, VC), Adapto Half-Shell/Low-Profile D (T), Adapto ITC, Adapto MIC, Adapto CIC

- Design optimized for size and cosmetics
- Programs for dedicated listening situations (Adapto HS/LP styles only)
- Fully configurable push-button operation (Adapto HS/LP styles only)

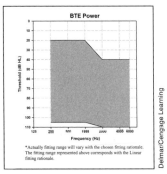

Fitting range for Adapto BTE Power

Options of Adapto Full-Shell Power (T), Adapto Full-Shell Power P1/P2 (T), Adapto Half-Shell/Low-Profile (T, VC), Adapto Half-Shell/Low-Profile P1/P2 (T, VC), Adapto Half-Shell/Low-Profile D (T), Adapto ITC, Adapto MIC, Adapto CIC

- Telecoil
- Automatic telecoil
- Manual override
- Colors: pink, tan, medium brown, and dark brown

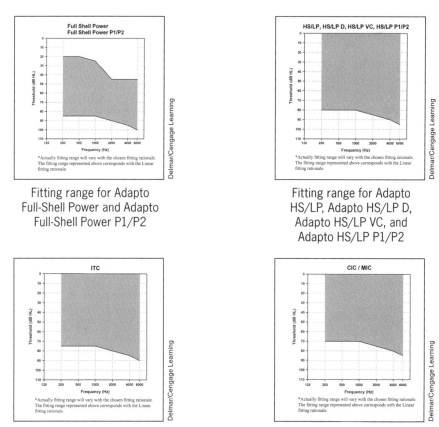

Fitting range for Adapto
Full-Shell Power and Adapto
Full-Shell Power P1/P2

Fitting range for Adapto
HS/LP, Adapto HS/LP D,
Adapto HS/LP VC, and
Adapto HS/LP P1/P2

Fitting range for Adapto ITC

Fitting range for Adapto CIC
and Adapto MIC

Typical Specifications		Adapto BTE	Adapto D BTE	Adapto Power BTE
Standard ANSI S3.22-2003 and S3.7 (1995)				
Output sound Pressure level	Max OSPL 90 (dB SPL)	115	115	131
	HFA OSPL 90 (dB SPL)	111	111	126
Full-on gain (50 dB SPL input)	Peak gain (dB)	57	57	71
	HFA (dB)	53	52	65
Total harmonic distortion (Hz)	500	1.0%	1.0%	2.0%
	800	1.0%	1.0%	2.0%
	1600	1.0%	1.0%	1.0%
Equivalent input noise (dB SPL)	Typical/maximum, Omni	16/20	16/20	15/19
	Typical/maximum, Dir	n/a	19/23	n/a
Telecoil sensitivity	SPLITS (dB SPL)	93.5	93.5	108.5
Battery	Operating current (mA)	0.95	1.1	1.3
	Battery type	13	13	13

Delmar/Cengage Learning

Typical Specifications		Adapto Full-Shell (13), T, Full-Shell Power (13) P1/ P2, T	Adapto Full-Shell Power (312), T, Full-Shell Power (312) P1/P2, T	Adapto HS/LP D (T)	Adapto HS/LP (T, VC), HS/LP P1/P2 (T, VC)	Adapto ITC	Adapto CIC, MIC
Standard ANSI S3.22-2003 and S3.7 (1995)							
Output sound Pressure level	Max OSPL 90 (dB SPL)	125	117	110	110	110	104
	HFA OSPL 90 (dB SPL)	122	112	106	107	107	100
Full-on gain (50 dB SPL input)	Peak gain (dB)	55	49	43	46	40	35
	HFA (dB)	52	42	41	42	37	32
Total harmonic distortion (Hz)	500	3.5%	2.0%	2.0%	2.5%	1.5%	1.0%
	800	3.5%	3.0%	2.0%	2.5%	1.5%	1.0%
	1600	1.0%	3.0%	2.0%	2.5%	1.5%	1.0%
Equivalent input noise (dB SPL)	Typical/ maximum, Omni	20/24	18/21	20/24	16/20	19/23	19/23
Telecoil sensitivity	SPLITS (dB SPL)	104	95	88	90	n/a	n/a
Battery	Operating current (mA)	1.5	1.15	0.95	0.9	0.8	0.7
	Battery type	13	312	312	312	312	10

Delmar/Cengage Learning

PRODUCT 10: SAFRAN

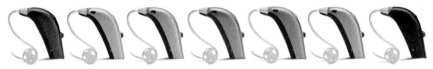

Safran BTE
Photos granted by Oticon, Inc.

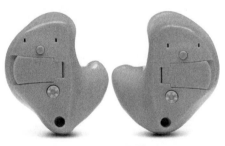

Safran ITE FS
Photos granted by Oticon, Inc.

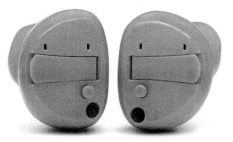

Safran ITE HS
Photos granted by Oticon, Inc.

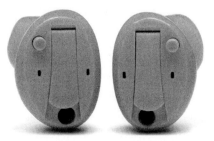

Safran ITC
Photos granted by Oticon, Inc.

OTICON

Product Application

Safran BTE
Safran BTE Power
Safran ITE
Safran ITC
Safran CIC/MIC

Features of All Safran products

- AI – automatically selects the best possible outcomes from multiple processing alternatives
- Trimode adaptive directionality – automatic adaptive directionality works in 3 modes: surround, split, and full
- Noise management (speech-weighted) – speech-weighted modulation index-based noise reduction in 8 frequency channels
- Voice-aligned compression – a proprietary compression system designed to make speech more intelligible and comfortable; available in dynamic, active, and gradual
- DSL v5.0 m[i/o]rationale for children and adults
- Wide-range bandwidth
- Activity analyzer – a data-logging feature that suggests adjustments to the hearing professional – displayed in an Envirogram

- Automatic adaptation manager – gradually increases gain to the prescribed level to facilitate acclimatization
- OpenEar Acoustics – a combination of an open fit with feedback cancellation, low-frequency emphasis, and a low processing delay; Safran can be fitted with Corda to provide open fittings
- Dynamic Feedback Cancellation – proprietary feedback cancellation algorithm
- Automatic microphone matching
- Fully automatic operation
- Up to 4 customizable programs
- Sound indicators for programs and low-battery warning
- Standby function
- Onset delay
- Programmable via the Oticon Genie software
- Recommended for all types of hearing losses, ranging from mild to severe for adults as well as children

Options of Safran BTE and Safran BTE Power

- Open dome, plus dome, and custom ear mold options are available
- Classic colors: beige, light brown, dark brown, light gray, and dark gray
- Cool colors: black, transparent, yellow, orange, pink, purple, blue, green
- New exclusive colors and baby colors: pearl white, silver-gray, steel gray, golden beige, copper, orchid, ice blue, baby blue, and baby pink
- Sound hooks
- Pediatric hooks
- Tamper-resistant battery door (available in all colors)
- DAI and FM shoes

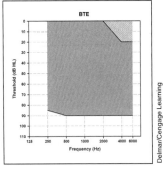

Fitting range for Safran BTE

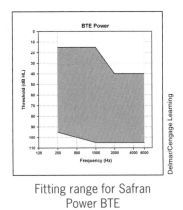

Fitting range for Safran Power BTE

Options of Safran ITE, ITC, CIC/MIC

- Colors: beige, light brown, medium brown, and dark brown
- Wax protection options – NoWax, MicroWaxBuster, and WaxBuster
- Tamper-resistant battery door (available in all custom colors)

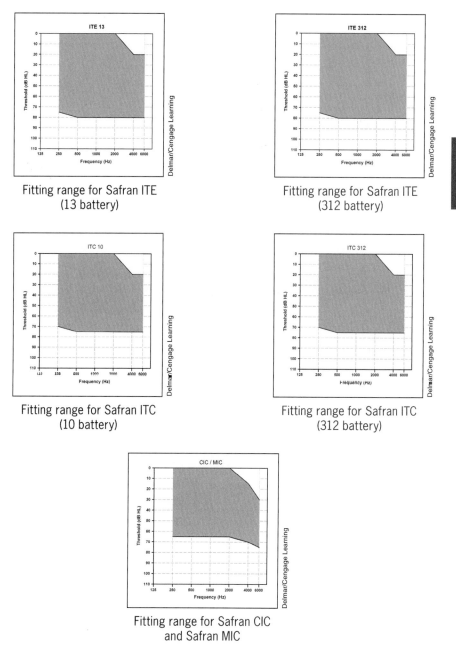

Fitting range for Safran ITE
(13 battery)

Fitting range for Safran ITE
(312 battery)

Fitting range for Safran ITC
(10 battery)

Fitting range for Safran ITC
(312 battery)

Fitting range for Safran CIC
and Safran MIC

Typical Specifications		Safran BTE	Safran Power BTE
Standard ANSI S3.22-2003 and S3.7 (1995)			
Output sound Pressure level	Max OSPL 90 (dB SPL)	112	126
	HFA OSPL 90 (dB SPL)	110	121
Full-on gain (50 dB SPL input)	Peak gain (dB)	54	62
	HFA (dB)	51	54
Total harmonic distortion (Hz)	500	0.5%	1.5%
	800	0.5%	1.0%
	1600	0.5%	0.5%
Equivalent input noise (dB SPL)	Typical/maximum, Omni	12	16
	Typical/maximum, Dir	20	26
Telecoil sensitivity	SPLITS (dB SPL)	93.5	99.5
Battery	Quiescent current drain (mA)	1.1	1.4
	Battery type	13	13

Delmar/Cengage Learning

Typical Specifications		Safran ITE (13)	Safran ITE (312)	Safran ITC (312)	Safran ITC (10)	Safran CIC/ MIC
Standard ANSI S3.22-2003 and S3.7 (1995)						
Output sound Pressure level	Max OSPL 90 (dB SPL)	113	112	110	104	103
	HFA OSPL 90 (dB SPL)	107	106	105	99	98
Full-on gain (50 dB SPL input)	Peak gain (dB)	52	47	41	37	37
	HFA (dB)	46	43	37	33	32
Total harmonic distortion (Hz)	500	1.5%	1.5%	0.5%	0.5%	1.0%
	800	1.0%	1.0%	0.5%	0.5%	0.5%
	1600	1.5%	1.0%	0.5%	0.5%	1.0%
Equivalent input noise (dB SPL)	Omni	17	19	20	18	20
	Dir	33	31	29	33	n/a
Telecoil sensitivity	SPLITS (dB SPL)	91	87	n/a	n/a	n/a
Battery	Quiescent current drain (mA)	1.1	1.1	1.1	1.0	0.7
	Battery type	13	312	312	10	10

Delmar/Cengage Learning

PRODUCT 11: GAIA

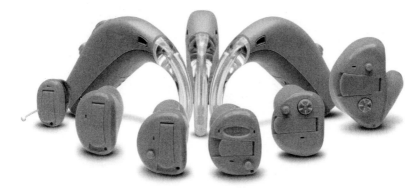

Gaia family line ranging from BTE through CIC
Photos granted by Oticon, Inc.

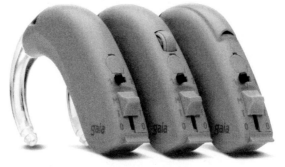

Gaia BTE, Gaia BTE Direct, and Gaia BTE Power
hearing aids
Photos granted by Oticon, Inc.

Product Application

Gaia BTE
Gaia BTE Direct
Gaia BTE Power
Gaia FS Power
Gaia FS Power P1/P2
Gaia HS/LP
Gaia HS/LP P1/P2
Gaia HS/LP Direct
Gaia HS/LP Power
Gaia HS/LP Power P1/P2
Gaia ITC
Gaia MIC
Gaia CIC

Features of All Gaia Products

- OpenEar Acoustics – a combination of an open fit with feedback cancellation, low-frequency emphasis, and a low processing delay; allows for open-ear fittings
- Choice of rationales:
  - Gaia
  - ASA^2
  - NAL – NL$_1$
  - DSL i/o
  - ASA^2p
- 7 frequency bands, 2 channels
- Multiple programs (Gaia BTE and ITE only)
- Dynamic Feedback Cancellation – proprietary feedback cancellation algorithm
- Low power consumption
- Fully automatic operation
- Adaptation manager – gradually increases gain to the prescribed level to facilitate acclimatization
- Optional volume control
- Optional programmable telecoil
- Feedback manager
- Directional BTE and ITE instruments
- Programmable via the Oticon Genie software

Features of Gaia BTE, Gaia BTE Direct, and Gaia BTE Power

- Multiple programs for dedicated listening environments
- Fully configurable function switches
- DAI
- FM-compatible
- Adjustable sound hook
- Low battery consumption
- Slim and light design

Options of Gaia BTE, Gaia BTE Direct, and Gaia BTE Power

- Volume control (manual override)
- 5 dB and undamped sound hooks
- Pediatric sound hook
- Tamper-resistant battery door
- Eyeglasses adapter
- CROS and BiCROS input via DAI
- 6 hair tone colors and 7 kids' colors
- Cool colors: transparent, yellow, orange, pink, purple, blue, green, and black

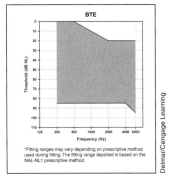

Fitting range for Gaia BTE

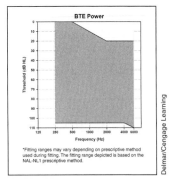

Fitting range for Gaia BTE Power

Features of Gaia FS Power P1/P2, Gaia FS Power, Gaia HS/LP Power P1/P2, Gaia HS/LP Power, Gaia HS/LP Direct, Gaia HS/LP P1/P2, Gaia HS/LP, Gaia ITC, Gaia MIC, and Gaia CIC

- Design optimized for size and cosmetics
- Selection of 3 wax-protection systems – NoWax, MicroWaxBuster, and WaxBuster
- Low battery consumption

Options of Gaia FS Power P1/P2, Gaia FS Power, Gaia HS/LP Power P1/P2, Gaia HS/LP Power, Gaia HS/LP Direct, Gaia HS/LP P1/P2, Gaia HS/LP, Gaia ITC, Gaia MIC, and Gaia CIC

- Manual override in ITE styles
- Directional models (HS/LP)
- Power models (HS/LP/FS)
- Manual or automatic telecoil in ITE styles
- Multiple programs for dedicated listening situations in ITE styles
- Fully configurable push-button operation in ITE styles
- Colors: pink, tan, medium brown, and dark brown

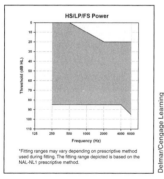

Fitting range for Gaia HS/LP/ FS Power

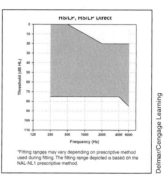

Fitting range for Gaia HS/LP and Gaia HS/LP Direct

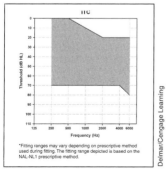

Fitting range for Gaia ITC

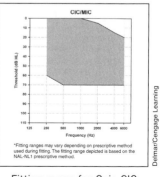

Fitting range for Gaia CIC and Gaia MIC

Typical Specifications		Gaia BTE/ BTE VC	Gaia BTE Direct	Gaia BTE Power
Standard ANSI S3.22-2003 and S3.7 (1995)				
Output sound Pressure level	Max OSPL 90 (dB SPL)	115	115	131
	HFA OSPL 90 (dB SPL)	111	111	126
Full-on gain (50 dB SPL input)	Peak gain (dB)	57	57	71
	HFA (dB)	52	52	65
Total harmonic distortion (Hz)	500	1.0%	1.0%	2.0%
	800	1.0%	1.0%	2.0%
	1600	1.0%	1.0%	1.0%
Equivalent input noise (dB SPL)	Typical/maximum, Omni	16/20	16/20	15/19
	Typical/maximum, Dir	n/a	19/23	n/a
Telecoil sensitivity	SPLITS (dB SPL)	93.5	93.5	108.5
Battery	Quiescent current drain (mA)	1.0	1.1	1.3
	Battery type	13	13	13

Delmar/Cengage Learning

Typical Specifications		Gaia FS Power (13)	Gaia HS/LP	Gaia HS/LP Direct	Gaia HS/LP Power (312)	Gaia ITC	Gaia CIC/ MIC
Standard ANSI S3.22-2003 and S3.7 (1995)							
Output sound Pressure level	Max OSPL 90 (dB SPL)	125	110	110	117	110	104
	HFA OSPL 90 (dB SPL)	122	107	106	112	106	100
Full-on gain (50 dB SPL input)	Peak gain (dB)	55	46	43	49	40	35
	HFA (dB)	52	42	41	42	37	32
Total harmonic distortion (Hz)	500	3.5%	2.5%	2.0%	2.0%	1.5%	1.0%
	800	3.5%	2.5%	2.0%	3.0%	1.5%	1.0%
	1600	1.0%	2.5%	2.0%	3.0%	1.5%	1.0%
Equivalent input noise (dB SPL)	Typical/ maximum, Omni	20/24	16/20	20/24	18/21	19/23	19/23
	Typical/ maximum, Dir	n/a	n/a	25/29	n/a	n/a	n/a
Telecoil sensitivity	SPLITS (dB SPL)	104	90	88	95	n/a	n/a
Battery	Operating current (mA)	1.5	0.9	1.0	1.15	0.8	0.7
	Battery type	13	312	312/10	312	312	10

Delmar/Cengage Learning

PRODUCT 12: TEGO PRO

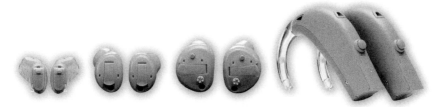

Tego Pro family product lines ranging from BTE through CIC
Photos granted by Oticon, Inc.

Product Application

Tego Pro BTE
Tego Pro BTE Power
Tego Pro HS/LP/FS
Tego Pro ITC
Tego Pro CIC/MIC

Features of All Tego Pro Products

- DecisionMaker – general program enabled by AI to ensure that the features are used at the right time and in the right combination for each situation
- Identities – active, gradual, or dynamic identity can be selected to make the fitting process fast and accurate
- Adaptive directionality – attenuates noise sources from the sides and behind (excludes Tego Pro CIC/MIC)
- Automatic directionality – automatically switches between HF Direct™ and surround modes
- HF Direct – speech-focused directionality
- Surround mode
- Noise management
- Wide-range bandwidth
- OpenEar Acoustics – a combination of an open fit with feedback cancellation, low-frequency emphasis, and a low processing delay; allows for open-ear fittings
- Dynamic Feedback Cancellation – proprietary feedback cancellation algorithm
- Many options and programs for phone use
- Up to 4 customizable programs
- Program sound indicators (beeps)
- Standby function
- Onset delay
- Programmable via the Oticon Genie software

Features of Tego Pro BTE and Tego Pro BTE Power

- DAI
- Fully programmable telecoil
- FM-compatible
- Adjustable sound hook

Options of Tego Pro BTE and Tego Pro BTE Power

- Volume control with audible indication
- 9 dB, 5 dB, and undamped sound hooks
- Pediatric sound hooks
- Thin-tube fitting (Oticon Corda)
- Tamper-resistant battery door
- DAI and FM shoes
- Eyeglasses adapter
- CROS and BiCROS
- Hair-tone colors: beige, light brown, dark brown, light gray, and dark gray
- Cool colors: black, transparent, yellow, orange, pink, purple, blue, and green

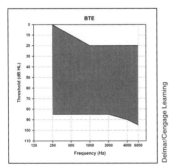

Fitting range for Tego Pro BTE

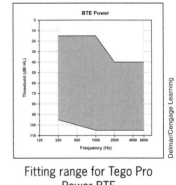

Fitting range for Tego Pro
Power BTE

Features of Tego Pro HS/LP/FS, Tego Pro ITC, and Tego Pro CIC/MIC

- Design optimized for size and cosmetics
- Selection of 3 wax-protection systems – NoWax, MicroWaxBuster, and WaxBuster

Options of Tego Pro HS/LP/FS, Tego Pro ITC, and Tego Pro CIC/MIC

- AutoPhone program – automatic shift to 1 of 2 dedicated phone programs, acoustic phone (AP): microphone or phone T (PT): telecoil
- Fully programmable telecoil
- Volume control with audible indication
- Colors: beige, light brown, medium brown, and dark brown

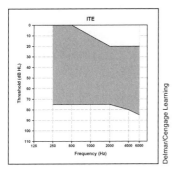

Fitting range for Tego Pro
HS/LP/FS

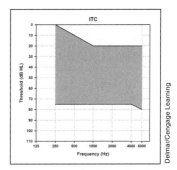

Fitting range for Tego Pro ITC

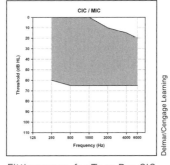

Fitting range for Tego Pro CIC
and Tego Pro MIC

Typical Specifications		Tego Pro BTE	Tego Pro BTE Power
Standard ANSI S3.22-2003 and S3.7 (1995)			
Output sound Pressure level	Max OSPL 90 (dB SPL)	112	126
	HFA OSPL 90 (dB SPL)	110	121
Full-on gain (50 dB SPL input)	Peak gain (dB)	54	62
	HFA (dB)	51	54
Total harmonic distortion (Hz)	500	0.5%	1.5%
	800	0.5%	1.0%
	1600	0.5%	0.5%
Equivalent input noise (dB SPL)	Typical/maximum, Omni	12/16	16/20
	Typical/maximum, Dir	20/24	26/30
Telecoil sensitivity	SPLITS (dB SPL)	93.5	99.5
Battery	Quiescent current drain (mA)	1.1	1.4
	Battery type	13	13

Delmar/Cengage Learning

Typical Specifications		Tego Pro Full-Shell (13)	Tego Pro Half-Shell/ Low-Profile (312)	Tego Pro ITC (312)	Tego Pro ITC (10)	Tego Pro CIC/ MIC
Standard ANSI S3.22-2003 and S3.7 (1995)						
Output sound Pressure level	Max OSPL 90 (dB SPL)	113	112	110	104	103
	HFA OSPL 90 (dB SPL)	107	106	105	99	98
Full-on gain (50 dB SPL input)	Peak gain (dB)	52	47	41	37	37
	HFA (dB)	46	43	37	33	32
Total harmonic distortion (Hz)	500	1.5%	1.5%	0.5%	0.5%	1.0%
	800	1.0%	1.0%	0.5%	0.5%	0.5%
	1600	1.5%	1.0%	0.5%	0.5%	1.0%
Equivalent input noise (dB SPL)	Typical/ maximum, Omni	17/21	19/23	20/24	18/22	20/24
	Typical/ maximum, Dir	33/37	31/35	29/33	33/37	n/a
Telecoil sensitivity	SPLITS (dB SPL)	91	87	n/a	n/a	n/a
Battery	Quiescent current drain (mA)	1.2	1.2	1.2	1.1	0.7
	Battery type	13	312	312	10	10

Delmar/Cengage Learning

PRODUCT 13: TEGO

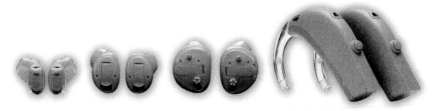

Tego family product lines ranging from BTE through CIC
Photos granted by Oticon, Inc.

Product Application

Tego BTE
Tego BTE Power
Tego (13) ITE
Tego (312) ITE
Tego (312) ITC
Tego (10) ITC
Tego CIC/MIC

Features of All Tego Products

- DecisionMaker – general program enabled by AI to ensure that the features are used at the right time and in the right combination for each situation
- Identities – active, gradual, or dynamic identity can be selected to make the fitting process fast and accurate
- Directionality (excludes Tego CIC/MIC)
- Automatic directionality – automatically switches between HF Direct and surround modes
- HF Direct – speech-focused directionality
- Surround mode – omnidirectional mode
- Noise management – controls noise depending on the presence/absence of speech/noise
- OpenEar Acoustics – a combination of an open fit with feedback cancellation, low-frequency emphasis, and a low processing delay; allows for open-ear fittings
- Dynamic Feedback Cancellation – proprietary feedback cancellation algorithm
- Many options and programs for phone use
- Up to 3 customizable programs
- Program sound indicators (beeps)
- Standby function
- Onset delay

Features of Tego BTE and Tego BTE Power

- DAI
- Fully programmable telecoil
- FM-compatible
- Adjustable sound hook
- Hair tone colors: beige, light brown, dark brown, light gray, and dark gray
- Cool colors: black, transparent, yellow, orange, pink, purple, blue, and green

Options of Tego BTE and Tego BTE Power

- Volume control with audible indication
- 9 dB, 5 dB, and undamped sound hooks
- Pediatric sound hooks
- Tamper-resistant battery door
- DAI and FM shoes
- Eyeglasses adapter
- CROS and BiCROS

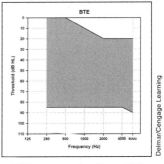
Fitting range for Tego BTE

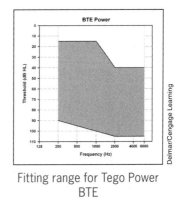
Fitting range for Tego Power BTE

Features of Tego (13) ITE, Tego (312) ITE, Tego (312) ITC, Tego (10) ITC, and Tego CIC/MIC

- Design optimized for size and cosmetics
- Colors: beige, light brown, medium brown, and dark brown
- Selection of 3 wax-protection systems – NoWax, MicroWaxBuster, and WaxBuster

Options of Tego (13) ITE, Tego (312) ITE, Tego (312) ITC, Tego (10) ITC, and Tego CIC/MIC

- AutoPhone program – automatic shift to 1 of 2 dedicated phone programs, acoustic phone (AP): microphone or phone T (PT): telecoil
- Fully programmable telecoil
- Volume control with audible indication

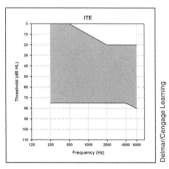

Fitting range for Tego ITE

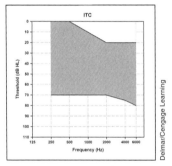

Fitting range for Tego ITC

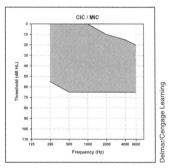

Fitting range for Tego CIC and Tego MIC

Typical Specifications		Tego BTE	Tego BTE Power
Standard ANSI S3.22-2003 and S3.7 (1995)			
Output sound Pressure level	Max OSPL 90 (dB SPL)	112	126
	HFA OSPL 90 (dB SPL)	110	121
Full-on gain (50 dB SPL input)	Peak gain (dB)	53	62
	HFA (dB)	51	55
Total harmonic distortion (Hz)	500	0.5%	2.0%
	800	0.5%	2.0%
	1600	0.5%	2.0%
Equivalent input noise (dB SPL)	Typical/maximum, Omni	12/16	16/20
	Typical/maximum, Dir	20/24	26/30
Telecoil sensitivity	SPLITS (dB SPL)	93.5	99.5
Battery	Operating current (mA)	1.1	1.4
	Battery type	13	13

Delmar/Cengage Learning

Typical Specifications		Tego ITE (13)	Tego ITE (312)	Tego ITC (312)	Tego ITC (10)	Tego CIC/ MIC
Standard ANSI S3.22-2003 and S3.7 (1995)						
Output sound Pressure level	Max OSPL 90 (dB SPL)	113	112	110	104	103
	HFA OSPL 90 (dB SPL)	108	106	105	99	98
Full-on gain (50 dB SPL input)	Peak gain (dB)	51	46	40	36	36
	HFA (dB)	46	43	37	32	33
Total harmonic distortion (Hz)	500	1.5%	1.5%	0.5%	0.5%	1.0%
	800	1.0%	1.0%	0.5%	0.5%	0.5%
	1600	1.5%	1.0%	1.0%	0.5%	1.0%
Equivalent input noise (dB SPL)	Typical/maximum, Omni	17/21	19/23	20/24	18/22	20/24
	Typical/maximum, Dir	33/37	31/35	29/33	33/37	n/a
Telecoil sensitivity	SPLITS (dB SPL)	91	87	n/a	n/a	n/a
Battery	Operating current (mA)	1.2	1.2	1.2	1.1	0.7
	Battery type	13	312	312	10	10

Delmar/Cengage Learning

PRODUCT 14: ATLASPLUS OPEN

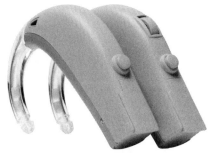

AtlasPlus BTE and AtlasPlus BTE with
volume control
Photos granted by Oticon, Inc.

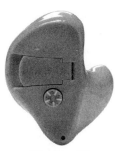

AtlasPlus FS
Photos granted by
Oticon, Inc.

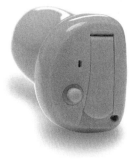

AtlasPlus HS with push button
Photos granted by Oticon, Inc.

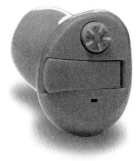

AtlasPlus HS with volume control
Photos granted by Oticon, Inc.

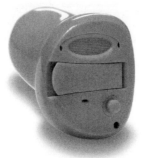

AtlasPlus HS Direct
Photos granted by Oticon, Inc.

Product Application

AtlasPlus Open BTE
AtlasPlus Open BTE Power
AtlasPlus Open BTE Directional
AtlasPlus Open FS Power
AtlasPlus Open FS Power P1/P2
AtlasPlus Open HS/LP
AtlasPlus Open HS/LP P1/P2
AtlasPlus Open HS/LP Direct
AtlasPlus Open HS/LP Power
AtlasPlus Open HS/LP Power P1/P2
AtlasPlus Open ITC
AtlasPlus Open MIC
AtlasPlus Open CIC

Features of All AtlasPlus Open Products

- 100% digital
- 2 channels, 4 frequency shaping bands
- OpenEar Acoustics – a combination of an open fit with feedback cancellation, low-frequency emphasis, and a low processing delay; allows for open-ear fittings
- Dynamic Feedback Cancellation – proprietary feedback cancellation algorithm
- 2 program options including standby
- NAL – NL_1, DSL i/o rationales
- NAL – RP, DSL i/o (LIN) available in power models
- Automatic feedback manager
- Adaptation manager – gradually increases gain to the prescribed level to facilitate acclimatization
- Programmable via the Oticon Genie software

Features of AtlasPlus Open BTE, AtlasPlus Open BTE Power, and AtlasPlus Open BTE Directional

- ON/OFF in battery drawer
- Push-button drawer
- Swing hook
- Slim and light design

Options of AtlasPlus Open BTE, AtlasPlus Open BTE Power, and AtlasPlus Open BTE Directional

- Volume control
- Swing hooks – undamped, 5 dB damped, 9 dB damped, and small size for children
- Eyeglasses adapter
- Tamper-resistant battery door
- Colors: beige, light brown, dark brown, light gray, dark gray, black, and kids' colors
- CROS and BiCROS input via DAI
- Compatible with DAI and wireless FM systems via DAI and FM adapters

Features of AtlasPlus Open FS Power P1/P2, AtlasPlus Open FS Power, AtlasPlus Open HS/LP Power P1/P2, AtlasPlus Open HS/LP Power, AtlasPlus Open HS/LP Direct, AtlasPlus Open HS/LP P1/P2, AtlasPlus Open HS/LP, AtlasPlus Open ITC, AtlasPlus Open MIC, and AtlasPlus Open CIC

- Fully automatic solutions
- Low battery consumption
- ON/OFF battery door
- Push-button telecoil
- Selection of 3 wax-protection systems – NoWax, MicroWaxBuster, and WaxBuster

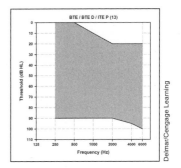

Fitting range for AtlasPlus Open BTE, AtlasPlus Open BTE-D, and AtlasPlus Open ITE-P (13 battery)

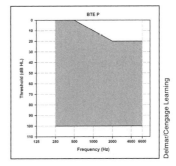

Fitting range for AtlasPlus Open BTE Power

Options of AtlasPlus Open FS Power P1/P2, AtlasPlus Open FS Power, AtlasPlus Open HS/LP Power P1/P2, AtlasPlus Open HS/LP Power, AtlasPlus Open HS/LP Direct, AtlasPlus Open HS/LP P1/P2, AtlasPlus Open HS/LP, AtlasPlus Open ITC, AtlasPlus Open MIC, and AtlasPlus Open CIC

- Volume control in ITE styles
- Programmable telecoil in ITE styles
- Selection of 4 faceplate colors

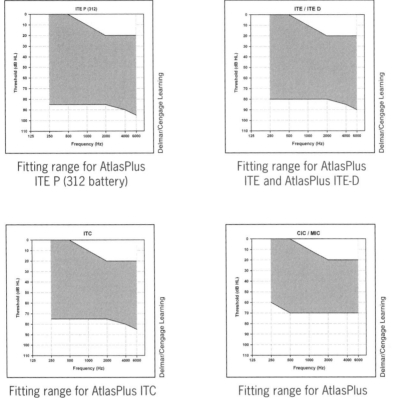

Fitting range for AtlasPlus
ITE P (312 battery)

Fitting range for AtlasPlus
ITE and AtlasPlus ITE-D

Fitting range for AtlasPlus ITC

Fitting range for AtlasPlus
CIC and AtlasPlus MIC

Typical Specifications		AtlasPlus Open BTE	AtlasPlus Open Directional	AtlasPlus Open BTE Power
Standard ANSI S3.22-2003 and S3.7 (1995)				
Output sound pressure level	Max OSPL 90 (dB SPL)	119	115	133
	HFA OSPL 90 (dB SPL)	114	111	127
Full-on gain (50 dB SPL input)	Peak gain (dB)	59	57	71
	HFA (dB)	54	52	65
Total harmonic distortion (Hz)	500	1.5%	1.0%	2.0%
	800	1.5%	1.0%	1.0%
	1600	1.0%	1.0%	0.5%
Equivalent input noise (dB SPL)	Typical/maximum, Omni	17/21	16/20	17/21
	Typical/maximum, Dir	n/a	19/23	n/a
Telecoil sensitivity	SPLITS (dB SPL)	93.5	93.5	110
Battery	Operating current (mA)	1.1	1.1	1.2
	Battery type	13	13	13

Typical Specifications		AtlasPlus Open Full-Shell Power (13)	Atlas-Plus Open HS/LP Power (312)	AtlasPlus Open HS/LP Directional	Atlas-Plus Open HS/LP	Atlas-Plus Open ITC	Atlas-Plus Open CIC/ MIC
Standard ANSI S3.22-2003 and S3.7 (1995)							
Output sound pressure level	Max OSPL 90 (dB SPL)	125	117	110	110	110	104
	HFA OSPL 90 (dB SPL)	122	112	106	107	106	100
Full-on gain (50 dB SPL input)	Peak gain (dB)	55	49	43	46	40	35
	HFA (dB)	52	42	41	42	37	35
Total harmonic distortion (Hz)	500	3.5%	0.2%	2.0%	2.5%	1.5%	1.0%
	800	3.5%	0.3%	2.0%	2.5%	1.5%	1.0%
	1600	1.0%	0.3%	2.0%	2.5%	1.5%	1.0%
Equivalent input noise (dB SPL)	Typical/ Maximum, Omni	20/24	21/25	16/20	16/20	19/23	19/23
Telecoil sensitivity	SPLITS (dB SPL)	104	95	88	90	n/a	n/a
Battery	Operating current (mA)	1.5	1.2	1.0	0.9	0.8	0.7
	Battery type	13	312	312	312	312	10

Delmar/Cengage Learning

PRODUCT 15: ATLAS

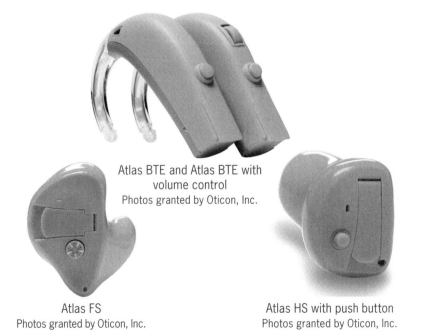

Atlas BTE and Atlas BTE with
volume control
Photos granted by Oticon, Inc.

Atlas FS
Photos granted by Oticon, Inc.

Atlas HS with push button
Photos granted by Oticon, Inc.

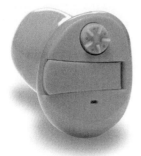

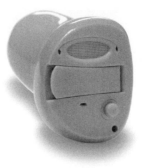

Atlas HS with volume control   Atlas HS Direct
Photos granted by Oticon, Inc.   Photos granted by Oticon, Inc.

Product Application

Atlas BTE
Atlas BTE Power
Atlas BTE Direct
Atlas FS/HS Power
Atlas HS/LP
Atlas HS/LP Direct
Atlas ITC
Atlas MIC
Atlas CIC

Features of All Atlas Products

- Fully digital
- Selection of nonlinear NAL – NL_1 and DSL i/o fitting algorithms
- Power instruments also offer linear NAL – RP and DSL i/o (LIN) fitting algorithms
- 2 channels, 4 frequency shaping bands
- Adaptation manager – gradually increases gain to the prescribed level to facilitate acclimatization
- Acoustic feedback manager
- Optional volume control
- Optional programmable telecoil
- Directional BTE and ITE instruments
- Programmable via the Oticon Genie software

Features of Atlas BTE, Atlas BTE Power, and Atlas BTE Direct

- ON/OFF in battery door
- Push-button telecoil
- Swing hook
- Slim and light design

Options of Atlas BTE, Atlas BTE Power, and Atlas BTE Direct

- Volume control
- Swing hooks – undamped, 5 dB damped, 9 dB damped, and pediatric hooks available
- Eyeglasses adapter
- Tamper-resistant battery door
- 6 hair tone colors and 7 kids' colors
- CROS and BiCROS input via DAI
- Compatible with DAI and wireless FM systems via DAI and FM adapters

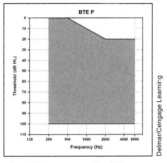

Fitting range for Atlas BTE, Atlas BTE-D and Atlas FSP

Features of Atlas FS/HS Power, Atlas HS/LP Direct, Atlas HS/LP, Atlas ITC, Atlas MIC, and Atlas CIC

- Compact, fully automatic solutions
- Excellent battery consumption
- ON/OFF in battery door
- Selection of wax-protection systems – NoWax or MicroWaxBuster

Fitting range for Atlas Power BTE

Options of Atlas FS/HS Power, Atlas HS/LP Direct, Atlas HS/LP, Atlas ITC, Atlas MIC, and Atlas CIC

- Volume control in ITE styles
- Programmable telecoil in ITE styles
- Selection of 4 faceplate colors

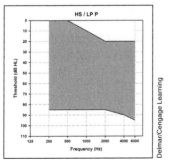

Fitting range for Atlas HS/LP

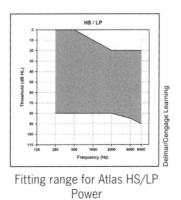

Fitting range for Atlas HS/LP Power

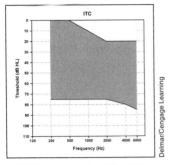

Fitting range for Atlas ITC

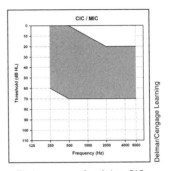

Fitting range for Atlas CIC
and Atlas MIC

Typical Specifications		Atlas BTE	Atlas BTE Direct	Atlas BTE Power
Standard ANSI S3.22-2003 and S3.7 (1995)				
Output sound pressure level	Max OSPL 90 (dB SPL)	119	115	133
	HFA OSPL 90 (dB SPL)	114	111	127
Full-on gain (50 dB SPL input)	Peak gain (dB)	59	57	71
	HFA (dB)	54	52	65
Total harmonic distortion (Hz)	500	1.5%	1.0%	2.0%
	800	1.5%	1.0%	1.0%
	1600	1.0%	1.0%	0.5%
Equivalent input noise (dB SPL)	Typical/maximum, Omni	17/21	16/20	18/22
	Typical/maximum, Dir	n/a	19/23	n/a
Telecoil sensitivity	SPLITS (dB SPL)	91.5	93.5	114
Battery	Operating current (mA)	0.9	1.1	1.2
	Battery type	13	13	13

Delmar/Cengage Learning

Typical Specifications		Atlas Full-Shell Power (13)	Atlas HS/LP Power (312)	Atlas HS/LP Direct	Atlas HS/LP	Atlas ITC	Atlas CIC/MIC
Standard ANSI S3.22-2003 and S3.7 (1995)							
Output sound pressure level	Max OSPL 90 (dB SPL)	124	117	110	110	110	104
	HFA OSPL 90 (dB SPL)	122	112	106	107	107	100

Delmar/Cengage Learning

continues

continued

Typical Specifications		Atlas Full-Shell Power (13)	Atlas HS/LP Power (312)	Atlas HS/LP Direct	Atlas HS/LP	Atlas ITC	Atlas CIC/MIC
Full-on gain (50 dB SPL input)	Peak gain (dB)	55	49	43	46	40	35
	HFA (dB)	51	42	41	42	37	35
Total harmonic distortion (Hz)	500 Hz	3.5%	0.2%	2.0%	2.5%	1.5%	1.0%
	800 Hz	3.5%	0.3%	2.0%	2.5%	1.5%	1.0%
	1600 Hz	1.0%	0.3%	2.0%	2.5%	1.5%	1.0%
Equivalent input noise (dB SPL)	Typical/ maximum, Omni	21/25	21/25	16/20	16/20	19/23	19/23
	Typical/ maximum, Dir	n/a	n/a	25/29	n/a	n/a	n/a
Telecoil sensitivity	SPLITS (dB SPL)	103	95	88	90	n/a	n/a
Battery	Operating current (mA)	1.4	1.2	0.95	0.9	0.8	0.7
	Battery type	13	312	312	312	312	10

Delmar/Cengage Learning

PRODUCT 16: SUMO

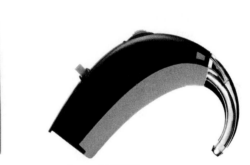

Sumo DM BTE
Photos granted by Oticon, Inc.

Product Application

Sumo DM BTE Super Power
Sumo XP BTE
Sumo E BTE

Features of Sumo DM BTE Super Power

- Fully digital
- Dynamic Feedback Cancellation – proprietary feedback cancellation algorithm

- Feedback management system
- TriState noise management – uses modulations in speech to determine speech and noise content in eight bands to improve the overall speech-to-noise ratio
- High-resolution fitting, 8 channels, and 3 input levels gain adjustments
- 4 identities for efficient fitting based on the DSEsp loudness model
- 4 additional linear rationales: SSL v5.0, DSL i/o (LIN), NAL – RP, and POGO II+BC
- Volume control with clear markings, end stop, and integrated OFF function
- Beep at preferred volume control setting
- Up to 3 customizable programs
- Audible program indicators (beeps)
- Visual status indicator (LED)
- Undamped sound hook
- DAI and FM-compatible
- Left/right identification
- Fully programmable 3-position switch with clear markings
- Programmable telecoil
- Programmable via the Oticon Genie software

Options of Sumo DM BTE Super Power

- Sound hooks – 5 dB damped and pediatric hooks, damped and undamped
- Interlocking DAI and FM shoes
- Tamper-resistant battery door
- Eyeglasses adapter
- CROS and BiCROS
- External microphone (MIC32)
- Hair-tone colors
- Kids' translucent colors, and new "baby pink" and "baby blue" opaque colors

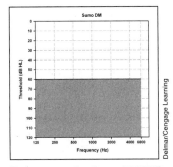

Fitting range for Sumo DM BTE

Features of Sumo XP BTE

- Digitally programmable
- Fitting rationales – POGO II+BC (default), NAL – RP, DSL i/o, SSM+, and Corell-2
- A-gram slope control (fourth-order LF/HF cut)
- Variable crossover frequency (0.5–2.0 kHz)
- Gain control (preset)
- UCL control with 3 output-limiting options: PC, AGCo fast, and AGCo slow
- Feedback manager (variable roll-off)
- Telecoil boost (+6 dB)
- Undamped sound hook

- FM- and DAI-compatible
- Left/right identification
- Programmable telecoil
- Programmable VC range – full (30 dB), half (15 dB), and disabled
- Programmable via the Oticon Genie software

Options of Sumo XP BTE

- Hooks – 5 dB damped and pediatric, damped and undamped
- Interlocking DAI and FM shoes
- Tamper-resistant battery door
- Eyeglasses adapter
- CROS and BiCROS
- Bone conduction modification/oscillator
- Colors: beige, light brown, dark brown, light gray, dark gray, and kids' colors

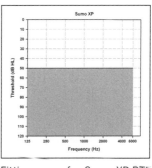

Fitting range for Sumo XP BTE

Features of Sumo E BTE

- Digitally programmable
- A-gram slope control (fourth-order LF/HF cut)
- Gain control (preset)
- UCL control
- Output limiting – PC or AGCo + PC
- Feedback manager
- Telecoil, M-MT-T with programmable disable function
- Volume control disable function
- Undamped sound hook
- DAI- and FM-compatible
- Fitting rationales – POGO II+BC (default), NAL – RP, DSL i/o (LIN), SSM+, and Corell-2
- Programmable via the Oticon Genie software

Options of Sumo E BTE

- Hooks – 5 dB damped and pediatric, damped and undamped
- Interlocking DAI and FM shoes
- Tamper-resistant battery door
- CROS and BiCROS
- Bone conduction oscillator
- Left/right identification

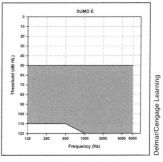

Fitting range for Sumo E BTE

Typical Specifications		Sumo DM BTE Super Power	Sumo XP BTE	Sumo E BTE
Standard ANSI S3.22-2003 and S3.7 (1995)				
Output sound pressure level	Max OSPL 90 (dB SPL)	140	142	140
	HFA OSPL 90 (dB SPL)	133	134	134
Full-on gain (50 dB SPL input)	Peak gain (dB)	82	82	80
	HFA (dB)	73	72	72
Total harmonic distortion (Hz)	500 Hz	1.0%	n/a	n/a
	800 Hz	0.5%	2.0%	2.0%
	1600 Hz	0.5%	2.0%	1.0%
Equivalent input noise (dB SPL)	Typical/maximum, Omni	27	28	7
	Typical/maximum, Dir	n/a	n/a	n/a
Telecoil sensitivity	SPLITS (dB SPL)	117	117	119
Battery	Operating current, typical/maximum (mA)	1.5	1.8/3.9	2.9
	Battery type	675	675	675

Delmar/Cengage Learning

PRODUCT 17: GO PRO

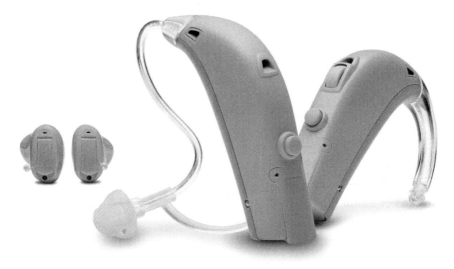

GO Pro standard BTE, open-ear BTE, and CIC hearing aids
Photos granted by Oticon, Inc.

Product Application

Go Pro BTE Power Omni
Go Pro BTE Power
Go Pro BTE Corda
Go Pro BTE

Go Pro ITE Power Omni
Go Pro ITE
Go Pro ITC
Go Pro CIC/MIC

Features of All Go Pro Products

- Fixed directionality
- 2 power omni styles
- Noise reduction
- OpenEar Acoustics – a combination of an open fit with feedback cancellation, low-frequency emphasis, and a low processing delay; allows for open-ear fittings
- Dynamic Feedback Cancellation – proprietary feedback cancellation algorithm
- 3 configurable programs
- NAL – NL$_1$
- 4 channels and 4 trimmers
- Sound indicator for programs and low-battery warning
- Standby function
- Onset delay and "jingle" sound indicator
- Recommended for any type of hearing loss, from mild to severe
- Programmable via the Oticon Genie software

OTICON

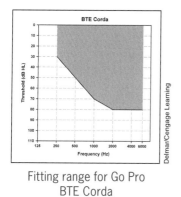

Fitting range for Go Pro BTE
Power Omni

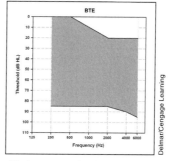

Fitting range for Go Pro
Power BTE

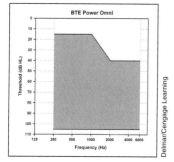

Fitting range for Go Pro
BTE Corda

Fitting range for Go Pro BTE

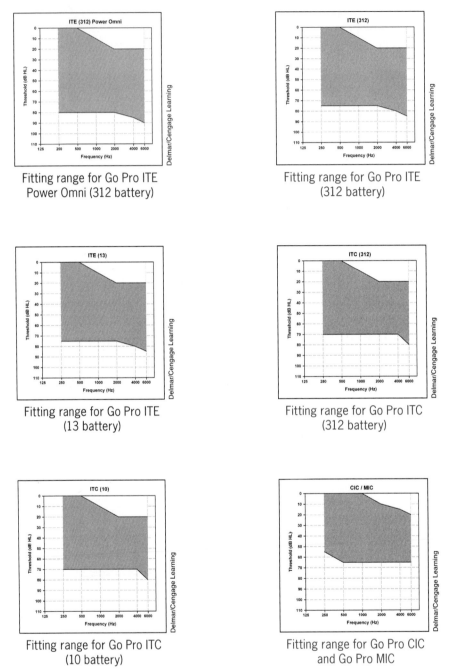

Fitting range for Go Pro ITE
Power Omni (312 battery)

Fitting range for Go Pro ITE
(312 battery)

Fitting range for Go Pro ITE
(13 battery)

Fitting range for Go Pro ITC
(312 battery)

Fitting range for Go Pro ITC
(10 battery)

Fitting range for Go Pro CIC
and Go Pro MIC

Typical Specifications		Go Pro BTE	Go Pro BTE Power	Go Pro BTE Power Omni
Standard ANSI S3.22-2003 and S3.7 (1995)				
Output sound pressure level	Max OSPL 90 (dB SPL)	112	126	133
	HFA OSPL 90 (dB SPL)	110	121	127
Full-on gain (50 dB SPL input)	Peak gain (dB)	53	62	70
	HFA (dB)	51	55	63
Total harmonic distortion (Hz)	500 Hz	0.5%	2.0%	1.0%
	800 Hz	0.5%	2.0%	0.5%
	1600 Hz	0.5%	2.0%	0.5%
Equivalent input noise (dB SPL)	Omni	12	16	17
	Dir	20	26	n/a
Telecoil sensitivity	SPLITS (dB SPL)	93.5	99.5	109
Battery	Current drain, quiescent/ typical (mA)	1.1/1.1	1.4/1.4	1.3/1.3
	Battery type	13	13	13

Delmar/Cengage Learning

Typical Specifications		Go Pro Power Omni ITE (312)	Go Pro ITE (13)	Go Pro ITE (312)	Go Pro ITC (312)	Go Pro ITC (10)	Go Pro CIC/ MIC
Standard ANSI S3.22-2003 and S3.7 (1995)							
Output sound pressure level	Max OSPL 90 (dB SPL)	118	113	112	110	104	103
	HFA OSPL 90 (dB SPL)	112	108	106	105	99	98
Full-on gain (50 dB SPL input)	Peak gain (dB)	51	51	46	40	36	36
	HFA (dB)	42	46	43	37	32	33
Total harmonic distortion (Hz)	500 Hz	1.5%	1.5%	1.5%	0.5%	0.5%	1.0%
	800 Hz	1.0%	1.0%	1.0%	0.5%	0.5%	0.5%
	1600 Hz	1.0%	1.5%	1.0%	1.0%	0.5%	1.0%
Equivalent input noise (dB SPL)	Omni	19	17	19	20	18	20
	Dir	n/a	33	31	29	33	n/a
Telecoil sensitivity	SPLITS (dB SPL)	93	91	87	n/a	n/a	n/a
	Current drain, quiescent/ typical (mA)	1.4/1.4	1.1/1.2	1.1/1.2	1.1/1.2	1.0/1.1	0.7/0.7
	Battery type	312	13	312	312	10	10

Delmar/Cengage Learning

PRODUCT 18: GO

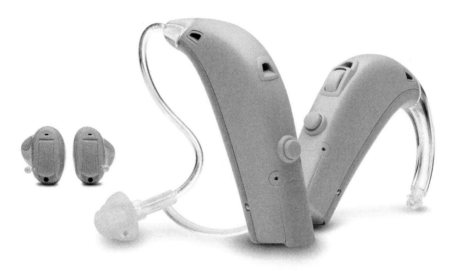

GO Standard BTE, open-ear BTE, and CIC hearing aids
Photos granted by Oticon, Inc.

Product Application

GO BTE Direct
GO BTE Power
GO BTE
GO Full-Shell Power
GO HS/LP Power
GO HS/LP Direct
GO HS/LP
GO ITC
GO MIC
GO CIC

Features of All GO Products

- 2-channel WDRC compression
- NAL – NL$_1$ rationale
- 6 fitting controls:
  - LF Soft
  - HF Soft
  - LF Loud
  - HF Loud
  - LF MPO
  - HF MPO

- Adaptation manager – gradually increases gain to the prescribed level to facilitate acclimatization
- Automatic feedback manager
- Optional programmable volume control and telecoil
- Directional BTE and ITE instruments
- Power BTE and ITE instruments
- Programmable via the Oticon Genie software

Features of GO BTE, GO BTE Direct, and GO BTE Power

- ON/OFF in battery door
- Push-button telecoil
- Swing hook
- Slim and light design

Options of GO BTE, GO BTE Direct, and GO BTE Power

- Volume control
- Swing hooks – undamped, 5 dB damped, 9 dB damped, and pediatric hooks
- Eyeglasses adapter
- Tamper-resistant battery door
- Colors: beige, light brown, dark brown, light gray, dark gray, black, and kids' colors
- CROS and BiCROS input via DAI
- Compatible with DAI and wireless FM systems via DAI and FM adapters

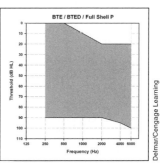

Fitting range for GO BTE, GO BTE-D, and GO FSP

Features of GO Full-Shell Power, GO HS/LP Power, GO HS/LP Direct, GO HS/LP, GO ITC, GO MIC, and GO CIC

- Fully automatic solutions
- Excellent battery consumption
- ON/OFF in battery door
- Push-button telecoil
- Selection of 3 wax-protection systems – NoWax, MicroWaxBuster, and WaxBuster

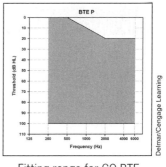

Fitting range for GO BTE Power

Options of GO Full-Shell Power, GO HS/LP Power, GO HS/LP Direct, GO HS/LP, GO ITC, GO MIC, and GO CIC

- Volume control in ITE styles
- Programmable telecoil in ITE styles
- Selection of 4 faceplate colors

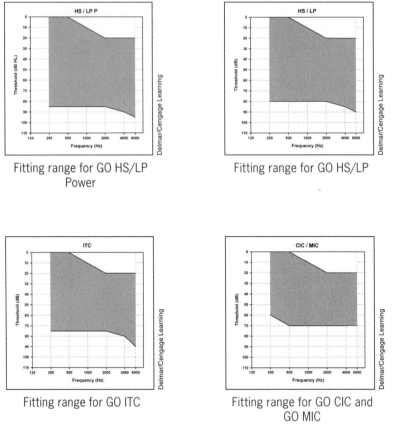

Fitting range for GO HS/LP Power

Fitting range for GO HS/LP

Fitting range for GO ITC

Fitting range for GO CIC and GO MIC

Typical Specifications		GO BTE	GO BTE Direct	GO BTE Power
Standard ANSI S3.22-2003 and S3.7 (1995)				
Output sound pressure level	Max OSPL 90 (dB SPL)	119	115	133
	HFA OSPL 90 (dB SPL)	114	111	127
Full-on gain (50 dB SPL input)	Peak gain (dB)	59	57	71
	HFA (dB)	54	52	65
Total harmonic distortion (Hz)	500 Hz	1.5%	1.0%	2.0%
	800 Hz	1.5%	1.0%	1.0%
	1600 Hz	1.0%	1.0%	0.5%
Equivalent input noise (dB SPL)	Typical/maximum, Omni	17/21	16/20	17/21
	Typical/maximum, Dir	n/a	19/23	n/a
Telecoil sensitivity	SPLITS (dB SPL)	93	93.5	110
Battery	Operating current (mA)	0.9	1.1	1.2
	Battery type	13	13	13

Delmar/Cengage Learning

Typical Specifications		GO Full-Shell Power (13)	GO HS/LP Power (312)	GO HS/LP Direct	GO HS/LP	GO ITC	GO CIC/ MIC
Standard ANSI S3.22-2003 and S3.7 (1995)							
Output sound pressure level	Max OSPL 90 (dB SPL)	125	117	110	110	110	104
	HFA OSPL 90 (dB SPL)	122	112	106	107	106	100
Full-on gain (50 dB SPL input)	Peak gain (dB)	55	49	43	46	40	35
	HFA (dB)	52	42	41	42	37	32
Total harmonic distortion (Hz)	500 Hz	3.5%	0.2%	2.0%	2.5%	1.5%	1.0%
	800 Hz	3.5%	0.3%	2.0%	2.5%	1.5%	1.0%
	1600 Hz	1.0%	0.3%	2.0%	2.5%	1.5%	1.0%
Equivalent input noise (dB SPL)	Typical/ maximum, Omni	20/24	21/25	16/20	16/20	19/23	19/23
	Typical/ maximum, Dir	n/a	n/a	25/29	n/a	n/a	n/a
Telecoil sensitivity	SPLITS (dB SPL)	104	91	88	90	n/a	n/a
	Operating current (mA)	1.5	1.2	1.0	0.9	0.8	0.7
	Battery type	13	312	312/10	312	312	10

Delmar/Cengage Learning

PRODUCT 19: ERGO

Product Application

Ergo BTE
Ergo BTE Power
Ergo Concha
Ergo Canal P
Ergo Canal
Ergo Mini Canal
Ergo CIC

Features of Ergo BTE and Ergo BTE Power

- Digitally programmable
- Class-D amplifier
- A-gram slope control (fourth-order LF/HF control)
- Gain control (preset)
- UCL control with 3 output-limiting options – PC, AGCO fast, and AGCO slow
- Feedback manager

- Programmable telecoil:
  - M-MT-T setting
  - Beep level control
  - Boost (+6 dB, Ergo BTE only)
- Swing hook – 9 dB damped
- DAI
- Programmable via NOAH/OtiSet PC-based software or the handheld EasyFit programming box

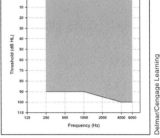

Fitting range for Ergo BTE

Options of Ergo BTE and Ergo BTE Power

- Hooks – undamped, 5 dB damped, small size for children
- Audio shoes for DAI and MLX/TMX
- Tamper-resistant battery drawer and volume control
- Eyeglasses adapter
- Colors: dark gray, light gray, dark brown, light brown, beige, black, and all OtiKids colors (except flips)

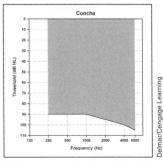

Fitting range for Ergo Power BTE

Features of Ergo Concha, Ergo Canal P, Ergo Canal, Ergo Mini Canal, and Ergo CIC

- Digitally programmable
- Class-D amplifier
- A-gram slope control (fourth-order LF or HF cut)
- UCL (uncomfortable loudness) control
- 3 output-limiting options – peak clipping (PC), AGCO fast, and AGCO slow
- Feedback manager
- MicroWaxBuster

Options of Ergo Concha, Ergo Canal P, Ergo Canal, Ergo Mini Canal, and Ergo CIC

- Programmable telecoil (not available in CIC):
- M-MT-T setting
- Beep level control
- Boost (+6 dB)
- Select-a-vent

Fitting range for Ergo Concha

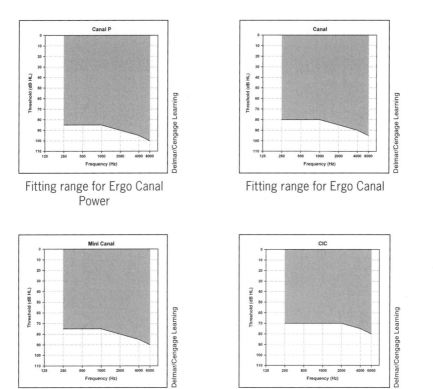

Fitting range for Ergo Canal Power

Fitting range for Ergo Canal

Fitting range for Ergo Mini Canal

Fitting range for Ergo CIC

Typical Specifications		Ergo BTE	Ergo BTE Power
Standard ANSI S3.22-2003 and S3.7 (1995)			
Output sound pressure level	Max OSPL 90 (dB SPL)	134	134
	HFA OSPL 90 (dB SPL)	127	127
Full-on gain (50 dB SPL input)	Peak gain (dB)	64	74
	HFA (dB)	58	68
Total harmonic distortion (Hz)	500 Hz	2.0%	2.0%
	800 Hz	1.0%	2.0%
	1600 Hz	0.5%	1.0%
	2000 Hz	0.5%	0.5%
Equivalent input noise (dB SPL)	Typical/maximum, Omni	22/25	22/25
Telecoil sensitivity	10 mA/m field, 1000 Hz (dB SPL)	110	118
Battery	Operating current, typical/maximum (mA)	0.8/1.0	1.5/2.0
	Battery type	13	13

Delmar/Cengage Learning

Typical Specifications		Ergo Concha	Ergo Canal P	Ergo Canal	Ergo Mini Canal	Ergo CIC
Standard ANSI S3.22-2003 and S3.7 (1995)						
Output sound pressure level	Max OSPL 90 (dB SPL)	121	120	118	115	110
	HFA OSPL 90 (dB SPL)	117	116	114	112	106
Full-on gain (50 dB SPL input)	Peak gain (dB)	55	45	45	40	33
	HFA (dB)	51	40	39	36	29
Total harmonic distortion (Hz)	500 Hz	1.5%	1.0%	1.0%	1.5%	1.0%
	800 Hz	1.5%	1.0%	1.0%	1.5%	1.0%
	1600 Hz	1.5%	0.5%	1.0%	1.0%	1.0%
	2000 Hz	0.5%	0.5%	0.5%	1.0%	0.5%
Equivalent input noise (dB SPL)	Typical/maximum, Omni	31/34	31/34	29/32	29/32	27/30
Telecoil sensitivity	10 mA/m field, 1000 Hz (dB SPL)	100	89	86	86	n/a
	Operating current, typical/ maximum (mA)	0.9/1.1	0.8/1.0	0.7/0.8	0.7/0.8	0.9/1.1
	Battery type	13	312	312	10	10

Delmar/Cengage Learning

PRODUCT 20: SWIFT

Product Application

Swift 70+ BTE
Swift 90+ BTE
Swift 100+ BTE
Swift Full-Shell+
Swift Canal+

Features of Swift 70+ BTE, Swift 90+ BTE, and Swift 100+ BTE

- Digitally programmable
- Class-D amplifier
- A-gram slope control (fourth-order LF or HF cut)
- Hearing-level control (simultaneous adjustment of gain and MPO)
- AGCo
- Swing hook (9 dB damped)
- DAI
- Beige color
- Programmable via NOAH/OtiSet PC-based software or the handheld EasyFit programming box
- Swift 70+ BTE recommended for mild to moderate hearing losses
- Swift 90+ BTE recommended for moderate to severe hearing losses
- Swift 100+ BTE recommended for severe to profound hearing losses

Options of Swift 70+ BTE, Swift 90+ BTE, and Swift 100+ BTE

- Telecoil
- Hooks – undamped, 5 dB damped, small size for children
- Audio shoes for DAI and MLx/TMX
- Tamper-resistant battery drawer
- Tamper-resistant volume control
- Hair-tone color top shell

Features of Swift Full-Shell+ and Swift Canal+

- Digitally programmable
- Class-D amplifier
- A-gram slope control (fourth-order LF or HF cut)
- Hearing level control (simultaneous adjustment of gain and MPO)
- AGCo
- MicroWaxBuster
- Recommended for most types of sensorineural and conductive hearing losses from mild to severe; first-time or experienced users; and people with high demands on cosmetics
- Programmable via the EasyFit unit or the Noah/OtiSet PC-based software

Options of Swift Full-Shell+ and Swift Canal+

- Telecoil
- Select-a-vent
- Colors: pink, tan, medium brown, and dark brown

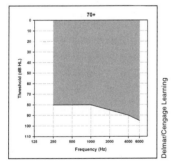

Fitting range for Swift 70+ BTE

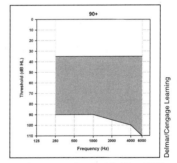

Fitting range for Swift 90+ BTE

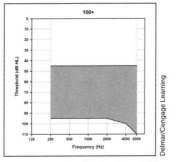

Fitting range for Swift 100+ BTE

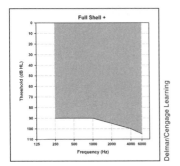

Fitting range for Swift FS+

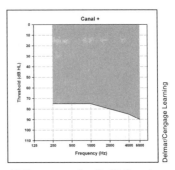

Fitting range for Swift Canal+

Typical Specifications		Swift 70+ BTE	Swift 90+ BTE	Swift 100+ BTE
Standard ANSI S3.22-2003 and S3.7 (1995)				
Output sound pressure level	Max OSPL 90 (dB SPL)	124	134	134
	HFA OSPL 90 (dB SPL)	119	127	127
Full-on gain (50 dB SPL input)	Peak gain (dB)	53	64	72
	HFA (dB)	47	58	66
Total harmonic distortion (Hz)	500 Hz	0.5%	2.0%	2.0%
	800 Hz	0.5%	1.0%	2.0%
	1600 Hz	0.5%	0.5%	1.0%
	2000 Hz	0.5%	0.5%	0.5%
Equivalent input noise (dB SPL)	Typical/maximum, Omni	22/25	22/25	22/25
Telecoil sensitivity	10 mA/m field, 1000 Hz (dB SPL)	100	110	116
Battery	Operating current, typical/maximum (mA)	0.8/1.0	0.8/1.0	1.2/2.0
	Battery type	13	13	13

Delmar/Cengage Learning

Typical Specifications		Swift Full-Shell+	Swift Canal+
Standard ANSI S3.22-2003 and S3.7 (1995)			
Output sound pressure level	Max OSPL 90 (dB SPL)	120	118
	HFA OSPL 90 (dB SPL)	116	114
Full-on gain (50 dB SPL input)	Peak gain (dB)	55	42
	HFA (dB)	51	35
Total harmonic distortion (Hz)	500 Hz	1.5%	1.0%
	800 Hz	1.5%	1.0%
	1600 Hz	1.5%	1.0%
	2000 Hz	0.5%	0.5%
Equivalent input noise (dB SPL)	Typical/maximum, Omni	31/34	31/34
Telecoil sensitivity	SPLITS (dB SPL)	92	90
	Operating current, typical/maximum (mA)	0.9/1.1	0.8/1.0
	Battery type	13	312

Delmar/Cengage Learning

CHAPTER SIX

Phonak

PHONAK: NOW HEAR THIS

International Headquarters
Phonak AG
Laubisrütistrasse 28
CH-8712 Stäfa
Switzerland
Phone: +41 44 928 01 01
Fax: +41 44 928 07 07
Email: contact@phonak.ch
Web site: http://www.phonak.com

U.S. Headquarters
Phonak Inc., USA
4520 Weaver Parkway
Warrenville, IL 60555-3927
Phone: 1 (630) 821-5000
Phone (alt): 1 (800) 679-4871
Fax: 1 (630) 393-7400
E-mail: info@phonak.com
Web site: www.phonak-us.com

Phonak's headquarters have been in or near Zurich, Switzerland, since it was founded in 1947. It was founded as AG fur Elektroakustik until 1965, when it was acquired by Ernst Rihs (Stursberg, 2005). In 1978, the first foreign distribution companies were founded in Germany and France (Phonak, 2007). Finally, in 1987, Phonak moved out of Zurich to the nearby town of Stäfa. Once going public in 1994, Phonak's business and product activities accelerated as follows (Phonak, 2007, unless otherwise cited):

- 1999: Launched a high-end digital hearing instrument, the Claro.
- 2000: Acquired Unitron Industries, Ltd., a Canadian-based hearing instrument manufacturer.
- 2001: Acquired Hansaton Akustische Gerate GmbH. Also merged Unitron, Argosy, and Lori into Unitron Hearing.
- 2003: Opened a manufacturing facility in China. Also introduced a new top-line product, the Perseo with PersonalLogic, and a new value-line digital product, the MAAX.

2004: Acquired Viennatone Horgerate GmbH to join Hansaton in Austria. Also launched the mid-level, digital Valeo.

2005: Acquired controlling interest in CAS Produtos Medicos in Brazil. Also introduced the Savia, which won the 2005 Medical Design Excellence Awards competition.

2007: Phonak Holding changed its name to Sonova Holding. The Phonak brand was maintained.

2008: Introduced new line of devices covering the full range of consumer products, Exélia micro, Naída SuperPower, and the Audéo III (Phonak, 2009).

2009: Introduced several new hearing instruments, Nios micro, Audéo YES, Certéna, Versáta, Exélia Art, Savia Art, Savia, Eleva, and the Naída IX

Phonak's business practices are as shrewd and well thought out as their product offering. Consolidation happens in any industry as it matures. As the industry develops, the product offering becomes more sophisticated and competition stiffer. Increased marketing and development is expensive, which naturally leads to consolidation. Having been described as a "well-managed growth story" (Gretler, 2006, p. 2), Phonak easily wins the "most companies acquired" award. As a business, they are driven by innovation and customer intimacy (Phonak, 2006a). Phonak's development cycles have decreased from three or more years down to two, or even fewer, years (Stursberg, 2005). In addition, Phonak aims to improve customer intimacy through general awareness programs, such as "Hear the World," brand awareness, and stronger distribution channels (Phonak, 2006a; Stursberg, 2006). Phonak's stated values and business practices promises it a strong future in the industry.

Generally, Phonak has passionately stated the desire to improve the quality of life through its research-motivated product offering (Phonak, 2006a). Phonak has a strong and well-articulated set of values in the world of hearing. It places great value on innovation that is driven by science, including pediatric and high-power fittings, strong audiology support, wireless communication, and remote controls (Phonak, 2006a; Stursberg, 2005).

Philanthropy

Phonak's main philanthropic efforts have been through the Hear the World initiative. Hear the World is an awareness campaign focusing on the importance of hearing, social/emotional effects of hearing impairment, importance of prevention, and how technology can help ameliorate hearing loss (Phonak, 2006a). Hear the World is a very active organization; readers are invited to visit their Web site for comprehensive coverage: http://www.hear-the-world.com.

PRODUCT INFORMATION

PRODUCT 1: NIOS MICRO™

Product Application
- Nios™ micro V
- Nios™ micro III

Features of Nios™ micro V
- Advanced sound flow: Allows individual fine-tuning of up to four base programs, setting the boundaries within which SoundFlow functions
- WhistleBlock Technology: Differentiates true feedback from naturally occurring tonal signals
- 4 manual programs
- Sound Recover: A nonlinear frequency compression system that allows subtle sounds to be heard without feedback
- Directionality, VoiceZoom 12 channels: Allows for suppression of multiple and moving noise sources
- Real Ear Sound: Maintains accurate localization of sound by applying discrete, frequency-specific directionality to restore the effect of the pinna
- NoiseBlock Processing, 16 channels: reduces uncomfortable environmental noises
- WindBlock Management: Identifies and suppresses noise caused by wind
- QuickSync
- Data logging
- CableFree Fitting (via iCube)
- iCom
- Click'nTalk
- myPilot
- iView
- KeyPilot2 / WatchPilot2
- FM system AS/ML12i

Features of Nios™ micro III
- SoundFlow: Allows individual fine-tuning of up to four base programs, setting the boundaries within which SoundFlow functions
- WhistleBlock Technology: Differentiates true feedback from naturally occurring tonal signals
- 2 manual programs
- Sound Recover: A nonlinear frequency compression system that allows subtle sounds to be heard without feedback
- Directionality, digital AudioZoom
- NoiseBlock Processing, 6 channels: reduces uncomfortable environmental noises

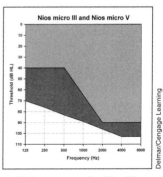

Fitting ranges for Nios™ micro V and Nios™ micro III: Micro tube (light gray), regular tubing (all shaded areas).

- Data Logging
- CableFree Fitting (via iCube)
- iCom
- Click'nTalk
- myPilot
- iView
- KeyPilot2 / WatchPilot2
- FM system AS/ML12i

Typical Specifications		Nios™ micro V	Nios™ micro III
Standard ANSI S3.22-2003			
Output sound pressure level (OSPL 90)	Peak (dB SPL)	127	127
	HF Average (dB SPL)	113	113
Full-on gain (input 50 dB SPL)	Peak (dB)	53	53
	HF Average (dB)	48	48
Total harmonic distortion (Hz)	500	0.5%	0.5%
	800	0.5%	0.5%
	1600	0.5%	0.5%
Equivalent input Noise (dB SPL)		19	19
Telecoil sensitivity (input 31.6 mA/m)	HFA-SPLIV (dB SPL)	97	97
Battery	Battery current Drain – Working (mA)	1.3	1.3
	Battery type	13	13
Compression	Attack (ms)	1	1
	Release (ms)	50	50

Delmar/Cengage Learning

PRODUCT 2: AUDÉO YES

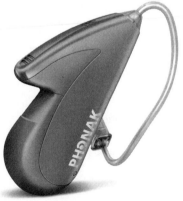

Audéo YES BTE
Phonak Hearing Systems

Product Application

Audéo YES IX
Audéo YES V
Audéo YES III

Features of Audéo YES IX

- Premium sound flow – allows individual fine-tuning of up to 4 base programs, setting the boundaries within which SoundFlow™ functions
- SoundRecover™ – a nonlinear frequency compression system that allows subtle sounds to be heard without feedback
- WhistleBlock™ technology – differentiates true feedback from naturally occurring tonal signals
- Directionality, VoiceZoom™ 33 channels – allows for suppression of multiple and moving noise sources
- NoiseBlock™ processing, 20 channels – reduces uncomfortable environmental noises
- WindBlock™ management – identifies and suppresses noise caused by wind
- RealEar Sound™ – maintains accurate localization of sound by applying discrete, frequency-specific directionality to restore the effect of the pinna
- SoundReflex™ – applies gain reduction relative to the original peak signal characteristics without altering MPO
- EchoBlock™ system – instantly removes reflections of the reverberant signal so sound remains natural and undistorted
- ZoomControl™ – combines real-audio streaming with directional beamforming that allows focus to the back or side
- DataLogging™
- Self-learning
- iCom™/myPilot™
- Cable-free fitting (via iCube™)

Options for Audéo YES IX

- Standard xReceiver units (4 different lengths for left and right: 0–3)
- Optional power xReceiver units (4 different lengths for left and right: 0–3)
- Standard xReceiver open dome (3 different sizes: 5/7/10, 2 lengths)
- Standard xReceiver/power xReceiver closed dome (2 lengths)
- Standard xReceiver/power xReceiver power dome (3 different sizes: 9/10/11, 2 lengths)
- Standard xReceiver SlimTip
- cShell/xShell standard xReceiver/power xReceiver

Features of Audéo YES V

- Advanced sound flow – allows individual fine-tuning of up to 4 base programs, setting the boundaries within which SoundFlow functions
- SoundRecover – a nonlinear frequency compression system that allows subtle sounds to be heard without feedback

- WhistleBlock technology – differentiates true feedback from naturally occurring tonal signals
- Directionality, VoiceZoom 12 channels – allows for suppression of multiple and moving noise sources
- NoiseBlock processing, 16 channels – reduces uncomfortable environmental noises
- WindBlock management – identifies and suppresses noise caused by wind
- RealEar Sound – maintains accurate localization of sound by applying discrete, frequency-specific directionality to restore the effect of the pinna
- DataLogging
- Self-learning
- iCom/myPilot
- Cable-free fitting (via iCube)

Options for Audéo YES V

- Standard xReceiver units (4 different lengths for left and right: 0 – 3)
- Optional power xReceiver units (4 different lengths for left and right: 0 – 3)
- Standard xReceiver open dome (3 different sizes: 5/7/10, 2 lengths)
- Standard xReceiver/power xReceiver closed dome (2 lengths)
- Standard xReceiver/power xReceiver power dome (3 different sizes: 9/10/11, 2 lengths)
- Standard xReceiver SlimTip
- cShell/xShell standard xReceiver/power xReceiver

Features of Audéo YES III

- Standard sound flow – allows individual fine-tuning of up to 4 base programs, setting the boundaries within which SoundFlow functions
- SoundRecover – a nonlinear frequency compression system that allows subtle sounds to be heard without feedback
- WhistleBlock technology – differentiates true feedback from naturally occurring tonal signals
- Directionality, adaptive digital AudioZoom – allows for suppression of multiple and moving noise sources
- NoiseBlock processing, 6 channels – reduces uncomfortable environmental noises
- DataLogging
- iCom/myPilot
- Cable-free fitting (via iCube)

Options for Audéo YES III

- Standard xReceiver units (4 different lengths for left and right: 0 – 3)
- Optional power xReceiver units (4 different lengths for left and right: 0 – 3)

- Standard xReceiver open dome (3 different sizes: 5/7/10, 2 lengths)
- Standard xReceiver/power xReceiver closed dome (2 lengths)
- Standard xReceiver/power xReceiver power dome (3 different sizes: 9/10/11, 2 lengths)
- Standard xReceiver SlimTip
- cShell/xShell standard xReceiver/power xReceiver

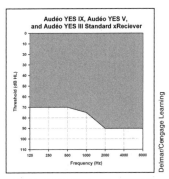

Audéo YES IX, Audéo YES V
and Audéo YES III standard
xReceiver BTE

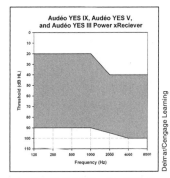

Audéo YES IX, Audéo YES V
and Audéo YES III power
xReceiver BTE

Typical Specifications		Audéo YES IX	Audéo YES V	Audéo YES III
Standard ANSI S3.22-2003				
Output sound pressure level (OSPL 90)	Peak (dB SPL)	112	112	112
	HF Average (dB SPL)	105	105	105
Full-on gain (input 50 dB SPL)	Peak (dB)	44	44	44
	HF Average (dB)	38	38	38
Total harmonic distortion (Hz)	500	1.0%	1.0%	1.0%
	800	0.5%	0.5%	0.5%
	1600	0.5%	0.5%	0.5%
Equivalent input noise (dB SPL)		19	19	19
Telecoil sensitivity (input 31.6 mA/m)	HFA-SPLIV (dB SPL)	n/a	n/a	n/a
Battery	Operating current (mA)	1.1	1.1	1.1
	Battery type	312	312	312
Compression	Attack (ms)	1	1	1
	Release (ms)	50	50	50

Delmar/Cengage Learning

PRODUCT 3: CERTÉNA

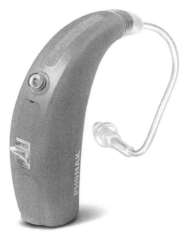

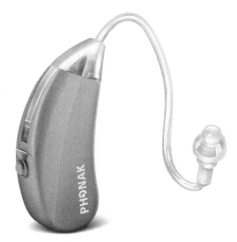

Certéna Power BTE
Phonak Hearing Systems

Certéna BTE
Phonak Hearing Systems

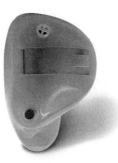

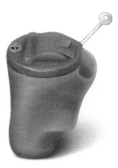

Certéna ITC
Phonak Hearing Systems

Certéna CIC/MC
Phonak Hearing Systems

Product Application

Certéna micro BTE
Certéna M BTE
Certéna P BTE
Certéna SP BTE
Certéna FS

Certéna Power FS
Certéna ITC/HS
Certéna ITC/HS Petite
Certéna CIC/MC Petite
Certéna CIC/MC P Petite

Features of Certéna micro BTE, Certéna M BTE, Certéna P BTE, and Certéna SP BTE

• Digital AudioZoom, 1 channel, adaptive – automatically activates when it is needed and zooms in on the speech while reducing noise

- SoundFlow Standard – automatically, continuously, and instantly adapts to changing sound environments, for a seamless transition between soundscapes
- WhistleBlock technology – accurately identifies and eliminates annoying whistling or squealing with more stable amplification without sound quality impact
- NoiseBlock processing – 6-channel signal-to-noise ratio–dependent noise canceller
- QuickSync™ – binaural volume and program control with one-touch simplicity

Options for Certéna micro BTE

- Standard HE9 680
- Optional mini hook HE9 680
- Optional battery door without switch
- Standard EasyPhone™ – automatic activation of telephone program
- Standard telecoil
- Optional micro tube (open/close) with SlimTip/dome
- Optional tamper-proof battery compartment

Options for Certéna M BTE

- Standard hook HE7 680
- Optional hook HE7
- Optional mini hook HE7 680
- Standard version 1 volume control
- Optional version 2 volume control
- Optional cover volume control
- Standard EasyPhone
- Standard telecoil
- Optional slim tube (open/close) with SlimTip/dome
- Optional tamper-proof battery compartment

Options for Certéna P BTE

- Standard hook HE7 680
- Optional hook HE7
- Optional mini hook HE7 680
- Standard version 1 volume control
- Optional version 2 volume control
- Optional cover volume control
- Standard EasyPhone
- Standard telecoil
- Optional tamper-proof battery compartment

PHONAK

Options for Certéna SP BTE

- Standard hook HE7 680
- Optional hook HE7
- Optional mini hook HE7 680
- Standard version 1 volume control
- Optional version 2 volume control
- Optional cover volume control
- Standard EasyPhone
- Standard telecoil
- Optional tamper-proof battery compartment

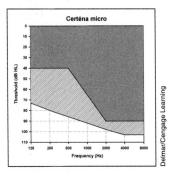

Fitting range for Certéna
Micro BTE with micro tube
(dark gray) and regular tubing
(all shaded areas)

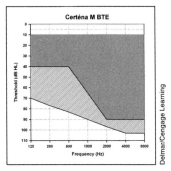

Fitting range for Certéna M
BTE with slim tube (dark gray)
and regular tubing (all shaded
areas)

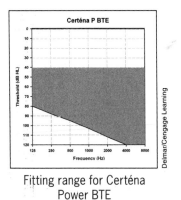

Fitting range for Certéna
Power BTE

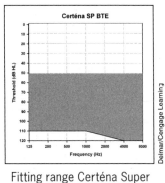

Fitting range Certéna Super
Power BTE

Features of Certéna FS and Certéna ITC/HS

- Digital AudioZoom, 1 channel, adaptive – automatically activates when it is
  needed and zooms in on the speech while reducing the noise
- SoundFlow Standard – automatically, continuously, and instantly adapts to
  changing sound environments, for a seamless transition between soundscapes

- WhistleBlock technology – accurately identifies and eliminates annoying whistling or squealing with more stable amplification without sound quality impact
- NoiseBlock processing – 6-channel signal-to-noise ratio–dependent noise canceller
- QuickSync – binaural volume and program control with one-touch simplicity
- Acoustically Optimized Vent (AOV) – freedom from occlusion for all custom products

Features of Certéna Power FS

- SoundFlow Standard – automatically, continuously, and instantly adapts to changing sound environments, for a seamless transition between soundscapes
- WhistleBlock technology – accurately identifies and eliminates annoying whistling or squealing with more stable amplification without sound quality impact
- NoiseBlock processing – 6-channel signal-to-noise ratio–dependent noise canceller
- QuickSync – binaural volume and program control with one-touch simplicity
- Acoustically Optimized Vent – freedom from occlusion for all custom products

Features of Certéna ITC/HS Petite

- Digital AudioZoom, 1 channel, adaptive – automatically activates when it is needed and zooms in on the speech while reducing the noise
- SoundFlow Standard – automatically, continuously, and instantly adapts to changing sound environments, for a seamless transition between soundscapes
- WhistleBlock technology – accurately identifies and eliminates annoying whistling or squealing with more stable amplification without sound quality impact
- NoiseBlock processing – 6-channel signal-to-noise ratio–dependent noise canceller
- Acoustically Optimized Vent – freedom from occlusion for all custom products

Options of Certéna FS, Certéna Power FS, Certéna ITC/HS, and Certéna ITC/HS Petite

- Optional volume control
- Optional TacTronic™ program switch
- Optional EasyPhone
- Optional telecoil
- Standard SmartGuard™

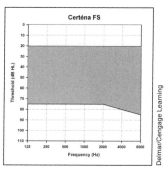

Fitting range for Certéna FS

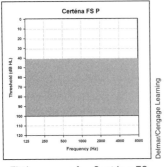

Fitting range for Certéna FS Power

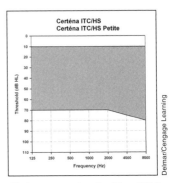

Fitting range for Certéna ITC/ HS and Certéna ITC/HS Petite

Features of Certéna CIC/MC Petite and Certéna CIC/MC P Petite

- SoundFlow Standard – automatically, continuously, and instantly adapts to changing sound environments, for a seamless transition between soundscapes
- WhistleBlock technology – accurately identifies and eliminates annoying whistling or squealing with more stable amplification without sound quality impact
- NoiseBlock processing – 6-channel signal-to-noise ratio–dependent noise canceller
- Acoustically Optimized Vent – freedom from occlusion for all custom product

Options of Certéna CIC/MC Petite and Certéna CIC/MC P Petite

- Optional volume control
- Optional TacTronic program switch
- Standard SmartGuard

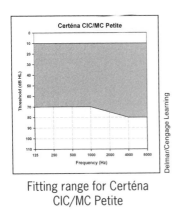

Fitting range for Certéna CIC/MC Petite

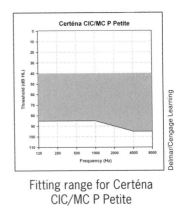

Fitting range for Certéna CIC/MC P Petite

Typical Specifications		Certéna micro BTE	Certéna M BTE	Certéna P BTE	Certéna SP BTE
Standard ANSI S3.22-2003					
Output sound pressure level (OSPL 90)	Peak (dB SPL)	127	128	133	134
	HF Average (dB SPL)	113	120	127	128
Full-on gain (input 50 dB SPL)	Peak (dB)	53	53	63	70
	HF Average (dB)	48	49	58	64
Total harmonic distortion (Hz)	500	0.5%	2.0%	2.5%	3.0%
	800	0.5%	1.0%	2.0%	2.0%
	1600	0.5%	1.0%	1.0%	1.0%
Equivalent input noise (dB SPL)		19	19	19	19
Telecoil sensitivity (input 31.6 mA/m)	HFA-SPLIV (dB SPL)	97	103	110	111
Battery	Operating current (mA)	1.3	1.1	1.2	1.2
	Battery type	13	13	13	13
Compression	Attack (ms)	1	1	1	1
	Release (ms)	50	50	50	50

Delmar/Cengage Learning

Typical Specifications		Certéna FS	Certéna Power FS	Certéna ITC/HC	Certéna ITC/HS Petite
Standard ANSI S3.22-2003					
Output sound pressure level (OSPL 90)	Peak (dB SPL)	118	125	116	116
	HF Average (dB SPL)	110	119	108	108
Full-on gain (input 50 dB SPL)	Peak (dB)	50	55	48	48
	HF Average (dB)	43	49	41	41
Total harmonic distortion (Hz)	500	1.5%	1.5%	1.5%	1.5%
	800	1.0%	1.0%	1.0%	1.0%
	1600	1.0%	1.0%	1.0%	1.0%
Equivalent input noise (dB SPL)		19	19	19	19
Telecoil sensitivity (input 31.6 mA/m)	HFA-SPLIV (dB SPL)	95	102	93	93
Battery	Operating current (mA)	1.2	1.2	1.2	1.2
	Battery type	13	13	312	312
Compression	Attack (ms)	1	1	1	1
	Release (ms)	50	50	50	50

Delmar/Cengage Learning

Typical Specifications		Certéna CIC/ MC Petite	Certéna CIC/ MC P Petite
Standard ANSI S3.22-2003			
Output sound pressure level (OSPL 90)	Peak (dB SPL)	116	118
	HF Average (dB SPL)	108	112
Full-on gain (input 50 dB SPL)	Peak (dB)	35	55
	HF Average (dB)	28	51
Total harmonic distortion (Hz)	500	1.5%	0.9%
	800	1.0%	1.2%
	1600	1.0%	0.3%
Equivalent input noise (dB SPL)		19	19
Telecoil sensitivity (input 31.6 mA/m)	HFA-SPLIV (dB SPL)	n/a	n/a
Battery	Operating current (mA)	0.9	1.1
	Battery type	10	10
Compression	Attack (ms)	1	1
	Release (ms)	10	50

Delmar/Cengage Learning

PRODUCT 4: VERSÁTA

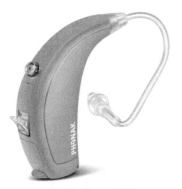

Versáta Power BTE
Phonak Hearing Systems

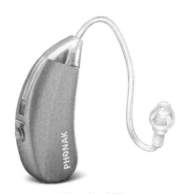

Versáta BTE
Phonak Hearing Systems

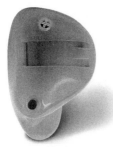

Versáta ITC
Phonak Hearing Systems

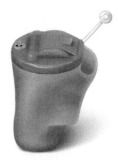

Versáta CIC/MC
Phonak Hearing Systems

Product Application

Versáta micro BTE   Versáta Power FS
Versáta M BTE   Versáta ITC/HS
Versáta P BTE   Versáta ITC/HS Petite
Versáta SP BTE   Versáta CIC/MC Petite
Versáta FS   Versáta CIC/MC P Petite

Features of Versáta micro BTE, Versáta M BTE, Versáta P BTE, and Versáta SP BTE

- VoiceZoom – 12-channel automatic adaptive directionality
- SoundFlow Advanced – automatically, continuously, and instantly adapts to changing sound environments, for a seamless transition between soundscapes
- WhistleBlock technology – accurately identifies and eliminates annoying whistling or squealing with more stable amplification without sound quality impact
- NoiseBlock processing – 6-channel signal-to-noise ratio–dependent noise canceller
- QuickSync – binaural volume and program control with one-touch simplicity

Options of Versáta micro BTE

- Standard HE9 680 hook
- Optional mini hook HE9 680
- Optional battery door without program switch
- Standard EasyPhone
- Standard telecoil
- Optional micro tube (open/close) with SlimTip/dome
- Optional tamper-proof battery door

Options of Versáta M BTE

- Standard HE7 680 hook
- Optional HE7 hook
- Optional mini hook HE 7 680
- Standard version 1 volume control
- Optional version 2 volume control
- Optional cover volume control
- Standard EasyPhone
- Standard telecoil
- Optional slim tube (open/close) with SlimTip/dome
- Optional tamper-proof battery door

Options of Versáta P and Versáta SP

- Standard HE7 680 hook
- Optional HE7 hook

- Optional mini hook HE 7 680
- Standard version 1 volume control
- Optional version 2 volume control
- Optional cover volume control
- Standard EasyPhone – automatically activates telephone program
- Standard telecoil
- Optional tamper-proof battery door

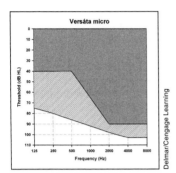

Fitting range for Versáta
Micro BTE with micro tube
(dark gray) and regular tubing
(all shaded areas)

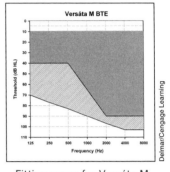

Fitting range for Versáta M
BTE for slim tube (dark gray)
and regular tubing (all shaded
areas)

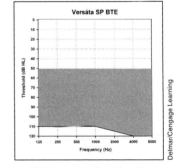

Fitting range for Versáta
Power BTE

Fitting range for Versáta
Super Power BTE

Features of Versáta FS and Versáta ITC/HS

- VoiceZoom – 12-channel automatic adaptive directionality
- SoundFlow Advanced – automatically, continuously, and instantly adapts
  to changing sound environments, for a seamless transition between
  soundscapes

- WhistleBlock technology – accurately identifies and eliminates annoying whistling or squealing with more stable amplification without sound quality impact
- NoiseBlock processing – 6-channel signal-to-noise ratio–dependent noise canceller
- QuickSync – binaural volume and program control with one-touch simplicity
- Acoustically Optimized Vent – freedom from occlusion for all custom product

Features of Versáta Power FS

- SoundFlow Advanced – automatically, continuously, and instantly adapts to changing sound environments, for a seamless transition between soundscapes
- WhistleBlock technology – accurately identifies and eliminates annoying whistling or squealing with more stable amplification without sound quality impact
- NoiseBlock processing – 6-channel signal-to-noise ratio–dependent noise canceller
- QuickSync – binaural volume and program control with one-touch simplicity
- Acoustically Optimized Vent – freedom from occlusion for all custom product

Features of Versáta ITC/HS Petite

- VoiceZoom – 12-channel automatic adaptive directionality
- SoundFlow Advanced – automatically, continuously, and instantly adapts to changing sound environments, for a seamless transition between soundscapes
- WhistleBlock technology – accurately identifies and eliminates annoying whistling or squealing with more stable amplification without sound quality impact
- NoiseBlock processing – 6-channel signal-to-noise ratio–dependent noise canceller
- Acoustically Optimized Vent – freedom from occlusion for all custom product

Options of Versáta FS, Versáta Power FS, Versáta ITC/HS, and Versáta ITC/HS Petite

- Optional volume control
- Optional TacTronic program switch
- Optional EasyPhone – automatically activates telephone program
- Optional telecoil
- Standard SmartGuard

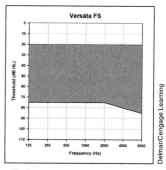

Fitting range for Versáta FS

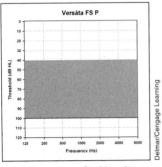

Fitting range for Versáta
FS Power

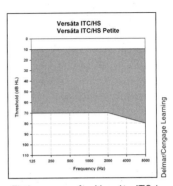

Fitting range for Versáta ITC/
HS and Versáta ITC/HS Petite

Features of Versáta CIC/MC Petite and Versáta CIC/MC P Petite

- SoundFlow Advanced – automatically, continuously, and instantly adapts to changing sound environments, for a seamless transition between soundscapes
- WhistleBlock technology – accurately identifies and eliminates annoying whistling or squealing with more stable amplification without sound quality impact
- NoiseBlock processing – 6-channel signal-to-noise ratio–dependent noise canceller
- Acoustically Optimized Vent – freedom from occlusion for all custom product

Options of Versáta CIC/MC Petite and Versáta CIC/MC P Petite

- Optional volume control
- Optional TacTronic program switch
- Optional SmartGuard

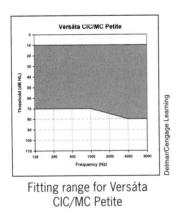

Fitting range for Versáta
CIC/MC Petite

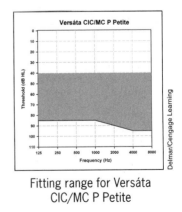

Fitting range for Versáta
CIC/MC P Petite

Typical Specifications		Versáta micro BTE	Versáta M BTE	Versáta P BTE	Versáta SP BTE
Standard ANSI S3.22-2003					
Output sound pressure level (OSPL 90)	Peak (dB SPL)	27	128	133	134
	HF Average (dB SPL)	113	120	126	128
Full-on gain (input 50 dB SPL)	Peak (dB)	53	53	63	70
	HF Average (dB)	48	49	58	63
Total harmonic distortion (Hz)	500	0.5%	2.0%	2.0%	3.0%
	800	0.5%	1.0%	1.0%	2.0%
	1600	0.5%	1.0%	1.0%	1.0%
Equivalent input noise (dB SPL)		19	19	19	19
Telecoil sensitivity (input 31.6 mA/m)	HFA-SPLIV (dB SPL)	97	103	109	111
Battery	Operating current (mA)	1.3	1.1	1.3	1.3
	Battery type	13	13	13	13
Compression	Attack (ms)	1	1	1	1
	Release (ms)	50	50	50	50

Delmar/Cengage Learning

Typical Specifications		Versáta FS	Versáta Power FS	Versáta ITC/HC	Versáta ITC/HS Petite
Standard ANSI S3.22-2003					
Output sound pressure level (OSPL 90)	Peak (dB SPL)	118	125	116	116
	HF Average (dB SPL)	110	119	108	108
Full-on gain (input 50 dB SPL)	Peak (dB)	50	55	48	48
	HF Average (dB)	43	49	41	41
Total harmonic distortion (Hz)	500	1.5%	1.5%	1.5%	1.5%
	800	1.0%	1.0%	1.0%	1.0%
	1600	1.0%	1.0%	1.0%	1.0%
Equivalent input noise (dB SPL)		19	19	19	19
Telecoil sensitivity (input 31.6 mA/m)	HFA-SPLIV (dB SPL)	95	102	93	93
Battery	Operating current (mA)	1.2	1.2	1.2	1.2
	Battery type	13	13	312	312
Compression	Attack (ms)	1	1	1	1
	Release (ms)	50	50	50	50

Delmar/Cengage Learning

PHONAK

Typical Specifications		Versáta CIC/MC Petite	Versáta CIC/MC P Petite
Standard ANSI S3.22-2003			
Output sound pressure level (OSPL 90)	Peak (dB SPL)	116	118
	HF Average (dB SPL)	108	112
Full-on gain (input 50 dB SPL)	Peak (dB)	35	55
	HF Average (dB)	28	51
Total harmonic distortion (Hz)	500	1.5%	0.9%
	800	1.0%	1.2%
	1600	1.0%	0.3%
Equivalent input noise (dB SPL)		19	19
Telecoil sensitivity (input 31.6 mA/m)	HFA-SPLIV (dB SPL)	n/a	n/a
Battery	Operating current (mA)	0.9	1.1
	Battery type	10	10
Compression	Attack (ms)	1	1
	Release (ms)	10	50

Delmar/Cengage Learning

PRODUCT 5: EXÉLIA ART

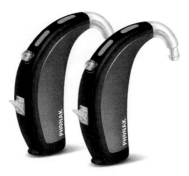

Exélia Art P BTE
Phonak Hearing Systems

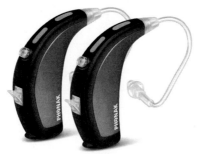

Exélia Art M BTE
Phonak Hearing Systems

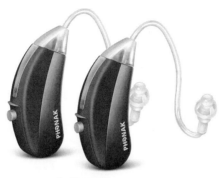

Exélia Art micro BTE
Phonak Hearing Systems

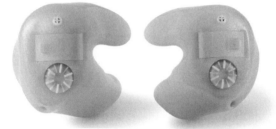

Exélia Art Wireless FS
Phonak Hearing Systems

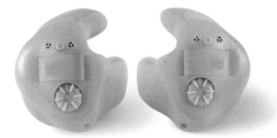

Exélia Art Wireless Power FS
Phonak Hearing Systems

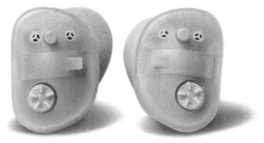

Exélia Art Petite HS and Exélia Art Petite Canal
Phonak Hearing Systems

PHONAK

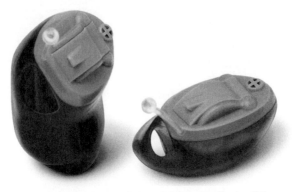

Exélia Art Petite CIC and Exélia Art Petite MC
Phonak Hearing Systems

Product Application

Exélia Art M BTE
Exélia Art P BTE
Exélia Art SP BTE
Exélia Art micro BTE
Exélia Art Wireless HS
Exélia Art Wireless FS
Exélia Art Wireless FS P
Exélia Art Petite HS
Exélia Art Petite Canal
Exélia Art Petite CIC
Exélia Art Petite MC

Features of All Exélia Art Products

- SoundFlow Premium – automatically, continuously, and instantly adapts to changing sound environments, for a seamless transition between soundscapes
- WhistleBlock – accurately identifies and eliminates annoying whistling or squealing with more stable amplification without sound quality impact
- VoiceZoom – automatic/adaptive directionality for optimum speech understanding in noise, cancels up to 33 unique noises (not available on CIC, MC, FS P)
- Fully programmable 20-channel digital hearing instrument
- SoundRelax™ – automatically detects and decreases unwanted sharp sounds
- WindBlock – automatically suppresses wind noise without changing microphone characteristics
- NoiseBlock – detects and reduces annoying sounds such as fans
- EchoBlock – reverberation canceller
- Feedback phase inverter
- Mute mode and delayed start-up
- Self-learning and DataLogging^{plus} with Smart Tips

- End-of-battery-life indicator (2 long beeps)
- RealEar Sound – restores effortless sound localization to determine the source of the sound (available on BTE models only)
- BassBoost™ (SP BTE and FS P only)

Features of Exélia Art M BTE, Exélia Art P BTE, and Exélia Art SP BTE

- Up to 3 manually accessible hearing programs plus SoundFlow Premium
- EasyPhone automatic activation of telephone program
- Telecoil
- EasyFM – automatic activation of FM program
- Exélia M – recommended for mild to moderate hearing losses
- Exélia P – recommended for moderate to severe hearing losses
- Exélia SP – recommended for severe to profound hearing losses

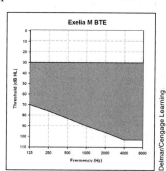

Fitting range for Exélia M BTE

Options of Exélia Art M BTE, Exélia Art P BTE, and Exélia Art SP BTE

- iCom binaural, hands-free wireless connection
- myPilot command center – access to instrument control
- ZoomControl for end-user–controlled directionality
- Cable-free fitting (via iCube)
- QuickSync – binaural volume and program control with one-touch simplicity
- EasyPhone Bluetooth – automatic program for hands-free binaural mobile phone use
- EasyAudio™ – automatic program for binaural stereo streaming
- Tamper-proof battery compartment
- Design-integrated FM
- FM-compatible – ML9i, MLxi, myLink™ receivers, and all Phonak transmitters
- Choice of 16 colors

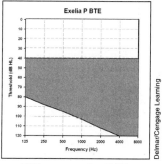

Fitting range for Exélia P BTE

Features of Exélia Art micro BTE

- Open fitting
- Telecoil
- EasyPhone with telecoil
- Recommended for mild to moderate losses that are high-frequency or "ski-slope"

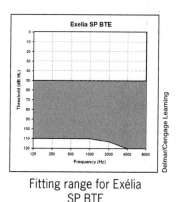

Fitting range for Exélia SP BTE

Options of Exélia Art micro BTE

- iCom binaural, hands-free wireless connection
- myPilot command center – access to instrument control
- Tamper-proof battery compartment
- FM-compatible – myLink receiver and all Phonak transmitters
- Choice of 11 colors

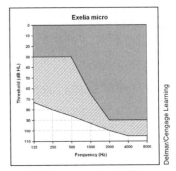

Fitting range for Exélia micro BTE with micro tube (dark gray) and ear hook (all shaded areas)

Features of Exélia Art Wireless HS, Exélia Art Wireless FS, and Exélia Art Wireless FS P

- Up to 5 manually accessible hearing programs plus SoundFlow Premium
- BassBoost (FS P only)
- Recommended for moderate to severe hearing losses

Options of Exélia Art Wireless HS, Exélia Art Wireless FS, and Exélia Art Wireless FS P

- iCom binaural, hands-free wireless connection
- myPilot command center – access to instrument control
- ZoomControl for end-user–controlled directionality
- Cable-free fitting (via iCube)
- QuickSync – binaural volume and program control with one-touch simplicity
- EasyPhone Bluetooth – automatic program for hands-free binaural mobile phone use
- EasyAudio – automatic program for binaural stereo streaming
- Tamper-proof battery compartment
- FM-compatible – myLink receiver and all Phonak transmitters

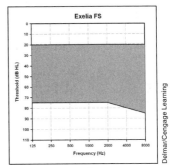
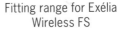

Fitting range for Exélia Wireless FS

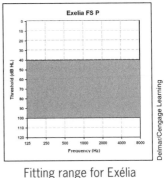

Fitting range for Exélia Wireless Power FS

Features of Exélia Art Petite Canal, Exélia Art Petite HS, Exélia Art Petite CIC, and Exélia Art Petite MC

- Up to 5 manually accessible hearing programs plus SoundFlow Premium
- Recommended for mild to moderate hearing losses
- Exélia Petite CIC and Exélia Petite MC recommended for high-frequency or "ski slope" hearing losses, and open fittings

Options of Exélia Art Petite Canal, Exélia Art Petite HS, Exélia Art Petite CIC, and Exélia Art Petite MC

- Digital volume control
- Acoustically Optimized Vent – provides individually based minimization of occlusion with maximum vent size (CIC only)
- EasyPhone telecoil (Canal and HS only)
- FM-compatible – myLink receiver and all Phonak transmitters (Canal/HS only)

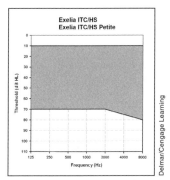

Fitting range for Exélia Art Petite HS and Exélia Art Petite Canal

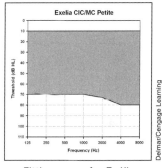

Fitting range for Exélia Petite CIC and Exélia Petite MC

Typical Specifications		Exélia M BTE	Exélia P BTE	Exélia SP BTE	Exélia micro BTE
Standard ANSI S3.22-1996					
Output sound pressure level (OSPL 90)	Peak (dB SPL)	115	122	122	127
	HF Average (dB SPL)	111	119	119	113
Full-on gain (input 50 dB SPL)	Peak (dB)	50	55	55	53
	HF Average (dB)	44	49	49	48
Total harmonic distortion (Hz)	500	1.5%	1.5%	1.5%	0.5%
	800	1.0%	1.0%	1.0%	0.5%
	1600	1.0%	1.0%	1.0%	0.5%
Equivalent input noise (dB SPL)		19	19	19	19
Telecoil sensitivity (input 31.6 mA/m)	HFA-SPLIV (dB SPL)	97	103	103	97
Battery	Operating current (mA)	1.1	1.1	1.1	1.3
	Battery type	13	13	13	13
Compression	Attack (ms)	1	1	1	1
	Release (ms)	10	10	10	50

Typical Specifications		Exélia FS	Exélia FS P	Exélia ITC & Exélia HS Petite	Exélia CIC & Exélia MC Petite
Standard ANSI S3.22-1996					
Output sound pressure level (OSPL 90)	Peak (dB SPL)	118	125	116	116
	HF Average (dB SPL)	110	119	108	108
Full-on gain (input 50 dB SPL)	Peak (dB)	50	55	48	35
	HF Average (dB)	43	49	41	28
Total harmonic distortion (Hz)	500	1.5%	1.5%	1.5%	1.5%
	800	1.0%	1.0%	1.0%	1.0%
	1600	1.0%	1.0%	1.0%	1.0%
Equivalent input noise (dB SPL)		19	19	19	19
Telecoil sensitivity (input 31.6 mA/m)	HFA-SPLIV (dB SPL)	95	102	93	n/a
Battery	Operating current (mA)	1.2	1.2	1.2	0.9
	Battery type	13	13	312	10
Compression	Attack (ms)	1	1	1	1
	Release (ms)	50	50	50	10

Delmar/Cengage Learning

PRODUCT 6: SAVIA ART

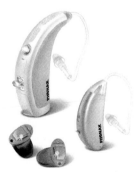

Savia Art BTE and CIC/
MC collection
Phonak Hearing Systems

Product Application

Savia Art 211 dSZ BTE

Savia Art 311 dSZ Forte BTE

Savia Art 411 dSZ Power BTE

microSavia Art 100 dSZ BTE

microSavia Art CRT dSZ BTE

Savia Art 33 FS

Savia Art 33 FS P

Savia Art 33 FS dSZ

Savia Art 22 ITC/HS

Savia Art 22 ITC/HS dSZ

Savia Art 11 CIC/MC

Savia Art 11 CIC/MC RC

Features* of All Savia Art Products

- Fully programmable digital hearing system
- 20-band digital Bionic Perception Processing (BPP) – a combination of features designed to emulate the natural processing of the ear
- AutoPilot™ – selects appropriate program for the listening environment
- EasyPhone^plus – automatically switches to telephone program when phone is used
- EasyFM – automatic activation of FM program
- SoundRelax – suppresses impulsive sounds
- RealEar Sound – an algorithm designed to improve localization by filtering sounds by location with an outer-ear–inspired filter
- NoWhistle™ technology – uses acoustic cancellation to reduce feedback
- Digital Surround Zoom (dSZ) – adaptive directional microphone system
- EchoBlock – reduces the effects of reverberation
- Wind Noise management – a 2-step process to reduce the effects of wind noise
- High-resolution noise canceller – reduces the gain in bands where a negative signal-to-noise ratio is measured
- Self-learning – learns preferred volume control settings for each program
- DataLogging^plus with User Preference Tuning
- Flexible fitting – choice of sound delivery systems
- BassBoost – up to 6 dB additional gain to improve audibility required in high-power applications
- Remote control for binaural functions
- OpenSound™ fitting – open fit
- Mute mode
- Up to 5 manually accessible hearing programs
- Acoustic confirmation when user changes device
- End-of-battery-life indicator
- Delayed start-up
- Fitting software – iPFG version 1.6 or higher, NOAH-compatible

PHONAK

*Some key features are product-dependent.

Features of All Savia Art BTE Products

• microSavia Art CRT dSZ BTE recommended for mild to moderate hearing losses, "ski-slope" hearing losses, open fittings
• microSavia Art 100 dSZ BTE and Savia Art 211 BTE recommended for mild to moderate hearing losses, all audiometric configurations
• Savia Art 311 dSZ Forte BTE recommended for moderate to severe hearing losses, all audiometric configurations
• Savia Art 411 dSZ BTE recommended for severe to profound hearing losses, all audiometric configurations
• dSZ
• Earhook – HE7 680 (standard on Savia Art 211 dSZ BTE, Savia Art 311 dSZ Forte BTE, and Savia Art 411dSZ BTE only)
• Version 1 volume control variation (standard on Savia Art 211 dSZ BTE, Savia Art 311 dSZ Forte BTE, and Savia Art 411 Power dSZ BTE only)
• Remote compatibility
• EasyPhone (plus) (excludes microSavia Art 100 dSZ BTE)
• T-coil
• Open fitting (standard on microSavia Art 100 CRT dSZ BTE and microSavia Art 100 dSZ BTE)
• Fit'n'Go™ canal receiver technology (CRT; open/closed) – open fitting (standard on microSavia Art 100 CRT dSZ BTE only)
• Fit'n'Go micro tube (open/closed) – open fitting (standard on microSavia Art 100 dSZ BTE)

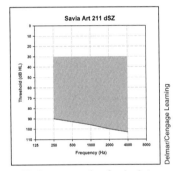

Fitting range for Savia Art 211 dSZ BTE

Options of Savia Art BTE Products

• Earhook – HE7 and mini hook HE7 680 (Savia Art 211 dSZ BTE, Savia Art 311 dSZ Forte BTE, and Savia Art 411 dSZ Power BTE only)
• Earhook – HE9 680 (microSavia Art 100 dSZ BTE only)
• Version 2 volume control variations and volume control cover (Savia Art 211 dSZ BTE, Savia Art 311 dSZ Forte BTE, and Savia Art 411 dSZ Power BTE only)
• Open fitting (Savia Art 211 dSZ BTE only)
• Fit'n'Go slim tube (open/closed) – open fitting (Savia Art 211 dSZ BTE only)

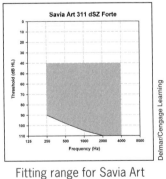

Fitting range for Savia Art 311 dSZ Forte BTE

- Tamper-proof battery compartment (Savia Art 211 dSZ BTE, Savia Art 311 dSZ Forte BTE, and Savia Art 411 dSZ Power BTE only)
- Choice of colors for Savia BTEs: palladium/pearl, palladium/black, palladium/red transparent, palladium/blue transparent, palladium/purple transparent, pearl, beige, taupe, brown, high-tech gray, light gray, light blue, light pink, blond, chestnut brown, and black
- Choice of colors for microSavia BTEs: palladium, pearl, transparent black, high-tech gray, beige, brown, taupe, blond, chestnut brown, black, and gray
- Remote controls – WatchPilot2, SoundPilot2, KeyPilot2
- Spectacles adaptor (Savia Art 211 dSZ BTE, Savia Art 311 dSZ Forte BTE, and Savia Art 411 dSZ Power BTE only)
- Audio shoe AS9-MLxS (Savia Art 211 dSZ BTE, Savia Art 311 dSZ Forte BTE, and Savia Art 411 dSZ Power BTE only)
- Multifrequency receiver – MyLink
- Multifrequency receiver – MLxS and ML9S (Savia Art 211 dSZ BTE, Savia Art 311 dSZ Forte BTE, and Savia Art 411 dSZ Power BTE only)
- Multifrequency transmitters – SmartLink™ SX, EasyLink™, Campus S (Savia Art 211 dSZ BTE, Savia Art 311 dSZ Forte BTE, and Savia Art 411 dSZ Power BTE only)
- CROS-adapter-M2 (Savia Art 211 dSZ BTE, Savia Art 311 dSZ Forte BTE, and Savia Art 411 dSZ Power BTE only)
- CROSLink (Savia Art 211 dSZ BTE, Savia Art 311 dSZ Forte BTE, and Savia Art 411 dSZ Power BTE only)

Note: Some options are country-dependent. Refer to order form.

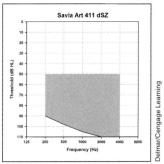

Fitting range for Savia Art 411 dSZ Power BTE

Features of All Savia Art Custom Products

- Savia 11 CIC/MC, Savia 11 CIC/MC RC, Savia Art 22 ITC/HS, and Savia Art 22 ITC/HS dSZ recommended for mild to moderate hearing losses, all audiometric configurations
- Savia Art 33 FS, Savia 33 FS dSZ, and Savia Art 33 FS P recommended for moderate to severe hearing losses, all audiometric configurations
- dSZ (Savia Art 22 ITC/HS dSZ and Savia Art 33 FS dSZ only)
- Remote compatibility (Savia Art MC/CIC RC only)

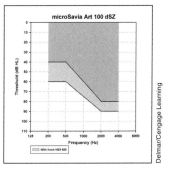

Fitting range for Savia Art 100dSZ BTE: Standard earhook (dark gray), HE9 680 earhook (all shaded areas)

Options of All Savia Art Custom Products

- Volume control
- Program switch TacTronic
- Remote compatibility (excludes Savia Art 11 CIC/MC)
- EasyPhone (plus) (excludes Savia Art 11 CIC/MC and Savia Art CIC/MC RC)
- T-coil (excludes Savia Art 11 CIC/MC and Savia Art CIC/MC RC)
- Remote controls – WatchPilot2, Sound-Pilot2, KeyPilot2 (excludes Savia Art 11 CIC/MC)
- Multifrequency receiver – MyLink (excludes Savia Art 11 CIC/MC and Savia Art CIC/MC RC)

Note: Some options are country-dependent. Refer to order form.

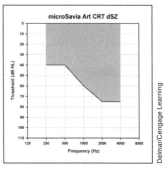

Fitting range for Savia
Art CRT dSZ BTE

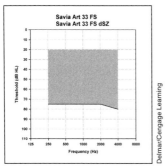

Fitting range for Savia Art
33 FS and 33 FS dSZ

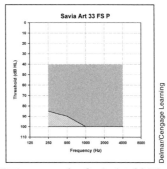

Fitting range for Savia Art 33 FS
P (dark gray) and with bass boost
extended range (all shaded regions)

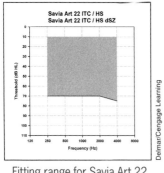

Fitting range for Savia Art 22
ITC/HS and 22 ITC/HS dSZ

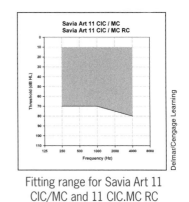

Fitting range for Savia Art 11
CIC/MC and 11 CIC.MC RC

Typical Specifications		Savia Art 211 dSZ BTE	Savia Art 311 dSZ Forte BTE	Savia Art 411 dSZ Power BTE
Standard ANSI S3.22-1996				
Output sound pressure level (OSPL 90)	Peak (dB SPL)	125	130	131
	HF Average (dB SPL)	120	127	127
Full-on gain (input 50 dB SPL)	Peak (dB)	53	63	70
	HF Average (dB)	49	60	62
Total harmonic distortion	500 Hz	2.0%	2.0%	3.0%
	800 Hz	1.0%	1.0%	2.0%
	1600 Hz	1.0%	1.0%	1.0%
Equivalent input noise (dB SPL)		19	19	19
Telecoil sensitivity (input 31.6 mA/m)	HFA-SPLIV (dB SPL)	103	110	110
Battery	Operating current (mA)	1.1	1.1	1.1
	Battery Type	13	13	13
Compression	Attack (ms)	1	1	1
	Release (ms)	10	10	10

Delmar/Cengage Learning

Typical Specifications		microSavia Art 100 dSZ BTE	microSavia Art CRT dSZ BTE
Standard ANSI S3.22-1996			
Output sound pressure level (OSPL 90)	Peak (dB SPL)	117	109
	HF Average (dB SPL)	107	105
Full-on gain (input 50 dB SPL)	Peak (dB)	45	44
	HF Average (dB)	37	38
Total harmonic distortion	500 Hz	0.5%	1.0%
	800 Hz	1.0%	0.5%
	1600 Hz	1.5%	0.5%
Equivalent input noise (dB SPL)		19	19
Telecoil sensitivity (input 31.6 mA/m)	HFA-SPLIV (dB SPL)	93	91
Battery	Operating current (mA)	1.0	1.0
	Battery type	312 (Optional 10)	312 (Optional 10)
Compression	Attack (ms)	1	1
	Release (ms)	10	10

Delmar/Cengage Learning

PHONAK

Typical Specifications		Savia Art 33 FS	Savia Art 33 FS P	Savia Art 33 FS dSZ
Standard ANSI S3.22-1996				
Output sound pressure level (OSPL 90)	Peak (dB SPL)	115	122	115
	HF Average (dB SPL)	111	119	111
Full-on gain (input 50 dB SPL)	Peak (dB)	50	55	50
	HF Average (dB)	44	49	44
Total harmonic distortion	500 Hz	1.5%	1.5%	1.5%
	800 Hz	1.0%	1.0%	1.0%
	1600 Hz	1.0%	1.0%	1.0%
Equivalent input noise (dB SPL)		19	19	19
Telecoil sensitivity (input 31.6 mA/m)	HFA-SPLIV (dB SPL)	97	103	97
Battery	Operating current (mA)	1.1	1.1	1.1
	Battery type	13	13	13
Compression	Attack (ms)	1	1	1
	Release (ms)	10	10	10

Delmar/Cengage Learning

Typical Specifications		Savia Art 22 ITC/HS	Savia Art 22 ITC/ HS dSZ	Savia Art 11 CIC/ MC and CIC/MC RC
Standard ANSI S3.22-1996				
Output sound pressure level (OSPL 90)	Peak (dB SPL)	113	113	113
	HF Average (dB SPL)	109	109	107
Full-on gain (input 50 dB SPL)	Peak (dB)	48	48	35
	HF Average (dB)	42	42	31
Total harmonic distortion	500 Hz	1.5%	1.5%	1.5%
	800 Hz	1.0%	1.0%	1.0%
	1600 Hz	1.0%	1.0%	1.0%
Equivalent input noise (dB SPL)		19	19	19
Telecoil sensitivity (input 31.6 mA/m)	HFA-SPLIV (dB SPL)	94	94	97
Battery	Operating current (mA)	1.1	1.1	0.9 (CIC/ MC) 1.1 (CIC/ MC RC)
	Battery type	312	312	10
Compression	Attack (ms)	1	1	1
	Release (ms)	10	10	10

Delmar/Cengage Learning

PRODUCT 7: SAVIA

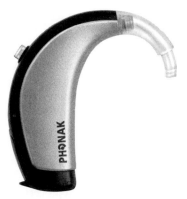

Savia BTE
Phonak Hearing Systems

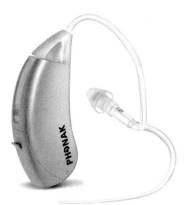

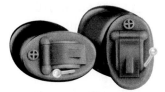

microSavia BTE
Phonak Hearing Systems

Savia CIC hearing aids
Phonak Hearing Systems

Product Application

Savia 111 dSZ BTE
Savia 211 dSZ BTE
Savia 311 dSZ Forte BTE
microSavia 100 dSZ BTE
Savia 33 FS
Savia 33 FS dSZ
Savia 22 ITC/HS
Savia 22 ITC/HS dSZ
Savia 11 CIC/MC
Savia 11 CIC/MC RC

Features of All Savia BTE and microBTE Products

- Fully programmable digital hearing system
- SoundNavigation™ – automatic sound scene analysis and dedicated base program selection
- dSZ – 20-band frequency-specific adaptive beamformer
- RealEar Sound – an algorithm designed to improve localization by filtering sounds by location with an outer-ear–inspired filter
- EchoBlock – reduces the effects of reverberation
- 20-band digital BPP – a combination of features designed to emulate the natural processing of the ear
- DataLogging with User Preference Tuning
- High-resolution noise canceller – reduces the gain in bands where a negative signal-to-noise ratio is measured
- Wind Noise Management™ – a 2-step process to reduce the effects of wind noise
- Feedback Phase Inverter™ – acoustic cancellation technology to reduce feedback
- Acoustic confirmation when user changes device
- Mute mode and delayed start-up
- End-of-battery-life indicator (1 long beep)
- Volume control variations
- Remote controllable for binaural functions

Features of Savia 111 dSZ BTE, Savia 211 dSZ BTE, and Savia 311 dSZ Forte BTE

- Savia 111 dSZ BTE and Savia 211 dSZ BTE recommended for mild to moderate hearing losses
- Savia 311 dSZ Forte BTE recommended for moderate to severe hearing losses
- EasyFM – automatic activation of FM program
- Configurable BTE user controls
- EasyPhone – automatically switches to telephone program when phone is used (only available on EasyPhone models)
- Program switch (TacTronic)
- Telecoil
- Up to 5 manually accessible hearing programs plus AutoPilot

Options of Savia 111 dSZ BTE, Savia 211 dSZ BTE, and Savia 311 dSZ Forte BTE

- Open fitting/Fit'n'Go (Savia 111 dSZ and Savia 211 dSZ BTE only)
- Tamper-proof battery compartment
- Multifrequency FM receivers ML9S or MLxS

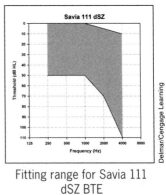

Fitting range for Savia 111 dSZ BTE

- Remote controls – WatchPilot2, Sound Pilot2, KeyPilot2
- Choice of colors: beige, taupe, brown, light gray, dark gray, anthracite, black, pearl, light pink, light blue, blond, chestnut brown, pall/black, pall/transparent red, pall/transparent blue, pall/transparent purple, and pall/pearl

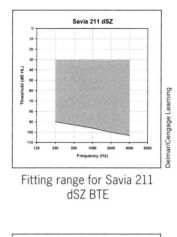

Fitting range for Savia 211 dSZ BTE

Features of microSavia 100 dSZ BTE

- Recommended for mild to moderate hearing losses, high-frequency or "ski-slope" hearing losses
- Open fitting/Fit'n'Go
- Up to 3 manually accessible hearing programs plus AutoPilot

Options of microSavia 100 dSZ BTE

- Remote controls – WatchPilot2, SoundPilot2, KeyPilot2
- Choice of colors: beige, taupe, brown, dark gray, anthracite, palladium, pearl, blond, and chestnut brown

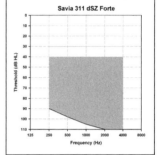

Fitting range for Savia 311 dSZ Forte BTE

Features of All Savia Custom Products

- Fully programmable digital hearing system
- SoundNavigation – automatic sound scene analysis and dedicated base program selection
- EchoBlock – reduces the effects of reverberation
- 20-band digital BPP – a combination of features designed to emulate the natural processing of the ear
- DataLogging with User Preference Tuning
- High-resolution noise canceller – reduces the gain in bands where a negative signal-to-noise ratio is measured
- Wind Noise Management – a 2-step process to reduce the effects of wind noise

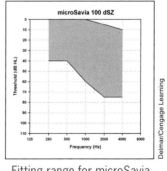

Fitting range for microSavia 100 dSZ BTE

- Feedback Phase Inverter – acoustic cancellation technology to reduce feedback
- Acoustic confirmation when user changes device
- Mute mode and delayed start-up
- End-of-battery-life indicator (1 long beep)

Features of Savia 33 FS, Savia 33 FS dSZ, Savia 22 ITC/HS, and Savia 22 ITC/HS dSZ

- Savia 33 FS and Savia 33 FS dSZ are recommended for moderate to severe hearing losses
- Savia 22 ITC/HS and Savia 22 ITC/HS dSZ are recommended for mild to moderate hearing losses, high-frequency or "ski-slope" hearing losses
- dSZ – 20-band frequency-specific adaptive beamformer (Savia 22 ITC/HS dSZ and Savia 33 FS dSZ only)
- Up to 5 manually accessible hearing programs plus AutoPilot
- Remote control for binaural functions
- Telecoil

Options of Savia 33 FS, Savia 33 FS dSZ, Savia 22 ITC/HS, and Savia 22 ITC/HS dSZ

- Remote controls – WatchPilot2, SoundPilot2, KeyPilot2
- EasyPhone – automatically switches to telephone program when phone is used
- Digital volume control
- Program selection switch (TacTronic)
- Digital "eShell" made with NemoTech™ laser sintering technology
- Colors: cocoa, pink, tan, and brown

Features of Savia 11 CIC/MC and Savia 11 CIC/MC RC

- Recommended for mild to moderate hearing losses, high-frequency or "ski-slope" hearing losses
- Up to 3 manually accessible hearing programs plus AutoPilot

Options of Savia 11 CIC/MC and Savia 11 CIC/MC RC

- Digital volume control
- Program selection switch (TacTronic)
- Remote control for binaural functions (Savia 11 RC MC/CIC only)
- Choice of colors: cocoa, pink, tan, and brown

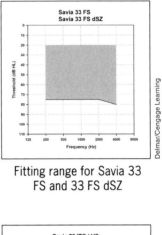

Fitting range for Savia 33 FS and 33 FS dSZ

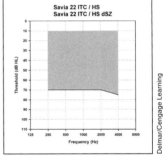

Fitting range for Savia 22 ITC/HS and 22 ITC/HS dSZ

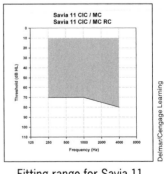

Fitting range for Savia 11 CIC/MC and 11 CIC/MC RC

Typical Specifications		Savia 111 dSZ BTE	Savia 211 dSZ BTE	Savia 311 dSZ Forte BTE	micro Savia 100 dSZ BTE
Standard ANSI S3.22-1996					
Output sound pressure level (OSPL 90)	Peak (dB SPL)	120	125	130	117
	HF Average (dB SPL)	116	120	127	107
Full-on gain (input 50 dB SPL)	Peak (dB)	43	53	63	45
	HF Average (dB)	40	49	60	37
Total harmonic distortion	500 Hz	1.5%	2.0%	2.0%	0.5%
	800 Hz	1.0%	1.0%	1.0%	1.0%
	1600 Hz	1.0%	1.0%	1.0%	1.5%
Equivalent input noise (dB SPL)		19	19	19	19
Telecoil sensitivity (input 31.6 mA/m)	HFA-SPLIV (dB SPL)	105	103	110	n/a
Battery	Operating current (mA)	1.14	1.1	1.1	1.0
	Battery type	13	13	13	312
Compression	Attack (ms)	1	1	1	1
	Release (ms)	10	10	10	10

Delmar/Cengage Learning

PHONAK

Typical Specifications		Savia 33 FS and Savia 33 FS dSZ	Savia 22 ITC/HS and Savia 22 ITC/HS dSZ	Savia 11 CIC/MC and Savia CIC/MC RC
Standard ANSI S3.22-1996				
Output sound pressure level (OSPL 90)	Peak (dB SPL)	115	113	113
	HF Average (dB SPL)	111	109	107
Full-on gain (input 50 dB SPL)	Peak (dB)	50	48	35
	HF Average (dB)	45	42	31
Total harmonic distortion	500 Hz	1.5%	1.5%	1.5%
	800 Hz	1.0%	1.0%	1.0%
	1600 Hz	1.0%	1.0%	1.0%
Equivalent input noise (dB SPL)		19	19	19
Telecoil sensitivity (input 31.6 mA/m)	HFA-SPLIV (dB SPL)	97	103	n/a
Battery	Operating current (mA)	1.1	1.1	0.6 (CIC/MC) 1.1 (CIC/MC RC)
	Battery type	13	312	10
Compression	Attack (ms)	1	1	1
	Release (ms)	10	10	10

Delmar/Cengage Learning

PRODUCT 8: ELEVA

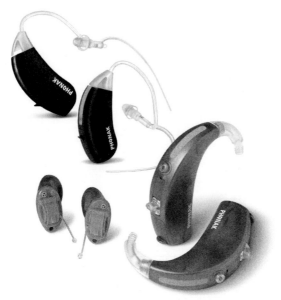

microEleva BTE, Eleva BTE, and Eleva CIC hearing aids
Phonak Hearing Systems

Product Application

Eleva 211 dAZ BTE
Eleva 311 dAZ BTE
Eleva 411 dAZ BTE
microEleva 100 dAZ BTE
Eleva 33 FS
Eleva 33 FS dAZ
Eleva 33 FS P
Eleva 22 ITC/HS
Eleva 22 ITC/HS dAZ
Eleva 11 CIC/MC
Eleva 11 CIC/MC RC

Features of All Eleva BTE and microBTE Products

- Fully programmable digital hearing system
- TriPilot™ – sound analysis and selection of 3 base automatic programs
- 16 channels with dual processing strategy, WDRC or dSC
- 16-channel high-resolution noise canceller
- Smart fitting with DataLogging[plus]
- Wind and weather protector
- Feedback Phase Inverter – acoustic cancellation technology to reduce feedback

- Acoustic confirmation when user changes device
- Mute mode and delayed start-up
- Smart design – including extended color line to match hair colors
- Adaptive Digital AudioZoom (dAZ) – adaptive directional microphone system
- Remote control for binaural functions
- End-of-battery-life indicator (1 long beep)

Features of Eleva 211 dAZ BTE, Eleva 311 dAZ BTE, and Eleva 411 dAZ BTE

- Eleva 211 dAZ BTE recommended for mild to moderate hearing losses
- Eleva 311 dAZ BTE recommended for moderate to severe hearing losses
- Eleva 411 dAZ BTE recommended for severe to profound hearing losses
- Up to 5 manually accessible hearing programs
- Program switch (TacTronic)
- Telecoil
- Fills pediatric requirements – mini earhook and tamper-proof battery door

Options of Eleva 211 dAZ BTE, Eleva 311 dAZ BTE, and Eleva 411 dAZ BTE

- Open fitting/Fit'n'Go (Eleva 211 dAZ BTE only)
- EasyPhone
- Tamper-proof battery compartment
- Multifrequency FM receivers ML9S or MLxS
- Remote controls – WatchPilot2, SoundPilot2, KeyPilot2
- Choice of colors: beige, taupe, brown, light gray, dark gray, anthracite, black, light pink, light blue, blond, chestnut brown, transparent red, transparent blue, and transparent purple

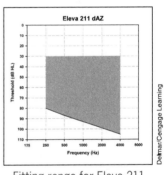

Fitting range for Eleva 211 dAZ BTE

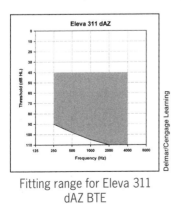

Fitting range for Eleva 311 dAZ BTE

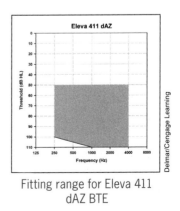

Fitting range for Eleva 411 dAZ BTE

Features of microEleva 100 dAZ BTE

- Open fitting/Fit'n'Go
- Up to 3 manually accessible hearing programs

Options of microEleva 100 dAZ BTE

- Remote controls: WatchPilot2, Sound-Pilot2, KeyPilot2
- Choice of colors: beige, taupe, brown, anthracite, black, pearl, blond, chestnut brown

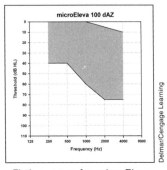

Fitting range for microEleva
100 dAZ BTE

Features of All Eleva Custom Products

- Fully programmable digital hearing system
- TriPilot – sound analysis and selection of 3 base automatic programs
- 16 channels with dual processing strategy, WDRC or dSC
- Smart fitting with DataLogging^{plus}
- 16-channel high-resolution noise canceller
- Feedback Noise Inverter – acoustic cancellation technology to reduce feedback
- Acoustic confirmation when user changes device
- Mute mode and delayed start-up
- End-of-battery-life indicator (1 long beep)

Features of Eleva 33 FS, Eleva 33 FS dAZ, Eleva 33 FS P, Eleva 22 ITC/HS, and Eleva 22 ITC/HS dAZ

- Eleva 33 FS, Eleva 33 FS dAZ, and Eleva 33 FS P recommended for moderate to severe hearing losses
- Eleva 22 ITC/HS and Eleva 22 ITC/HS dAZ recommended for mild to moderate hearing losses, high-frequency or "ski-slope" hearing losses
- Automatically activated, adaptive dAZ – adaptive directional microphone system (Eleva 22 ITC/HS dAZ and Eleva 33 FS dAZ only)
- Up to 5 manually accessible hearing programs
- Remote control for binaural functions
- Telecoil

Options of Eleva 33 FS, Eleva 33 FS dAZ, Eleva 33 FS P, Eleva 22 ITC/HS, and Eleva 22 ITC/HS dAZ

- Remote controls: WatchPilot2, SoundPilot2, KeyPilot2
- EasyPhone
- Program selection switch (TacTronic)
- Volume control

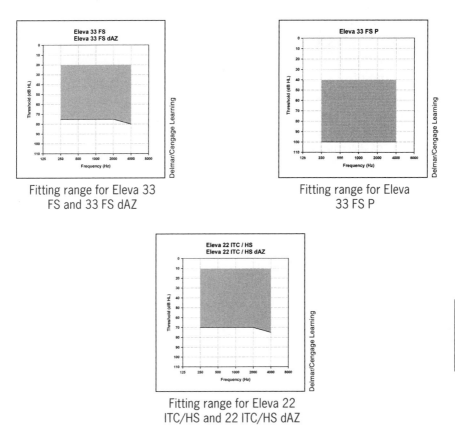

Fitting range for Eleva 33
FS and 33 FS dAZ

Fitting range for Eleva
33 FS P

Fitting range for Eleva 22
ITC/HS and 22 ITC/HS dAZ

- Digital "eShell" made with NemoTech laser sintering technology
- Colors: cocoa, pink, tan, and brown

Features of Eleva 11 CIC/MC and Eleva 11 CIC/MC RC

- Recommended for mild to moderate hearing losses, high-frequency or "ski-slope" hearing losses
- Up to 3 manually accessible hearing programs

Options of Eleva 11 CIC/MC and Eleva 11 CIC/MC RC

- Digital volume control
- Remote control for binaural functions (Eleva 11 CIC/MC RC only)
- Colors: cocoa, pink, tan, and brown

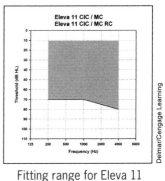

Fitting range for Eleva 11
CIC/MC and 11 CIC/MC RC

Typical Specifications		Eleva 211 dAZ BTE	Eleva 311 dAZ BTE	Eleva 411 daZ BTE	micro-Eleva 100 dAZ BTE
Standard ANSI S3.22-1996					
Output sound pressure level (OSPL 90)	Peak (dB SPL)	125	130	131	117
	HF Average (dB SPL)	120	127	127	107
Full-on gain (input 50 dB SPL)	Peak (dB)	53	63	70	45
	HF Average (dB)	49	58	62	37
Total harmonic distortion	500 Hz	2.0%	2.0%	3.0%	0.5%
	800 Hz	1.0%	1.0%	2.0%	1.0%
	1600 Hz	1.0%	1.0%	1.0%	1.5%
Equivalent input noise (dB SPL)		19	19	19	19
Telecoil sensitivity (input 31.6 mA/m)	HFA-SPLIV (dB SPL)	103	110	110	n/a
Battery	Operating current (mA)	1.1	1.1	1.1	1.0
	Battery Type	13	13	13	312
Compression	Attack (ms)	1	1	1	1
	Release (ms)	10	10	10	10

Delmar/Cengage Learning

Typical Specifications		Eleva 33 FS and Eleva 33 FS dAZ	Eleva 33 FS P
Standard ANSI S3.22-1996			
Output sound pressure level (OSPL 90)	Peak (dB SPL)	115	122
	HF Average (dB SPL)	111	119
Full-on gain (input 50 dB SPL)	Peak (dB)	50	55
	HF Average (dB)	44	49
Total harmonic distortion	500 Hz	1.5%	1.5%
	800 Hz	1.0%	1.0%
	1600 Hz	1.0%	1.0%
Equivalent input noise (dB SPL)		19	19
Telecoil sensitivity (input 31.6 mA/m)	HFA-SPLIV (dB SPL)	97	103
Battery	Operating current (mA)	1.1	1.1
	Battery type	13	13
Compression	Attack (ms)	1	1
	Release (ms)	10	10

Delmar/Cengage Learning

Typical Specifications	Standard ANSI S3.22-1996	Eleva 22 ITC/ HS and Eleva 22 ITC/HS dAZ	Eleva 11 CIC/ MC and Eleva 11 CIC/MC RC
Output sound pressure level (OSPL 90)	Peak (dB SPL)	113	113
	HF Average (dB SPL)	109	107
Full-on gain (input 50 dB SPL)	Peak (dB)	48	35
	HF Average (dB)	42	31
Total harmonic distortion	500 Hz	1.5%	1.5%
	800 Hz	1.0%	1.0%
	1600 Hz	1.0%	1.0%
Equivalent input noise (dB SPL)		19	19
Telecoil sensitivity (input 31.6 mA/m)	HFA-SPLIV (dB SPL)	94	n/a
Battery	Operating current (mA)	1.1	0.6 CIC/MC 1.1 CIC/MC RC
	Battery type	312	10
Compression	Attack (ms)	1	1
	Release (ms)	10	10

Delmar/Cengage Learning

PRODUCT 9: NAÍDA

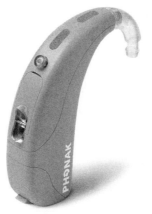

Naída Adult BTE and Naída Junior BTE
Phonak Hearing Systems

Product Application

Naída IX UP Adult BTE	Naída IX SP Adult BTE
Naída V UP Adult BTE	Naída V SP Adult BTE
Naída III UP Adult BTE	Naída III SP Adult BTE
Naída V UP Junior BTE	Naída V SP Junior BTE
Naída III UP Junior BTE	Naída III SP Junior BTE

Features of All Naída Products

- Power solution for optimal sound experience
- Junior mode makes pediatric fittings easy
- SoundRecover – nonlinear frequency compression algorithm
- 2 levels of power
- Adult and junior models
- Slim design – 35% smaller than competition
- Water-resistant
- Power processing and BassBoost
- WhistleBlock technology
- QuickSync
- EasyPhone – automatic telephone
- NoiseBlock processing
- Telecoil
- EasyFM
- Universal FM receiver

Features of Naída™ IX UP Adult BTE

- Directionality Voice Zoom
- SoundFlow Premium
- 20 channels
- 5 manual programs
- EchoBlock System
- SoundRelax
- Zoom Control
- DuoPhone
- WindBlock Management
- QuickSync
- RealEar Sound

Options of all Naída products

- FM-compatible
- Multifrequency FM receiver
- Dynamic FM with inspire transmitter
- Choice of 17 colors
- FM transmitters – inspiro, SmartLink, EasyLink, ZoomLink™

- iCom – wireless Bluetooth, FM
- iView™
- Remote – myPilot
- Secure'n'Stay™
- Cable-free fitting (via iCube)

Features of Naída V UP Adult and Naída V UP Junior

- Microphone mode dAZ
- SoundFlow Advanced
- 16 channels
- Design-integrated FM receiver ML10i
- 4 manual programs
- 16 noise-canceller channels
- RealEar Sound

Options of Naída V UP Junior

- Minihook
- Tamper-proof battery door
- Volume control lock
- iPFG Junior mode

Features of Naída III UP Adult and Naída III UP Junior

- SoundFlow Standard
- Omnidirectional microphone mode
- 6 channels
- 6 noise-canceller channels
- 2 manual programs and 2 dedicated T/FM
- Design-integrated FM receiver ML10i

Options of Naída III UP Junior

- Minihook
- Tamper-proof battery door
- Volume control lock
- iPFG Junior mode

Features of Naída™ IX SP Adult BTE

- Directionality Voice Zoom
- SoundFlow Premium
- 20 channels
- 5 manual programs
- EchoBlock System
- SoundRelax
- Zoom Control

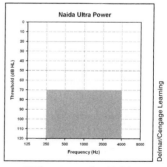

Fitting range for Naída V UP Adult BTE, Naída III UP Adult BTE, Naída V UP Junior BTE, and Naída III UP Junior BTE

- DuoPhone
- WindBlock Management
- QuickSync
- RealEar Sound

Features of Naída V SP Adult and Naída V SP Junior

- Microphone mode dAZ
- 16 channels
- Design-integrated FM receiver ML11i
- 4 manual programs
- 16 noise-canceller channels
- RealEar Sound
- SoundFlow Advanced

Options of Naída V SP Junior

- Minihook
- Tamper-proof battery door
- Volume control lock
- iPFG Junior mode

Features of Naída III SP Adult and Naída III SP Junior

- SoundFlow Standard
- Omnidirectional microphone mode
- 6 channels
- 6 noise-canceller channels
- 2 manual programs and 2 dedicated T/FM
- Design-integrated FM receiver ML11i

Options of Naída III SP Junior

- Minihook
- Tamper-proof battery door
- Volume control lock
- iPFG Junior mode

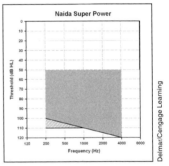

Fitting range for Naída V SP Adult BTE, Naída III SP Adult BTE, Naída V SP Junior BTE, and Naída III SP Junior BTE (all shaded regions)

Typical Specifications		Naída™ IX SP Adult	Naída™ IX UP Adult
Standard ANSI S3.22-1996			
Output sound pressure level (OSPL 90)	Peak (dB SPL)	140	142
	HF Average (dB SPL)	131	133
Full-on gain (input 50 dB SPL)	Peak (dB)	75	82
	HF Average (dB)	67	73

continues

continued

Typical Specifications		Naída™ IX SP Adult	Naída™ IX UP Adult
Total harmonic distortion (Hz)	500	4.0%	3.0%
	800	2.0%	2.0%
	1600	1.0%	1.0%
Equivalent input noise (dB SPL)		19	19
Telecoil sensitivity (input 31.6 mA/m)	HFA-SPLIV (dB SPL)	114	117
Battery	Battery current drain – working (mA)	1.1	1.3
	Battery type	13	675
Compression	Attack (ms)	1	1
	Release (ms)	50	70

Delmar/Cengage Learning

Typical Specifications		Naída V UP Adult	Naída V UP Junior
Standard ANSI S3.22-1996			
Output sound pressure level (OSPL 90)	Peak (dB SPL)	141	141
	HF Average (dB SPL)	133	133
Full-on gain (input 50 dB SPL)	Peak (dB)	82	82
	HF Average (dB)	73	73
Total harmonic distortion (Hz)	500	3.0%	3.0%
	800	2.0%	2.0%
	1600	1.0%	1.0%
Equivalent input noise (dB SPL)		19	19
Telecoil sensitivity (input 31.6 mA/m)	HFA-SPLIV (dB SPL)	117	117
Battery	Operating current (mA)	1.3	1.3
	Battery type	675	675
Compression	Attack (ms)	1	1
	Release (ms)	70	70

Delmar/Cengage Learning

Typical Specifications		Naída III UP Adult	Naída III UP Junior
Standard ANSI S3.22-1996			
Output sound pressure level (OSPL 90)	Peak (dB SPL)	141	141
	HF Average (dB SPL)	133	133
Full-on gain (input 50 dB SPL)	Peak (dB)	82	82
	HF Average (dB)	73	73

PHONAK

continues

continued

Typical Specifications		Naída III UP Adult	Naída III UP Junior
Total harmonic distortion (Hz)	500	3.0%	3.0%
	800	2.0%	2.0%
	1600	1.0%	1.0%
Equivalent input noise (dB SPL)		19	19
Telecoil sensitivity (input 31.6 mA/m)	HFA-SPLIV (dB SPL)	117	117
Battery	Operating current (mA)	1.3	1.3
	Battery type	675	675
Compression	Attack (ms)	1	1
	Release (ms)	70	70

Delmar/Cengage Learning

Typical Specifications		Naída V SP Adult	Naída V SP Junior
Standard ANSI S3.22-1996			
Output sound pressure level (OSPL 90)	Peak (dB SPL)	140	140
	HF Average (dB SPL)	131	131
Full-on gain (input 50 dB SPL)	Peak (dB)	75	75
	HF Average (dB)	67	67
Total harmonic distortion (Hz)	500	4.0%	4.0%
	800	2.0%	2.0%
	1600	1.0%	1.0%
Equivalent input noise (dB SPL)		19	19
Telecoil sensitivity (input 31.6 mA/m)	HFA-SPLIV (dB SPL)	114	114
Battery	Operating current (mA)	1.3	1.3
	Battery type	13	13
Compression	Attack (ms)	1	1
	Release (ms)	50	50

Delmar/Cengage Learning

Typical Specifications		Naída III SP Adult	Naída III SP Junior
Standard ANSI S3.22-1996			
Output sound pressure level (OSPL 90)	Peak (dB SPL)	140	140
	HF Average (dB SPL)	131	131
Full-on gain (input 50 dB SPL)	Peak (dB)	75	75
	HF Average (dB)	67	67
Total harmonic distortion (Hz)	500	4.0%	4.0%
	800	2.0%	2.0%
	1600	1.0%	1.0%

continues

continued

Typical Specifications		Naída III SP Adult	Naída III SP Junior
Equivalent input noise (dB SPL)		19	19
Telecoil sensitivity (input 31.6 mA/m)	HFA-SPLIV (dB SPL)	114	114
Battery	Operating current (mA)	1.3	1.3
	Battery type	13	13
Compression	Attack (ms)	1	1
	Release (ms)	50	50

Delmar/Cengage Learning

PRODUCT 10: AUDÉO PERSONAL COMMUNICATION ASSISTANT

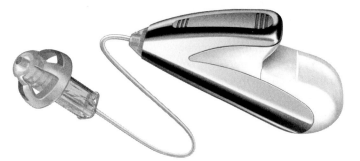

Audéo Personal Communication Assistant
Phonak Hearing Systems

Product Application

Audéo IX dSZ BTE
Audéo V dAZ BTE
Audéo III BTE

Features of All Audéo Products

- Recommended to fit mild to moderate hearing losses
- Optimal performance in noise
- CRT
- Up to 5 manually accessible hearing programs (Audéo IX & V only)
- Telecoil for MyLink and telephone use (Audéo IX & V only)
- Low battery indicator

Options of All Audéo Products

- Multifrequency FM receiver with MyLink
- Remote controls – WatchPilot2, SoundPilot2, KeyPilot2 (Audéo IX & V only)
- Closed/open fitting or new C-Tip

PHONAK

- Choice of colors: royal velvet, pinot noir, green with envy, solar flare, pure passion, back in black, lunar eclipse, precious metal, antique mahogany, flower power, crème brûlée, fiery temper, raku glaze, classic caddy, snow blade, beige, and taupe

Features of Audéo IX dSZ BTE

- For patients who are highly demanding of exceptional cosmetics, sound quality, and assistance in noise
- BPP signal-processing strategy – a combination of features designed to emulate the natural processing of the ear
- Calm situation
- Speech in noise
- Noise only
- Music
- Resolution of sound processing: 20
- RealEar Sound – an algorithm designed to improve localization by filtering sounds by location with an outer-ear–inspired filter
- dSZ automatic directional microphone
- SoundRelax – suppresses impulsive sounds
- 20 noise-canceller channels
- Reduces echoing
- NoWhistle technology
- Effective feedback suppression
- Wind noise suppressor – electronic suppression of wind noise
- Wind and weather protector

Options of Audéo IX dSZ BTE

- Records and stores personal use and listening preferences
- Self-learning – learns preferred volume control settings for each program
- Records actual usage, with one-click correction, reducing time in office
- Remote control
- 5 manual programs
- Telecoil
- Manual access to the right settings for telephone use
- Manual access to the right settings for wireless use

Features of Audéo V dAZ BTE

- For patients who are demanding of exceptional cosmetics, sound quality, and assistance in noise
- dWDRC and dSC signal-processing strategy
- Calm situation
- Speech in noise
- Noise only
- Resolution of sound processing: 20
- Adaptive dAZ – adaptive directional microphone system

- 16 noise-canceller channels
- NoWhistle technology
- Effective feedback suppression
- Wind and weather protector

Options of Audéo V dAZ BTE

- Records actual usage, with one-click correction, reducing time in office
- Remote control
- 5 manual programs
- Telecoil
- Manual access to the right settings for telephone use
- Manual access to the right settings for wireless use

Features of Audéo III

- For patients who are seeking exceptional cosmetics, sound quality, and assistance in noise
- Uses dWDRC and dSC as a signal-processing strategy
- Calm situation
- Speech in noise
- 6 channels
- AudioZoom automatic directional microphone
- 6 noise-canceller channels
- NoWhistle technology
- Effective feedback suppression
- Wind and weather protector
- DataLogging

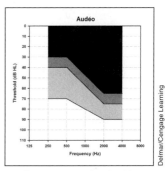

Fitting range for Audéo IX dSZ BTE: open dome (black), closed dome (dark gray and black), and power dome (all shaded regions)

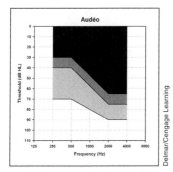

Fitting range for Audéo V dAZ BTE: open dome (black), closed dome (dark gray and black), and power dome (all shaded regions)

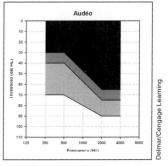

Fitting range for Audéo III BTE: open dome (black), closed dome (dark gray and black), and power dome (all shaded regions)

Typical Specifications		Audéo IX dSZ BTE	Audéo V dAZ BTE	Audéo III BTE
Standard ANSI S3.22-1996				
Output sound pressure level (OSPL 90)	Peak (dB SPL)	121	121	112
	1600 Hz (dB SPL)	113	113	105
Full-on gain (input 50 dB SPL)	Peak (dB)	56	56	44
	1600 Hz(dB)	46	46	38
Total harmonic distortion	500 Hz	1.0%	1.0%	1.0%
	800 Hz	1.0%	1.0%	0.5%
	1600 Hz	0.5%	0.5%	0.5%
Equivalent input noise (dB SPL)		19	19	19
Telecoil sensitivity (input 31.6 mA/m)	Maximum (dB SPL)	87	87	88
Battery	Operating current (mA)	1.0	1.0	1.0
	Battery type	312	312	312
Compression	Attack (ms)	1	1	1
	Release (ms)	10	10	10

Delmar/Cengage Learning

PRODUCT 11: MICROPOWER

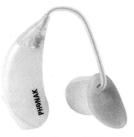

microPower BTE
Phonak Hearing Systems

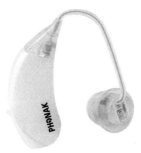

microPower BTE with dome
Phonak Hearing Systems

Product Application

microPower IX dSZ BTE
microPower V dAZ BTE
microPower III AZ BTE

Features of All microPower BTE Products

• Recommended to fit moderate to severe hearing losses
• Optimal performance in noise
• CRT

- Up to 5 manually accessible hearing programs (excludes microPower III AZ BTE)
- EasyPhone – automatically switches to telephone program when phone is used
- Low-battery indicator

Options of All microPower BTE Products

- Multifrequency FM receiver with MyLink (excludes microPower III AZ BTE)
- Remote controls – WatchPilot2, SoundPilot2, KeyPilot2 (excludes micro-Power III AZ BTE)
- Power dome fitting or xShell
- Choice of colors: beige, taupe, brown, dark gray, anthracite, black, pearl, palladium, transparent black, blond, and chestnut brown

Features of microPower IX dSZ BTE

- For patients who are highly demanding in terms of comfort, sound quality, and assistance in noise
- BPP – a combination of features designed to emulate the natural processing of the ear
- Speech in noise
- Noise only
- Music
- Automatic telephone
- Resolution of sound processing: 20
- RealEar Sound – an algorithm designed to improve localization by filtering sounds by location with an outer-ear–inspired filter
- dSZ – automatic directional microphones
- SoundRelax – suppresses impulsive sounds
- 20 noise-canceller channels
- Reduces echoing
- NoWhistle technology
- Effective feedback suppression
- Wind noise suppressor – electronic suppression of wind noise
- Wind and weather protector

Options of microPower IX dSZ BTE

- Records and stores use and listening preferences
- Self-learning
- Records actual usage, with one-click correction, reducing time in office
- Remote control
- 5 manual programs

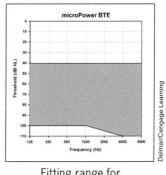

Fitting range for
microPower IX dSZ BTE

- Telecoil
- Manual access to the right settings for telephone use
- Manual access to the right settings for wireless use

Features of microPower V dAZ BTE

- For patients who are demanding in terms of comfort, sound quality, and assistance in noise
- dWDRC and dSC signal-processing strategy
- Calm situation
- Speech in noise
- Noise only
- Automatic telephone
- Resolution of sound processing: 16
- Adaptive dAZ – adaptive directional microphone system
- 16 noise-canceller channels
- Effective feedback suppression
- Wind and weather protector

Options of microPower V dAZ BTE

- Records and stores personal use and listening preferences
- Records actual usage, with one-click correction, reducing time in office
- Remote control
- 5 manual programs
- Telecoil
- Manual access to the right settings for telephone use
- Manual access to the right settings for wireless use

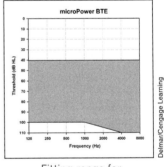

Fitting range for microPower V dAZ BTE

Features of microPower III AZ BTE

- For patients who are interested in full natural sound quality and effortless hearing
- dWDRC and dSC signal-processing strategy
- Calm situation
- Speech in noise
- Automatic telephone
- Resolution of sound processing: 6
- AudioZoom – automatic directional microphones
- 6 noise-canceller channels
- Effective feedback suppression
- Wind and weather protector

Options of microPower III AZ BTE

- Records and stores personal use and listening preferences
- Telecoil

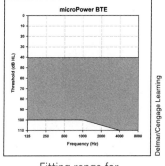

Fitting range for
microPower III dAZ BTE

Typical Specifications		microPower IX dSZ BTE	microPower V dAZ BTE	microPower III AZ BTE
Standard ANSI S3.22-1996				
Output sound pressure level (OSPL 90)	Peak (dB SPL)	123	123	126
	HF Average (dB SPL)	118	118	118
Full-on gain (input 50 dB SPL)	Peak (dB)	55	55	55
	HF Average (dB)	48	48	48
Total harmonic distortion	500 Hz	1.5%	1.5%	1.5%
	800 Hz	1.0%	1.0%	1.0%
	1600 Hz	0.5%	0.5%	0.5%
Equivalent input noise (dB SPL)		19	19	19
Telecoil sensitivity (input 31.6 mA/m)	HFA-SPLIV (dB SPL)	104	104	104
Battery	Operating current (mA)	1.1	1.1	1.1
	Battery type	312	312	312
Compression	Attack (ms)	1	1	1
	Release (ms)	6	6	6

Delmar/Cengage Learning

PRODUCT 12: EXTRA

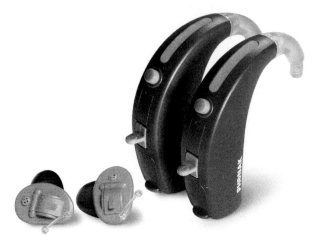

eXtra and Una BTE and CIC collection
Phonak Hearing Systems

Product Application

eXtra 211 AZ BTE	eXtra 33 Power FS
eXtra 311 AZ Forte BTE	eXtra 22 ITC/HS
eXtra 411 AZ Power BTE	eXtra 22 ITC/HS AZ
eXtra 33 FS	eXtra 11 CIC/MC
eXtra 33 FS AZ	

Features of All eXtra BTE and Custom Products

- Fully programmable digital hearing system
- SoundManager™ – automatic feature activation for noise and quiet
- 6 channels
- DataLogging
- eXtraSound™ – eXtra broadband frequency response
- 6-channel digital Noise Canceller
- Feedback Phase Inverter – acoustic cancellation technology to reduce feedback
- Mute mode and delayed start-up
- Up to 2 manually accessible hearing programs
- Acoustic confirmation when user changes device
- End-of-battery-life indicator

Features of eXtra 211 AZ BTE, eXtra 311 AZ Forte BTE, eXtra 411 AZ Power BTE

- eXtra 211 AZ BTE recommended for mild to moderate hearing losses
- eXtra 311 AZ Forte BTE recommended for moderate to severe hearing losses

- eXtra 411 AZ Power BTE recommended for severe to profound hearing losses
- Wind and weather protector
- Telecoil
- AudioZoom dual microphone beamformer
- Program switch (TacTronic)

Options of eXtra 211 AZ BTE, eXtra 311 AZ Forte BTE, eXtra 411 AZ Power BTE

- Volume control variations
- EasyPhone
- Open fitting/Fit'n'Go (eXtra 211 AZ BTE only)
- Tamper-proof battery compartment
- Multifrequency FM receivers ML9S or MLxS
- Choice of colors: beige, taupe, brown, light gray, dark gray, anthracite, black, light pink, light blue, blond, chestnut brown, transparent red, transparent blue, and transparent purple

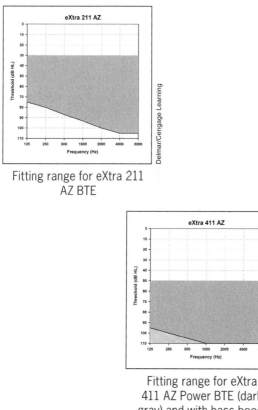

Fitting range for eXtra 211 AZ BTE

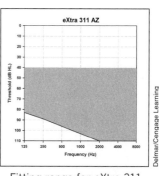

Fitting range for eXtra 311 AZ Forte BTE

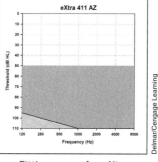

Fitting range for eXtra 411 AZ Power BTE (dark gray) and with bass boost extended range (all shaded regions)

Features of eXtra 33 FS, eXtra 33 FS AZ, eXtra 33 Power FS, eXtra 22 ITC/HS, eXtra 22 ITC/HS AZ, and eXtra 11 CIC/MC

- Recommended for mild to moderate hearing losses, high-frequency or "ski-slope" hearing losses
- Telecoil (excludes eXtra 11 CIC/MC)
- AudioZoom dual microphone beamformer (eXtra 33 FS AZ and eXtra ITC/HS only)

Options of eXtra 33 FS, eXtra 33 FS AZ, eXtra 33 Power FS, eXtra 22 ITC/HS, eXtra 22 ITC/HS AZ, and eXtra 11 CIC/MC

- Analog volume control
- EasyPhone (excludes eXtra 11 CIC/MC)
- Program selection switch (TacTronic)
- Digital "eShell" made with NemoTech laser sintering technology
- Choice of colors: cocoa, pink, tan, and brown

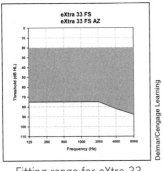

Fitting range for eXtra 33 FS and 33 FS AZ

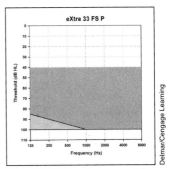

Fitting range for eXtra 33 Power FS (dark gray) and with bass boost extended range (all shaded regions)

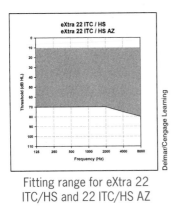

Fitting range for eXtra 22 ITC/HS and 22 ITC/HS AZ

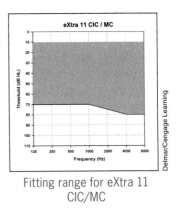

Fitting range for eXtra 11 CIC/MC

Typical Specifications		eXtra 211 AZ BTE	eXtra 311 AZ Forte	eXtra 411 AZ Power BTE
Standard ANSI S3.22-1996				
Output sound pressure level (OSPL 90)	Peak (dB SPL)	125	130	131
	HF Average (dB SPL)	120	127	127
Full-on gain (input 50 dB SPL)	Peak (dB)	53	63	70
	HF Average (dB)	49	58	62
Total harmonic distortion	500 Hz	2.0%	2.0%	3.0%
	800 Hz	1.0%	1.0%	2.0%
	1600 Hz	1.0%	1.0%	1.0%
Equivalent input noise (dB SPL)		19	19	19
Telecoil sensitivity (input 31.6 mA/m)	HFA-SPLIV (dB SPL)	103	110	110
Battery	Operating current (mA)	0.9	0.9	0.9
	Battery type	13	13	13
Compression	Attack (ms)	1	1	1
	Release (ms)	10	10	10

Delmar/Cengage Learning

Typical Specifications		eXtra 33 FS and eXtra 33 FS AZ	eXtra 33 Power FS
Standard ANSI S3.22-1996			
Output sound pressure level (OSPL 90)	Peak (dB SPL)	115	122
	HF Average (dB SPL)	111	119
Full-on gain (input 50 dB SPL)	Peak (dB)	50	55
	HF Average (dB)	44	49
Total harmonic distortion	500 Hz	1.5%	1.5%
	800 Hz	1.0%	1.0%
	1600 Hz	1.0%	1.0%
Equivalent input noise (dB SPL)		19	19
Telecoil sensitivity (input 31.6 mA/m)	HFA-SPLIV (dB SPL)	97	103
Battery	Operating current (mA)	1.1	1.1
	Battery type	13	13
Compression	Attack (ms)	1	1
	Release (ms)	10	10

Delmar/Cengage Learning

PHONAK

Typical Specifications		eXtra 22 ITC/ HS and eXtra 22 ITC/HS AZ	eXtra 11 CIC/MC
Standard ANSI S3.22-1996			
Output sound pressure level (OSPL 90)	Peak (dB SPL)	113	113
	HF Average (dB SPL)	109	107
Full-on gain (input 50 dB SPL)	Peak (dB)	48	35
	HF Average (dB)	42	31
Total harmonic distortion	500 Hz	1.5%	1.5%
	800 Hz	1.0%	1.0%
	1600 Hz	1.0%	1.0%
Equivalent input noise (dB SPL)		19	19
Telecoil sensitivity (input 31.6 mA/m)	HFA-SPLIV (dB SPL)	94	n/a
Battery	Operating current (mA)	1.1	0.6
	Battery type	312	10
Compression	Attack (ms)	1	1
	Release (ms)	10	10

Delmar/Cengage Learning

PRODUCT 13: UNA

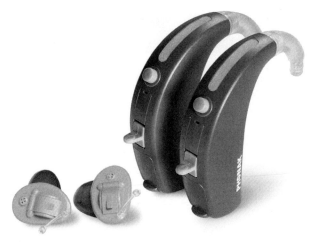

eXtra and Una BTE and CIC collection
Phonak Hearing Systems

Product Application

Una M BTE
Una M AZ BTE
Una SP BTE

Una AZ FS
Una P FS
Una ITC/HS

Una SP AZ BTE   Una AZ ITC/HS
Una FS   Una CIC/MC

Features of All Una BTE and Custom Products

- Fully programmable digital hearing system
- 2 flexible listening programs (2 separate programs for telecoil or FM)
- 4-channel gain and MPO shaping
- dWDRC signal processing
- DataLogging
- 4-channel noise canceller
- Feedback Phase Inverter – acoustic cancellation technology to reduce feedback
- Mute mode and delayed start-up
- Acoustic confirmation when user changes device
- End-of-battery-life indicator

Features of Una M BTE and Una M AZ BTE

- Recommended to fit mild to moderate hearing losses, high-frequency or "ski-slope" hearing losses
- Telecoil
- AudioZoom dual microphone beamformer (Una M AZ BTE only)
- Program switch (TacTronic)
- Wind and weather protector

Options of Una M BTE and Una M AZ BTE

- Volume control variations
- Open fitting/Fit'n'Go
- Tamper-proof battery compartment
- Multifrequency FM receivers ML9S or MLxS
- Choice of colors: beige, taupe, brown, light gray, dark gray, anthracite, black, light pink, light blue, pearl, transparent red, transparent blue, transparent purple, palladium, transparent black, blond, and chestnut brown

Features of Una SP BTE and Una SP AZ BTE

- Recommended to fit severe to profound hearing losses
- Telecoil
- AudioZoom dual microphone beamformer (Una SP AZ BTE only)
- Program switch (TacTronic)
- Wind and weather protector
- BassBoost – up to 6 dB additional gain to improve audibility required in high-power applications

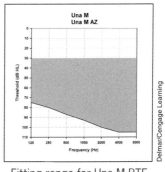

Fitting range for Una M BTE and Una M AZ BTE

Options of Una SP BTE and Una SP AZ BTE

- Volume control variations
- Tamper-proof battery compartment
- Multifrequency FM receivers ML9S or MLxS
- Choice of colors: beige, taupe, brown, light gray, dark gray, anthracite, black, light pink, light blue, pearl, transparent red, transparent blue, transparent purple, palladium, transparent black, blond, and chestnut brown

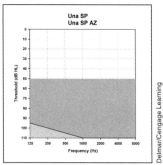

Fitting range for Una SP BTE and Una SP AZ BTE (dark gray) and with bass boost extended range (all shaded regions)

Features of Una FS, Una AZ FS, and Una P FS

- Recommended to fit moderate to severe hearing losses
- Telecoil
- AudioZoom dual microphone beamformer (Una AZ FS only)
- BassBoost – up to 6 dB additional gain to improve audibility required in high-power applications (Una P FS only)

Options of Una FS, Una AZ FS, and Una P FS

- Analog volume control
- Program switch (TacTronic)
- EasyPhone

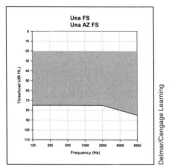

Fitting range for Una FS and Una AZ FS

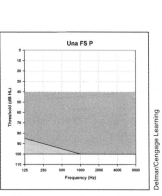

Fitting range for Una P FS (dark gray) and with bass boost extended range (all shaded regions)

Features of Una ITC/HS, Una AZ ITC/HS, and Una CIC/MC

- Recommended to fit mild to moderate hearing losses, high-frequency or "ski-slope" hearing losses
- Telecoil (Una ITC/HS and Una AZ ITC/HS only)
- AudioZoom dual microphone beamformer (Una AZ ITC/HS only)

Options of Una ITC/HS, Una AZ ITC/HS, and Una CIC/MC

- Analog volume control
- Program switch (TacTronic)
- EasyPhone (Una ITC/HS and Una AZ ITC/HS only)

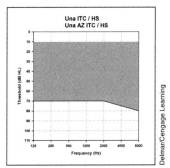

Fitting range for Una ITC/
HS and Una AZ ITC/HS

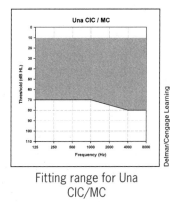

Fitting range for Una
CIC/MC

Typical Specifications		Una M BTE and Una M AZ BTE	Una SP BTE and Una SP AZ BTE
Standard ANSI S3.22-1996			
Output sound pressure level (OSPL 90)	Peak (dB SPL)	128	134
	HF Average (dB SPL)	120	127
Full-on gain (input 50 dB SPL)	Peak (dB)	53	70
	HF Average (dB)	49	62
Total harmonic distortion	500 Hz	2.0%	3.0%
	800 Hz	1.0%	2.0%
	1600 Hz	1.0%	1.0%
Equivalent input noise (dB SPL)		19	19
Telecoil sensitivity (input 31.6 mA/m)	HFA-SPLIV (dB SPL)	103	110
Battery	Operating current (mA)	0.9	0.9
	Battery type	13	13
Compression	Attack (ms)	1	1
	Release (ms)	10	10

Delmar/Cengage Learning

Typical Specifications		Una FS and Una AZ FS	Una FS P
Standard ANSI S3.22-1996			
Output sound pressure level (OSPL 90)	Peak (dB SPL)	118	122
	HF Average (dB SPL)	111	119
Full-on gain (input 50 dB SPL)	Peak (dB)	50	55
	HF Average (dB)	44	49
Total harmonic distortion	500 Hz	1.5%	1.5%
	800 Hz	1.0%	1.0%
	1600 Hz	1.0%	1.0%
Equivalent input noise (dB SPL)		19	19
Telecoil sensitivity (input 31.6 mA/m)	HFA-SPLIV (dB SPL)	97	103
Battery	Operating current (mA)	1.1	1.1
	Battery type	13	13
Compression	Attack (ms)	1	1
	Release (ms)	10	10

Delmar/Cengage Learning

Typical Specifications		Una ITC/HS and Una AZ ITC/HS	Una CIC/MC
Standard ANSI S3.22-1996			
Output sound pressure level (OSPL 90)	Peak (dB SPL)	116	116
	HF Average (dB SPL)	109	107
Full-on gain (input 50 dB SPL)	Peak (dB)	48	35
	HF Average (dB)	42	31
Total harmonic distortion	500 Hz	1.5%	1.5%
	800 Hz	1.0%	1.0%
	1600 Hz	1.0%	1.0%
Equivalent input noise (dB SPL)		19	19
Telecoil sensitivity (input 31.6 mA/m)	HFA-SPLIV (dB SPL)	94	103
Battery	Operating current (mA)	1.1	0.9
	Battery type	312	10
Compression	Attack (ms)	1	1
	Release (ms)	10	10

Delmar/Cengage Learning

PRODUCT 14: PERSEO

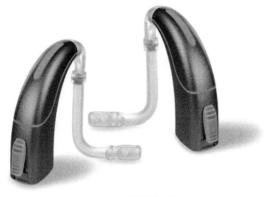

Perseo BTE Fit'n'Go
Phonak Hearing Systems

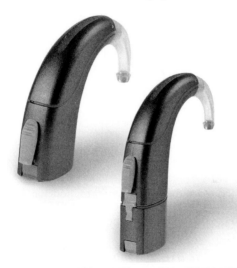

Perseo 111 and Perseo 211 dAZ-FM BTE
Phonak Hearing Systems

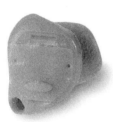

Perseo 23 dAZ HS
Phonak Hearing Systems

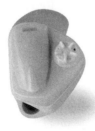

Perseo Open
Phonak Hearing
Systems

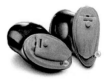

Perseo 12 MC
Phonak Hearing
Systems

Product Application

Perseo 111 dAZ BTE
Perseo 111 dAZ Open BTE
Perseo 211 dAZ BTE
Perseo 311 dAZ Forte BTE
Perseo 23 dAZ ITE/ITC
Perseo 12 Open MC
Perseo 11 CIC

Features of Perseo 111 dAZ BTE, Perseo 111 dAZ Open BTE, Perseo 211 dAZ BTE, and Perseo 311 dAZ Forte BTE

- Personal*Logic*™ – programmable automatic program selection
- Digital Perception Processing[2] (DPP[2]) – frequency-based analysis in 20 dynamically overlapping critical bands
- 20 adjustable channels
- Personal system managers
- Listening situation manager
- Occlusion manager
- Adaptive dAZ – adaptive directional microphone system
- Fine-scale noise canceller (FNC) – for precise, effective reduction of steady-state noise with 3 levels of reduction
- Programmable telecoil with preamplifier
- TacTronic switch – on-board access to manual programs
- Dynamic feedback manager
- Telecoil
- Perseo 111 dAZ BTE and Perseo 111 dAZ Open BTE recommended for mild to moderate hearing losses, high-frequency hearing losses ("ski-slope")
- Perseo 211 dAZ BTE recommended for mild to moderate hearing losses
- Perseo 311 dAZ Forte BTE recommended for moderate to severe hearing losses
- Open fitting/Fit'n'Go (Perseo 111 dAZ Open BTE only)

Options of Perseo 111 dAZ BTE, Perseo 111 dAZ Open BTE, Perseo 211 dAZ BTE, and Perseo 311 dAZ Forte BTE

- Remote controls: WatchPilot2, SoundPilot2, KeyPilot2
- Integrated MicroLink™ ML85 FM Receiver
- Choice of colors: beige, tank, brown, light gray, dark gray, anthracite, blue, violet, red, green, yellow, silver, light pink, and light blue

Features of Perseo 23 dAZ ITE/ITC, Perseo 12 Open MC, and Perseo 11 CIC Custom Products

- Personal*Logic* – programmable automatic program selection
- DPP[2] – frequency-based analysis in 20 dynamically overlapping critical bands
- 20 adjustable channels
- Personal system manager

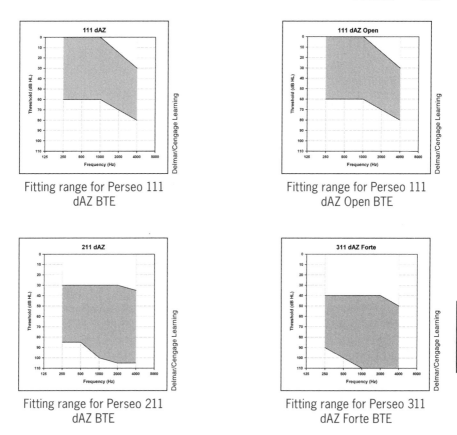

Fitting range for Perseo 111 dAZ BTE

Fitting range for Perseo 111 dAZ Open BTE

Fitting range for Perseo 211 dAZ BTE

Fitting range for Perseo 311 dAZ Forte BTE

- Listening situation manager
- Occlusion manager
- FNC – for precise, effective reduction of steady-state noise
- Dynamic feedback manager
- Adaptive dAZ – adaptive directional microphone system (Perseo 23 dAZ ITE/ITC only)
- Programmable telecoil with preamplifier (Perseo 23 dAZ ITE/ITC only)
- Low-battery indicator (4 beeps, 2 times) (Perseo 12 Open MC and Perseo 11 CIC only)
- Perseo 23 dAZ ITE/ITC is recommended for mild to moderate hearing losses
- Perseo 12 Open MC and Perseo 11 CIC are recommended for mild to moderate hearing losses, high-frequency or "ski-slope" hearing losses

Options of Perseo 23 dAZ ITE/ITC

- Digital "eShell" made with NemoTech laser sintering technology
- Program selection switch (TacTronic)
- Remote controls – WatchPilot2, SoundPilot2, KeyPilot2
- Choice of colors: pink, cocoa, tan, and brown

Options of Perseo 12 Open MC and Perseo 11 CIC

- Custom CIC faceplate available for difficult-to-fit ears (Perseo 11 CIC only)
- Digital "eShell" made with NemoTech laser sintering technology
- Program selection switch (TacTronic)
- Choice of colors: pink, cocoa, tan, and brown

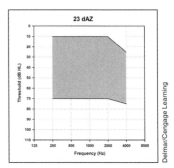

Fitting range for Perseo 23 dAZ ITE/ITC

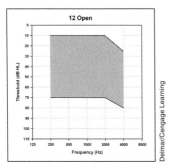

Fitting range for Perseo 12 Open (Mini Canal)

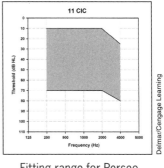

Fitting range for Perseo 11 CIC

Typical Specifications		Perseo 111 dAZ BTE and Perseo 111 dAZ Open BTE	Perseo 211 dAZ BTE	Perseo 311 dAZ Forte BTE
Standard ANSI S3.22-1996				
Output sound pressure level (OSPL 90)	Peak (dB SPL)	115	119	125
	HF Average (dB SPL)	113	117	123
Full-on gain (Input 50 dB SPL)	Peak (dB)	44	53	64
	HF Average (dB)	40	49	58
Total harmonic distortion (Hz)	500 Hz	0.5%	0.5%	1.0%
	800 Hz	0.5%	0.5%	0.5%
	1600 Hz	0.5%	0.5%	0.5%
Equivalent input noise (dB SPL)		20	22	20
Telecoil sensitivity (input 31.6 mA/m)	HFA-SPLIV (dB SPL)	96	101	108
Battery	Operating current (mA)	1.3	1.35	1.35
	Battery type	13	13	13
Compression	Attack (ms)	6	6	6
	Release (ms)	60	60	60

Typical Specifications		Perseo 23 dAZ ITE/ITC	Perseo 12 Open MC (Mini Canal)	Perseo 11 CIC
Standard ANSI S3.22-1996				
Output sound pressure level (OSPL 90)	Peak (dB SPL)	108	108	108
	HF Average (dB SPL)	104	103	103
Full-on gain (Input 50 dB SPL)	Peak (dB)	48	40	35
	HF Average (dB)	43	35	28
Total harmonic distortion (Hz)	500 Hz	1.0%	0.3%	0.3%
	800 Hz	0.5%	0.3%	0.3%
	1600 Hz	0.5%	0.3%	0.3%
Equivalent input noise (dB SPL)		20	19	19
Telecoil sensitivity (input 31.6 mA/m)	HFA-SPLIV (dB SPL)	187	n/a	n/a
Battery	Operating current (mA)	1.35	0.6	00.6
	Battery type	312	10	10
Compression	Attack (ms)	6	6	6
	Release (ms)	60	60	60

Delmar/Cengage Learning

PRODUCT 15: VALEO

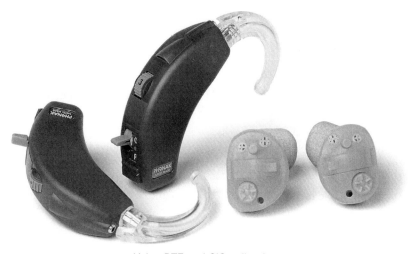

Valeo BTE and CIC collection
Phonak Hearing Systems

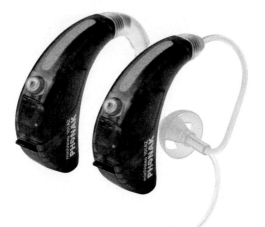

miniValeo BTE
Phonak Hearing Systems

Product Application

Valeo 211 BTE
Valeo 211 AZ BTE
Valeo 311 BTE
Valeo 311 AZ Forte BTE
miniValeo 101 AZ BTE
Valeo 33 P (Forte) FS
Valeo 23 AZ ITE/ITC
Valeo 22 ITE/ITC
Valeo 11 CIC

Features of Valeo 211 BTE, Valeo 211 AZ BTE, Valeo 311 BTE, Valeo 311 AZ Forte BTE, and miniValeo 101 AZ BTE

- 15 adjustable channels
- SoundSelect™ with digital Multimode Signal Processing (dMSP2) – choose from dWDRC, dSC, or dLimiting in each memory
- AudioZoom directional microphone system in AZ instruments
- 3 programmable memories with on-board memory switch
- Digital Noise Canceller (dNC) with 2 levels of noise reduction
- Multimode feedback manager
- Push-button program switch
- Wind and weather protection
- Low-battery indicator (1 long beep)
- Standard telecoil

- Valeo 211 BTE and Valeo 211 AZ BTE recommended for mild to moderate hearing losses
- Valeo 311 BTE and Valeo 311 AZ BTE recommended for moderate to severe hearing losses
- miniValeo 101 AZ BTE recommended for mild to moderate hearing losses, high-frequency hearing losses ("ski-slope") and for patients desiring optional performance in noise, patients requiring the comfort of an open fit, and patients desiring advanced technology in a discreet size
- AudioZoom directional microphone system (Valeo 211 AZ BTE, Valeo 311 AZ BTE, and miniValeo 101 AZ BTE)

Options of Valeo 211 BTE, Valeo 211 AZ BTE, Valeo 311 BTE, and Valeo 311 AZ Forte BTE

- MicroLink FM system
- Mini ear hooks
- Choice of colors: beige, tan, brown, light gray, dark gray, anthracite, blue, violet, red, green, yellow, light pink, and light blue

Options of miniValeo 101 AZ BTE

- Fit'n'Go slim tube
- Choice of colors: beige, taupe, brown, light gray, dark gray, anthracite, transparent red, transparent blue, transparent purple, and transparent black

Features of Valeo 33 P (Forte) FS, Valeo 23 AZ ITE/ITC, Valeo 22 ITE/ITC, and Valeo CIC

- 15 adjustable channels
- SoundSelect with dMSP2: choose from dWDRC, dSC, or dLimiting in each memory
- 2 programmable memories with on-board memory switch
- dNC with 2 levels of noise reductions
- Multimode feedback manager
- Low-battery indicator (1 long beep)
- Faceplate with swing-out battery door

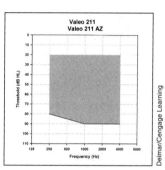

Fitting range for Valeo 211 BTE and Valeo 211 AZ BTE

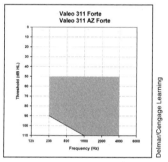

Fitting range for Valeo 311 BTE and Valeo 311 AZ Forte BTE

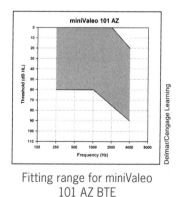

Fitting range for miniValeo 101 AZ BTE

- Manual volume control
- Valeo 33 P (Forte) FS is a power ITE and is recommended for moderate to severe hearing losses
- Valeo 23 AZ ITE/ITC, Valeo 22 ITE/ITC, and Valeo CIC are recommended for mild to moderate hearing losses
- AudioZoom directional microphone system (Valeo 23 AZ ITE/ITC only)

Options of Valeo 33 P (Forte) FS, Valeo 23 AZ ITE/ITC, Valeo 22 ITE/ITC, and Valeo CIC

- Telecoil on full-shell to canal models (space permitting)
- EasyPhone on full-shell to canal models (space permitting)
- Digital "eShell" made with NemoTech technology
- Can remove volume control and/or memory switch
- Choice of colors: cocoa, brown, and pink

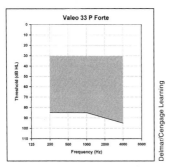

Fitting range for Valeo 33 P (Forte) FS

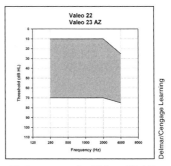

Fitting range for Valeo 23 AZ ITE/ITC and Valeo 22 ITE/ITC

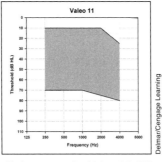

Fitting range for Valeo 11 CIC

Typical Specifications		Valeo 211 BTE	Valeo 211 AZ BTE	Valeo 311 BTE	Valeo 311 AZ Forte BTE	mini Valeo 101 AZ BTE
Standard ANSI S3.22-1996						
Output sound pressure level (OSPL 90)	Peak (dB SPL)	121	121	132	132	115
	HF Average (dB SPL)	117	116	127	127	113
Full-on gain (input 50 dB SPL)	Peak (dB)	55	56	68	65	40
	HF Average (dB)	50	46	65	61	37
Total harmonic distortion (Hz)	500 Hz	2.0%	3.0%	1.5%	2.0%	1.0%
	800 Hz	1.0%	2.0%	1.0%	1.0%	0.5%
	1600 Hz	1.5%	2.0%	1.0%	1.0%	0.5%
Equivalent input noise (dB SPL)		18	16	18	16	19
Telecoil sensitivity (input 31.6 mA/m)	HFA-SPLIV (dB SPL)	100	100	112	110	99
Battery	Operating current (mA)	0.9	0.9	1.10	1.10	0.9
	Battery type	13	13	13	13	10
Compression	Attack (ms)	1	1	1	1	1
	Release (ms)	10	10	9	8	15

Delmar/Cengage Learning

Typical Specifications		Valeo 33 P Forte FS	Valeo 23 AC ITE/ITC	Valeo 22 ITE/ITC	Valeo 11 CIC
Standard ANSI S3.22-1996					
Output sound pressure level (OSPL 90)	Peak (dB SPL)	120	114	114	114
	HF Average (dB SPL)	114	109	108	110
Full-on gain (input 50 dB SPL)	Peak (dB)	55	45	46	40
	HF Average (dB)	50	37	37	34
Total harmonic distortion (Hz)	500 Hz	2.5%	2.5%	2.5%	2.0%
	800 Hz	2.0%	2.5%	2.5%	2.0%
	1600 Hz	2.0%	2.0%	2.0%	1.0%
Equivalent input noise (dB SPL)		20	24	24	23
Telecoil sensitivity (input 31.6 mA/m)	HFA-SPLIV (dB SPL)	96	92	90	n/a
Battery	Operating current (mA)	1.0	1.0	1.0	1.0
	Battery type	13	312	312	10
Compression	Attack (ms)	2	2	2	2
	Release (ms)	40	10	40	40

Delmar/Cengage Learning

PRODUCT 16: SUPERO+

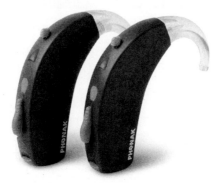

Supero+ BTE
Phonak Hearing Systems

Product Application

Supero+ 411 BTE
Supero+ 412 BTE
Supero+ 413 AZ BTE

Features of Supero+ 411 BTE, Supero+ 412 BTE, and Supero+ 413 AZ BTE

- Fully programmable digital hearing system
- dMSP
- Variable start-up program (including FM program)
- Feedback manager
- Programmable telecoil with preamplifier
- ON/OFF program switch
- Supero+ fitting formulas
- Low-battery indicator (4 beeps, 2 tones)
- Telecoil
- Supero+ 411 BTE and Supero+ 412 BTE recommended for severe to profound hearing losses where power is priority
- Supero+413 AZ BTE recommended for severe to profound hearing losses where power and performance in noise are priorities
- Fully programmable digital hearing system
- dMSP – choose from dWDRC, dSC, or dLimiting (Supero+ 412 BTE and Supero+ 413 AZ BTE only)
- Supero+ 411 BTE comes standard with dLimiting

- dNC (Supero+ 412 BTE and Supero+ 413 AZ BTE only)
- 3 programmable memories (Supero+ 412 BTE and Supero+ 413 AZ BTE) plus telecoil and FM

Options of Supero+ 411 BTE, Supero+ 412 BTE, and Supero+ 413 AZ BTE

- Remote controls – SoundPilot, WatchPilot2, KeyPilot2 (Supero+ 412 BTE and Supero+ 413 AZ BTE)
- RECD direct-fitting verification
- MicroLink FM system
- Tamper-resistant battery door and VC covers
- Mini earhooks
- Choice of colors: beige, tan, brown, light gray, dark gray, anthracite, blue, violet, red, green, yellow, light pink, and light blue

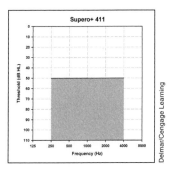

Fitting range for Supero+
411 BTE

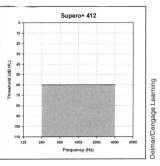

Fitting range for Supero+
412 BTE

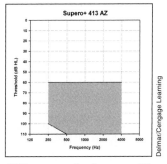

Fitting range for Supero+ AZ
BTE (digital super-power BTE)

Typical Specifications		Supero+ 411 BTE	Supero+ 412 BTE	Supero+ 413 AZ BTE
Standard ANSI S3.22-1996				
Output sound pressure level (OSPL 90)	Peak (dB SPL)	138	140	140
	HF Average (dB SPL)	130	132	132
Full-on gain (input 50 dB SPL)	Peak (dB)	75	80	75
	HF Average (dB)	69	73	69
Total harmonic distortion (Hz)	500 Hz	0.9%	1.5%	1.0%
	800 Hz	0.7%	0.6%	0.7%
	1600 Hz	0.2%	0.4%	0.3%
Equivalent input noise (dB SPL)		20	20	20
Telecoil sensitivity (input 31.6 mA/m)	HFA-SPLIV (dB SPL)	114	115	116
Battery	Operating current (mA)	1.4	1.9	1.9
	Battery type	675	675	675
Compression	Attack (ms)	5	5	1
	Release (ms)	5	8	10

Delmar/Cengage Learning

PRODUCT 17: AMIO

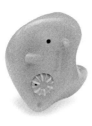

Amio FS
Phonak Hearing
Systems

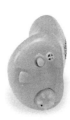

Amio ITC
Phonak Hearing
Systems

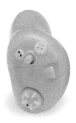

Amio ITC with
miniZoom
directional system
Phonak Hearing
Systems

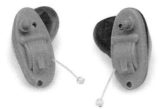

Amio CIC
Phonak Hearing Systems

Product Application
Amio 22 FS
Amio 22 ITC
Amio 22 mZ ITC
Amio 11 CIC

Features of Amio 22 FS, Amio 22 ITC, Amio 22 mZ ITC, and Amio 11 CIC

- 5-channel digital signal processing
- Choice of signal-processing strategy at time of order (dSC, dLim, dWDRC)
- Feedback manager
- Low-battery indicator (1 long beep)
- Standard with digital "eShell" made with NemoTech technology
- Digital noise canceller
- Amio 11 CIC and Amio 22 recommended for mild to moderate hearing losses
- Amio 22 mZ recommended for mild to moderate hearing losses and a desire to hear better in background noise
- Manual volume control (excludes Amio 11 CIC)

Options of Amio 22 FS, Amio 22 ITC, Amio 22 mZ ITC, and Amio 11 CIC

- Multiple memories
- MiniZoom™ directional system (excludes Amio 11 CIC)
- Telecoil (space permitting) (excludes Amio 11 CIC)
- Can remove volume control and/or memory switch

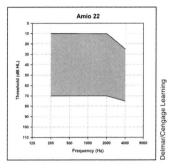

Fitting range for Amio 22 FS, Amio 22 ITC, and Amio 22 nZ ITC

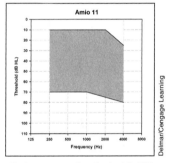

Fitting range for Amio 11 CIC

Typical Specifications		Amio 22 FS, 22 ITC, and 22 mZ ITC	Amio 11 CIC
Standard ANSI S3.22-1996			
Output sound pressure level (OSPL 90)	Peak (dB SPL)	110	110
	HF Average (dB SPL)	107	107
Full-on gain (input 50 dB SPL)	Peak (dB)	46	40
	HF Average (dB)	42	35
Total harmonic distortion (Hz)	500 Hz	1.5%	2.0%
	800 Hz	2.5%	2.0%
	1600 Hz	1.0%	1.0%

continues

continued

Typical Specifications		Amio 22 FS, 22 ITC, and 22 mZ ITC	Amio 11 CIC
Equivalent input noise (dB SPL)		27	27
Telecoil sensitivity (input 31.6 mA/m)	HFA-SPLIV (dB SPL)	95	n/a
Battery	Operating current (mA)	1.05	0.95
	Battery type	13 or 312	10
Compression	Attack (ms)	1	2
	Release (ms)	10	40

Delmar/Cengage Learning

PRODUCT 18: MAXX

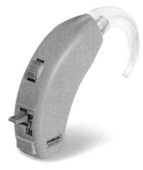

MAXX BTE
Phonak Hearing Systems

Product Application

MAXX 211 BTE
MAXX 211D BTE
MAXX 311 Forte BTE
PowerMAXX BTE

Features of MAXX 211 BTE, MAXX 211D BTE, MAXX 311 Forte BTE, and PowerMAXX BTE

- 6-channel digital signal processing (PowerMAXX BTE has 5 channels)
- digital Wide Dynamic Range Compression (dWDRC) signal processing
- dNC
- Feedback manager
- Manual volume control
- Telecoil
- MicroLink-compatible

- Low-battery indicator (4 beeps, 2 tones)
- MAXX 211 BTE and MAXX 211D BTE recommended for mild to moderate hearing losses
- MAXX 311 Forte BTE recommended for moderate to severe hearing losses
- PowerMAXX BTE recommended for severe to profound hearing losses
- MAXX 211D BTE includes a directional microphone
- Bass frequency boost (PowerMAXX BTE only)
- Choice of dSC or dWDRC (PowerMAXX BTE only)

Options of MAXX 211 BTE, MAXX 211D BTE, MAXX 311 Forte BTE, and Power MAXX BTE Products

- Directional microphone switch (MAXX 211D BTE only)
- Tamper-resistant battery door and VC covers
- Mini earhooks
- Choice of colors: beige, tan, brown, light gray, dark gray, anthracite, blue, violet, red, green, yellow, light pink, and light blue

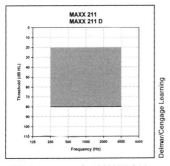

Fitting range for MAXX 211 BTE and MAXX 211D BTE

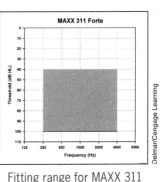

Fitting range for MAXX 311 Forte BTE

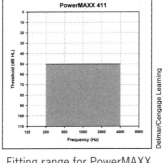

Fitting range for PowerMAXX 411 BTE

Typical Specifications		MAXX 211 BTE	MAXX 211 D BTE	MAXX 311 Forte BTE	Power MAXX BTE
Standard ANSI S3.22-1996					
Output sound pressure level (OSPL 90)	Peak (dB SPL)	126	125	130	133
	HF Average (dB SPL)	120	119	122	127
Full-on gain (input 50 dB SPL)	Peak (dB)	55	55	65	74
	HF Average (dB)	52	50	62	69
Total harmonic distortion (Hz)	500 Hz	1.0%	1.0%	1.0%	1.5%
	800 Hz	0.5%	0.5%	0.5%	1.2%
	1600 Hz	0.5%	0.5%	0.5%	0.5%
Equivalent input noise (dB SPL)		20	21	22	20
Telecoil sensitivity (input 31.6 mA/m)	HFA-SPLIV (dB SPL)	102	103	105	110
Battery	Operating current (mA)	0.6	0.65	0.7	1.35
	Battery type	13	13	13	13
Compression	Attack (ms)	6	6	6	5
	Release (ms)	60	60	60	30

Delmar/Cengage Learning

CHAPTER SEVEN

ReSound

RESOUND: RE-SOUND PRODUCTS FOR RE-HEARING

International Headquarters
ReSound A/S
Lautrupbjerg 7
P.O. Box 99
DK – 2750 Ballerup
Denmark
Phone: +45 75 11 11 11
Fax: +45 75 11 11 88
Web site: http://www.resound.com

U.S. Headquarters
ReSound North America
8001 Bloomington Freeway
Bloomington, MN 55420
Phone: 1 (952) 769-8000
Fax: 1 (952) 769-8001
E-mail: consumerhelp@gnresound.com
Web site: http://www.gnresound.com

GN ReSound (hereafter ReSound) has gone through several corporate meta-morphoses in its short life since its start in 1984. In 1996, ReSound established a formal working relationship with GN Danavox. With its combined research and development capabilities, it developed its first digital hearing aid. In 1999, the two companies became one when GN Store Nord, GN Danavox's parent company, acquired ReSound. The very next year, GN Store Nord acquired Beltone, a name that has been around since 1940. Beltone and ReSound have both maintained their own branding throughout their histories.

In 2003, GN launched "The New GN" in which specific goals were stated claiming its future stake as the global leader in each of its core areas (AudiologyOnline, 2006b). However, a certain capacity and investment in research, development, sales, marketing, and so on are required to achieve this ambition. GN worked to consolidate in its core areas of headsets and hearing instruments to improve its internal structures. As a result, its headset efforts paid off well, while its hearing instrument division could not keep up with the shorter product cycles (AudiologyOnline, 2006b). Therefore, in mid-2006, GN investigated the possibility of spinning off its hearing instrument activities. As of this writing, no acquisition has been successful.

Philanthropy

In recent years, ReSound has assisted audiology in its transition to a doctorate-level degree by providing scholarships for practicing audiologists seeking to transition from a lower degree to an AuD. In 2006, ReSound donated funds to the Audiology Foundation of America (AFA) providing five distance-enrolled AuD students with $1,000 scholarships (AudiologyOnline, 2006a). In 2005, ReSound donated $10,000 to the AFA in support of professionals transitioning to the AuD (Hearing Review, 2005).

Warranty

ReSound offers a 2-year warranty for the device and for loss and damage of its Canta7, Canta4, and ReSoundAIR™ hearing instruments. Similarly, it offers a 1-year product and loss-and-damage warranty for its Canta2 and NewTone hearing instruments. An additional 1 or 2 years of warranty can be purchased. If a ReSound product is out of warranty, ReSound will repair it for a nominal fee so long as the hearing instrument is less than 60 months old. If the instrument is older than 60 months, then it will be repaired based on the availability of parts (ReSound, 2003).

PRODUCT INFORMATION

PRODUCT 1: LIVE™

Product Application

A0970-DIVR RIE BTE
LV70-DVIR RIE BTE
LV70-DVIR High Power RIE BTE
A0971-DVI Silhouette BTE
LV81-DVI Silhouette Power BTE
LV71-DVI Silhouette BTE
LV61-DVI Silhouette mini BTE
LV40/D ITE half shell
LV40P/DP Power ITE half shell
LV50/D ITE full shell
LV50-P/DP Power ITE full shell
LV30-D ITC
LV30-DP Power ITC
LV30 ITC
LV30-P Power ITC
LV20 mini canal

LV20-P Power mini canal
LV10 CIC
LV10 Power CIC
LV10-B CIC
LV10-PB Power CIC
LV10-M CIC
LV10-MP Power CIC

Features of A0970-DIVR RIE BTE

- Tinnitus sound generator
- Environmental steering – compression characteristics adapt according to listening situation
- Amplitude modulation and frequency shaping
- Full-featured receiver-in-the-ear technology
- Surround sound processor with integrated wind noise suppression – sound streams are split into low- and high-frequency bands for independent processing
- Personalized blending point – the cutoff frequency between bands is adjustable
- 17-Band warp compression, expanded bandwidth to 7 kHz-high resolution compression
- Dual stabilizer II DFS with whistle control – proprietary feedback cancellation algorithm designed to reduce false cancellations
- Noise tracker II noise reduction – a proprietary algorithm employing spectral subtraction in order to improve the speech-to-noise ratio
- Natural directionality II – bilateral fitting strategy employing a directional microphone on one ear and an Omnidirectional microphone on the other
- Auto scope adaptive directionality – directional microphone system that also adapts the size of the preferred listening direction
- Multi scope adaptive directionality – lets you select different beam widths to effectively reduce multiple competing background sounds; 2 beam widths
- Soft switching – automatically switches between omnidirectional and directional modes
- Fixed directionality
- Echo stop – reduces room reverberation and echo
- Environmental optimizer – delivers automatic, personally optimized gain in 7 different environments
- Environmental learner – an algorithm that learns user preferences based on usage patterns in up to 7 different listening environments
- Onboard analyzer II data logging – stores usage data and provides efficient troubleshooting and customization
- Smart start power-up timer
- 9 Gain handles
- iSolate humidity and shock protection
- Replaceable GORE filters

- Duel microphone technology
- Power saving chip technology
- Push button program selector
- Programmable telecoil with T/MT modes
- Programmable volume control
- Compatible with Beetle Bluetooth device
- Direct audio input (DIA)

Options of A0970-DIVR RIE BTE

- Up to 4 programs
- Open fitting capabilities
- Choice of multiple domes and custom micro-mold
- Low power (LP) and high power (HP) receiver options
- Available in 14 colors

Features of LV70-DVIR RIE BTE

- Full-featured receiver-in-the-ear (RIE) BTE
- Surround sound processor with integrated wind noise suppression – sound streams are split into low- and high-frequency bands for independent processing
- 17-Band warp compression, expanded bandwidth to 7 kHz-high resolution compression
- 9 Gain handles
- Natural directionality II – bilateral fitting strategy employing a directional microphone on one ear and an Omnidirectional microphone on the other
- Auto scope adaptive directionality – directional microphone system that also adapts the size of the preferred listening direction
- Soft switching – automatically switches between omnidirectional and directional modes
- Integrated microphone matching – allows for increased precision of MultiScope™ adaptive directionality
- Dual stabilizer II DFS with whistle control – proprietary feedback cancellation algorithm designed to reduce false cancellations
- Environmental optimizer – delivers automatic, personally optimized gain in 7 different environments

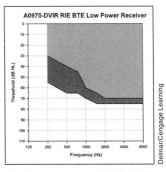

Fitting range for A0970-DVIR RIE BTE Low Power Receiver (light gray open configuration, all shaded regions closed configuration)

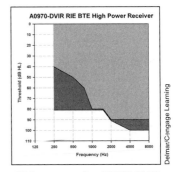

Fitting range for A0970-DVIR RIE BTE High Power Receiver (light gray open configuration, all shaded regions closed configuration)

- Environmental learner – an algorithm that learns user preferences based on usage patterns in up to 7 different listening environments
- Noise tracker II noise reduction – a proprietary algorithm employing spectral subtraction in order to improve the speech-to-noise ratio
- Onboard analyzer II data logging – stores usage data and provides efficient troubleshooting and customization
- Echo stop – reduces room reverberation and echo
- Smart start power-up timer
- iSolate humidity and shock protection
- Compatible with Beetle Bluetooth device
- Power saving chip technology
- Battery door with integrated on/off switch
- Push button program selector
- Programmable volume control with acoustic indicator
- Programmable telecoil with T/MT modes
- Direct audio input (DIA)
- Low battery warning

Options of LV70-DVIR RIE BTE

- Up to 4 customizable programs with acoustic indicator for program selection
- Open fitting capabilities
- Supports standard dome, tulip-dome, flex vent, and standard earmold
- 3 Earhook sizes and thin tube adaptor
- Available in 14 colors

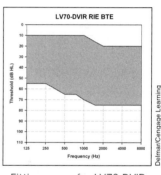

Fitting range for LV70-DVIR RIE BTE

Features of LV70-DVIR High Power RIE BTE

- High-power, full-featured receiver-in-the-ear (RIE) BTE
- 17-Band warp with extended bandwidth – high resolution compression
- 9 Gain handles
- Natural directionality II – bilateral fitting strategy employing a directional microphone on one ear and an Omnidirectional microphone on the other
- Auto scope adaptive directionality – directional microphone system that also adapts the size of the preferred listening direction
- Soft switching – automatically switches between omnidirectional and directional modes
- Integrated Microphone Matching – allows for increased precision of multi scope adaptive directionality
- Dual stabilizer II DFS with whistle control – proprietary feedback cancellation algorithm designed to reduce false cancellations
- Environmental optimizer – delivers automatic, personally optimized gain in 7 different environments

- Environmental learner – an algorithm that learns user preferences based on usage patterns in up to 7 different listening environments
- Noise tracker II noise reduction – a proprietary algorithm employing spectral subtraction in order to improve the speech-to-noise ratio Onboard analyzer II data logging – stores usage data and provides efficient troubleshooting and customization
- Echo stop – reduces room reverberation and echo
- Surround sound processor with integrated wind noise management – sound streams are split into low- and high-frequency bands for independent processing
- Smart start power-up timer
- iSolate humidity and shock protection
- Compatible with Beetle Bluetooth device
- Power saving chip technology
- Battery door with integrated on/off switch
- Push button program selector
- Programmable volume control with acoustic indicator
- Programmable telecoil with T/MT modes
- Direct audio input (DIA)
- Low battery warning

Options of LV70-DVIR High Power RIE BTE

- Up to 4 customizable programs with acoustic indicator for program selection
- Open fitting capabilities
- Supports standard dome, tulip-dome, flex vent and standard earmold
- 3 Earhook sizes and thin tube adaptor
- Available in 14 colors

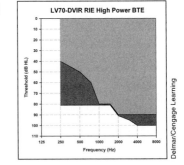

Fitting range for LV70-DVIR RIE High Power BTE (light gray open configuration, all shaded regions closed configuration)

Features of A0971-DVI Silhouette BTE

- Tinnitus sound generator
- Environmental steering – Compression characteristics adapt according to listening situation
- Amplitude modulation and frequency shaping
- Surround sound processor with integrated wind noise management – sound streams are split into low- and high-frequency bands for independent processing
- Personalized blending point – the cutoff frequency between bands is adjustable
- 17-Band warp compression – extended bandwidth to 7 kHz-high resolution compression

- Dual stabilizer II DFS – proprietary feedback cancellation algorithm designed to reduce false cancellations
- Auto scope adaptive directionality – directional microphone system that also adapts the size of the preferred listening direction
- MultiScope™ adaptive directionality – lets you select different beam widths to effectively reduce multiple competing background sounds; 2 beam widths
- Soft switching – automatically switches between omnidirectional and directional modes
- Fixed directionality
- Echo stop – reduces room reverberation and echo
- Environmental optimizer – delivers automatic, personally optimized gain in 7 different environments
- Environmental learner – an algorithm that learns user preferences based on usage patterns in up to 7 different listening environments
- Onboard analyzer II data logging – stores usage data and provides efficient troubleshooting and customization
- Smart start power-up timer
- 9 gain handles
- iSolate humidity and shock protection
- Duel microphone technology
- Power saving chip technology
- Push button program selector
- Programmable telecoil with T/MT modes
- Programmable volume control
- Compatible with Beetle Bluetooth device
- Direct Audio Input (DIA)

Options of A0971-DVI Silhouette BTE

- Up to 4 customizable programs
- Open fitting capabilities
- Supports multiple domes and custom earmolds
- 3 Earhook sizes and thin tube adaptor
- Available in 14 colors

Features of LV81-DVI Silhouette Power BTE

- 17-Band warp compression – extended bandwidth to 7 kHz-high resolution compression
- 9 gain handles
- Natural directionality II – bilateral fitting strategy employing a directional microphone on one ear and an Omnidirectional microphone on the other
- Auto scope adaptive directionality – directional microphone system that also adapts the size of the preferred listening direction

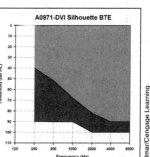

Fitting range for A0971-DVI Silhouette BTE (light gray open configuration, all shaded regions classic configuration)

- Soft switching automatic program – automatically switches between omni-directional and directional modes
- Integrated microphone matching – allows for increased precision of MultiScope™ adaptive directionality
- Dual stabilizer II DFS with whistle control – proprietary feedback cancellation algorithm designed to reduce false cancellations
- Environmental optimizer – delivers automatic, personally optimized gain in 7 different environments
- Environmental learner – an algorithm that learns user preferences based on usage patterns in up to 7 different listening environments
- Noise tracker II noise reduction – a proprietary algorithm employing spectral subtraction in order to improve the speech-to-noise ratio
- Onboard analyzer II data logging – stores usage data and provides efficient troubleshooting and customization
- Echo stop – reduces room reverberation and echo
- Surround sound processor with integrated wind noise management – sound streams are split into low- and high-frequency bands for independent processing
- Smart start power-up timer
- iSolate humidity and shock protection
- Compatible with Beetle Bluetooth device
- Power saving chip technology
- Battery door with integrated on/off switch
- Push button program selector
- Programmable volume control with acoustic indicator
- Programmable telecoil with T/MT modes
- Direct audio input (DIA)
- Low battery warning

Options of LV81-DVI Silhouette Power BTE

- Up to 4 customizable programs with acoustic indicator for program selection
- Available in 14 colors

Features of LV71-DVI Silhouette BTE

- 17-Band warp compression – extended bandwidth to 7 kHz-high resolution compression
- 9 gain handles
- Natural directionality II – bilateral fitting strategy employing a directional microphone on one ear and an Omnidirectional microphone on the other
- Auto scope adaptive directionality – directional microphone system that also adapts the size of the preferred listening direction

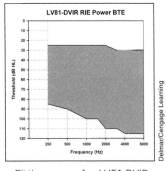

Fitting range for LV81-DVIR RIE Power BTE

- Soft switching – automatically switches between omnidirectional and directional modes
- Integrated microphone matching – allows for increased precision of multi scope adaptive directionality
- Dual stabilizer II DFS with whistle control – proprietary feedback cancellation algorithm designed to reduce false cancellations
- Environmental optimizer – delivers automatic, personally optimized gain in 7 different environments
- Environmental learner – an algorithm that learns user preferences based on usage patterns in up to 7 different listening environments
- Noise tracker II noise reduction – a proprietary algorithm employing spectral subtraction in order to improve the speech-to-noise ratio
- Onboard analyzer II data logging – stores usage data and provides efficient troubleshooting and customization
- Echo stop – reduces room reverberation and echo
- Surround sound processor with integrated wind noise management – sound streams are split into low- and high-frequency bands for independent processing
- Smart start power-up timer
- iSolate humidity and shock protection
- Compatible with Beetle Bluetooth device
- Power saving chip technology
- Battery door with integrated on/off switch
- Push button program selector
- Programmable volume control with acoustic indicator
- Programmable telecoil with T/MT modes
- Direct audio input (DIA)
- Low battery warning

Options of LV71-DVI Silhouette BTE

- Up to 4 customizable programs with acoustic indicator for program selection
- Open fitting capabilities
- Supports standard dome, tulip-dome, flex vent and standard earmold
- 3 Earhook sizes with thin tube adaptor
- Available in 14 colors

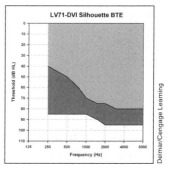

Fitting range for LV71-DVI Silhouette BTE (light gray open configuration, all shaded regions classic configuration)

Features of LV61-DVI Silhouette mini BTE

- 17-Band warp compression – extended bandwidth to 7 kHz-high resolution compression
- 9 gain handles
- Natural directionality II – bilateral fitting strategy employing a directional microphone on one ear and an Omnidirectional microphone on the other

- Auto scope adaptive directionality – directional microphone system that also adapts the size of the preferred listening direction
- Soft switching automatic program – automatically switches between omni-directional and directional modes
- Integrated microphone matching – allows for increased precision of MultiScope™ adaptive directionality
- Dual stabilizer II DFS with whistle control – proprietary feedback cancellation algorithm designed to reduce false cancellations
- Environmental optimizer – delivers automatic, personally optimized gain in 7 different environments
- Noise tracker II noise reduction – a proprietary algorithm employing spectral subtraction in order to improve the speech-to-noise ratio
- Onboard analyzer II data logging – stores usage data and provides efficient troubleshooting and customization
- Echo stop – reduces room reverberation and echo
- Surround sound processor with integrated wind noise management – sound streams are split into low- and high-frequency bands for independent processing
- Smart start power-up timer
- iSolate humidity and shock protection
- Compatible with Beetle Bluetooth device
- Power saving chip technology
- Battery door with integrated on/off switch
- Push button program selector
- Programmable telecoil with T/MT modes
- Direct audio input (DIA)
- Low battery warning

Options of LV61-DVI Silhouette mini BTE

- Up to 4 customizable programs with acoustic indicator for program selection
- Open fitting capabilities
- Supports standard dome, tulip-dome, flex vent, and standard earmold
- 3 Earhook sizes with thin tube adaptor
- Available in 14 colors

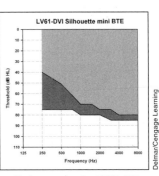

Fitting range for LV61-DVI Silhouette mini BTE (light gray open configuration, all shaded regions classic configuration)

Features of LV40/D ITE half shell and LV50/D ITE full shell

- 17-Band warp compression – extended bandwidth to 7 kHz-high resolution compression
- 9 gain handles
- Natural directionality II – bilateral fitting strategy employing a directional microphone on one ear and an Omnidirectional microphone on the other

- Auto scope adaptive directionality – directional microphone system that also adapts the size of the preferred listening direction
- Soft switching automatic program – automatically switches between omni-directional and directional modes
- Integrated microphone matching – allows for increased precision of MultiScope™ adaptive directionality
- Stabilizer II or dual stabilizer II DFS with whistle control – proprietary feedback cancellation algorithm designed to reduce false cancellations
- Environmental optimizer – delivers automatic, personally optimized gain in 7 different environments
- Environmental learner – an algorithm that learns user preferences based on usage patterns in up to 7 different listening environments
- Noise tracker II noise reduction – a proprietary algorithm employing spectral subtraction in order to improve the speech-to-noise ratio
- Onboard analyzer II data logging – stores usage data and provides efficient troubleshooting and customization
- Echo stop – reduces room reverberation and echo
- Surround sound processor with integrated wind noise management – sound streams are split into low- and high-frequency bands for independent processing
- Smart start power-up timer
- Compatible with Beetle Bluetooth device
- Power saving chip technology
- Battery door with integrated on/off switch
- Push button program selector
- Programmable telecoil with T/MT modes
- Low battery warning

Options of LV40/D ITE half shell and LV50/D ITE full shell

- Up to 4 customizable programs with acoustic indicator for program selection
- Programmable volume control with acoustic indicator
- Available in 5 colors

Features of LV40P/DP Power ITE half shell and LV50-P/DP Power ITE full shell

- 17-Band warp compression – extended bandwidth to 7 kHz-high resolution compression
- 9 gain handles
- Environmental optimizer – delivers automatic, personally optimized gain in 7 different environments
- Environmental learner – an algorithm that learns user preferences based on usage patterns in up to 7 different listening environments
- Noise tracker II noise reduction – a proprietary algorithm employing spectral subtraction in order to improve the speech-to-noise ratio
- Onboard analyzer II data logging – stores usage data and provides efficient troubleshooting and customization

- Echo stop – reduces room reverberation and echo
- Smart start power-up timer
- Compatible with Beetle Bluetooth device
- Power saving chip technology
- Battery door with integrated on/off switch
- Push button program selector
- Programmable telecoil with T/MT modes
- Low battery warning

Options of LV40P/DP Power ITE half shell and LV50-P/DP Power ITE full shell

- Up to 4 customizable programs with acoustic indicator for program selection
- Programmable volume control with acoustic indicator
- Available in 5 colors

Features of LV30/D ITC and LV30/DP Power ITC

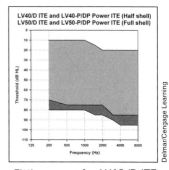

Fitting range for LV40/D ITE and LV40-P/DP Power ITE Half Shell (light gray region) and LV50/D and LV50-P/DP Power ITE Full Shell (all shaded regions)

- 17-Band warp compression – extended bandwidth to 7 kHz-high resolution compression
- 9 gain handles
- Natural directionality II – bilateral fitting strategy employing a directional microphone on one ear and an Omnidirectional microphone on the other
- Auto scope adaptive directionality – directional microphone system that also adapts the size of the preferred listening direction
- Soft switching – automatically switches between omnidirectional and directional modes
- Integrated microphone matching – allows for increased precision of MultiScope™ adaptive directionality
- Dual stabilizer II DFS with whistle control – proprietary feedback cancellation algorithm designed to reduce false cancellations
- Environmental optimizer – delivers automatic, personally optimized gain in 7 different environments
- Environmental learner – an algorithm that learns user preferences based on usage patterns in up to 7 different listening environments
- Noise tracker II noise reduction – a proprietary algorithm employing spectral subtraction in order to improve the speech-to-noise ratio
- Onboard analyzer II data logging – stores usage data and provides efficient troubleshooting and customization
- Echo stop – reduces room reverberation and echo
- Surround sound processor with integrated wind noise management – sound streams are split into low- and high-frequency bands for independent processing

- Smart start power-up timer
- Compatible with Beetle Bluetooth device
- Power saving chip technology
- Battery door with integrated on/off switch
- Push button program selector
- Programmable telecoil with T/MT modes
- Low battery warning

Options of LV30/D ITC and LV30/DP Power ITC

- Up to 4 customizable programs with acoustic indicator for program selection
- Programmable volume control with acoustic indicator
- Available in 5 colors

Features of LV30 ITC and LV30-P Power ITC

- 17-Band warp compression – extended bandwidth to 7 kHz-high resolution compression
- 9 gain handles
- Stabilizer II DFS with whistle control – delivers fewer artifacts and distortion-free feedback emergency brake
- Environmental optimizer – delivers automatic, personally optimized gain in 7 different environments
- Environmental learner – an algorithm that learns user preferences based on usage patterns in up to 7 different listening environments
- Noise tracker II noise reduction – a proprietary algorithm employing spectral subtraction in order to improve the speech-to-noise ratio
- Onboard analyzer II data logging – stores usage data and provides efficient troubleshooting and customization
- Smart start power-up timer
- Compatible with Beetle Bluetooth device
- Power saving chip technology
- Battery door with integrated on/off switch
- Push button program selector
- Programmable telecoil with T/MT modes
- Low battery warning

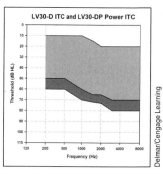

Fitting range for LV30-D ITC (light gray region) and LV30-DP Power ITC (all shaded regions)

Delmar/Cengage Learning

Options of LV30 ITC and LV30-P Power ITC

- Up to 4 customizable programs with acoustic indicator for program selection
- Programmable volume control with acoustic indicator
- Available in 5 colors

Features of LV20 mini Canal and LV20-P Power mini Canal

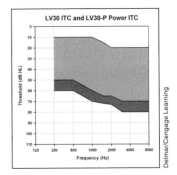

- 17-Band warp compression – extended bandwidth to 7 kHz-high resolution compression
- 9 gain handles
- Stabilizer II DFS with whistle control-delivers fewer artifacts and distortion-free feedback emergency brake
- Environmental optimizer – delivers automatic, personally optimized gain in 7 different environments
- Environmental learner – an algorithm that learns user preferences based on usage patterns in up to 7 different listening environments

Fitting range for LV30 ITC (light gray region) and LV30-P Power ITC (all shaded regions)

- Noise tracker II noise reduction – a proprietary algorithm employing spectral subtraction in order to improve the speech-to-noise ratio
- Onboard analyzer II Data logging – stores usage data and provides efficient troubleshooting and customization
- Smart start power-up timer
- Power saving chip technology
- Battery door with integrated on/off switch
- Push button program selector
- Low battery warning

Options of LV20 mini Canal and LV20-P Power mini Canal

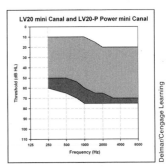

- Up to 4 customizable programs with acoustic indicator for program selection
- Programmable volume control with acoustic indicator
- Available in 5 colors

Features of LV10 CIC and LV10-P Power CIC

- 17-Band warp compression – extended bandwidth to 7 kHz-high resolution compression
- 9 gain handles
- Stabilizer II DFS with whistle control-delivers fewer artifacts and distortion-free feedback emergency brake

Fitting range for LV20 mini canal (light gray region) and LV20-P Power mini canal (all shaded regions)

- Environmental optimizer – delivers automatic, personally optimized gain in 7 different environments
- Noise tracker II noise reduction – a proprietary algorithm employing spectral subtraction in order to improve the speech-to-noise ratio

- Onboard analyzer II data logging – stores usage data and provides efficient troubleshooting and customization
- Smart start power-up timer
- Power saving chip technology
- Battery door with integrated on/off switch
- Low battery warning

Options of LV10 CIC and LV10-P Power CIC

- Available in 5 colors

Features of LV10-B CIC and LV10-BP Power CIC

- 17-Band warp compression – extended bandwidth to 7 kHz-high resolution compression
- 9 gain handles
- Stabilizer II DFS with whistle control-delivers fewer artifacts and distortion-free feedback emergency brake
- Environmental optimizer – delivers automatic, personally optimized gain in 7 different environments
- Noise tracker II noise reduction – a proprietary algorithm employing spectral subtraction in order to improve the speech-to-noise ratio
- Onboard analyzer II data logging – stores usage data and provides efficient troubleshooting and customization
- Smart start power-up timer
- Power saving chip technology
- Battery door with integrated on/off switch
- Push button program selector
- Low battery warning

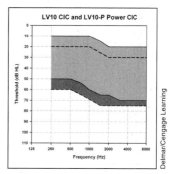

Fitting range for LV10 CIC (area within the dotted lines) and LV10-P Power CIC (light gray region only)

Options of LV10-B CIC and LV10-BP Power CIC

- Up to 4 customizable programs with acoustic indicator for program selection
- Available in 5 colors

Features of LV10-M CIC and LV10-MP Power CIC

- 17-Band warp compression – extended bandwidth to 7 kHz-high resolution compression
- 9 gain handles
- Stabilizer II DFS with whistle control-delivers fewer artifacts and distortion-free feedback emergency brake

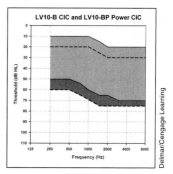

Fitting range for LV10-B CIC (area within the dotted lines) and LV10-BP Power CIC (light gray region only)

ReSOUND

- Environmental Optimizer – delivers automatic, personally optimized gain in 7 different environments
- Noise tracker II noise reduction – a proprietary algorithm employing spectral subtraction in order to improve the speech-to-noise ratio
- Onboard analyzer II data logging – stores usage data and provides efficient trouble-shooting and customization
- Smart start power-up timer
- Power saving chip technology
- Battery door with integrated on/off switch
- Low battery warning

Options of LV10-M CIC

- Open fitting capabilities
- Available in 5 colors

Options of LV10-MP Power CIC

- Available in 5 colors

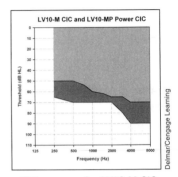

Fitting range for LV10-M CIC (light gray region) and LV10-MP Power CIC (all shaded regions)

Typical Specifications		A0970-DIVR RIE BTE Low Power Receiver-Closed	A0970-DIVR RIE BTE Low Power Receiver-Open	A0970-DIVR RIE BTE High Power Receiver-Closed	A0970-DIVR RIE BTE High Power Receiver-Open
Standard ANSI S3.22-2003					
Output sound pressure level	Max OSPL 90 (dB SPL)	108	107	119	118
	HFA OSPL 90 (dB SPL)	101	101	113	114
Full-on gain (50 dB SPL input)	Peak gain (dB)	42	41	57	52
	HFA (dB)	35	35	46	46
Total harmonic distortion (Hz)	500	1.1%	1.1%	1.0%	0.9%
	800	0.7%	0.7%	0.8%	0.6%
	1600	0.7%	0.7%	1.0%	0.8%
Equivalent input noise (dB SPL), without noise reduction		27	27	27	27
Telecoil sensitivity	31.6 mA/m Input HFA (dB SPL)	84	85	96	96
Battery	Battery current drain (mA)	0.89	0.93	0.88	.093
	Battery type	312	312	312	312
Compression characteristics	Attack (ms)	12	12	12	12
	Release (ms)	70	70	70	70

Typical Specifications		LV70-DVIR RIE BTE	LV70-DVIR High Power RIE BTE Closed	LV70-DVIR High Power RIE BTE Open
Standard ANSI S3.22-2003				
Output sound pressure level	Max OSPL 90 (dB SPL)	108	119	118
	HFA OSPL 90 (dB SPL)	101	113	114
Full-on gain (50 dB SPL input)	Peak gain (dB)	42	57	52
	HFA (dB)	35	46	46
Total harmonic distortion (Hz)	500	1.1%	1.0%	0.9%
	800	0.7%	0.8%	0.6%
	1600	0.7%	1.0%	.08%
Equivalent input noise (dB SPL), without noise reduction		27	27	27
Telecoil sensitivity	31.6 mA/m Input HFA (dB SPL)	85	96	97
Battery	Battery current drain (mA)	0.89	0.88	0.93
	Battery type	312	312	312
Compression characteristics	Attack (ms)	12	12	12
	Release (ms)	70	70	70

Delmar/Cengage Learning

Typical Specifications		A0971-DVI Silhouette BTE- Classic	A0971-DVI Silhouette BTE- Open	LV81-DVI Silhouette Power BTE
Standard ANSI S3.22-2003				
Output sound pressure level	Max OSPL 90 (dB SPL)	126	129	133
	HFA OSPL 90 (dB SPL)	125	120	130
Full-on gain (50 dB SPL input)	Peak gain (dB)	56	49	65
	HFA (dB)	51	45	60
Total harmonic distortion (Hz)	500	1.7%	0.5%	1.0%
	800	1.2%	0.2%	0.3%
	1600	0.5%	0.8%	0.6%
Equivalent input noise (dB SPL), without noise reduction		25	26	22
Telecoil sensitivity	31.6 mA/m Input HFA (dB SPL)	108	105	114

ReSOUND

continues

continued

Typical Specifications		A0971-DVI Silhouette BTE- Classic	A0971-DVI Silhouette BTE- Open	LV81-DVI Silhouette Power BTE
Battery	Battery current drain (mA)	0.88	0.9	1.09
	Battery type	13	13	13
Compression characteristics	Attack (ms)	12	12	12
	Release (ms)	70	70	70

Delmar/Cengage Learning

Typical Specifications		LV71-DVI Silhouette BTE- Classic (Standard Tube)	LV71-DVI Silhouette BTE- Open (Thin Tube)	LV61-DVI Silhouette mini BTE Classic (Standard Tube)	LV61-DVI Silhouette mini BTE- Open (Thin Tube)
Standard ANSI S3.22-2003					
Output sound pressure level	Max OSPL 90 (dB SPL)	126	129	123	123
	HFA OSPL 90 (dB SPL)	125	120	120	116
Full-on gain (50 dB SPL input)	Peak gain (dB)	56	45	54	48
	HFA (dB)	51	45	47	42
Total harmonic distortion (Hz)	500	1.8%	0.5%	3.1%	2.1%
	800	1.2%	0.2%	3.5%	0.4%
	1600	0.5%	0.8%	0.8%	1.9%
Equivalent input noise (dB SPL), without noise reduction		25	27	27	28
Telecoil sensitivity	31.6 mA/m input HFA (dB SPL)	108	105	104	100
Battery	Battery current drain (mA)	0.9	0.9	0.9	0.9
	Battery type	13	13	312	312
Compression characteristics	Attack (ms)	12	12	12	12
	Release (ms)	70	70	70	70

Delmar/Cengage Learning

Typical Specifications		LV40/D ITE half shell and LV50/D ITE full shell	LV40P/DP Power ITE half shell and LV50-P/ DP Power ITE full shell
Standard ANSI S3.22-2003			
Output sound pressure level	Max OSPL 90 (dB SPL)	119	125
	HFA OSPL 90 (dB SPL)	115	125

continues

continued

Typical Specifications		LV40/D ITE half shell and LV50/D ITE full shell	LV40P/DP Power ITE half shell and LV50-P/DP Power ITE full shell
Full-on gain (50 dB SPL input)	Peak gain (dB)	52	58
	HFA (dB)	45	53
Total harmonic distortion (Hz)	500	1.6%	0.5%
	800	1.1%	0.4%
	1600	1.0%	0.5%
Equivalent input noise (dB SPL), without noise reduction		22	25/37
Telecoil sensitivity	31.6 mA/m input HFA (dB SPL)	97	106
Battery	Battery current drain (mA)	1.04	1.1
	Battery type	13 (half shell) 312 (full shell)	13 (half shell) 312 (full shell)
Compression characteristics	Attack (ms)	12	12
	Release (ms)	70	70

Delmar/Cengage Learning

Typical Specifications		LV30-D ITC	LV30-DP Power ITC
Standard ANSI S3.22-2003			
Output sound pressure level	Max OSPL 90 (dB SPL)	112	118
	HFA OSPL 90 (dB SPL)	110	115
Full-on gain (50 dB SPL input)	Peak gain (dB)	42	49
	HFA (dB)	38	43
Total harmonic distortion (Hz)	500	1.3%	1.4%
	800	0.9%	1.0%
	1600	0.9%	1.0%
Equivalent Input Noise (dB SPL), Without Noise Reduction		25	27
Telecoil sensitivity	31.6 mA/m input HFA (dB SPL)	93	98
Battery	Battery current drain (mA)	1.09	1.104
	Battery type	10A	10A
Compression characteristics	Attack (ms)	12	12
	Release (ms)	70	70

Delmar/Cengage Learning

ReSOUND

Typical Specifications		LV30 ITC	LV30-P Power ITC
Standard ANSI S3.22-2003			
Output sound pressure level	Max OSPL 90 (dB SPL)	112	118
	HFA OSPL 90 (dB SPL)	108	115
Full-on gain (50 dB SPL input)	Peak gain (dB)	43	50
	HFA (dB)	37	44
Total harmonic distortion (Hz)	500	1.2%	1.1%
	800	0.9%	0.9%
	1600	0.8%	0.9%
Equivalent input noise (dB SPL), without noise reduction		24	24
Telecoil sensitivity	31.6 mA/m input HFA (dB SPL)	91	97
Battery	Battery current drain (mA)	1.12	1.08
	Battery type	10A	10A
Compression characteristics	Attack (ms)	12	12
	Release (ms)	70	70

Delmar/Cengage Learning

Typical Specifications		LV20 mini canal	LV20-P Power mini canal
Standard ANSI S3.22-2003			
Output sound pressure level	Max OSPL 90 (dB SPL)	108	111
	HFA OSPL 90 (dB SPL)	103	108
Full-on gain (50 dB SPL input)	Peak gain (dB)	33	38
	HFA (dB)	27	32
Total harmonic distortion (Hz)	500	0.5%	1.25%
	800	0.4%	0.8%
	1600	0.5%	1.1%
Equivalent input noise (dB SPL), without noise reduction		25	26
Telecoil sensitivity	31.6 mA/m input HFA (dB SPL)	n/a	n/a
Battery	Battery current drain (mA)	0.96	1.02
	Battery type	10A	10A
Compression characteristics	Attack (ms)	12	12
	Release (ms)	70	70

Delmar/Cengage Learning

Typical Specifications		LV10 CIC	LV10 Power CIC
Standard ANSI S3.22-2003			
Output sound pressure level	Max OSPL 90 (dB SPL)	112	111
	HFA OSPL 90 (dB SPL)	107	108
Full-on gain (50 dB SPL input)	Peak gain (dB)	31	38
	HFA (dB)	28	33
Total harmonic distortion (Hz)	500	0.7%	1.2%
	800	0.7%	0.8%
	1600	0.5%	1.1%
Equivalent input noise (dB SPL), without noise reduction		25	26
Telecoil sensitivity	31.6 mA/m input HFA (dB SPL)	n/a	n/a
Battery	Battery current drain (mA)	0.93	1.02
	Battery type	10A	10A
Compression characteristics	Attack (ms)	12	12
	Release (ms)	70	70

Delmar/Cengage Learning

Typical Specifications		LV10-B CIC	LV10-PB Power CIC
Standard ANSI S3.22-2003			
Output sound pressure level	Max OSPL 90 (dB SPL)	109	113
	HFA OSPL 90 (dB SPL)	105	110
Full-on gain (50 dB SPL input)	Peak gain (dB)	31	40
	HFA (dB)	27	34
Total harmonic distortion (Hz)	500	0.4%	1.0%
	800	0.3%	0.8%
	1600	0.4%	0.9%
Equivalent input noise (dB SPL), without noise reduction		27	28
Telecoil sensitivity	31.6 mA/m input HFA (dB SPL)	n/a	n/a
Battery	Battery current drain (mA)	0.86	0.89
	Battery type	10A	10A
Compression characteristics	Attack (ms)	12	12
	Release (ms)	70	70

Delmar/Cengage Learning

ReSOUND

Typical Specifications		LV10-M CIC	LV10-MP Power CIC
Standard ANSI S3.22-2003			
Output sound pressure level	Max OSPL 90 (dB SPL)	109	118
	HFA OSPL 90 (dB SPL)	106	115
Full-on gain (50 dB SPL input)	Peak gain (dB)	43	50
	HFA (dB)	38	46
Total harmonic distortion (Hz)	500	1.1%	1.3%
	800	0.8%	1.3%
	1600	0.9%	0.8%
Equivalent input noise (dB SPL), without noise reduction			
Telecoil sensitivity	31.6 mA/m input HFA (dB SPL)	n/a	n/a
Battery	Battery current drain (mA)	0.88	0.98
	Battery type	10A	10A
Compression characteristics	Attack (ms)	12	12
	Release (ms)	70	70

Delmar/Cengage Learning

PRODUCT 2: X-PLORE

Product Application

XE 80-DVI Power BTE
XE71-DVI Silhouette BTE
XE60-DI Mini BTE
XE50/D FS
XE50-P/DP FS Power
XE40/D HS
XE40-P/DP HS Power
XE30/D ITC

XE30-P/DP ITC Power
XE20 MC
XE20-P MC Power
XE10 CIC
XE10-B CIC
XE10-BP CIC Power
XE10-P CIC Power

Features of XE80-DVI Power BTE

- MultiScope Adaptive Directionality™ – lets you select different beam widths to effectively reduce multiple competing background sounds; 2 beam widths
- SoftSwitching™ – automatically switches between omnidirectional and directional modes
- Integrated Microphone Matching™ – allows for increased precision of MultiScope Adaptive Directionality
- Acceptance Manager™ – gradually increases gain over time to allow patients to adapt to amplification

- Active Wind Stop™ – reduces wind noise
- 17-band WARP™ compression – provides superb sound quality based on fast processing and accurate resolution
- NoiseTracker™ II – a proprietary algorithm employing spectral subtraction in order to improve the speech-to-noise ratio
- EchoStop™ – reduces room reverberation and echo
- Dual Stabilizer™ II DFS feedback management – proprietary feedback cancellation algorithm designed to reduce false cancellations
- Advanced data-logging – stores usage data and provides efficient troubleshooting and customization
- SmartStart™ power-up timer
- Up to 4 customizable programs
- Acoustic indicator for program selection
- Acoustic indicator for volume control
- Low-battery warning indicator
- Power-saving chip technology

Options of XE80-DVI Power BTE

- Dual microphone technology
- Push button
- Programmable volume control
- Programmable telecoil with T/MT modes
- Direct audio input (DAI)
- Available in 13 different colors

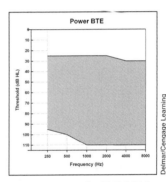

Fitting range for XE80-DVI Power BTE

Features of XE71-DVI Silhouette BTE

- MultiScope Adaptive Directionality – lets you select different beam widths to effectively reduce multiple competing background sounds; 2 beam widths
- SoftSwitching – automatically switches between omnidirectional and directional modes
- Integrated Microphone Matching – allows for increased precision of MultiScope Adaptive Directionality
- Acceptance Manager – gradually increases gain over time to allow patients to adapt to amplification
- Active Wind Stop – reduces wind noise
- 17-band WARP compression – provides superb sound quality based on fast processing and accurate resolution
- NoiseTracker II – a proprietary algorithm employing spectral subtraction in order to improve the speech-to-noise ratio
- EchoStop – reduces room reverberation and echo
- Dual Stabilizer II DFS feedback management – proprietary feedback cancellation algorithm designed to reduce false cancellations

- Advanced data-logging – stores usage data and provides efficient troubleshooting and customization
- SmartStart power-up timer
- Up to 4 customizable programs
- Acoustic indicator for program selection
- Acoustic indicator for volume control
- Low-battery warning indicator
- Power-saving chip technology
- Open-fitting capabilities

Options of XE71-DVI Silhouette BTE

- Dual microphone technology
- Push button
- Programmable volume control
- Programmable telecoil with T/MT modes
- Direct audio input
- Supports standard dome, Tulip-Dome™, FlexVent™, and standard ear molds
- 3 Earhook sizes and thin-tube adapter
- Available in 16 different colors

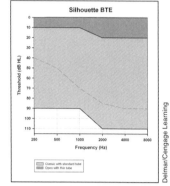

Fitting range for the XE71-DVI Silhouette BTE: open with thin tube (dark gray and light gray to dashed line), classic with thin tube (dashed down to light gray) and classic with standard tube (entire light gray region)

Features of XE60-DI Mini BTE

- MultiScope Adaptive Directionality – lets you select different beam widths to effectively reduce multiple competing background sounds; 2 beam widths
- SoftSwitching – automatically switches between omnidirectional and directional modes
- Integrated Microphone Matching – allows for increased precision of MultiScope Adaptive Directionality
- Acceptance Manager – gradually increases gain over time to allow patients to adapt to amplification
- Active Wind Stop – reduces wind noise
- 17-band WARP compression – provides superb sound quality based on fast processing and accurate resolution
- NoiseTracker II – a proprietary algorithm employing spectral subtraction in order to improve the speech-to-noise ratio
- EchoStop – reduces room reverberation and echo
- Dual Stabilizer II DFS feedback management – proprietary feedback cancellation algorithm designed to reduce false cancellations
- Advanced data-logging – stores usage data and provides efficient troubleshooting and customization
- SmartStart power-up timer
- Up to 4 customizable programs
- Acoustic indicator for program selection

- Low-battery warning indicator
- Power-saving chip technology
- Open-fitting capabilities

Options of XE60-DI Mini BTE

- Dual microphone technology
- Push button
- Programmable telecoil with T/MT modes
- Direct audio input
- Supports standard dome, Tulip-Dome, FlexVent, and standard ear molds
- 3 Earhook sizes and thin-tube adapter
- Available in 13 different colors

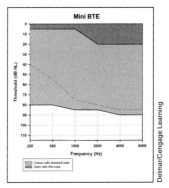

Delmar/Cengage Learning

Fitting range for XE60-DI Mini BTE: open with thin tube (dark gray and light gray to dashed line), classic with thin tube (dashed line down to light gray), and classic with standard tube (entire light gray region)

Features of XE50/D FS

- MultiScope Adaptive Directionality – lets you select different beam widths to effectively reduce multiple competing background sounds; 2 beam widths
- SoftSwitching – automatically switches between omnidirectional and directional modes
- Integrated Microphone Matching – allows for increased precision of MultiScope Adaptive Directionality
- Acceptance Manager – gradually increases gain over time to allow patients to adapt to amplification
- Active Wind Stop – reduces wind noise
- 17-band WARP compression – provides superb sound quality based on fast processing and accurate resolution
- NoiseTracker II – a proprietary algorithm employing spectral subtraction in order to improve the speech-to-noise ratio
- EchoStop – reduces room reverberation and echo
- Stabilizer™ or Dual Stabilizer II DFS feedback management – proprietary feedback cancellation algorithm designed to reduce false cancellations
- Advanced data-logging – stores usage data and provides efficient troubleshooting and customization
- SmartStart power-up timer
- Up to 4 customizable programs
- Acoustic indicator for program selection
- Acoustic indicator for volume control
- Low-battery warning indicator
- Power-saving chip technology

Options of XE50/D FS

- Dual microphone technology
- Push button

- Programmable volume control
- Programmable telecoil with T/MT modes
- Available in 3 different colors
- Supports StepVent™
- Open-fitting capabilities with an IROS vent

Features of XE50-P/DP FS Power

- MultiScope Adaptive Directionality – lets you select different beam widths to effectively reduce multiple competing background sounds; 2 beam widths
- SoftSwitching – automatically switches between omnidirectional and directional modes
- Integrated Microphone Matching – allows for increased precision of MultiScope Adaptive Directionality
- Acceptance Manager – gradually increases gain over time to allow patients to adapt to amplification
- Active Wind Stop – reduces wind noise
- 17-band WARP compression – provides superb sound quality based on fast processing and accurate resolution
- NoiseTracker II – a proprietary algorithm employing spectral subtraction in order to improve the speech-to-noise ratio
- EchoStop – reduces room reverberation and echo
- Stabilizer or Dual Stabilizer II DFS feedback management – proprietary feedback cancellation algorithm designed to reduce false cancellations
- Advanced data-logging – stores usage data and provides efficient trouble-shooting and customization
- SmartStart power-up timer
- Up to 4 customizable programs
- Acoustic indicator for program selection
- Acoustic indicator for volume control
- Low-battery warning indicator
- Power-saving chip technology

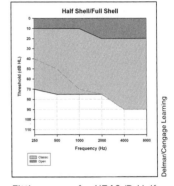

Fitting range for XE40/D Half-Shell and XE50/D Full-Shell ITE: open (dark and light gray to dashed line) and classic (entire light gray region)

Options of XE50-P/DP FS Power

- Dual microphone technology
- Push button
- Programmable volume control
- Programmable telecoil with T/MT modes
- Available in 3 different colors
- Supports StepVent

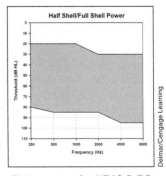

Fitting range for XE40-P/DP Half-Shell and XE50-P/DP Full-Shell Power ITE

Features of XE40/D HS

- MultiScope Adaptive Directionality – lets you select different beam widths to effectively reduce multiple competing background sounds; 2 beam widths
- SoftSwitching – automatically switches between omnidirectional and directional modes
- Integrated Microphone Matching – allows for increased precision of MultiScope Adaptive Directionality
- Acceptance Manager – gradually increases gain over time to allow patients to adapt to amplification
- Active Wind Stop – reduces wind noise
- 17-band WARP compression – provides superb sound quality based on fast processing and accurate resolution
- NoiseTracker II – a proprietary algorithm employing spectral subtraction in order to improve the speech-to-noise ratio
- EchoStop – reduces room reverberation and echo
- Stabilizer or Dual Stabilizer II DFS feedback management – proprietary feedback cancellation algorithm designed to reduce false cancellations
- Advanced data-logging – stores usage data and provides efficient trouble-shooting and customization
- SmartStart power-up timer
- Up to 4 customizable programs
- Acoustic indicator for program selection
- Acoustic indicator for volume control
- Low-battery warning indicator
- Power-saving chip technology

Options of XE40/D HS

- Dual microphone technology
- Push button
- Programmable volume control
- Programmable telecoil with T/MT modes
- Available in 3 different colors
- Supports StepVent
- Open-fitting capabilities with an IROS vent

Features of XE40-P/DP HS Power

- MultiScope Adaptive Directionality – lets you select different beam widths to effectively reduce multiple competing background sounds; 2 beam widths
- SoftSwitching – automatically switches between omnidirectional and directional modes
- Integrated Microphone Matching – allows for increased precision of MultiScope Adaptive Directionality
- Acceptance Manager – gradually increases gain over time to allow patients to adapt to amplification

- Active Wind Stop – reduces wind noise
- 17-band WARP compression – provides superb sound quality based on fast processing and accurate resolution
- NoiseTracker II – a proprietary algorithm employing spectral subtraction in order to improve the speech-to-noise ratio
- EchoStop – reduces room reverberation and echo
- Stabilizer or Dual Stabilizer II DFS feedback management – proprietary feedback cancellation algorithm designed to reduce false cancellations
- Advanced data-logging – stores usage data and provides efficient trouble-shooting and customization
- SmartStart power-up timer
- Up to 4 customizable programs
- Acoustic indicator for program selection
- Acoustic indicator for volume control
- Low-battery warning indicator
- Power-saving chip technology

Options of XE40-P/DP HS Power
- Dual microphone technology
- Push button
- Programmable volume control
- Programmable telecoil with T/MT modes
- Available in 3 different colors
- Supports StepVent

Features of XE30/D ITC
- MultiScope Adaptive Directionality – lets you select different beam widths to effectively reduce multiple competing background sounds; 2 beam widths
- SoftSwitching – automatically switches between omnidirectional and directional modes
- Integrated Microphone Matching – allows for increased precision of MultiScope Adaptive Directionality
- Acceptance Manager – gradually increases gain over time to allow patients to adapt to amplification
- Active Wind Stop – reduces wind noise
- 17-band WARP compression – provides superb sound quality based on fast processing and accurate resolution
- NoiseTracker II – a proprietary algorithm employing spectral subtraction in order to improve the speech-to-noise ratio
- EchoStop – reduces room reverberation and echo
- Stabilizer or Dual Stabilizer II DFS feedback management – proprietary feedback cancellation algorithm designed to reduce false cancellations
- Advanced data-logging – stores usage data and provides efficient trouble-shooting and customization

- SmartStart power-up timer
- Up to 4 customizable programs
- Acoustic indicator for program selection
- Acoustic indicator for volume control
- Low-battery warning indicator
- Power-saving chip technology

Options of XE30/D ITC

- Dual microphone technology
- Push button
- Choice of 312 or 10 battery size
- Programmable volume control
- Programmable telecoil with T/MT modes
- Available in 3 different colors
- Supports StepVent
- Open-fitting capabilities with an IROS vent

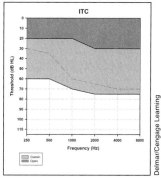

Fitting range for XE30/D ITC:
open (dark and light gray
to dashed line) and classic
(entire light gray region)

Features of XE30-P/DP ITC Power

- MultiScope Adaptive Directionality – lets you select different beam widths to effectively reduce multiple competing background sounds; 2 beam widths
- SoftSwitching – automatically switches between omnidirectional and directional modes
- Integrated Microphone Matching – allows for increased precision of MultiScope Adaptive Directionality
- Acceptance Manager – gradually increases gain over time to allow patients to adapt to amplification
- Active Wind Stop – reduces wind noise
- 17-band WARP compression – provides superb sound quality based on fast processing and accurate resolution
- NoiseTracker II – a proprietary algorithm employing spectral subtraction in order to improve the speech-to-noise ratio
- EchoStop – reduces room reverberation and echo
- Stabilizer or Dual Stabilizer II DFS feedback management – proprietary feedback cancellation algorithm designed to reduce false cancellations
- Advanced data-logging – stores usage data and provides efficient troubleshooting and customization
- SmartStart power-up timer
- Up to 4 customizable programs
- Acoustic indicator for program selection
- Acoustic indicator for volume control
- Low-battery warning indicator
- Power-saving chip technology

Options of XE30-P/DP ITC Power

- Dual microphone technology
- Push button
- Programmable volume control
- Programmable telecoil with T/MT modes
- Available in 3 different colors
- Supports StepVent

Features of XE20 MC

- Acceptance Manager – gradually increases gain over time to allow patients to adapt to amplification
- Active Wind Stop – reduces wind noise
- 17-band WARP compression – provides superb sound quality based on fast processing and accurate resolution
- NoiseTracker II – a proprietary algorithm employing spectral subtraction in order to improve the speech-to-noise ratio
- Stabilizer II DFS feedback management – provides more usable gain with virtually no artifacts
- Advanced data-logging – stores usage data and provides efficient troubleshooting and customization
- SmartStart power-up timer
- Up to 4 customizable programs
- Acoustic indicator for program selection
- Acoustic indicator for volume control
- Low-battery warning indicator
- Power-saving chip technology

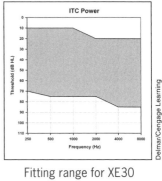

Fitting range for XE30 Power ITC

Options of XE20 MC

- Push button
- Programmable volume control
- Available in 3 different colors
- Supports StepVent
- Open-fitting capabilities with an IROS vent

Features of XE20-P MC Power

- Acceptance Manager – gradually increases gain over time to allow patients to adapt to amplification
- Active Wind Stop – reduces wind noise

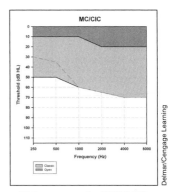

Fitting range for XE20 MC, XE10 CIC, and XE10 B CIC: open (dark and light gray to dashed line) and classic (entire light gray region)

- 17-band WARP compression – provides superb sound quality based on fast processing and accurate resolution
- NoiseTracker II – a proprietary algorithm employing spectral subtraction in order to improve the speech-to-noise ratio
- Stabilizer II DFS feedback management – provides more usable gain with virtually no artifacts
- Advanced data-logging – stores usage data and provides efficient trouble-shooting and customization
- SmartStart power-up timer
- Up to 4 customizable programs
- Acoustic indicator for program selection
- Acoustic indicator for volume control
- Low-battery warning indicator
- Power-saving chip technology

Options of XE20-P MC Power

- Push button
- Programmable volume control
- Available in 3 different colors
- Supports StepVent

Features of XE10 CIC

- Acceptance Manager – gradually increases gain over time to allow patients to adapt to amplification
- Active Wind Stop – reduces wind noise
- 17-band WARP compression – provides superb sound quality based on fast processing and accurate resolution
- NoiseTracker II – a proprietary algorithm employing spectral subtraction in order to improve the speech-to-noise ratio
- Stabilizer II DFS feedback management – provides more usable gain with virtually no artifacts
- Advanced data-logging – stores usage data and provides efficient trouble-shooting and customization
- SmartStart power-up timer
- Low-battery warning indicator
- Power-saving chip technology

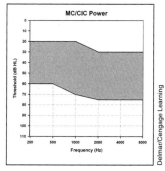

Fitting range for XE20 Power MC, XE10 B Power CIC, and XE10 Power CIC

Options of XE10 CIC

- Available in 3 different colors
- Supports StepVent
- Open-fitting capabilities with an IROS vent

Features of XE10-B CIC

- Acceptance Manager – gradually increases gain over time to allow patients to adapt to amplification
- Active Wind Stop – reduces wind noise
- 17-band WARP compression – provides superb sound quality based on fast processing and accurate resolution
- NoiseTracker II – a proprietary algorithm employing spectral subtraction in order to improve the speech-to-noise ratio
- Stabilizer II DFS feedback management – provides more usable gain with virtually no artifacts
- Advanced data-logging – stores usage data and provides efficient trouble-shooting and customization
- SmartStart power-up timer
- Up to 4 customizable programs
- Acoustic indicator for program selection
- Low-battery warning indicator
- Power-saving chip technology

Options of XE10-B CIC

- Push button
- Available in 3 different colors
- Supports StepVent
- Open-fitting capabilities with an IROS vent

Features of XE10-BP CIC Power

- Acceptance Manager – gradually increases gain over time to allow patients to adapt to amplification
- Active Wind Stop – reduces wind noise
- 17-band WARP compression – provides superb sound quality based on fast processing and accurate resolution
- NoiseTracker II – a proprietary algorithm employing spectral subtraction in order to improve the speech-to-noise ratio
- Stabilizer II DFS feedback management – provides more usable gain with virtually no artifacts
- Advanced data-logging – stores usage data and provides efficient trouble-shooting and customization
- SmartStart power-up timer
- Up to 4 customizable programs
- Acoustic indicator for program selection
- Low-battery warning indicator
- Power-saving chip technology

Options of XE10-BP CIC Power

- Push button
- Available in 3 different colors
- Supports StepVent

Features of XE10-P CIC Power

- Acceptance Manager – gradually increases gain over time to allow patients to adapt to amplification
- Active Wind Stop – reduces wind noise
- 17-band WARP compression – provides superb sound quality based on fast processing and accurate resolution
- NoiseTracker II – a proprietary algorithm employing spectral subtraction in order to improve the speech-to-noise ratio
- Stabilizer II DFS feedback management – provides more usable gain with virtually no artifacts
- Advanced data-logging – stores usage data and provides efficient trouble-shooting and customization
- SmartStart power-up timer
- Low-battery warning indicator
- Power-saving chip technology

Options of XE10-P CIC Power

- Available in 3 different colors
- Supports StepVent

Typical Specifications		XE80-DVI Power BTE	XE71-DVI Silhouette BTE Classic/ Thin Tube Open	XE60-DI Mini BTE Classic/Thin Tube Open
Standard ANSI S3.22-1996				
Output sound pressure level	Max OSPL 90 (dB SPL)	136	126/129	126/127
	HFA OSPL 90 (dB SPL)	129	125/120	120/117
Full-on gain (50 dB SPL input)	Peak gain (dB)	65	56/51	53/50
	HFA (dB)	60	51/45	46/41
Total harmonic distortion (Hz)	500	1.8%	1.7%/0.5%	0.9%
	800	0.6%	1.2%/0.1%	1.0%/0.1%
	1600	0.4%	0.5%/0.7%	0.6%/0.7%
Equivalent input noise (dB SPL), without noise reduction		22	25/37	26/28
Telecoil sensitivity	10 mA/m input max (dB SPL)	113	108/102	105/100
Battery	Operating current (mA)	0.85	0.9	0.9/0.85
	Battery type	13	13	13
Compression characteristics	Attack (ms)	12	12	12
	Release (ms)	70	70	70

Delmar/Cengage Learning

Typical Specifications		XE40/D HS XE50/D FS	XE40-P/DP Power HS XE50-P/DP Power FS	XE30/D ITC	XE30-P/ DP Power ITC
Standard ANSI S3.22-1996					
Output sound pressure level	Max OSPL 90 (dB SPL)	120	126	112	119
	HFA OSPL 90 (dB SPL)	116	123	110	115
Full-on gain (50 dB SPL input)	Peak gain (dB)	52	59	43	50
	HFA (dB)	46	53	39	44
Total harmonic distortion (Hz)	500	1.2%	0.6%	1.1%	1.0%
	800	1.1%	0.9%	1.1%	0.8%
	1600	1.9%	1.0%	1.3%	1.3%
Equivalent input noise (dB SPL), without noise reduction		26	24	25	26
Telecoil sensitivity	10 mA/m input max (dB SPL)	102	109	93	100
Battery	Operating current (mA)	1.04	1.05	0.95	1.0
	Battery type	13/312	13/312	312/10	312
Compression characteristics	Attack (ms)	12	12	12	12
	Release (ms)	70	70	70	70

Delmar/Cengage Learning

Typical Specifications		XE20 MC	XE20-P Power MC	XE10 CIC	XE10-B CIC
Standard ANSI S3.22-1996					
Output sound pressure level	Max OSPL 90 (dB SPL)	108	113	108	108
	HFA OSPL 90 (dB SPL)	106	110	106	105
Full-on gain (50 dB SPL input)	Peak gain (dB)	31	39	31	31
	HFA (dB)	28	33%	28	28
Total harmonic distortion (Hz)	500	0.5%	1.1%	0.5%	0.5%
	800	0.5%	1.2%	0.5%	0.4%
	1600	0.4%	1.6%	0.4%	0.9%
Equivalent input noise (dB SPL), without noise reduction		24	25	24	29

continues

continued

Typical Specifications		XE20 MC	XE20-P Power MC	XE10 CIC	XE10-B CIC
Telecoil sensitivity	10 mA/m input max (dB SPL)	n/a	n/a	n/a	n/a
Battery	Operating current (mA)	0.87	0.94	0.87	0.85
	Battery type	10	10	10	10
Compression characteristics	Attack (ms)	12	12	12	12
	Release (ms)	70	70	70	70

Delmar/Cengage Learning

Typical Specifications		XE10-BP Power CIC	XE10-P Power CIC
Standard ANSI S3.22-1996			
Output sound pressure level	Max OSPL 90 (dB SPL)	114	113
	HFA OSPL 90 (dB SPL)	111	110
Full-on gain (50 dB SPL input)	Peak gain (dB)	39	39
	HFA (dB)	35	33
Total harmonic distortion (Hz)	500	1.2%	1.1%
	800	0.8%	1.2%
	1600	1.1%	1.6%
Equivalent input noise (dB SPL), without noise reduction		28	25
Telecoil sensitivity	10 mA/m input max (dB SPL)	n/a	n/a
Battery	Operating current drain (mA)	0.92	0.94
	Battery type	10	10
Compression characteristics	Attack (ms)	12	12
	Release (ms)	70	70

Delmar/Cengage Learning

PRODUCT 3: ZIGA

Product Application

ZG71-DVI BTE
ZG71-DI BTE
ZG71-VI BTE
ZG60-DI Mini BTE
ZG60-VI Mini BTE
ZG80-DVI Power BTE

ZG80-VI Power BTE
ZG40/40-D ITE
ZG50/50-D ITE
ZG40-P Power ITE
ZG40-DP Power ITE
ZG50-P Power ITE

ZG50-DP Power ITE   ZG20 MC
ZG30 ITC   ZG20-P Power MC
ZG30-D ITC   ZG10-B CIC
ZG30-P Power ITC   ZG10-P Power CIC
ZG30-DP Power ITC   ZG10-BP Power CIC

Features of ZG71-DVI BTE
- Ergonomic and slim tube
- 9-band WARP sound processing (6 gain handles) – wide dynamic range compression system
- Wide-scope adaptive directionality
- Fixed directionality
- SoftSwitching automatic program
- NoiseTracker noise reduction
- Impulse noise smoother
- Integrated Microphone Matching
- Dual Stabilizer II DFS feedback cancellation – proprietary feedback cancellation algorithm designed to reduce false cancellations
- Open-fitting capabilities
- Data-logging
- SmartStart power-up timer
- Acoustic indicator for program selection
- Acoustic indicator for volume control
- Low-battery warning indicator
- 2 flexible environment programs plus telecoil options
- Low-battery consumption chip technology
- Dual microphone technology
- Best for mild to severe hearing losses

Options of ZG71-DVI BTE
- Push button
- Rechargeable solution
- Programmable volume control
- Programmable telecoil with T and MT modes
- Direct audio input
- Standard hook, mini hook, cosmetic hook, and thin-tube adapter
- Supports dome, Tulip-Dome, FlexVent, and standard ear molds
- Easy reconfiguration between hook and thin-tube adapter
- Available in wide variety of colors

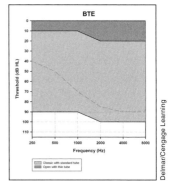

Fitting range for ZG71-DI BTE, ZG71-VI BTE, and ZG71-DVI BTE: open with thin tube (dark and light gray to the dashed line) and classic with standard tube (entire light gray region)

Features of ZG71-DI BTE

- Ergonomic and slim tube
- 9-band WARP sound processing (6 gain handles) – wide dynamic range compression system
- Wide-scope adaptive directionality
- Fixed directionality
- SoftSwitching automatic program
- NoiseTracker noise reduction
- Impulse noise smoother
- Integrated Microphone Matching
- Dual Stabilizer II DFS feedback cancellation – proprietary feedback cancellation algorithm designed to reduce false cancellations
- Open-fitting capabilities
- Data-logging
- SmartStart power-up timer
- Acoustic indicator for program selection
- Low-battery warning indicator
- 2 flexible environment programs plus telecoil options
- Low-battery consumption chip technology
- Dual microphone technology
- Best for mild to severe hearing losses

Options of ZG71-DI BTE

- Push button
- Rechargeable solution
- Programmable telecoil with T and MT modes
- Direct audio input
- Standard hook, mini hook, cosmetic hook, and thin-tube adapter
- Supports dome, Tulip-Dome, FlexVent, and standard ear molds
- Easy reconfiguration between hook and thin-tube adapter
- Available in wide variety of colors

Features of ZG71-VI BTE

- Ergonomic and slim tube
- 9-band WARP sound processing (6 gain handles) – wide dynamic range compression system
- NoiseTracker noise reduction
- Impulse noise smoother
- Integrated Microphone Matching
- Dual Stabilizer II DFS feedback cancellation – proprietary feedback cancellation algorithm designed to reduce false cancellations
- Open-fitting capabilities
- Data-logging

- SmartStart power-up timer
- Acoustic indicator for program selection
- Acoustic indicator for volume control
- Low-battery warning indicator
- 2 flexible environment programs plus telecoil options
- Low-battery consumption chip technology
- Best for mild to severe hearing losses

Options of ZG71-VI BTE

- Push button
- Rechargeable solution
- Programmable volume control
- Programmable telecoil with T and MT modes
- Direct audio input
- Standard hook, mini hook, cosmetic hook, and thin-tube adapter
- Supports dome, Tulip-Dome, FlexVent, and standard ear molds
- Easy reconfiguration between hook and thin-tube adapter
- Available in wide variety of colors

Features of ZG60-DI Mini BTE

- Mini BTE design
- 9-band WARP sound processing (6 gain handles) – wide dynamic range compression system
- Wide-scope adaptive directionality
- Fixed directionality
- SoftSwitching automatic program
- NoiseTracker noise reduction
- Impulse noise smoother
- Integrated Microphone Matching
- Dual Stabilizer II DFS feedback cancellation – proprietary feedback cancellation algorithm designed to reduce false cancellations
- Open-fitting capabilities
- Data-logging
- SmartStart power-up timer
- Acoustic indicator for program selection
- Low-battery warning indicator
- 2 flexible environment programs plus telecoil options
- Low-battery consumption chip technology
- Dual microphone technology
- Best for mild to severe hearing losses

Options of ZG60-DI Mini BTE

- Bluetooth wireless headset
- Rechargeable solution

- Push button
- Programmable telecoil with T and MT modes
- Direct audio input
- Standard hook, mini hook, cosmetic hook, and thin-tube adapter
- Supports dome, Tulip-Dome, FlexVent, and standard ear molds
- Available in wide variety of colors

Features of ZG60-VI Mini BTE

- Mini BTE design
- 9-band WARP sound processing (6 gain handles) – wide dynamic range compression system
- NoiseTracker noise reduction
- Impulse noise smoother
- Dual Stabilizer II DFS feedback cancellation – proprietary feedback cancellation algorithm designed to reduce false cancellations
- Open-fitting capabilities
- Data-logging
- SmartStart power-up timer
- Acoustic indicator for program selection
- Acoustic indicator for volume control
- Low-battery warning indicator
- 2 flexible environment programs plus telecoil options
- Low-battery consumption chip technology
- Best for mild to severe hearing losses

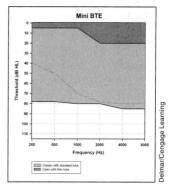

Fitting range for ZG60-DI Mini BTE and ZG60-VI Mini BTE: open with thin tube (dark and light gray to the dashed line) and classic with standard tube (entire light gray region)

Options of ZG60-VI Mini BTE

- Push button
- Bluetooth wireless headset
- Rechargeable solution
- Programmable volume control
- Programmable telecoil with T and MT modes
- Direct audio input
- Standard hook, mini hook, cosmetic hook, and thin-tube adapter
- Supports dome, Tulip-Dome, FlexVent, and standard ear molds
- Available in wide variety of colors

Features of ZG80-DVI Power BTE

- Power BTE
- 9-band WARP sound processing (6 gain handles) – wide dynamic range compression system

- Wide-scope adaptive directionality
- Fixed directionality
- SoftSwitching automatic program
- NoiseTracker noise reduction
- Impulse noise smoother
- Integrated Microphone Matching
- Dual Stabilizer II DFS feedback cancellation – proprietary feedback cancellation algorithm designed to reduce false cancellations
- Open-fitting capabilities
- Data-logging
- SmartStart power-up timer
- Acoustic indicator for program selection
- Acoustic indicator for volume control
- Low-battery warning indicator
- 2 flexible environment programs plus telecoil options
- Low-battery consumption chip technology
- Best for moderate to severe hearing losses

Options of ZG80-DVI Power BTE

- Dual microphone technology
- Push button
- Programmable volume control
- Programmable telecoil with T and MT modes
- Direct audio input
- Available in wide variety of colors

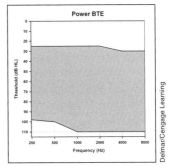

Fitting range for ZG80-DVI Power BTE and ZG80-VI Power BTE

Features of ZG80-VI Power BTE

- Power BTE
- 9-band WARP sound processing (6 gain handles) – wide dynamic range compression system
- NoiseTracker noise reduction
- Impulse noise smoother
- Dual Stabilizer II DFS feedback cancellation – proprietary feedback cancellation algorithm designed to reduce false cancellations
- Data-logging
- SmartStart power-up timer
- Acoustic indicator for program selection
- Acoustic indicator for volume control
- Low-battery warning indicator
- 2 flexible environment programs plus telecoil options
- Low-battery consumption chip technology
- Best for moderate to severe hearing losses

Options of ZG80-VI Power BTE

- Push button
- Programmable volume control
- Programmable telecoil with T and MT modes
- Direct audio input
- Available in wide variety of colors

Features of ZG40/40-D ITE

- In-the-ear (ITE)
- 9-band WARP sound processing (6 gain handles) – wide dynamic range compression system
- Wide-scope adaptive directionality (ZG40-D only)
- Fixed directionality (ZG40-D only)
- SoftSwitching automatic program (ZG40-D only)
- NoiseTracker noise reduction
- Impulse noise smoother
- Integrated Microphone Matching (ZG40-D only)
- Dual Stabilizer II DFS feedback cancellation – proprietary feedback cancellation algorithm designed to reduce false cancellations
- Data-logging
- SmartStart power-up timer
- Acoustic indicator for program selection
- Acoustic indicator for volume control
- Low-battery warning indicator
- 2 flexible environment programs plus telecoil options
- Low-battery consumption chip technology
- Best for mild to severe hearing losses

Options of ZG40/40-D ITE

- Dual microphone technology (ZG40-D only)
- Push button
- Programmable volume control (optional)
- Programmable telecoil with T and MT modes (optional)
- Available in 3 colors
- Supports StepVent

Features of ZG50/50-D ITE

- ITE
- 9-band WARP sound processing (6 gain handles) – wide dynamic range compression system
- Wide-scope adaptive directionality (ZG50-D only)

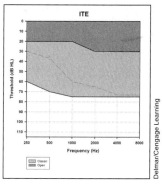

Fitting range for ZG40-D ITE and ZG50-D ITE: open (dark and light gray to the dashed line) and classic (entire light gray region)

- Fixed directionality (ZG50-D only)
- SoftSwitching automatic program (ZG50-D only)
- NoiseTracker noise reduction
- Impulse noise smoother
- Integrated Microphone Matching (ZG50-D only)
- Dual Stabilizer II DFS feedback cancellation – proprietary feedback cancellation algorithm designed to reduce false cancellations
- Data-logging
- SmartStart power-up timer
- Acoustic indicator for program selection
- Acoustic indicator for volume control
- Low-battery warning indicator
- 2 flexible environment programs plus telecoil options
- Low-battery consumption chip technology
- Best for mild to severe hearing losses

Options of ZG50/50-D ITE

- Dual microphone technology (ZG50-D only)
- Push button
- Programmable volume control (optional)
- Programmable telecoil with T and MT modes (optional)
- Available in 3 colors
- Supports StepVent

Features of ZG40-P Power ITE

- Power ITE
- 9-band WARP sound processing (6 gain handles) – wide dynamic range compression system
- NoiseTracker noise reduction
- Impulse noise smoother
- Dual Stabilizer II DFS feedback cancellation – proprietary feedback cancellation algorithm designed to reduce false cancellations
- Data-logging
- SmartStart power-up timer
- Acoustic indicator for program selection
- Acoustic indicator for volume control
- Low-battery warning indicator
- 2 flexible environment programs plus telecoil options
- Low-battery consumption chip technology
- Best for mild to severe hearing losses

Options of ZG40-P Power ITE

- Push button
- Programmable volume control (optional)

- Programmable telecoil with T and MT modes (optional)
- Available in 3 colors

Features of ZG40-DP Power ITE

- Power ITE
- 9-band WARP sound processing (6 gain handles) – wide dynamic range compression system
- Wide-scope adaptive directionality
- Fixed directionality
- SoftSwitching automatic program
- NoiseTracker noise reduction
- Impulse noise smoother
- Integrated Microphone Matching
- Dual Stabilizer II DFS feedback cancellation – proprietary feedback cancellation algorithm designed to reduce false cancellations Data-logging
- SmartStart power-up timer
- Acoustic indicator for program selection
- Acoustic indicator for volume control
- Low-battery warning indicator
- 2 flexible environment programs plus telecoil options
- Low-battery consumption chip technology
- Best for mild to severe hearing losses

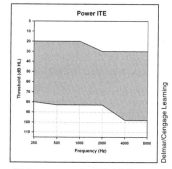

Fitting range for ZG40 Power ITE and ZG50 Power ITE

Options of ZG50-DP Power ITE

- Dual microphone technology
- Push button
- Programmable volume control (optional)
- Programmable telecoil with T and MT modes (optional)
- Available in 3 colors

Features of ZG50-P Power ITE

- Power ITE
- 9-band WARP sound processing (6 gain handles) – wide dynamic range compression system
- NoiseTracker noise reduction
- Impulse noise smoother
- Dual Stabilizer II DFS feedback cancellation – proprietary feedback cancellation algorithm designed to reduce false cancellations
- Data-logging
- SmartStart power-up timer
- Acoustic indicator for program selection
- Acoustic indicator for volume control

- Low-battery warning indicator
- 2 flexible environment programs plus telecoil options
- Low-battery consumption chip technology
- Best for mild to severe hearing losses

Options of ZG50-P Power ITE

- Push button
- Programmable volume control (optional)
- Programmable telecoil with T and MT modes (optional)
- Available in 3 colors

Features of ZG50-DP Power ITE

- Power ITE
- 9-band WARP sound processing (6 gain handles) – wide dynamic range compression system
- Wide-scope adaptive directionality
- Fixed directionality
- SoftSwitching automatic program
- NoiseTracker noise reduction
- Impulse noise smoother
- Integrated Microphone Matching
- Dual Stabilizer II DFS feedback cancellation – proprietary feedback cancellation algorithm designed to reduce false cancellations
- Data-logging
- SmartStart power-up timer
- Acoustic indicator for program selection
- Acoustic indicator for volume control
- Low-battery warning indicator
- 2 flexible environment programs plus telecoil options
- Low-battery consumption chip technology
- Best for mild to severe hearing losses

Options of ZG50-DP Power ITE

- Dual microphone technology
- Push button
- Programmable volume control (optional)
- Programmable telecoil with T and MT modes (optional)
- Available in 3 colors

Features of ZG30 ITC

- In-the-canal (ITC)
- 9-band WARP sound processing (6 gain handles) – wide dynamic range compression system
- NoiseTracker noise reduction
- Impulse noise smoother

- Dual Stabilizer II DFS feedback cancellation – proprietary feedback cancellation algorithm designed to reduce false cancellations
- Open-fitting capabilities
- Data-logging
- SmartStart power-up timer
- Acoustic indicator for program selection
- Acoustic indicator for volume control
- Low-battery warning indicator
- 2 flexible environment programs plus telecoil options
- Low-battery consumption chip technology
- Best for mild to severe hearing losses

Options of ZG30 ITC

- Push button
- Programmable volume control (optional)
- Programmable telecoil with T and MT modes (optional)
- Available in 3 colors

Features of ZG30-D ITC

- ITC
- 9-band WARP sound processing (6 gain handles) – wide dynamic range compression system
- Wide-scope adaptive directionality
- Fixed directionality
- SoftSwitching automatic program
- NoiseTracker noise reduction
- Impulse noise smoother
- Integrated Microphone Matching
- Dual Stabilizer II DFS feedback cancellation – proprietary feedback cancellation algorithm designed to reduce false cancellations
- Open-fitting capabilities
- Data-logging
- SmartStart power-up timer
- Acoustic indicator for program selection
- Acoustic indicator for volume control
- Low-battery warning indicator
- 2 flexible environment programs plus telecoil options
- Low-battery consumption chip technology
- Best for mild to severe hearing losses

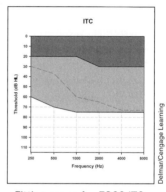

Fitting range for ZG30 ITC: open with thin tube (dark and light gray to dotted line) and classic with standard tube (entire light gray region)

Options of ZG30-D ITC

- Dual microphone technology
- Push button

- Programmable volume control (optional)
- Programmable telecoil with T and MT modes (optional)
- Available in 3 colors

Features of ZG30-P Power ITC

- Power ITC
- 9-band WARP sound processing (6 gain handles) – wide dynamic range compression system
- NoiseTracker noise reduction
- Impulse noise smoother
- Dual Stabilizer II DFS feedback cancellation – proprietary feedback cancellation algorithm designed to reduce false cancellations
- Data-logging
- SmartStart power-up timer
- Acoustic indicator for program selection
- Acoustic indicator for volume control
- Low-battery warning indicator
- 2 flexible environment programs plus telecoil options
- Low-battery consumption chip technology
- Best for mild to severe hearing losses

Options of ZG30-P Power ITC

- Push button (optional)
- Programmable volume control (optional)
- Programmable telecoil with T and MT modes (optional)
- Available in 3 colors

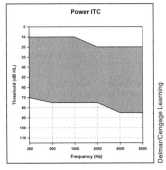

Fitting range for ZG30 Power ITC

Features of ZG30-DP Power ITC

- Power ITC
- 9-band WARP sound processing (6 gain handles) – wide dynamic range compression system
- Wide-scope adaptive directionality
- Fixed directionality
- SoftSwitching Automatic Program
- NoiseTracker noise reduction
- Impulse noise smoother
- Integrated Microphone Matching
- Dual Stabilizer II DFS feedback cancellation – proprietary feedback cancellation algorithm designed to reduce false cancellations
- Data-logging
- SmartStart power-up timer
- Acoustic indicator for program selection

- Acoustic indicator for volume control
- Low-battery warning indicator
- 2 flexible environment programs plus telecoil options
- Low-battery consumption chip technology
- Best for mild to severe hearing losses

Options of ZG30-DP Power ITC

- Dual microphone technology
- Push button (optional)
- Programmable volume control (optional)
- Programmable telecoil with T and MT modes (optional)
- Available in 3 colors

Features of ZG20 MC

- Mini-canal (MC)
- 9-band WARP sound processing (6 gain handles) – wide dynamic range compression system
- NoiseTracker noise reduction
- Impulse noise smoother
- Dual Stabilizer II DFS feedback cancellation – proprietary feedback cancellation algorithm designed to reduce false cancellations
- Open-fitting capabilities
- Data-logging
- SmartStart power-up timer
- Acoustic indicator for program selection
- Acoustic indicator for volume control
- Low-battery warning indicator
- 2 flexible environment programs plus telecoil options
- Low-battery consumption chip technology
- Best for mild to severe hearing losses

Options of ZG20 MC

- Push button (optional)
- Programmable volume control (optional)
- Available in 3 colors
- Supports StepVent

Features of ZG20-P Power MC

- Power mini-canal (MC)
- 9-band WARP sound processing (6 gain handles) – wide dynamic range compression system
- NoiseTracker noise reduction
- Impulse noise smoother

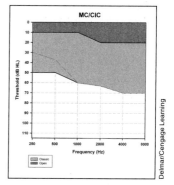

Fitting range for ZG20 MC and ZG10 CIC: open (dark and light gray to dashed line) and classic (entire light gray region)

ReSOUND

Delmar/Cengage Learning

- Dual Stabilizer II DFS feedback cancellation – proprietary feedback cancellation algorithm designed to reduce false cancellations
- Data-logging
- SmartStart power-up timer
- Acoustic indicator for program selection
- Acoustic indicator for volume control
- Low-battery warning indicator
- 2 flexible environment programs plus telecoil options
- Low-battery consumption chip technology
- Best for mild to severe hearing losses

Options of ZG20-P Power MC

- Push button (optional)
- Programmable volume control (optional)
- Available in 3 colors

Features of ZG10-B CIC

- Completely-in-the-canal (CIC)
- 9-band WARP sound processing (6 gain handles) – wide dynamic range compression system
- NoiseTracker noise reduction
- Impulse noise smoother
- Dual Stabilizer II DFS feedback cancellation – proprietary feedback cancellation algorithm designed to reduce false cancellations
- Open-fitting capabilities
- Data-logging
- SmartStart power-up timer
- Acoustic indicator for program selection
- Low-battery warning indicator
- 2 flexible environment programs plus telecoil options
- Low-battery consumption chip technology
- Best for mild to severe hearing losses

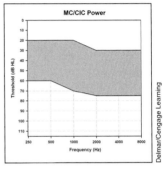

Fitting range for ZG20 MC Power and ZG10 CIC Power

Options of ZG10-B CIC

- Push button
- Available in 3 colors
- Supports StepVent

Features of ZG10-P Power CIC

- Power CIC
- 9-band WARP sound processing (6 gain handles) – wide dynamic range compression system
- NoiseTracker noise reduction

- Impulse noise smoother
- Dual Stabilizer II DFS feedback cancellation – proprietary feedback cancellation algorithm designed to reduce false cancellations
- Data-logging
- SmartStart power-up timer
- Low-battery warning indicator
- Low-battery consumption chip technology
- Best for mild to severe hearing losses

Options of ZG10-P Power CIC

- Available in 3 colors

Features of ZG10-BP Power CIC

- Power CIC
- 9-band WARP sound processing (6 gain handles) – wide dynamic range compression system
- NoiseTracker noise reduction
- Impulse noise smoother
- Dual Stabilizer II DFS feedback cancellation – proprietary feedback cancellation algorithm designed to reduce false cancellations
- Data-logging
- SmartStart power-up timer
- Acoustic indicator for program selection
- Low-battery warning indicator
- Low-battery consumption chip technology
- Best for mild to severe hearing losses

Options of ZG10-BP Power CIC

- Push button
- Available in 3 colors

Typical Specifications		ZG71-DVI BTE, ZG71-DI BTE, ZG71-VI BTE Classic	ZG71-DVI BTE, ZG71-DI BTE, ZG71-VI BTE Open	ZG60-DI Mini BTE, ZG60-VI Mini BTE Classic	ZG60-DI Mini BTE, ZG60-VI Mini BTE Open
IEC 60118-7 2CC coupler					
Output sound pressure level	Max OSPL 90 (dB SPL)	126	129	126	127
	HFA OSPL 90 (dB SPL)	125	120	120	117
Full-on gain (50 dB SPL input)	Peak gain (dB)	56	51	53	50
	HFA (dB)	51	45	46	41

continues

continued

Typical Specifications		ZG71-DVI BTE, ZG71-DI BTE, ZG71-VI BTE Classic	ZG71-DVI BTE, ZG71-DI BTE, ZG71-VI BTE Open	ZG60-DI Mini BTE, ZG60-VI Mini BTE Classic	ZG60-DI Mini BTE, ZG60-VI Mini BTE Open
Total harmonic distortion (Hz)	500	n/a	n/a	n/a	n/a
	800	1.2%	0.1%	1.0%	0.1%
	1600	0.5%	0.7%	0.6%	0.7%
Equivalent Input noise (dB SPL), without noise reduction		25	37	26	28
Telecoil sensitivity	31.6 mA/m input max (dB SPL)	108	102	105	100
Battery	Operating current (mA)	0.9	0.9	0.9	0.85
	Battery type	13	13	13	13

Delmar/Cengage Learning

Typical Specifications		ZG80-DVI Power BTE, ZG80-VI Power BTE	ZG40/40-D ITE, ZG50/50-D ITE	ZG40-P Power ITE, ZG40-DP Power ITE, ZG50-P Power ITE, ZG50-DP Power ITE	ZG30 ITC, ZG30-D ITC
IEC 60118-7 2CC coupler					
Output sound pressure level	Max OSPL 90 (dB SPL)	136	120	126	112
	HFA OSPL 90 (dB SPL)	129	116	123	110
Full-on gain (50 dB SPL input)	Peak gain (dB)	65	52	59	43
	HFA (dB)	60	46	53	39
Total harmonic distortion (Hz)	500	n/a	n/a	n/a	n/a
	800	0.6%	1.1%	0.9%	1.1%
	1600	0.4%	1.9%	1.0%	1.3%
Equivalent input noise (dB SPL), without noise reduction		22	26	24	25
Telecoil sensitivity	31.6 mA/m input max (dB SPL)	113	99	107	90
Battery	Operating current (mA)	0.85	1.04	1.05	0.95
	Battery type	13	13, 312	13, 312	312

Delmar/Cengage Learning

Typical Specifications		ZG30-P Power ITC, ZG30-DP Power ITC	ZG20 MC	ZG20-P Power MC	ZG10-B CIC
IEC 60118-7 2CC coupler					
Output sound pressure level	Max OSPL 90 (dB SPL)	119	108	113	108
	HFA OSPL 90 (dB SPL)	115	106	110	105
Full-on gain (50 dB SPL input)	Peak gain (dB)	50	31	39	31
	HFA (dB)	44	28	33	28
Total harmonic distortion (Hz)	500	n/a	n/a	n/a	n/a
	800	0.8%	0.5%	1.2%	0.4%
	1600	1.3%	0.4%	0.6%	0.9%
Equivalent input noise (dB SPL), without noise reduction		26	24	25	29
Telecoil sensitivity	31.6 mA/m input max (dB SPL)	98	n/a	n/a	n/a
Battery	Operating current (mA)	1.00	0.87	0.94	0.85
	Battery type	312	10	10	10

Delmar/Cengage Learning

Typical Specifications		ZG10-P Power CIC, ZG10-BP Power CIC	ZG10-P Power CIC	ZG10-BP Power CIC
IEC 60118-7 2CC coupler				
Output sound pressure level	Max OSPL 90 (dB SPL)	108	113	114
	HFA OSPL 90 (dB SPL)	105	110	111
Full-on gain (50 dB SPL input)	Peak gain (dB)	31	39	39
	HFA (dB)	28	33	35
Total harmonic distortion (Hz)	500	n/a	n/a	n/a
	800	0.4%	1.2%	0.8%
	1600	0.9%	1.6%	1.1%
Equivalent input noise (dB SPL), without noise reduction		29	25	29
Telecoil sensitivity	31.6 mA/m input max (dB SPL)	n/a	n/a	n/a
Battery	Operating current (mA)	0.85	0.94	0.92
	Battery type	10	10	10

Delmar/Cengage Learning

ReSOUND

PRODUCT 4: DOT²

Product Application

DTT 360 RITE	DTT 260 Low Power RITE
DTT 360 High Power RITE	DTT 160 RITE
DTT 360 Low Power RITE	DTT 160 High Power RITE
DTT 260 RITE	DTT 160 Low Power RITE
DTT 260 High Power RITE	

Features of DTT 360 RITE, DTT 360 High Power RITE, and DTT 360 Low Power RITE

- Ultimate Surround sound processor with integrated wind noise suppression – sound streams are split into low- and high-frequency bands for independent processing
- Ultimate Personalized blending point – the cutoff frequency between bands is adjustable
- Ultimate 17-Band warp compression, expanded bandwidth to 7 kHz-high resolution compression
- Ultimate Dual stabilizer II DFS with whistle control – proprietary feedback cancellation algorithm designed to reduce false cancellations
- Ultimate Noise tracker II noise reduction – a proprietary algorithm employing spectral subtraction in order to improve the speech-to-noise ratio
- Ultimate Natural directionality II – bilateral fitting strategy employing a directional microphone on one ear and an omnidirectional microphone on the other
- Ultimate Auto scope adaptive directionality – directional microphone system that also adapts the size of the preferred listening direction
- Ultimate Multi scope adaptive directionality – lets you select different beam widths to effectively reduce multiple competing background sounds; 2 beam widths
- Ultimate Soft switching – automatically switches between omnidirectional and directional modes
- Ultimate Fixed directionality
- Ultimate Echo stop – reduces room reverberation and echo
- Ultimate Environmental optimizer – delivers automatic, personally optimized gain in 7 different environments
- Ultimate Onboard analyzer II data logging – stores usage data and provides efficient troubleshooting and customization
- Ultimate Smart start power-up timer
- 9 Gain handles

Options of DTT 360 RITE, DTT 360 High Power RITE, and DTT 360 Low Power RITE

- Up to 4 programs
- Open fitting capabilities

- Choice of multiple domes and custom micro-mold
- Low power (LP) and high power (HP) receiver options
- Available in 15 colors

Features of DTT 260 RITE, DTT 260 High Power RITE, and DTT 260 Low Power RITE

- Ultimate Surround sound processor with integrated wind noise suppression – sound streams are split into low- and high-frequency bands for independent processing
- Advanced Personalized blending point – the cutoff frequency between bands is adjustable
- Ultimate 17-Band warp compression, expanded bandwidth to 7 kHz-high resolution compression
- Ultimate Dual stabilizer II DFS with advanced whistle control – proprietary feedback cancellation algorithm designed to reduce false cancellations
- Advanced Noise tracker II noise reduction – a proprietary algorithm employing spectral subtraction in order to improve the speech-to-noise ratio
- Advanced Multi scope adaptive directionality – lets you select different beam widths to effectively reduce multiple competing background sounds; 2 beam widths
- Ultimate Soft switching – automatically switches between omnidirectional and directional modes
- Ultimate Fixed directionality
- Ultimate Echo stop – reduces room reverberation and echo
- Advanced Onboard analyzer II data logging – stores usage data and provides efficient troubleshooting and customization
- Ultimate Smart start power-up timer
- 7 Gain handles

Options of DTT 260 RITE, DTT 260 High Power RITE, and DTT 260 Low Power RITE

- Up to 4 programs
- Open fitting capabilities
- Choice of multiple domes and custom micro-mold
- Low power (LP) and high power (HP) receiver options
- Available in 15 colors

Features of DTT 160 RITE, DTT 160 High Power RITE, and DTT 160 Low Power RITE

- Ultimate Surround sound processor with integrated wind noise suppression – sound streams are split into low- and high-frequency bands for independent processing
- Advanced Personalized blending point – the cutoff frequency between bands is adjustable

- Advanced 9-Band warp compression, expanded bandwidth to 7 kHz-high resolution compression
- Ultimate Dual stabilizer II DFS with whistle control – proprietary feedback cancellation algorithm designed to reduce false cancellations
- Standard Noise tracker II noise reduction – a proprietary algorithm employing spectral subtraction in order to improve the speech-to-noise ratio
- Standard Adaptive directionality
- Ultimate Soft switching – automatically switches between omnidirectional and directional modes
- Ultimate Fixed directionality
- Ultimate Echo stop – reduces room reverberation and echo
- Advanced Onboard analyzer II data logging – stores usage data and provides efficient troubleshooting and customization
- Ultimate Smart start power-up timer
- 6 Gain handles

Options of DTT 160 RITE, DTT 160 High Power RITE, and DTT 160 Low Power RITE

- Up to 4 programs
- Open fitting capabilities
- Choice of multiple domes and custom micro-mold
- Low power (LP) and high power (HP) receiver options
- Available in 15 colors

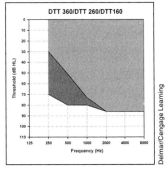

Fitting range for DTT360 RITE, DTT 260 RITE, and DTT 160 RITE open (light gray) and closed (all shaded regions)

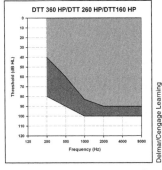

Fitting range for DTT360 HP RITE, DTT 260 HP RITE, and DTT 160 HP RITE open (light gray) and closed (all shaded regions)

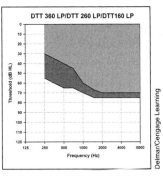

Fitting range for DTT360 LP RITE, DTT 260 LP RITE, and DTT 160 LP RITE open (light gray) and closed (all shaded regions)

Typical Specifications		DTT360 RITE (closed), DTT260 RITE (closed), DTT160 RITE (closed)	DTT360 RITE (open), DTT260 RITE (open), DTT160 RITE (open)	DTT360 RITE HP (closed), DTT260 RITE HP (closed), DT160 RITE HP (closed)	DTT360 RITE HP (open), DTT260 RITE HP (open), DTT160 RITE HP (open)
Standard ANSI S3.22-2003					
Output sound pressure level	Max OSPL 90 (dB SPL)	115	114	119	117
	HFA OSPL 90 (dB SPL)	110	110	113	114
Full-on gain (50 dB SPL input)	Peak gain (dB)	50	49	57	52
	HFA (dB)	42	42	46	47
Total harmonic distortion (Hz)	500	1.1%	1.1%	1.1%	1%
	800	0.9%	0.7%	0.9%	0.6%
	1600	1%	0.9%	1.3%	0.8%
Equivalent input noise (dB SPL), without noise reduction		29	28	27	26
Telecoil sensitivity	10 mA/m input max (dB SPL)	n/a	n/a	n/a	n/a
Battery	Operating current (mA)	0.9	0.9	0.9	0.9
	Battery type	10A	10A	10A	10A
Compression characteristics	Attack (ms)	12	12	12	12
	Release (ms)	70	70	70	70

Delmar/Cengage Learning

Typical Specifications		DTT360 RITE LP (closed), DTT260 RITE LP (closed), DTT160 RITE LP (closed)	DTT360 RITE LP (open), DTT260 RITE LP (open), DTT160 RITE LP (open)
Standard ANSI S3.22-2003			
Output sound pressure level	Max OSPL 90 (dB SPL)	108	107
	HFA OSPL 90 (dB SPL)	104	104
Full-on gain (50 dB SPL input)	Peak gain (dB)	43	42
	HFA (dB)	35	35
Total harmonic distortion (Hz)	500	1.1%	1.1%
	800	0.8%	0.8%
	1600	0.8%	0.7%
Equivalent input noise (dB SPL), without noise reduction		26	26

ReSOUND

continues

continued

Typical Specifications		DTT360 RITE LP (closed), DTT260 RITE LP (closed), DTT160 RITE LP (closed)	DTT360 RITE LP (open), DTT260 RITE LP (open), DTT160 RITE LP (open)
Telecoil sensitivity	10 mA/m input max (dB SPL)	n/a	n/a
Battery	Operating current (mA)	0.9	0.9
	Battery type	10A	10A
Compression characteristics	Attack (ms)	12	12
	Release (ms)	70	70

Delmar/Cengage Learning

PRODUCT 5: DOT

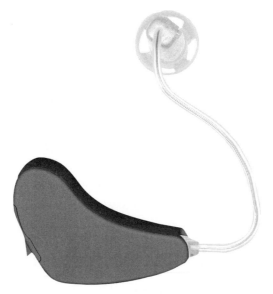

Dot BTE
Courtesy of ReSound

Product Application

DT3060 RITE
DT3060 RITE High Power
DT2060 RITE
DT2060 RITE High Power
DT1060 RITE
DT1060 RITE High Power

Features of DT3060 RITE/DT3060 RITE High Power

- Receiver-in-the-ear (RITE) and RITE high-power
- Ultimate 17-band WARP sound processing
- 9 gain handles in Aventa™
- Dual Stabilizer II DFS feedback cancellation – proprietary feedback cancellation algorithm designed to reduce false cancellations
- Open-fitting
- Ultimate Environmental Optimizer™ – allows for independent adjustment in specific environments
- Ultimate Natural Directionality™ – a combination of maximum speech clarity while maintaining full peripheral awareness
- Ultimate MultiScope Adaptive Directionality – directional microphone system with 3 different beam-width options
- SoftSwitching automatic program
- Ultimate NoiseTracker II noise reduction – reduces background noise
- Ultimate Acceptance Manager – gradual adaptation of gain levels
- EchoStop – reduces echo
- WindRush Manager™ – wind noise-suppression
- Ultimate Onboard Analyzer™ data-logging

Options of DT3060 RITE/DT3060 RITE High Power

- Dual microphone technology
- Integrated Microphone Matching
- Low-level expansion
- SmartStart power-up timer
- Low-battery warning indicator
- Available in 14 colors

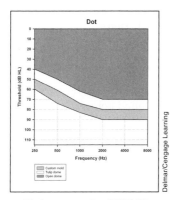

Fitting range for DT3060 RITE, DT2060 RITE, and DT1060 RITE: open dome (dark gray), tulip dome (white), and custom mold (light gray)

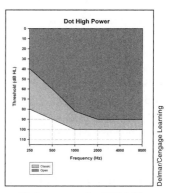

Fitting range for DT3060 HP RITE, DT2060 HP RITE, and DT1060 HP RITE: open fit (dark gray) and classic (light gray)

Features of DT2060 RITE/DT2060 RITE High Power

- RITE and RITE high power
- Ultimate 17-band WARP sound processing
- 7 gain handles in Aventa
- Dual Stabilizer II DFS feedback cancellation – proprietary feedback cancellation algorithm designed to reduce false cancellations
- Open-fitting
- Advanced MultiScope Adaptive Directionality – directional microphone system with 3 different beam-width options
- SoftSwitching automatic program
- Advanced NoiseTracker II noise reduction – reduces background noise
- Ultimate Acceptance Manager – gradual adaptation of gain levels
- EchoStop – reduces echo
- WindRush Manager – wind noise-suppression
- Advanced Onboard Analyzer data-logging

Options of DT2060 RITE/DT2060 RITE High Power

- Dual microphone technology
- Integrated Microphone Matching
- Low-level expansion
- SmartStart power-up timer
- Low-battery warning indicator
- Available in 14 colors

Features of DT1060 RITE/DT1060 RITE High Power

- RITE and RITE high-power
- 6 gain handles in Aventa
- Dual Stabilizer II DFS feedback cancellation – proprietary feedback cancellation algorithm designed to reduce false cancellations
- Open-fitting
- Basic Adaptive Directionality – directional microphone system with 3 different beam-width options
- SoftSwitching automatic program
- Basic NoiseTracker noise reduction – reduces background noise
- EchoStop – reduces echo
- WindRush Manager – wind noise-suppression
- Basic Onboard Analyzer data-logging

Options of DT1060 RITE/DT1060 RITE High Power

- Dual microphone technology
- Integrated Microphone Matching
- Low-level expansion
- SmartStart power-up timer
- Low-battery warning indicator
- Available in 14 colors

Typical Specifications		DT3060 RITE, DT2060 RITE, DT1060 RITE	DT3060 RITE HP, DT2060 RITE HP, DT1060 RITE HP
Standard ANSI S3.22-2003			
Output sound pressure level	Max OSPL 90 (dB SPL)	114	119
	HFA OSPL 90 (dB SPL)	110	113
Full-on gain (50 dB SPL input)	Peak gain (dB)	49	57
	HFA (dB)	42	46
Total harmonic distortion (Hz)	500	1.1%	1.1%
	800	0.7%	0.9%
	1600	0.9%	1.3%
Equivalent input noise (dB SPL), without noise reduction		28	27
Telecoil sensitivity	10 mA/m input max (dB SPL)	n/a	n/a
Battery	Operating current (mA)	0.8	0.88
	Battery type	10	10
Compression characteristics	Attack (ms)	5	5
	Release (ms)	60	60

Delmar/Cengage Learning

PRODUCT 6: BE

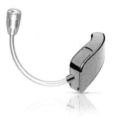

BE BTE
Courtesy of ReSound

Product Application

BE900
BE700

Features of BE900

- Invisible Open Technology™ (IOT)
- 17-band WARP sound processing
- 9 gain handles in Aventa
- Stabilizer II DFS feedback suppression – produces fewer sound artifacts
- Ultimate Environmental Optimizer – allows for independent adjustment in different specific environments
- Ultimate NoiseTracker II noise reduction – reduces background noise

- Ultimate Acceptance Manager – gradual adaptation of gain levels
- Ultimate Onboard Analyzer data-logging
- Best for mild to moderate hearing losses

Options of BE900

- Coyote 3.1 chip technology for extended battery life
- Low-level expansion
- SmartStart power-up timer
- Low-battery warning indicator

Features of BE700

- Invisible Open Technology
- 17-band WARP sound processing
- 7 gain handles in Aventa
- Stabilizer II DFS Feedback suppression – produces fewer sound artifacts
- Advanced NoiseTracker II noise reduction – reduces background noise
- Advanced Onboard Analyzer data-logging
- Best for mild to moderate hearing losses

Options of BE700

- Coyote 3.1 chip technology for extended battery life
- Low-level expansion
- SmartStart power-up timer
- Low-battery warning indicator

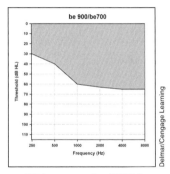

Fitting range for BE900 IOT and BE700 IOT

Typical Specifications		BE900 / BE700
Standard ANSI S3.22-2003		
Output sound pressure level	Max OSPL 90 (dB SPL)	109
	HFA OSPL 90 (dB SPL)	106
Full-on gain (50 dB SPL input)	Peak gain (dB)	34
	HFA (dB)	32
Total harmonic distortion (Hz)	500	1.4%
	800	0.9%
	1600	1.3%
Equivalent input noise (dB SPL), without noise reduction		24
Telecoil sensitivity	10 mA/m input max (dB SPL)	n/a
Battery	Operating current (mA)	0.9
	Battery type	10
Compression characteristics	Attack (ms)	2
	Release (ms)	40

Delmar/Cengage Learning

PRODUCT 7: SPARX

Product Application

SP90-VI Super Power BTE

Features of SP90-VI Super Power BTE

- 9-band WARP sound processing
- 6 gain handles in Aventa
- Sixth-generation DFS feedback manager
- Choice of linear or WDRC amplification strategy
- Multi-channel MPO
- Improved receiver for low-frequency optimization
- NoiseTracker II noise reduction – a proprietary algorithm employing spectral subtraction in order to improve the speech-to-noise ratio
- Low-battery consumption chip technology
- Analog volume control (software configurable)
- Up to 3 customizable programs
- Direct audio input
- Telecoil options
- Battery door with integrated ON/OFF switch
- Push-button program selector
- Acoustic indicator for program selection
- Low-battery warning

Options of SP90-VI Super Power BTE

- Programmable telecoil
- Standard and pediatric earhooks (filtered and unfiltered)
- 5 color options

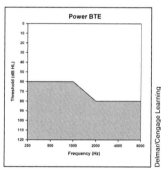

Fitting range for SP90-VI
Super Power BTE

Typical Specifications		SP90-VI Super Power BTE
Standard ANSI S3.22-1996		
Output sound pressure level	Max OSPL 90 (dB SPL)	135
	HFA OSPL 90 (dB SPL)	131
Full-on gain (50 dB SPL input)	Peak gain (dB)	78
	HFA (dB)	71
Total harmonic distortion (Hz)	500	2.0%
	800	0.6%
	1600	1.0%

continues

continued

Typical Specifications		SP90-VI Super Power BTE
Equivalent input noise (dB SPL), without noise reduction		27
Telecoil sensitivity	10 mA/m input max (dB SPL)	116/114 (unfiltered earhook/ filtered earhook)
Battery	Operating current (mA)	2.5
	Battery type	675
Compression characteristics	Attack (ms)	12
	Release (ms)	70

Delmar/Cengage Learning

PRODUCT 8: ESSENCE

| BTE (Behind-the-Ear) | ITE (In-the Ear) —Full shell | ITE (In-the Ear) —Half shell | ITC (In-the-Canal) | CIC (Completely-in-the-Canal) |

Essence family
Courtesy of ReSound

Product Application

ES70-DVI BTE
ES80-DVI Power BTE
ES50/D ITE
ES50 HS/D ITE
ES50-P/DP Power ITE
ES50 HS-P/DP Power ITE
ES30/D ITC
ES30-P/DP Power ITC
ES10 CIC
ES10-P Power CIC

Features of ES70-DVI BTE and ES80-DVI Power BTE

• Ergonomic BTE design
• 6-band WARP sound processing – 6 gain handles
• Dual Stabilizer DFS feedback suppression – proprietary feedback cancellation algorithm designed to reduce false cancellations
• NoiseTracker noise reduction

- Fixed directionality
- Open-fitting capabilities
- Numbered volume control
- 2 flexible environmental programs plus telecoil options
- Acoustic indicator for program selection
- Low-battery warning indicator
- Power-saving chip technology
- Dual microphone technology
- Push-button program selector
- Programmable telecoil with T/MT modes
- DAI capability

Options of ES70-DVI BTE and ES80-DVI Power BTE

- Standard and pediatric hooks
- Volume control cover
- CROS/BiCROS
- 5 color options

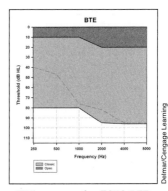

Fitting range for ES70 BTE: open (dark and light gray to dashed line) and classic (entire light gray region)

Features of ES50/D ITE, ES50 HS/D ITE, ES50-P/DP Power ITE, and ES50HS-P/DP Power ITE

- Standard and power full-shell and half-shell models
- 6-band WARP sound processing – 6 gain handles
- Stabilizer or Dual Stabilizer** DFS feedback suppression – proprietary feedback cancellation algorithm designed to reduce false cancellations
- NoiseTracker noise reduction
- Fixed directionality**
- 2 flexible environmental programs plus telecoil options
- Acoustic indicator for program selection
- Low-battery warning indicator
- Power-saving chip technology
- Dual microphone technology**
- Push-button program selector
- Programmable telecoil with T/MT modes

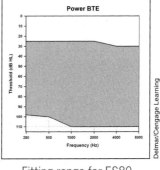

Fitting range for ES80 Power BTE

Options of ES50/D ITE, ES50 HS/D ITE, ES50-P/DP Power ITE, and ES50HS-P/DP Power ITE

- Analog volume control
- 3 color options

**ES50-D, ES50 HS-D, ES50-DP, and ES50 HS-DP only

Features of ES30/D ITC and ES30-P/DP Power ITC

- Standard and power ITC
- 6-band WARP sound processing – 6 gain handles
- Stabilizer or Dual Stabilizer** DFS feedback suppression – proprietary feedback cancellation algorithm designed to reduce false cancellations
- NoiseTracker noise reduction
- Fixed directionality**
- 2 flexible environmental programs plus telecoil options
- Acoustic indicator for program selection
- Low-battery warning indicator
- Power-saving chip technology
- Dual microphone technology**
- Push-button program selector
- Programmable telecoil with T/MT modes

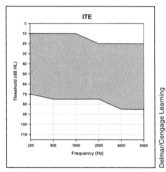

Fitting range for ES50 ITE

Options of ES30/D ITC and ES30-P/DP Power ITC

- Analog volume control
- 3 color options

**ES30-D and ES30-DP only

Features of ES10 CIC and ES10-P Power CIC

- Standard and power CIC
- 6-band WARP sound processing – 6 gain handles
- Stabilizer DFS feedback suppression
- NoiseTracker noise reduction
- Low-battery warning indicator
- Power-saving chip technology

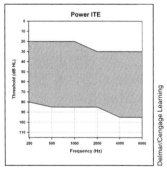

Fitting range for ES50 Power ITE

Options of ES10 CIC and ES10-P Power CIC

- 3 color options

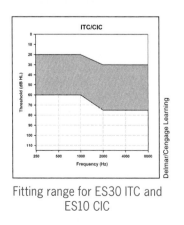

Fitting range for ES30 ITC and ES10 CIC

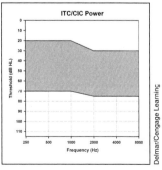

Fitting range for ES30 Power ITC and ES10 Power CIC

Typical Specifications		ES70-DVI BTE Classic	ES70-DVI BTE Open	ES80-DVI Power BTE
Standard ANSI S3.22-1996				
Output sound pressure level	Max OSPL 90 (dB SPL)	125	118	137
	HFA OSPL 90 (dB SPL)	120	109	131
Full-on gain (50 dB SPL input)	Peak gain (dB)	52	44	66
	HFA (dB)	47	36	61
Total harmonic distortion	500 Hz	0.6%	0.1%	1.8%
	800 Hz	0.3%	0.2%	0.4%
	1600 Hz	0.4%	0.2%	0.4%
Equivalent input noise (dB SPL), without noise reduction		24	31	22
Telecoil sensitivity	10 mA/m input max (dB SPL)	102	92	114
Battery	Operating current (mA)	0.92	0.83	0.99
	Battery type	13	13	13
Compression characteristics	Attack (ms)	12	12	12
	Release (ms)	70	70	70

Delmar/Cengage Learning

Typical Specifications		ES50/D ITE and ES50 HS/D ITE	ES50-P/DP Power ITE and ES50 HS-P/ DP Power ITE	ES 30/D ITC
Standard ANSI S3.22-1996				
Output sound pressure level	Max OSPL 90 (dB SPL)	120	125	112
	HFA OSPL 90 (dB SPL)	116	122	109
Full-on gain (50 dB SPL input)	Peak gain (dB)	52	60	43
	HFA (dB)	45	54	38
Total harmonic distortion	500 Hz	1.0%	0.6%	1.2%
	800 Hz	1.0%	0.9%	0.8%
	1600 Hz	1.0%	0.7%	1.2%
Equivalent input noise (dB SPL), without noise reduction		26	30	24
Telecoil sensitivity	10 mA/m input max (dB SPL)	99	108	93
Battery	Operating current (mA)	1.05	1.05	1.0
	Battery type	Full Shell 13 Half Shell 312	Full Shell 13 Half Shell 312	312
Compression characteristics	Attack (ms)	12	12	12
	Release (ms)	70	70	70

Delmar/Cengage Learning

ReSOUND

Typical Specifications		ES30-P/DP Power ITC	ES10 CIC	ES10-P Power CIC
Standard ANSI S3.22-1996				
Output sound pressure level	Max OSPL 90 (dB SPL)	120	110	116
	HFA OSPL 90 (dB SPL)	116	105	112
Full-on gain (50 dB SPL input)	Peak gain (dB)	50	34	45
	HFA (dB)	44	29	38
Total harmonic distortion	500 Hz	1.2%	0.6%	0.8%
	800 Hz	0.9%	0.7%	0.5%
	1600 Hz	1.2%	1.2%	1.5%
Equivalent input noise (dB SPL), without noise reduction		26	23	28
Telecoil sensitivity	10 mA/m input max (dB SPL)	99	n/a	n/a
Battery	Operating current (mA)	1.0	0.9	0.9
	Battery type	312	10	10
Compression characteristics	Attack (ms)	12	12	12
	Release (ms)	70	70	70

Delmar/Cengage Learning

PRODUCT 9: AZURE

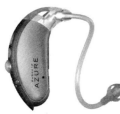

Azure 60 Mini BTE with thin tube
Courtesy of ReSound

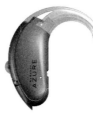

Azure 60 Mini BTE with standard ear hook
Courtesy of ReSound

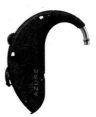

Azure 80 Power BTE
Courtesy of ReSound

Azure 40 Full-Shell
Courtesy of ReSound

Azure 30 ITC
Courtesy of ReSound

Azure 20 Mini-Canal
Courtesy of ReSound

Azure 10 CIC
Courtesy of ReSound

Product Application

AZ60-VI/DI Mini BTE
AZ70-DVI BTE
AZ80-DVI Power BTE
AZ40 HS ITE
AZ40 D HS ITE
AZ40 P HS ITE
AZ40 DP HS ITE
AZ50 FS ITE
AZ50 D HS ITE
AZ50 P HS ITE
AZ50 DP HS ITE
AZ30 ITC
AZ30 D ITC
AZ30 P Power ITC
AZ30 DP Power ITC
AZ20 Mini-Canal
AZ20-P Power Mini-Canal
AZ10-P Power CIC
AZ10-BP Power CIC
AZ10 CIC
AZ10-B CIC

Features of AZ60 VI/DI Mini BTE with Classic/Open and Thin Tube VI

- Environmental Optimizer – automatically adjusts gain for up to 7 different listening environments
- Environmental Learner™ – an algorithm that learns user preferences based on usage patterns in up to 7 different listening environments
- 17-band WARP compression – fast processing compression for 17 bands
- NoiseTracker II – tracks speech-to-noise ratio in each band to help improve overall speech-to-noise ratio
- Stabilizer DFS – cancellation system to reduce the occurrence of feedback
- Open-fitting capabilities allow for maximum cosmetics and comfort
- Onboard Analyzer II data-logging – tracks usage data as well as time spent in various listening situations
- Acceptance Manager – helps new users acclimate by slowly adjusting parameters over the first weeks/months
- 4 customizable programs
- Direct audio input
- Telecoil option
- SmartStart power-up timer
- Acoustic indicator for program selection
- Acoustic indicator for volume control
- Low-battery warning indicator

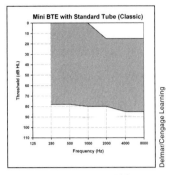

Fitting range for AZ60-VI
Mini BTE Standard Tubing
(Classic)

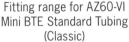

Fitting range for AZ60-VI
Mini BTE Standard Tubing
(Open)

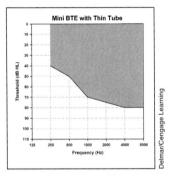

Fitting range for AZ60-VI Mini
BTE Thin Tube

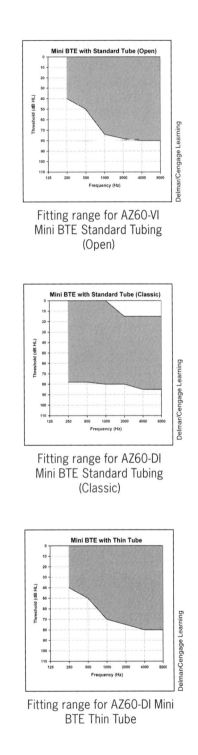

Fitting range for AZ60-DI
Mini BTE Standard Tubing
(Classic)

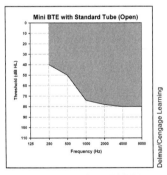

Fitting range for AZ60-DI
Mini BTE Standard Tubing
(Open)

Fitting range for AZ60-DI Mini
BTE Thin Tube

Features of AZ60 VI/DI Mini BTE with Classic/Open and Thin Tube DI

- Natural Directionality – a proprietary directional system that is designed to maintain audibility of off-axis sounds while simultaneously enhancing directionality
- MultiScope Adaptive Directionality – provides adaptive directionality with 2 beam-width options
- SoftSwitching automatic program – automatically changes from omnidirectional mode to MultiScope Adaptive Directionality
- Integrated Microphone Matching – calibrates microphones to match response across all frequencies
- Environmental Optimizer – delivers automatic, personally optimized gain in 7 different environments
- 17-band WARP compression – fast processing compression for 17 bands
- NoiseTracker II – tracks speech-to-noise ratio in each band to help improve overall speech-to-noise ratio
- Dual Stabilizer II DFS – cancellation system to reduce the occurrence of feedback
- EchoStop – helps reduce the effects of reverberation
- WindRush Manager – reduces the level of hiss and pops caused by wind
- Open-fitting capabilities allow for maximum cosmetics and comfort
- Onboard Analyzer II data-logging – tracks usage data as well as time spent in various listening situations
- Acceptance Manager – helps new users acclimate by slowly adjusting parameters over the first weeks/months
- 4 customizable programs
- DAI
- Telecoil option
- SmartStart power-up timer
- Acoustic indicator for program selection
- Low-battery warning indicator

Features of AZ70-DVI Standard BTE Classic/Open and FlexTube and AZ80-DVI Power BTE

- Natural Directionality – a proprietary directional system that is designed to maintain audibility of off-axis sounds while simultaneously enhancing directionality
- MultiScope Adaptive Directionality – provides adaptive directionality with 2 beam-width options
- SoftSwitching automatic program – automatically changes from omnidirectional mode to MultiScope Adaptive Directionality
- Integrated Microphone Matching – calibrates microphones to match response across all frequencies
- Environmental Optimizer – automatically adjusts gain for up to 7 different listening environments
- Environmental Learner – an algorithm that learns user preferences based on usage patterns in up to 7 different listening environments

- 17-band WARP – fast processing compression for 17 bands
- NoiseTracker II – tracks speech-to-noise ratio in each band to help improve overall speech-to-noise ratio
- Dual Stabilizer II DFS – cancellation system to reduce the occurrence of feedback
- EchoStop – helps reduce the effects of reverberation
- WindRush Manager – reduces the level of hiss and pops caused by wind
- Open-fitting capabilities allow for maximum cosmetics and comfort
- Onboard Analyzer II data-logging – tracks usage data as well as time spent in various listening situations
- Acceptance Manager – helps new users acclimate by slowly adjusting parameters over the first weeks/months
- 4 customizable programs
- DAI
- Telecoil option
- SmartStart power-up timer
- Acoustic indicator for program selection
- Acoustic indicator for volume control
- Low-battery warning indicator

Features of AZ40 D HS ITE, AZ40 DP HS ITE, AZ50 D HS ITE, and AZ50 DP HS ITE

- Natural Directionality – a proprietary directional system that is designed to maintain audibility of off-axis sounds while simultaneously enhancing directionality
- MultiScope Adaptive Directionality – provides adaptive directionality with 2 beam-width options
- SoftSwitching automatic program – automatically changes from omnidirectional mode to MultiScope Adaptive Directionality
- Integrated Microphone Matching – calibrates microphones to match response across all frequencies
- Environmental Optimizer – automatically adjusts gain for up to 7 different listening environments
- Environmental Learner – an algorithm that learns user preferences based on usage patterns in up to 7 different listening environments
- 17-band WARP compression – fast processing compression for 17 bands

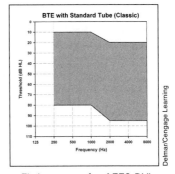

Fitting range for AZ70-DVI BTE Standard Tubing (Classic)

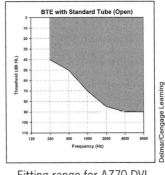

Fitting range for AZ70-DVI BTE Standard Tubing (Open)

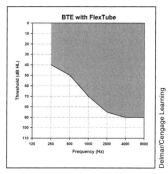

Fitting range for AZ70-DVI
BTE with Flex Tube

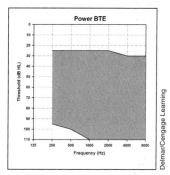

Fitting range for AZ80-DVI
Power BTE

- NoiseTracker II – tracks speech-to-noise ratio in each band to help improve overall speech-to-noise ratio
- Dual Stabilizer II DFS – cancellation system to reduce the occurrence of feedback
- EchoStop – helps reduce the effects of reverberation
- WindRush Manager – reduces the level of hiss and pops caused by wind
- Open-fitting capabilities allow for maximum cosmetics and comfort
- Onboard Analyzer II data-logging – tracks usage data as well as time spent in various listening situations
- Acceptance Manager – helps new users acclimate by slowly adjusting parameters over the first weeks/months
- 4 customizable programs
- Telecoil option
- SmartStart power-up timer
- Acoustic indicator for program selection
- Acoustic indicator for volume control
- Low-battery warning indicator

ReSOUND

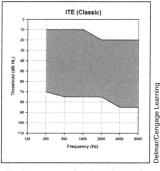

Fitting range for AZ40-D HS/
ITE Classic and AZ50-D HS/
ITE Classic

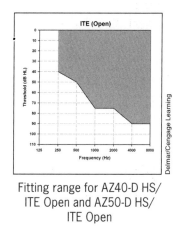

Fitting range for AZ40-D HS/
ITE Open and AZ50-D HS/
ITE Open

Features of AZ40 HS ITE, AZ40 P HS ITE, AZ50 FS ITE, and AZ50 P HS ITE

- Environmental Optimizer – automatically adjusts gain for up to 7 different listening environments
- Environmental Learner – an algorithm that learns user preferences based on usage patterns in up to 7 different listening environments
- 17-band WARP compression – fast processing compression for 17 bands
- NoiseTracker II – tracks speech-to-noise ratio in each band to help improve overall speech-to-noise ratio
- Stabilizer DFS – cancellation system to reduce the occurrence of feedback
- Onboard Analyzer II data-logging – tracks usage data as well as time spent in various listening situations
- Acceptance Manager – helps new users acclimate by slowly adjusting parameters over the first weeks/months
- 4 customizable programs
- Telecoil option
- SmartStart power-up timer
- Acoustic indicator for program selection
- Acoustic indicator for volume control
- Low-battery warning indicator

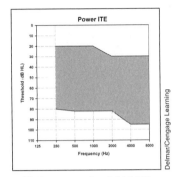

Fitting range for AZ40-DP Power HS/ITE and AZ50-DP Power HS/ITE

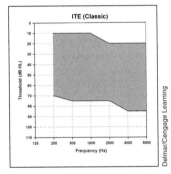

Fitting range for AZ40 HS/ITE Classic and AZ50 HS/ITE Classic

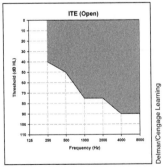

Fitting range for AZ40 HS/ITE Open and AZ50 HS/ITE Open

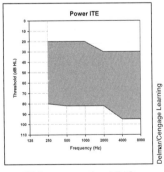

Fitting range for AZ40 Power HS/ITE and AZ50 Power HS/ITE

Features of AZ30 D ITC and AZ30 DP Power ITC

- Natural Directionality – a proprietary directional system that is designed to maintain audibility of off-axis sounds while simultaneously enhancing directionality
- MultiScope Adaptive Directionality – provides adaptive directionality with 2 beam-width options
- SoftSwitching automatic program – automatically changes from omnidirectional mode to MultiScope Adaptive Directionality
- Integrated Microphone Matching – calibrates microphones to match response across all frequencies
- Environmental Optimizer – automatically adjusts gain for up to 7 different listening environments
- Environmental Learner – an algorithm that learns user preferences based on usage patterns in up to 7 different listening environments
- 17-band WARP compression – fast processing compression for 17 bands
- NoiseTracker II – tracks speech-to-noise ratio in each band to help improve overall speech-to-noise ratio
- Dual Stabilizer II DFS – cancellation system to reduce the occurrence of feedback
- EchoStop – helps reduce the effects of reverberation
- WindRush Manager – reduces the level of hiss and pops caused by wind
- Open-fitting capabilities allow for maximum cosmetics and comfort
- Onboard Analyzer II data-logging – tracks usage data as well as time spent in various listening situations
- Acceptance Manager – helps new users acclimate by slowly adjusting parameters over the first weeks/months
- 4 customizable programs
- Telecoil option
- SmartStart power-up timer
- Acoustic indicator for program selection
- Acoustic indicator for volume control
- Low-battery warning indicator

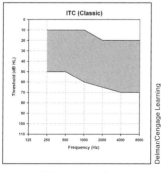

Fitting range for
AZ30-D ITC Classic

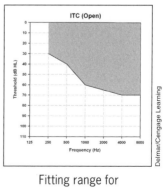

Fitting range for
AZ30-D ITC Open

Features of AZ30 ITC and AZ30 P Power ITC

- Environmental Optimizer – automatically adjusts gain for up to 7 different listening environments
- Environmental Learner – an algorithm that learns user preferences based on usage patterns in up to 7 different listening environments
- 17-band WARP compression – fast processing compression for 17 bands
- NoiseTracker II – tracks speech-to-noise ratio in each band to help improve overall speech-to-noise ratio
- Stabilizer DFS – cancellation system to reduce the occurrence of feedback
- Onboard Analyzer II data-logging – tracks usage data as well as time spent in various listening situations
- Acceptance Manager – helps new users acclimate by slowly adjusting parameters over the first weeks/months
- 4 customizable programs
- Telecoil option
- SmartStart power-up timer
- Acoustic indicator for program selection
- Acoustic indicator for volume control
- Low-battery warning indicator

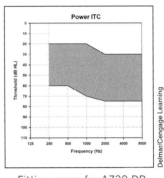

Fitting range for AZ30-DP Power ITC

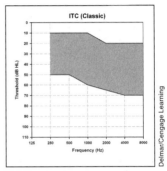

Fitting range for AZ30 ITC Classic

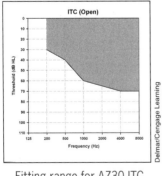

Fitting range for AZ30 ITC Open

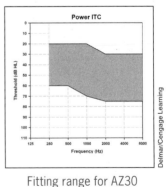

Fitting range for AZ30 Power ITC

Features of AZ20 Mini-Canal and AZ20-P Power Mini-Canal

- Environmental Optimizer – automatically adjusts gain for up to 7 different listening environments
- Environmental Learner – an algorithm that learns user preferences based on usage patterns in up to 7 different listening environments
- 17-band WARP compression – fast processing compression for 17 bands
- NoiseTracker II – tracks speech-to-noise ratio in each band to help improve overall speech-to-noise ratio
- Stabilizer DFS – cancellation system to reduce the occurrence of feedback
- Open-fitting capabilities allow for maximum cosmetics and comfort (AZ20 Mini-Canal only)
- Onboard Analyzer II data-logging – tracks usage data as well as time spent in various listening situations
- Acceptance Manager – helps new users acclimate by slowly adjusting parameters over the first weeks/months
- 4 customizable programs
- SmartStart power-up timer
- Acoustic indicator for program selection
- Acoustic indicator for volume control
- Low-battery warning indicator

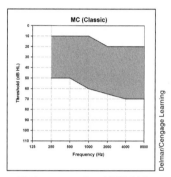

Fitting range for AZ20 MC Classic

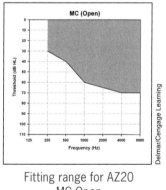

Fitting range for AZ20 MC Open

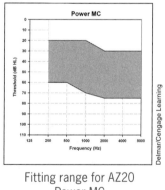

Fitting range for AZ20 Power MC

Features of AZ10-P Power CIC and AZ10-BP Power CIC

- Environmental Optimizer – automatically adjusts gain for up to 7 different listening environments
- 17-band WARP compression – fast processing compression for 17 bands
- NoiseTracker II – tracks speech-to-noise ratio in each band to help improve overall speech-to-noise ratio

- Stabilizer DFS – cancellation system to reduce the occurrence of feedback
- Onboard Analyzer II data-logging – tracks usage data as well as time spent in various listening situations
- Acceptance Manager – helps new users acclimate by slowly adjusting parameters over the first weeks/months
- 4 customizable programs (AZ10-BP Power CIC only)
- SmartStart power-up timer
- Acoustic indicator for program selection (AZ10-BP Power CIC only)
- Low-battery warning indicator

Fitting range for AZ10 Power CIC and AZ10-B Power CIC

Features of AZ10 CIC and AZ10-B CIC

- Environmental Optimizer – automatically adjusts gain for up to 7 different listening environments
- 17-band WARP compression – fast processing compression for 17 bands
- NoiseTracker II – tracks speech-to-noise ratio in each band to help improve overall speech-to-noise ratio
- Stabilizer DFS – cancellation system to reduce the occurrence of feedback
- Open-fitting capabilities allow for maximum cosmetics and comfort
- Onboard Analyzer II data-logging – tracks usage data as well as time spent in various listening situations
- Acceptance Manager – helps new users acclimate by slowly adjusting parameters over the first weeks/months
- 4 customizable programs (AZ10-B CIC only)
- SmartStart power-up timer
- Acoustic indicator for program selection (AZ10-B CIC only)
- Low-battery warning indicator

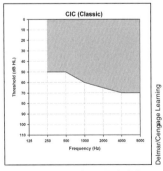

Fitting range for AZ10 CIC Classic and AZ10-B CIC Classic

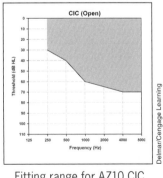

Fitting range for AZ10 CIC Open and AZ10-B CIC Open

Typical Specifications		AZ60-VI/DI Mini BTE Classic / Open	AZ60-VI/DI Mini BTE Thin Tube
Standard ANSI S3.22-1996			
Output sound pressure level	Max OSPL 90 (dB SPL)	126	127
	HFA OSPL 90 (dB SPL)	120	117
Full-on gain (50 dB SPL input)	Peak gain (dB)	53	50
	HFA (dB)	46	41
Total harmonic distortion	500 Hz	0.9%	0.2%
	800 Hz	1.0%	0.1%
	1600 Hz	0.6%	0.4%
Equivalent input noise (dB SPL), without noise reduction		26	28
Telecoil sensitivity	10 mA/m input max (dB SPL)	105	100
Battery	Operating current (mA)	0.9	0.85
	Battery type	13	13
Compression characteristics	Attack (ms)	12	12
	Release (ms)	70	70

Delmar/Cengage Learning

Typical Specifications		AZ70-DVI Standard BTE Classic/ Open	AZ70-DVI Standard BTE FlexTube	AZ80-DVI Power BTE
Standard ANSI S3.22-1996				
Output sound pressure level	Max OSPL 90 (dB SPL)	127	117	136
	HFA OSPL 90 (dB SPL)	118	112	129
Full-on gain (50 dB SPL input)	Peak gain (dB)	55	43	65
	HFA (dB)	43	38	60
Total harmonic distortion	500 Hz	0.2%	0.5%	1.8%
	800 Hz	0.6%	0.3%	0.6%
	1600 Hz	0.7%	0.6%	0.4%
Equivalent input noise (dB SPL), without noise reduction		29	29	22
Telecoil sensitivity	10 mA/m input max (dB SPL)	102	96	113
Battery	Operating current (mA)	0.85	0.85	0.85
	Battery type	13	13	13
Compression characteristics	Attack (ms)	12	12	12
	Release (ms)	70	70	70

Delmar/Cengage Learning

ReSOUND

Typical Specifications		AZ40/D, AZ50/D ITE	AZ40-P/DP, AZ50-P/DP Power ITE	AZ30/D ITC	AZ30-P/ DP Power ITC
Standard ANSI S3.22-1996					
Output sound pressure level	Max OSPL 90 (dB SPL)	120	126	112	119
	HFA OSPL 90 (dB SPL)	116	123	110	115
Full-on gain (50 dB SPL input)	Peak gain (dB)	52	59	43	50
	HFA (dB)	46	53	39	44
Total harmonic distortion	500 Hz	1.2%	0.6%	1.1%	1.0%
	800 Hz	1.1%	0.9%	1.1%	0.8%
	1600 Hz	1.9%	1.0%	1.3%	1.3%
Equivalent input noise (dB SPL), without noise reduction		26	24	25	26
Telecoil sensitivity	10 mA/m input max (dB SPL)	102	109	93	100
Battery	Operating current (mA)	1.04	1.05	0.95	1.0
	Battery type	13 or 312	13 or 312	10 or 12	312
Compression characteristics	Attack (ms)	12	12	12	12
	Release (ms)	70	70	70	70

Delmar/Cengage Learning

Typical Specifications		AZ20 Mini-Canal	AZ20-P Power Mini-Canal
Standard ANSI S3.22-1996			
Output sound pressure level	Max OSPL 90 (dB SPL)	108	113
	HFA OSPL 90 (dB SPL)	106	110
Full-on gain (50 dB SPL input)	Peak gain (dB)	31	39
	HFA (dB)	28	33
Total harmonic distortion	500 Hz	0.5%	1.1%
	800 Hz	0.5%	1.2%
	1600 Hz	0.4%	1.6%
Equivalent input noise (dB SPL), without noise reduction		24	25
Telecoil sensitivity	10 mA/m input max (dB SPL)	n/a	n/a
Battery	Operating current (mA)	0.87	0.94
	Battery type	10	10
Compression characteristics	Attack (ms)	12	12
	Release (ms)	70	70

Delmar/Cengage Learning

Typical Specifications		AZ10-P Power CIC	AZ10-BP Power CIC	AZ10 CIC	AZ10-B CIC
Standard ANSI S3.22-1996					
Output sound pressure level	Max OSPL 90 (dB SPL)	113	114	108	108
	HFA OSPL 90 (dB SPL)	110	111	106	105
Full-on gain (50 dB SPL input)	Peak gain (dB)	39	39	31	31
	HFA (dB)	33	35	28	28
Total harmonic distortion	500 Hz	1.1%	1.2%	0.5%	0.5%
	800 Hz	1.2%	0.8%	0.5%	0.4%
	1600 Hz	1.6%	1.1%	0.4%	0.9%
Equivalent input noise (dB SPL), without noise reduction		25	28	24	29
Telecoil sensitivity	10 mA/m input max (dB SPL)	n/a	n/a	n/a	n/a
Battery	Operating current (mA)	0.94	0.92	0.87	0.85
	Battery type	10	10	10	10
Compression characteristics	Attack (ms)	12	12	12	12
	Release (ms)	70	70	70	70

Delmar/Cengage Learning

PRODUCT 10: PIXEL

Product Application

PL60-DI Mini BTE
PL70 D/DI BTE
PL70-DV/DVI BTE
PL80-DVI Power BTE
PL40-D ITE
PL50-D ITE
PL40-DP Power ITE
PL50-DP Power ITE
PL30 ITC
PL30-P Power ITC
PL30-D ITC
PL30-DP Power ITC
PL10 CIC
PL10-B CIC
PL10-P CIC
PL10-BP CIC

FEATURES OF PL60-DI MINI BTE

- Small, cosmetic mini BTE design
- Recommended for mild to severe hearing losses
- Reconfigurable from standard hook to thin-tube (interchangeable by hearing healthcare professional)
- 17-band WARP – fast processing compression for 17 bands
- Noise reduction – 2 options
- Enhanced Adaptive Directionality
- SoftSwitching automatic program
- Dual Stabilizer DFS – cancellation system to reduce the occurrence of feedback
- Advanced data-logging
- SmartStart power-up timer
- Up to 3 customizable programs plus telecoil option
- Acoustic indicator for program selection
- Low-battery warning indicator
- DAI
- Fitting requirements: Aventa fitting software (Version 2.2 or higher), CS44 BTE socket cable, and HI-PRO™ or NOAHlink™ interface (NOAHlink recommended)
- Programmable telecoil

Options of PL60-DI Mini BTE

- Thin-tube, Tulip-Dome, and FlexVent standard domes, and standard ear molds
- Standard hook, cosmetic hook, and mini hook
- 10 color options available

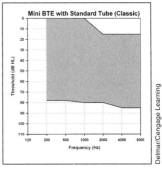

Fitting range for PL60-DI
Mini BTE Standard Tubing
(Classic)

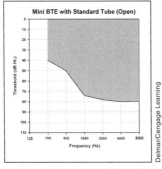

Fitting range for PL60-DI Mini
BTE Standard Tubing (Open)

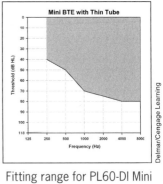

Fitting range for PL60-DI Mini
BTE Thin Tube

Features of PL70-D/DI BTE and PL70-DV/DVI BTE

- 17-band WARP – fast processing compression for 17 bands
- Noise reduction – 2 options
- Low-level expansion
- Enhanced Adaptive Directionality
- SoftSwitching automatic program
- Dual Stabilizer DFS – cancellation system to reduce the occurrence of feedback
- Advanced data-logging
- SmartStart power-up timer
- Up to 3 customizable programs plus telecoil option
- Open-fitting capabilities
- Acoustic indicator for program selection
- Acoustic indicator for volume control (PL70-DV/DVI BTE only)
- Low-battery warning indicator
- Fitting requirements: Aventa fitting software (Version 2.2 or higher), CS44 BTE socket cable, and HI-PRO or NOAHlink interface (NOAHlink recommended)

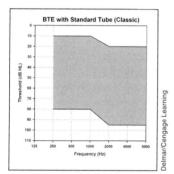

Fitting range for PL70-D BTE Classic, PL70-DI BTE Classic, PL70-DV BTE Classic, and PL70-DVI BTE Classic

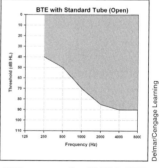

Fitting range for PL70-D BTE Open, PL70-DI BTE Open, PL70-DV BTE Open, and PL70-DVI BTE Open

Features of PL80-DVI Power BTE

- Ergonomic BTE design
- Recommended for severe to profound hearing losses
- 17-band WARP – fast processing compression for 17 bands
- Noise reduction – 2 options
- Enhanced Adaptive Directionality
- SoftSwitching automatic program
- Dual Stabilizer DFS – cancellation system to reduce the occurrence of feedback

- Advanced data-logging
- SmartStart power-up timer
- Up to 3 customizable programs plus telecoil option
- Acoustic indicator for program selection
- Acoustic indicator for volume control
- Low-battery warning indicator
- Volume control
- DAI
- Fitting requirements: Aventa fitting software (Version 2.2 or higher), CS44 BTE socket cable, and HI-PRO or NOAHlink interface (NOAHlink recommended)
- Programmable telecoil

Options of PL80-DVI Power BTE

- 20 color options available

Features of PL40-D/PL50-D ITE and PL40-DP/PL50-DP Power ITE

- 17-band WARP – fast processing compression for 17 bands
- Noise reduction – 2 options
- Low-level expansion
- Enhanced Adaptive Directionality
- SoftSwitching Automatic Programs
- Dual Stabilizer DFS – cancellation system to reduce the occurrence of feedback
- Advanced data-logging
- SmartStart power-up timer
- Up to 3 customizable programs plus telecoil option
- Open-fitting capabilities (PL40-D/ PL50-D ITE only)
- Acoustic indicator for program selection
- Acoustic indicator for volume control
- Low-battery warning indicator
- Power versions (PL40-DP/PL50-DP Power ITE only)
- Fitting requirements: Aventa fitting software (Version 2.2 or higher), CS63 FlexStrip cable (3 pin), and HI-PRO or NOAHlink interface (NOAHlink recommended)

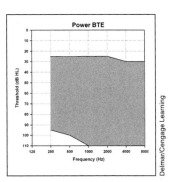

Fitting range for PL80-DVI Power BTE

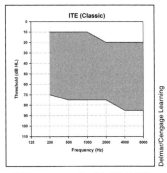

Fitting range for PL40-D ITE Classic and PL50-D ITE Classic

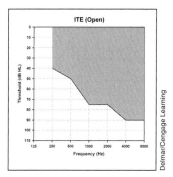

Fitting range for PL40-D ITE
Open and PL50-D ITE Open

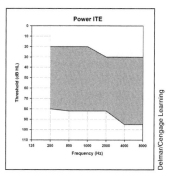

Fitting range for PL40-DP Power
ITE and PL50-DP Power ITE

Features of PL30-D ITC and PL30-DP Power ITC

- 17-band WARP – fast processing compression for 17 bands
- Noise reduction – 2 options
- Low-level expansion
- Enhanced Adaptive Directionality
- SoftSwitching Automatic Programs
- Dual Stabilizer DFS – cancellation system to reduce the occurrence of feedback
- Advanced data-logging
- SmartStart power-up timer
- Up to 3 customizable programs plus telecoil option
- Open-fitting capabilities (PL30-D ITC only)
- Acoustic indicator for program selection
- Acoustic indicator for volume control
- Low-battery warning indicator
- Power version (PL30-DP Power ITC only)
- Fitting requirements: Aventa fitting software (Version 2.2 or higher), CS63 FlexStrip cable (3 pin), and HI-PRO or NOAHlink interface (NOAHlink recommended)

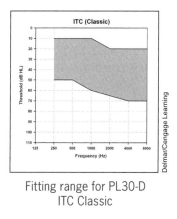

Fitting range for PL30-D
ITC Classic

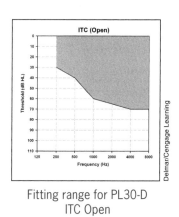

Fitting range for PL30-D
ITC Open

Features of PL30 ITC and PL30-P Power ITC

- 17-band WARP – fast processing compression for 17 bands
- Noise reduction – 2 options
- Stabilizer DFS – cancellation system to reduce the occurrence of feedback
- Advanced data-logging
- SmartStart power-up timer
- Up to 3 customizable programs plus telecoil option
- Open-fitting capabilities (PL30 ITC only)
- Acoustic indicator for program selection
- Acoustic indicator for volume control
- Low-battery warning indicator
- Power version (PL30-P ITC only)
- Fitting requirements: Aventa fitting software (Version 2.2 or higher), CS63 FlexStrip cable (3 pin), and HI-PRO or NOAHlink interface (NOAHlink recommended)

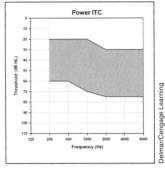

Fitting range for PL30-DP Power ITC and PL30-P Power ITC

FEATURES OF PL10 CIC, PL10-B CIC, PL10-P CIC, AND PL10-BP CIC

- 17-band WARP – fast processing compression for 17 bands
- Noise reduction – 2 options
- Low-level expansion
- Stabilizer DFS – cancellation system to reduce the occurrence of feedback
- Advanced data-logging
- SmartStart power-up timer
- Up to 3 customizable programs (PL10-B CIC and PL10-BP CIC only)
- Open-fitting capabilities (PL10 CIC and PL10-B CIC only)
- Acoustic indicator for program selection (PL10-B CIC and PL10-BP CIC only)
- Low-battery warning indicator
- Power versions (Pl10-P CIC and PL10-BP CIC only)
- Fitting requirements: Aventa fitting software (Version 2.2 or higher), CS63 FlexStrip cable (3 pin), and HI-PRO or NOAHlink interface (NOAHlink recommended)

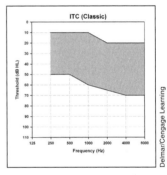

Fitting range for PL30 ITC Classic

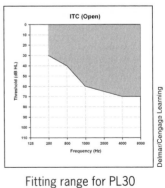

Fitting range for PL30 ITC Open

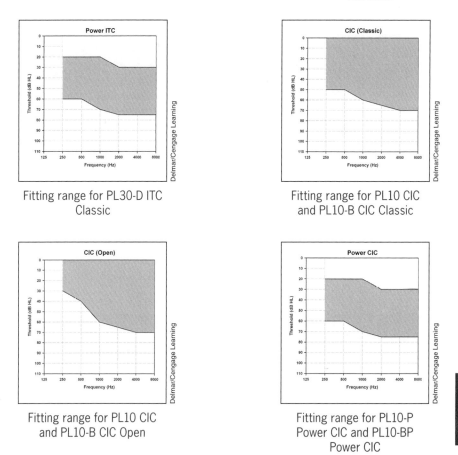

Fitting range for PL30-D ITC Classic

Fitting range for PL10 CIC and PL10-B CIC Classic

Fitting range for PL10 CIC and PL10-B CIC Open

Fitting range for PL10-P Power CIC and PL10-BP Power CIC

Typical Specifications		PL60-DI Mini BTE Classic / Open	PL60-DI Mini BTE Thin Tube	PL70-D/ DI BTE and PL70-DV/ DVI BTE	PL80-DVI Power BTE
Standard ANSI S3.22-1996					
Output sound pressure level	Max OSPL 90 (dB SPL)	125	128	127	135
	HFA OSPL 90 (dB SPL)	119	118	118	129
Full-on gain (50 dB SPL input)	Peak gain (dB)	53	50	55	65
	HFA (dB)	46	43	43	62
Total harmonic distortion	500 Hz	0.4%	0.2%	0.4%	1.2%
	800 Hz	0.6%	0.1%	0.4%	0.5%
	1600 Hz	0.5%	0.4%	0.7%	0.7%

continues

continued

Typical Specifications		PL60-DI Mini BTE Classic / Open	PL60-DI Mini BTE Thin Tube	PL70-D/ DI BTE and PL70-DV/ DVI BTE	PL80-DVI Power BTE
Equivalent input noise (dB SPL), without noise reduction		26	26	30	23
Telecoil sensitivity	10 mA/m input max (dB SPL)	103	100	107	118
Battery	Operating current (mA)	1.32	1.32	1.15	1.35
	Battery type	13	13	13	13
Compression characteristics	Attack (ms)	2	2	n/a	3
	Release (ms)	50	50	n/a	60

Delmar/Cengage Learning

Typical Specifications		PL30-P ITC and PL 30-DP ITC	PL40-DP ITE and PL 50-DP ITE	PL30 ITC and PL30-D ITC	PL30-P ITC and PL 30-DP ITC
Standard ANSI S3.22-1996					
Output sound pressure level	Max OSPL 90 (dB SPL)	121	125	111	118
	HFA OSPL 90 (dB SPL)	116	122	110	115
Full-on gain (50 dB SPL input)	Peak gain (dB)	53	59	43	49
	HFA (dB)	46	53	38	43
Total harmonic distortion	500 Hz	1.7%	0.7%	1.5%	1.7%
	800 Hz	1.7%	0.8%	1.3%	1.3%
	1600 Hz	1.4%	0.7%	1.2%	1.1%
Equivalent input noise (dB SPL), without noise reduction		26	25	26	25
Telecoil sensitivity	10 mA/m input max (dB SPL)	102	109	93	98
Battery	Operating current (mA)	1.3	1.3	1.1	1.3
	Battery type	13 or 312	13 or 312	312 or 10	312

Delmar/Cengage Learning

Typical Specifications		PL10 CIC and PL10-B CIC	PL10-P CIC and PL10-BP CIC
Standard ANSI S3.22-1996			
Output sound pressure level	Max OSPL 90 (dB SPL)	108	114
	HFA OSPL 90 (dB SPL)	105	110
Full-on gain (50 dB SPL input)	Peak gain (dB)	31	40
	HFA (dB)	29	35
Total harmonic distortion	500 Hz	0.9%	1.6%
	800 Hz	1.0%	1.5%
	1600 Hz	1.2%	1.5%
Equivalent input noise (dB SPL), without noise reduction		24	24
Telecoil sensitivity	10 mA/m input max (dB SPL)	n/a	n/a
Battery	Operating current (mA)	1.0	1.1
	Battery type (A)	10	10

Delmar/Cengage Learning

PRODUCT 11: PULSE

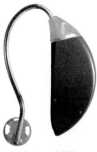

Pulse BTE
Courtesy of ReSound

Product Application

Model PS60

Features of Model PS60

- Small, cosmetic micro open-fit BTE design
- Receiver-in-the-canal (RIC) technology
- WARP high-resolution sound processing
- New Stabilizer DFS system – cancellation system to reduce the occurrence of feedback

- SuperTune™ intelligent recharger
- Directionality
- Environmental steering – compression characteristics adapt according to listening situation
- Virtual WindShield™ wind noise reduction
- Multiband noise reduction
- Low-battery warning indicator
- Onboard Analyzer data-logging – tracks usage data as well as time spent in various listening situations
- SmartStart power-up timer
- Battery door with integrated ON/OFF switch
- Fitting requirements: Aventa fitting software (Version 2.3 or higher), CS53 or CS63 FlexStrip programming cable, and HI-PRO, NOAHlink, or Speedlink interface (Speedlink recommended)

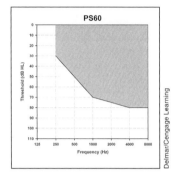

Fitting range for PS60

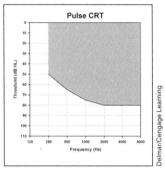

Fitting range for Pulse CRT

Options of Model PS60

- Sound tubes and domes in different sizes
- 8 standard, 5 chromatic, and 4 chameleon colors

Typical Specifications		Model PS60
Standard ANSI S3.22-1996		
Output sound pressure level	Max OSPL 90 (dB SPL)	107
	HFA OSPL 90 (dB SPL)	100
Full-on gain (50 dB SPL input)	Peak gain (dB)	41
	HFA (dB)	34
Total harmonic distortion (Hz)	500 Hz	0.5%
	800 Hz	0.1%
	1600 Hz	0.4%
Equivalent input noise (dB SPL), without noise reduction		27
Telecoil sensitivity	10 mA/m input max (dB SPL)	n/a
Battery	Operating current (mA)	0.78
	Battery type	10 or 312
Compression characteristics	Attack (ms)	7
	Release (ms)	91

Delmar/Cengage Learning

PRODUCT 12: PLUS 5

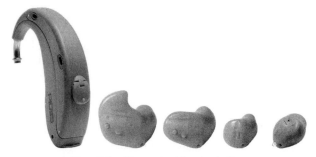

Plus 5 family product line including
BTE through CIC collection
Courtesy of ReSound

Product Application

RP60-VI Mini BTE
RP70-I/VI BTE
RP70-DI/DVI BTE
RP80-VI/DVI Power BTE
RP40/50 ITE
RP40-D/50-D ITE
RP40-P/50-P Power ITE
RP40-DP/50-DP Power ITE
RP30 ITC
RP30-P ITC
RP30-D ITC
RP30-DP ITC
RP10 CIC
RP10-B CIC
RP10-P Power CIC
RP10-BP Power CIC

Features of RP60-VI Mini BTE

- Small, cosmetic mini BTE design
- Recommended for mild to severe hearing losses
- Reconfigurable from standard hook to thin-tube (interchangeable by hearing healthcare professional)
- 6-band WARP sound processing
- Stabilizer DFS – cancellation system to reduce the occurrence of feedback
- Noise reduction
- Data-logging
- SmartStart power-up timer
- 2 customizable programs plus telecoil option

- Acoustic indicator for program selection
- Low-battery warning indicator
- Volume control
- DAI
- Fitting requirements: Aventa fitting software (Version 2.2 or higher), CS44 BTE socket cable, and HI-PRO or NOAHlink interface (NOAHlink recommended)
- Programmable telecoil

Options of RP60-VI Mini BTE

- Standard hook, cosmetic hook, and mini hook
- Supports thin-tube, Tulip-Dome, and FlexVent standard domes, and standard ear molds
- 10 color options available

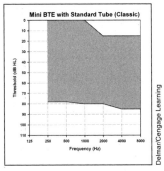

Fitting range for RP60-VI
Mini BTE Standard Tubing
(Classic)

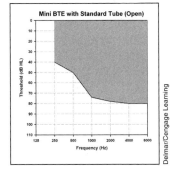

Fitting range for RP60-VI
Mini BTE Standard Tubing
(Open)

Features of RP70-I/VI BTE and RP70-DI/ DVI BTE

- 6-band WARP compression
- Stabilizer DFS – cancellation system to reduce the occurrence of feedback
- Dual microphone directionality (RP70-DI/ DVI BTE only)
- NoiseTracker – tracks speech-to-noise ratio in each band to help improve overall speech-to-noise ratio
- Data-logging
- Open-fitting capabilities
- SmartStart power-up timer
- Acoustic indicator for program selection
- Low-battery warning indicator

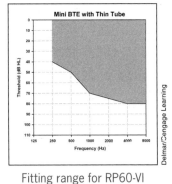

Fitting range for RP60-VI
Mini BTE Thin Tube

- 2 flexible environmental programs plus telecoil option
- Fitting requirements: Aventa fitting software (Version 2.2 or higher), CS44 BTE socket cable, and HI-PRO or NOAHlink interface (NOAHlink recommended)

Options of RP70-I/VI BTE and RP70-DI/DVI BTE

- DAI
- Volume control (RP70-VI BTE and RP70-DVI only)

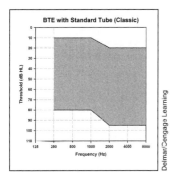

Fitting range for RP70-I BTE Classic, RP70-VI BTE Classic, RP70-DI BTE Classic, and RP70-DVI BTE Classic

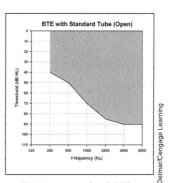

Fitting range for RP70-I BTE Open, RP70-VI BTE Open, RP70-DI BTE Open, and RP70-DVI BTE Open

Features of RP80-VI/DVI Power BTE

- Ergonomic BTE design
- Recommended for severe to profound hearing losses
- 6-band WARP compression
- Fixed directionality (RP80-DVI Power BTE only)
- Dual microphone technology (RP80-DVI Power BTE only)
- Stabilizer DFS – cancellation system to reduce the occurrence of feedback
- Noise reduction
- Data-logging
- SmartStart power-up timer
- 2 flexible environmental programs plus telecoil option
- Acoustic indicator for program selection
- Low-battery warning indicator
- DAI
- Volume control

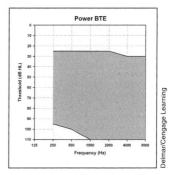

Fitting range for RP80-VI Power BTE and RP80-DVI Power BTE

- Fitting requirements: Aventa fitting software (Version 2.2 or higher), CS44 BTE socket cable, and HI-PRO or NOAHlink interface (NOAHlink recommended)
- Programmable telecoil
- 20 color options available

Features of RP40/50 ITE, RP40-D/50-D ITE, RP40-P/50-P ITE, and RP40-DP/50-DP ITE

- 6-band WARP compression
- Stabilizer DFS – cancellation system to reduce the occurrence of feedback
- Dual microphone directionality (RP40-D/50-D ITE and RP40-DP/50-DP ITE only)
- NoiseTracker – tracks speech-to-noise ratio in each band to help improve overall speech-to-noise ratio
- Low-level expansion
- Data-logging
- SmartStart power-up timer
- Open-fitting capabilities (RP40/50 ITE and RP40-D/50-D ITE only)
- Acoustic indicator for program selection
- Low-battery warning indicator
- 2 flexible environmental programs plus telecoil option
- Fitting requirements: Aventa fitting software (Version 2.2 or higher), CS63 FlexStrip cable (3 pin), and HI-PRO or NOAHlink interface (NOAHlink recommended)

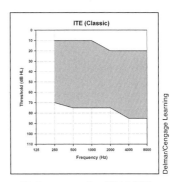

Fitting range for RP40 ITE Classic, RP50 ITE Classic, RP40-D ITE Classic, and RP50-D ITE Classic

Options of RP40/50 ITE, RP40-D/50-D ITE, RP40-P/50-P ITE, and RP40-DP/50-DP ITE

- Volume control

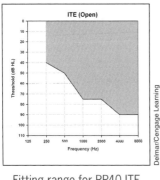

Fitting range for RP40 ITE Open, RP50 ITE Open, RP40-D ITE Open, and RP50-D ITE Open

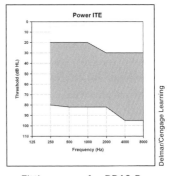

Fitting range for RP40-P Power ITE, RP50-P Power ITE, RP40-DP Power ITE, and RP50-DP Power ITE

Features of RP30 ITC, RP30-D ITC, RP30-P ITC, and RP30-DP ITC

- 6-band WARP compression
- Stabilizer DFS – cancellation system to reduce the occurrence of feedback
- Dual microphone directionality (RP30-D ITC and RP30-DP ITC only)
- NoiseTracker – tracks speech-to-noise ratio in each band to help improve overall speech-to-noise ratio
- Low-level expansion
- Data-logging
- Open-fitting capabilities (RP30 ITC and RP30-D ITC only)
- SmartStart power-up timer
- Acoustic indicator for program selection
- Low-battery warning indicator
- 2 flexible environmental programs plus telecoil option
- Fitting requirements: Aventa fitting software (Version 2.2 or higher), CS63 FlexStrip cable (3 pin), and HI-PRO or NOAHlink interface (NOAHlink recommended)

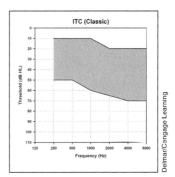

Options of RP30 ITC, RP30-D ITC, RP30-P ITC, and RP30-DP ITC

- Volume control

Fitting range for RP 30 ITC Classic and RP30-DI ITC Classic

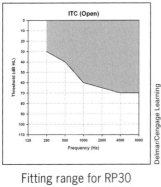

Fitting range for RP30 ITC Open and RP30-DI ITC Open

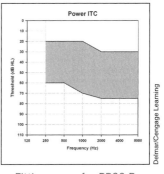

Fitting range for RP30-P Power ITC and RP30-DP Power ITC

Features of RP10 CIC, RP10-B CIC, RP10-P Power CIC, and RP10-BP Power CIC

- 6-band WARP compression
- Stabilizer DFS – cancellation system to reduce the occurrence of feedback
- NoiseTracker – tracks speech-to-noise ratio in each band to help improve overall speech-to-noise ratio

- Low-level expansion
- Data-logging
- Open-fitting capabilities (RP10 CIC and RP10-B CIC only)
- SmartStart power-up timer
- Acoustic indicator for program selection (RP10-B CIC and RP10-BP CIC only)
- Fitting requirements: Aventa fitting software (Version 2.2 or higher), CS63 FlexStrip cable (3 pin), and HI-PRO or NOAHlink interface (NOAHlink recommended)

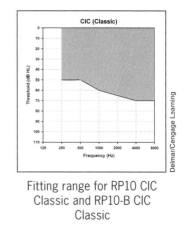

Fitting range for RP10 CIC
Classic and RP10-B CIC
Classic

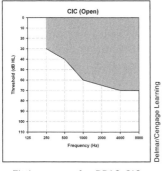

Fitting range for RP10 CIC
Open and RP10-B
CIC Open

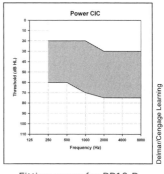

Fitting range for RP10-P
Power CIC and RP10-BP
Power CIC

Typical Specifications		RP60-DI Mini BTE Classic / Open	RP60-DI Mini BTE Thin Tube	RP70-I/ VI BTE and RP70-DI/ DVI BTE	RP80-VI Power BTE and RP80-DVI Power BTE
Standard ANSI S3.22-1996					
Output sound pressure level	Max OSPL 90 (dB SPL)	125	128	127	135
	HFA OSPL 90 (dB SPL)	119	118	118	129
Full-on gain (50 dB SPL input)	Peak gain (dB)	53	50	55	65
	HFA (dB)	46	43	43	62
Total harmonic distortion	500 Hz	0.4%	0.2%	0.4%	1.2%
	800 Hz	0.6%	0.1%	0.4%	0.5%
	1600 Hz	0.5%	0.4%	0.7%	0.7%

continues

continued

Typical Specifications		RP60-DI Mini BTE Classic / Open	RP60-DI Mini BTE Thin Tube	RP70-I/ VI BTE and RP70-DI/ DVI BTE	RP80-VI Power BTE and RP80-DVI Power BTE
Equivalent input noise (dB SPL), without noise reduction		26	26	30	23
Telecoil sensitivity	10 mA/m input max (dB SPL)	103	100	107	118
Battery	Operating current (mA)	1.32	1.32	1.15	1.35
	Battery type	13	13	13	13
Compression characteristics	Attack (ms)	2	2	n/a	3
	Release (ms)	50	50	n/a	60

Delmar/Cengage Learning

Typical Specifications		RP40/50 ITE and RP40-D/50-D ITE	RP40-P/50-P ITE and RP40-DP/50-DP ITE	RP30 ITC and RP30-D ITC	RP30-P ITC and RP30-DP ITC
Standard ANSI S3.22-1996					
Output sound pressure level	Max OSPL 90 (dB SPL)	121	125	111	118
	HFA OSPL 90 (dB SPL)	116	122	110	115
Full-on gain (50 dB SPL input)	Peak gain (dB)	53	59	38	43
	HFA (dB)	46	53	43	49
Total harmonic distortion	500 Hz	1.7%	0.7%	1.5%	1.7%
	800 Hz	1.7%	0.8%	1.3%	1.3%
	1600 Hz	1.4%	0.7%	1.2%	1.1%
Equivalent input noise (dB SPL), without noise reduction		26	25	26	25
Telecoil sensitivity	10 mA/m input max (dB SPL)	102	109	93	98
Battery	Operating current (mA)	1.3	1.3	1.1	1.3
	Battery type	13 or 312	13 or 312	312 or 10	312

Delmar/Cengage Learning

ReSOUND

Typical Specifications		RP10 CIC and RP10-B CIC	RP10-P CIC and RP10-BP CIC
Standard ANSI S3.22-1996			
Output sound pressure level	Max OSPL 90 (dB SPL)	108	114
	HFA OSPL 90 (dB SPL)	105	110
Full-on gain (50 dB SPL input)	Peak gain (dB)	31	40
	HFA (dB)	29	35
Total harmonic distortion	500 Hz	0.9%	1.6%
	800 Hz	1.0%	1.5%
	1600 Hz	1.2%	1.5%
Equivalent input noise (dB SPL), without noise reduction		24	24
Telecoil sensitivity	10 mA/m input max (dB SPL)	n/a	n/a
Battery	Operating current (mA)	1.0	1.1
	Battery type (A)	10	10

Delmar/Cengage Learning

CHAPTER EIGHT

Siemens Hearing

SIEMENS HEARING: NUMBER ONE

Hearing Division U.S. Headquarters
Siemens Hearing Instruments, Inc.
10 Constitution Ave.
P.O. Box 1397
Piscataway, NJ 08855-1397
Phone: 1 (800) 766-4500
Web site: http://www.siemens-hearing.com

> *Personal accomplishments of any kind should only be recognized or valued for the benefit they bring to others.*
> — Werner von Siemens, 1872 (Siemens, 2006d)

Siemens (Munich, Germany; http://www.siemens.com) has been in the business of health-care products for over 125 years (Siemens, 2006d). In fact, it has grown from a one-man operation to being the world's ninth-largest employer, employing over 427,000 people (Siemens, 2009b). Siemens is a customer-focused company. Its strength has been and remains at the forefront of innovation in product development. In fact, part of its vision is to have "leading positions in all our business [and] to remain at the forefront of technological progress" (Siemens, 2005, p. 5).

Siemens has several business foci, including automation and control information, communication, transportation, power, medical, and lighting. Overall, 19 percent of sales are to Germany (worldwide headquarters), 31 percent to the rest of Europe, and 26 percent to the Americas (Siemens, 2006f). Of over 87 billion euros in sales in 2006, Siemens has invested 7 billion euros in research and development, $400 million of which went into the medical division in the United States (Siemens, 2006f). Overall, Siemens invests over 9 percent of its annual revenue in research and development. In doing so, they dedicate over 5,000 employees who, in turn, produce about five patents per day (Siemens, 2009a).

Siemens Hearing Instruments is a wholly owned subsidiary of Siemens Medical Solutions. Although Siemens Hearing Instruments represents only a small percentage of Siemens's worldwide sales (0.5 percent), with the immense size of Siemens, the hearing instrument division is acknowledged as one of the largest hearing instrument manufacturers in the world (Parkhøi & Jessen, 2003). Throughout its growth as a company, involvement in hearing systems has grown exponentially. Currently located in Piscataway, New Jersey, Siemens Hearing Instruments (hereafter Siemens) offers a complete line of hearing instruments in all the expected form factors (CIC, ITC, etc.). Some of the major historical landmarks including its first product are as follows (Siemens, 2009a; Siemens, 2006e):

1878: Introduced the PHONOPHOR, a type of telephone receiver for the hearing impaired

1929: First portable hearing aid-type device

1949: A body-worn hearing instrument was introduced – PHONOPHOR ALPHA

1959: Siemens's first BTE – AURICULETTE 326

1966: Siemens's first ITE – SIRETTA 339

1991: Siemens's first three-channel programmable hearing instruments in BTE and ITE form factors – TRITON 3000

1997: Siemens introduced its first fully digital hearing instrument – PRISMA

2004: Siemens introduced technology to allow the two hearing instruments in a binaural fitting to communicate with each other – ACURIS with e2e wireless™

2005: Introduction of iScan allows for electronic scans of ear impressions to be made

2008: New "lifestyle" series of devices introduced, including the Explorer, Vibe, Pure, and Tek

2009: Expanded model line with Life and Motion

All Siemens' product lines are fully digital, and the main differentiating factor is no longer "digital" versus "digitally programmable" versus "analog," but rather the level of sophistication in the signal processing and directional microphones, as well as the number of independent channels in each instrument.

Philanthropy

Siemens' service is channeled through the Siemens Foundation, which donates approximately $2,000,000 annually to high-achieving college students for college tuition in the United States (Siemens Foundation, 2005a). Through various competitive student programs, including the Siemens Competition in Math, Science, and Technology and the Siemens Awards for Advance Placement, talented individuals are selected for scholarships (Siemens Foundation, 2005a). In 2005, the Siemens Foundation started the Siemens Teacher Scholarship to guide more minority students into teaching in the areas of math and science (Siemens Foundation, 2005b). It promised $1,000,000, spread over five years, to the Thurgood Marshall Scholarship Fund and the United Negro College Fund, which will be administering the donations (Siemens Foundation, 2005b). The decision criteria for the Siemens Teacher Scholarship are academic merit and financial need. As far as could be researched, Siemens does not have a philanthropy program specific to its hearing division; however, all divisions participate in the corporate programs.

Warranty

Siemens hearing instruments generally carry standard coverage consisting of a 1-year warranty with loss and damage. However, depending on the purchasing volume of the clinic, a 2-year warranty is standard. Extended warrantees with the same basic coverage can be purchased for up to 3 years. A deductible applies for loss and damage claims, and varies by model (Siemens, 2005).

PRODUCT INFORMATION

PRODUCT 1: LIFE

Product Application

Life 700 BTE
Life 500 BTE
Life 300 BTE

Features of Life 700 BTE

- Appropriate for mild to moderate hearing losses
- Highly flexible 16-channel digital signal processing and programming
- 16-channel AGC-I and AGC-O system
- SoundSmoothing™ – transient noise suppression
- Binaural synchronization with e2e wireless 2.0
- SoundLearning™ – remembers your loudness settings and automatically adjusts for volume, compression, and frequency shape
- Automatic and multichannel adaptive directional microphone system
- FeedbackBlocker™ – automatically and quickly reduces or eliminates annoying feedback noise without affecting sound quality
- Speech and noise management in 16 channels

- SoundBrilliance™ – enhances your perception of high pitches for a richer, fuller sound
- TruEar™ – simulates the acoustical functions of the outer ear and helps you distinguish sounds in front and back
- Compatible with ConnexxLink™ wireless programming system
- eWindScreen™ – constantly analyzes incoming signals to detect wind noise, then automatically adjusts signal processing to reduce it
- Automatic adaptive directional microphone systems transition automatically between omni, TruEar, and directional modes
- Adaptive melody beeps – tones that verify your manual settings

Options of Life 700 BTE

- Compatible with Tek wireless enhancement system
- Compatible with ePen™ remote control
- Compatible with ProPocket™ remote control
- LifeTubes and LifeTips in different sizes
- Earhook
- Exchangeable housing in 16 colors

Features of Life 500 BTE

- Appropriate for mild to moderate hearing losses
- Highly flexible 12-channel digital signal processing and programming
- 12-channel AGC-I and AGC-O system
- SoundSmoothing – transient noise suppression
- Binaural synchronization with e2e wireless 2.0
- DataLearning™ – automatically learns and adapts to your volume preferences in different environments
- Automatic and multichannel adaptive directional microphone system
- FeedbackBlocker – automatically and quickly reduces or eliminates annoying feedback noise without affecting sound quality
- Speech and noise management in 12 channels
- Compatible with ConnexxLink wireless programming system
- eWindScreen – constantly analyzes incoming signals to detect wind noise, then automatically adjusts signal processing to reduce it
- Automatic adaptive directional microphone systems transition automatically between omni, TruEar, and directional modes
- Adaptive melody beeps – tones that verify your manual settings

Options of Life 500 BTE

- Compatible with Tek wireless enhancement system
- Compatible with ePen remote control
- Compatible with ProPocket remote control
- LifeTubes and LifeTips in different sizes

- Earhook
- Exchangeable housing in 16 colors

Features of Life 300 BTE

- Appropriate for mild to moderate hearing losses
- Highly flexible 8-channel digital signal processing and programming
- 8-channel AGC-I and AGC-O system
- SoundSmoothing – transient noise suppression
- Binaural synchronization with e2e wireless 2.0
- Data-logging – tracks information such as program use and wearing time for faster, more precise fine-tuning and better counseling
- Automatic and multichannel adaptive directional microphone system
- FeedbackBlocker – automatically and quickly reduces or eliminates annoying feedback noise without affecting sound quality
- Speech and noise management in 8 channels
- Compatible with ConnexxLink wireless programming system
- eWindScreen – constantly analyzes incoming signals to detect wind noise, then automatically adjusts signal processing to reduce it
- Automatic adaptive directional microphone systems transition automatically between omni, TruEar, and directional modes
- Adaptive melody beeps – tones that verify your manual settings

Options of Life 300 BTE

- Compatible with Tek wireless enhancement system
- Compatible with ePen remote control
- Compatible with ProPocket remote control
- LifeTubes and LifeTips in different sizes
- Earhook
- Exchangeable housing in 16 colors

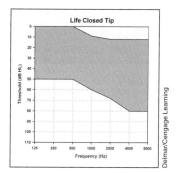

Fitting range for Life 700, Life 500, and Life 300 BTE with Closed Tip

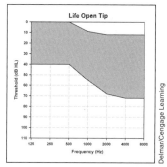

Fitting range for Life 700, Life 500, and Life 300 BTE with Open Tip

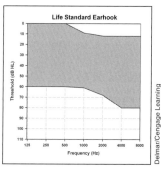

Fitting range for Life 700, Life 500, and Life 300 BTE with Earhook

Typical Specifications		Life 700 BTE, Life 500 BTE, Life 300 BTE, LifeTube	Life 700 BTE, Life 500 BTE, Life 300 BTE, Earhook
Standard ANSI S3.22-2003			
Output sound pressure level	Max OSPL 90 (dB)	124	124
	HF-Average OSPL 90 (dB)	114	120
Full-on gain	Peak gain (dB)	40	51
	HF-Average full-on gain (dB)	35	40
Total harmonic distortion	500 Hz	1%	2%
	800 Hz	1%	1%
	1600 Hz	1%	1%
Equivalent input noise (dB)		17	22
Telecoil sensitivity	HFA-SPLITS (dB)	n/a	n/a
Battery	Operating current (mA)	0.8	0.8
	Battery type	312	312
Compression characteristics – channel AGC-O (CK= –21 dB)	Attack (ms)	5	5
	Release (ms)	600	600

Delmar/Cengage Learning

PRODUCT 2: MOTION SERIES 700 AND 500

Product Application

Motion 700 P BTE
Motion 700 M VC BTE
Motion 700 Motion M BTE
Motion 700 ITE (118/50, 123/55, 123/60)
Motion 700 HS/ITC (113/40, 118/45, 118/50)
Motion 700 CIC (113/40, 113/47)
Motion 700 MC (113/47, 113/40)

Features of Motion 700 P BTE

- Appropriate for moderate to severe hearing losses
- Highly flexible, 16-channel digital signal processing
- 16-channel AGC-I and AGC-O system
- Automatic and multichannel adaptive directional microphone system
- SoundSmoothing – transient noise reduction
- Speech and noise management
- FeedbackBlocker – automatically and quickly reduces or eliminates annoying feedback noise without affecting sound quality

- Binaural synchronization with e2e wireless 2.0
- SoundLearning
- eWindScreen – constantly analyzes incoming signals to detect wind noise, then automatically adjusts signal processing to reduce it
- Push button for program selection with alert tones for program change
- Volume control
- AutoPhone
- Telecoil
- Digital Audio Input (DAI)
- Battery compartment with ON/OFF function and battery compartment lock
- Nanocoated housing
- Charger for batteries
- Compatible with ConnexxLink

Options of Motion 700 P BTE

- Compatible with Tek wireless enhancement system
- Compatible with ePen remote control
- Compatible with ProPocket remote control
- LifeTubes and LifeTips in different sizes
- Earhook
- Choice of 14 different colors

Features of Motion 700 M VC BTE

- Appropriate for moderate to severe hearing losses
- Highly flexible, 16-channel digital signal processing
- 16-channel AGC-I and AGC-O system
- Automatic and multichannel adaptive directional microphone system
- SoundBrilliance enhances your perception of high pitches for a richer, fuller sound
- TruEar simulates the acoustical functions of the outer ear and helps you distinguish sounds in front and back
- SoundSmoothing – transient noise reduction
- Speech and noise management
- FeedbackBlocker – automatically and quickly reduces or eliminates annoying feedback noise without affecting sound quality
- Binaural synchronization with e2e wireless 2.0
- SoundLearning
- eWindScreen – constantly analyzes incoming signals to detect wind noise, then automatically adjusts signal processing to reduce it
- Push button for program selection with alert tones for program change
- Volume control

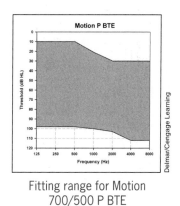

Fitting range for Motion 700/500 P BTE

Delmar/Cengage Learning

- AutoPhone
- Telecoil
- Digital audio input
- Battery compartment with ON/OFF function and battery compartment lock
- Nanocoated housing
- Charger for batteries
- Compatible with ConnexxLink

Options of Motion 700 M VC BTE

- Compatible with Tek wireless enhancement system
- Compatible with ePen remote control
- Compatible with ProPocket remote control
- LifeTubes and LifeTips in different sizes
- Earhook
- Choice of 14 different colors

Features of Motion 700 M BTE

- Appropriate for moderate to severe hearing losses
- Highly flexible, 16-channel digital signal processing
- 16-channel AGC-I and AGC-O system
- Automatic and multichannel adaptive directional microphone system
- SoundBrilliance enhances your perception of high pitches for a richer, fuller sound
- TruEar simulates the acoustical functions of the outer ear and helps you distinguish sounds in front and back
- SoundSmoothing – transient noise reduction
- Speech and noise management
- FeedbackBlocker – automatically and quickly reduces or eliminates annoying feedback noise without affecting sound quality
- Binaural synchronization with e2e wireless 2.0
- SoundLearning
- eWindScreen – constantly analyzes incoming signals to detect wind noise, then automatically adjusts signal processing to reduce it
- Push button for program selection with alert tones for program change
- AutoPhone
- Telecoil

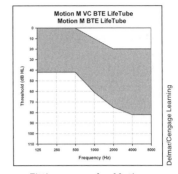

Fitting range for Motion 700/500 M and M VC BTE with LifeTube

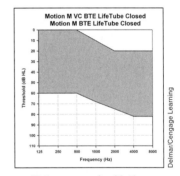

Fitting range for Motion 700/500 M and M VC BTE with LifeTube Closed

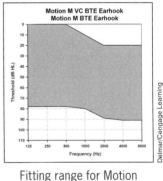

Fitting range for Motion 700/500 M and M VC BTE with Earhook

- Digital audio input
- Battery compartment with ON/OFF function and battery compartment lock
- Nanocoated housing
- Charger for batteries
- Compatible with ConnexxLink

Options of Motion 700 M BTE

- Compatible with Tek wireless enhancement system
- Compatible with ePen remote control
- Compatible with ProPocket remote control
- LifeTubes and LifeTips in different sizes
- Earhook
- Choice of 14 different colors

Features of Motion 700 ITE (118/50, 123/55, 123/60), Motion 700 HS/ITC (113/40, 118/45, 118/50), Motion 700 CIC (113/40, 113/47), and Motion 700 MC (113/47, 113/40)

- Appropriate for mild to moderate hearing losses
- Highly flexible, 16-channel digital signal processing
- 16-channel AGC-I and AGC-O system
- Automatic and multichannel adaptive directional microphone system
- SoundBrilliance enhances your perception of high pitches for a richer, fuller sound
- SoundSmoothing – transient noise reduction
- Speech and noise management
- FeedbackBlocker – automatically and quickly reduces or eliminates annoying feedback noise without affecting sound quality
- Binaural synchronization with e2e wireless 2.0
- SoundLearning
- eWindScreen – constantly analyzes incoming signals to detect wind noise, then automatically adjusts signal processing to reduce it (only for TwinMic™)
- Push button for program selection with alert tones for program change
- AutoPhone
- Telecoil
- Compatible with ConnexxLink

Options of Motion 700 ITE (118/50, 123/55, 123/60), Motion 700 HS/ITC (113/40, 118/45, 118/50), Motion 700 CIC (113/40, 113/47), and Motion 700 MC (113/47, 113/40)

- Compatible with Tek wireless enhancement system
- Compatible with ePen remote control
- Compatible with ProPocket remote control
- Volume control

SIEMENS HEARING

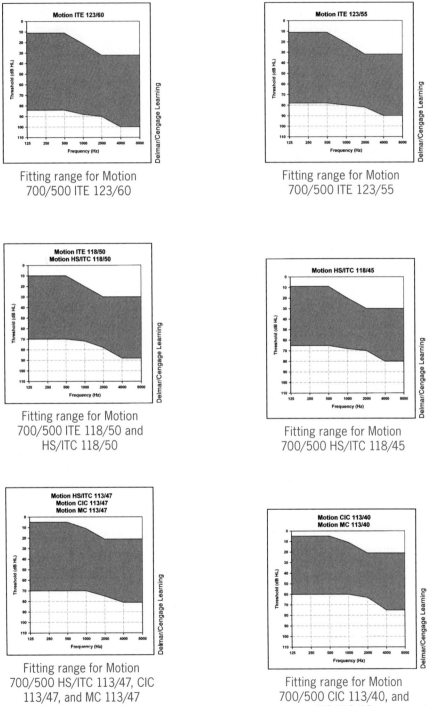

Fitting range for Motion
700/500 ITE 123/60

Fitting range for Motion
700/500 ITE 123/55

Fitting range for Motion
700/500 ITE 118/50 and
HS/ITC 118/50

Fitting range for Motion
700/500 HS/ITC 118/45

Fitting range for Motion
700/500 HS/ITC 113/47, CIC
113/47, and MC 113/47

Fitting range for Motion
700/500 CIC 113/40, and
MC 113/40

Typical Specifications		Motion 700 P BTE
Standard IEC 60118-7:2005		
Output sound pressure level	Max OSPL 90 (dB)	130
	HF-Average OSPL 90 (dB)	124
Full-on gain	Peak gain (dB)	70
	HF-Average full-on gain (dB)	61
Total harmonic distortion	500 Hz	2%
	800 Hz	1%
	1600 Hz	1%
Equivalent input noise (dB)		16
Telecoil sensitivity	HFA-SPLITS (dB) (left/right)	104/107
Battery	Operating current (mA)	1.0
	Battery type	13
Compression characteristics – channel AGC-O	Attack (ms)	5
	Release (ms)	600

Delmar/Cengage Learning

Typical Specifications		Motion 700 M VC BTE, Motion 700 M BTE Earhook	Motion 700 M VC BTE, Motion 700 M BTE S-LifeTube
Standard ANSI S3.22-2003			
Output sound pressure level	Max OSPL 90 (dB)	124	123
	HF-Average OSPL 90 (dB)	121	111
Full-on gain	Peak gain (dB)	55	55
	HF-Average full-on gain (dB)	47	40
Total harmonic distortion	500 Hz	4%	1 %
	800 Hz	3%	1%
	1600 Hz	1%	1%
Equivalent input noise (dB)		17	17
Telecoil sensitivity	HFA-SPLITS (dB) (left/right)	105/102	95/92
Battery	Operating current (mA)	1.0	1.1
	Battery type	13	13
Compression characteristics – channel AGC-O	Attack (ms)	5	5
	Release (ms)	600	600

Delmar/Cengage Learning

SIEMENS HEARING

Typical Specifications		Motion 700 ITE 123-55	Motion 700 ITE 123-60
Standard ANSI S3.22-2003			
Output sound pressure level	Max OSPL 90 (dB)	123	123
	HF-Average OSPL 90 (dB)	118	118
Full-on gain	Peak gain (dB)	55	60
	HF-Average full-on gain (dB)	49	54
Battery	Operating current (mA)	1.0	1.0
	Battery type	13	13

Delmar/Cengage Learning

Typical Specifications		Motion 700 HS/ITC 113/40	Motion 700 HS/ITC 118/45	Motion 700 HS/ITC 118/50
Standard ANSI S3.22-2003				
Output sound pressure level	Max OSPL 90 (dB)	113	118	118
	HF-Average OSPL 90 (dB)	111	114	115
Full-on gain	Peak gain (dB)	40	45	50
	HF-Average full-on gain (dB)	33	38	44
Battery	Operating current (mA)	1.0	1.0	1.0
	Battery type	312	312	312

Delmar/Cengage Learning

Typical Specifications		Motion 700 CIC 113/40	Motion 700 CIC 113/47	Motion 700 MC 113/40	Motion 700 MC 113/47
Standard ANSI S3.22-2003					
Output sound pressure level	Max OSPL 90 (dB)	113	113	113	113
	HF-Average OSPL 90 (dB)	108	109	111	110
Full-on gain	Peak gain (dB)	40	47	40	47
	HF-Average full-on gain (dB)	35	43	33	38
Battery	Operating current (mA)	0.8	0.8	0.8	0.8
	Battery type	10	10	10	10

Delmar/Cengage Learning

Product Application

Motion 500 P BTE
Motion 500 M VC BTE
Motion 500 M BTE
Motion 500 ITE (118/50, 123/55, 123/60)
Motion 500 HS/ITC (113/40, 118/45, 118/50)
Motion 500 CIC (113/40, 113/47)
Motion 500 MC (113/47, 113/40)

Features of Motion 500 P BTE

- Appropriate for moderate to severe hearing losses
- Highly flexible, 12-channel digital signal processing
- 12-channel AGC-I and AGC-O system
- Automatic and multichannel adaptive directional microphone system
- SoundSmoothing – transient noise reduction
- Speech and noise management
- FeedbackBlocker – automatically and quickly reduces or eliminates annoying feedback noise without affecting sound quality
- Binaural synchronization with e2e wireless 2.0
- DataLearning
- eWindScreen – constantly analyzes incoming signals to detect wind noise, then automatically adjusts signal processing to reduce it
- Push button for program selection with alert tones for program change
- Volume control
- AutoPhone
- Telecoil
- Digital audio input
- Battery compartment with ON/OFF function and battery compartment lock
- Nanocoated housing
- Charger for batteries
- Compatible with ConnexxLink

Options of Motion 500 P BTE

- Compatible with Tek wireless enhancement system
- Compatible with ePen remote control
- Compatible with ProPocket remote control
- LifeTubes and LifeTips in different sizes
- Earhook
- Choice of 14 different colors

Features of Motion 500 M VC BTE

- Appropriate for moderate to severe hearing losses
- Highly flexible, 12-channel digital signal processing

- 12-channel AGC-I and AGC-O system
- Automatic and multichannel adaptive directional microphone system
- SoundSmoothing – transient noise reduction
- Speech and noise management
- FeedbackBlocker – automatically and quickly reduces or eliminates annoying feedback noise without affecting sound quality
- Binaural synchronization with e2e wireless 2.0
- DataLearning
- eWindScreen – constantly analyzes incoming signals to detect wind noise, then automatically adjusts signal processing to reduce it
- Push button for program selection with alert tones for program change
- Volume control
- AutoPhone
- Telecoil
- Digital audio input
- Battery compartment with ON/OFF function and battery compartment lock
- Nanocoated housing
- Charger for batteries
- Compatible with ConnexxLink

Options of Motion 500 M VC BTE

- Compatible with Tek wireless enhancement system
- Compatible with ePen remote control
- Compatible with ProPocket remote control
- LifeTubes and LifeTips in different sizes
- Earhook
- Choice of 14 different colors

Features of Motion 500 M BTE

- Appropriate for moderate to severe hearing losses
- Highly flexible, 12-channel digital signal processing
- 12-channel AGC-I and AGC-O system
- Automatic and multichannel adaptive directional microphone system
- SoundSmoothing – transient noise reduction
- Speech and noise management
- FeedbackBlocker – automatically and quickly reduces or eliminates annoying feedback noise without affecting sound quality
- Binaural synchronization with e2e wireless 2.0
- DataLearning
- eWindScreen – constantly analyzes incoming signals to detect wind noise, then automatically adjusts signal processing to reduce it
- Push button for program selection with alert tones for program change
- AutoPhone
- Telecoil

- Digital audio input
- Battery compartment with ON/OFF function and battery compartment lock
- Nanocoated housing
- Charger for batteries
- Compatible with ConnexxLink

Options of Motion 500 M BTE

- Compatible with Tek wireless enhancement system
- Compatible with ePen remote control
- Compatible with ProPocket remote control
- LifeTubes and LifeTips in different sizes
- Earhook
- Choice of 14 different colors

Features of Motion 500 ITE (118/50, 123/55, 123/60), Motion 500 HS/ITC (113/40, 118/45, 118/50), Motion 500 CIC (113/40, 113/47), and Motion 500 MC (113/47, 113/40)

- Appropriate for mild to moderate hearing losses
- Highly flexible, 12-channel digital signal processing
- 12-channel AGC-I and AGC-O system
- Automatic and multichannel adaptive directional microphone system
- SoundSmoothing – transient noise reduction
- Speech and noise management
- FeedbackBlocker – automatically and quickly reduces or eliminates annoying feedback noise without affecting sound quality
- Binaural synchronization with e2e wireless 2.0
- DataLearning
- eWindScreen – constantly analyzes incoming signals to detect wind noise, then automatically adjusts signal processing to reduce it (only for TwinMic)
- Push button for program selection with alert tones for program change
- AutoPhone
- Telecoil
- Compatible with ConnexxLink

Options of Motion 500 ITE (118/50, 123/55, 123/60), Motion 500 HS/ITC (113/40, 118/45, 118/50), Motion 500 CIC (113/40, 113/47), and Motion 500 MC (113/47, 113/40)

- Compatible with Tek wireless enhancement system
- Compatible with ePen remote control
- Compatible with ProPocket remote control
- Volume control

Typical Specifications		Motion 500 P BTE	Motion 500 M VC BTE, Motion 500 M BTE Earhook	Motion 500 M VC BTE, Motion 500 M BTE S-LifeTube
Standard ANSI S3.22-2003				
Output sound pressure level	Max OSPL 90 (dB)	130	124	123
	HF-Average OSPL 90 (dB)	124	121	111
Full-on gain	Peak gain (dB)	70	55	55
	HF-Average full-on gain (dB)	61	47	40
Total harmonic distortion	500 Hz	2%	4%	1 %
	800 Hz	1%	3%	1%
	1600 Hz	1%	1%	1%
Equivalent input noise (dB)		16	17	17
Telecoil sensitivity	HFA-SPLITS (dB) (left/right)	104/107	105/102	95/92
Battery	Operating current (mA)	1.0	1.0	1.1
	Battery type	13	13	13
Compression characteristics – channel AGC-O	Attack (ms)	5	5	5
	Release (ms)	600	600	600

Delmar/Cengage Learning

Typical Specifications		Motion 500 ITE 118/50	Motion 500 ITE 123-55	Motion 500 ITE 123-60
Standard ANSI S3.22-2003				
Output sound pressure level	Max OSPL 90 (dB)	118	123	123
	HF-Average OSPL 90 (dB)	115	118	118
Full-on gain	Peak gain (dB)	50	55	60
	HF-Average full-on gain (dB)	43	49	54
Battery	Operating current (mA)	1.0	1.0	1.0
	Battery type	13	13	13

Delmar/Cengage Learning

Typical Specifications		Motion 500 HS/ITC 113/40	Motion 500 HS/ITC 118/45	Motion 500 HS/ITC 118/50
Standard ANSI S3.22-2003				
Output sound pressure level	Max OSPL 90 (dB)	113	118	118
	HF-Average OSPL 90 (dB)	111	114	115
Full-on gain	Peak gain (dB)	40	45	50
	HF-Average full-on gain (dB)	33	38	44
Battery	Operating current (mA)	1.0	1.0	1.0
	Battery type	312	312	312

Delmar/Cengage Learning

Typical Specifications		Motion 500 CIC 113/40	Motion 500 CIC 113/47	Motion 500 MC 113/40	Motion 500 MC 113/47
Standard ANSI S3.22-2003					
Output sound pressure level	Max OSPL 90 (dB)	113	113	113	113
	HF-Average OSPL 90 (dB)	108	109	111	110
Full-on gain	Peak gain (dB)	40	47	40	47
	HF-Average full-on gain (dB)	35	43	33	38
Battery	Operating current (mA)	0.8	0.8	0.8	0.8
	Battery type	10	10	10	10

Delmar/Cengage Learning

PRODUCT 3: PURE SERIES 700 AND 500

Product Application

Pure RIC 700 S 108/45
Pure RIC 700 M 119/55
Pure RIC 700 P 122/65
Pure RIC 500 S 108/45
Pure RIC 500 M 119/55
Pure RIC 500 P 122/65
Pure CIC 700 113/35
Pure CIC 700 113/40
Pure CIC 500 113/35
Pure CIC 500 113/40

Features of Pure RIC 700 series

- SoundLearning – remembers volume preferences and learns sound quality preferences independently for soft, medium, and loud sounds, as well as treble preferences
- SoundBrilliance – provides acoustic stimulation of up to 12 kHz, enhancing the perception of higher-pitched sounds, creating a richer, fuller sound
- FeedbackBlocker – automatically and quickly eliminates or reduces feedback noise without affecting sound quality
- e2e wireless 2.0 – synchronizes the signal processing of both hearing instruments in binaural fittings and provides "touch one, control both" functionality
- TruEar – available in the RIC BTE models; simulates the acoustical functions of the outer ear and helps distinguish sounds in front from those from behind
- Rechargeable – available in RIC BTE configurations; 2 instruments at a time can be placed in the easy-to-use charger, and 5 hours of charging is all that's necessary for all-day use
- Speech and noise management – automatically identifies and reduces environmental background noise to a comfortable level, while isolating and softening annoying sudden noises without affecting the quality of speech
- eWindScreen – constantly monitors the environment for wind noise and automatically softens it
- ProPocket – small, optional remote control provides easy fingertip control over virtually all instrument functions
- Tek option – wireless enhancement allows for streaming audio content in from stereos, mobile phones, MP3 players, television, and other sources directly into the hearing instrument
- Multichannel adaptive directional microphone – available in RIC BTE configurations, this feature has been clinically proven to improve speech clarity in noisy situations like parties or restaurants
- Loudness and recognition – an intuitive two-component amplification system automatically reduces the amplification for loud sounds while increasing it for soft sounds
- Exchangeable housing – with a number of colors to choose from, you can easily exchange the housing to suit your patients' needs
- Adaptive melody beeps – ensures that the acoustical signals are always audible to the wearer
- 16-channel digital signal processing
- AGC-I compression system 16 channels
- AGC-O output limitation 16/4

Features of Pure RIC 500 series

- DataLearning – automatically learns overall volume preferences in different environments for fewer manual adjustments

- FeedbackBlocker – automatically and quickly eliminates or reduces feedback noise without affecting sound quality
- e2e wireless 2.0 – synchronizes the signal processing of both hearing instruments in binaural fittings and provides "touch one, control both" functionality
- Rechargeable – available in RIC BTE configurations; 2 instruments at a time can be placed in the easy-to-use charger, and 5 hours of charging is all that's necessary for all-day use
- Speech and noise management – automatically identifies and reduces environmental background noise to a comfortable level, while isolating and softening annoying sudden noises without affecting the quality of speech
- eWindScreen – constantly monitors the environment for wind noise and automatically softens it
- ProPocket – small, optional remote control provides easy fingertip control over virtually all instrument functions
- Tek option – wireless enhancement allows for streaming audio content in from stereos, mobile phones, MP3 players, television, and other sources directly into the hearing instrument
- Multichannel adaptive directional microphone – available in RIC BTE configurations , this feature has been clinically proven to improve speech clarity in noisy situations like parties or restaurants
- Loudness and recognition – an intuitive two-component amplification system automatically reduces the amplification for loud sounds while increasing it for soft sounds
- Exchangeable housing – with a number of colors to choose from, you can easily exchange the housing to suit your patients' needs
- Adaptive melody beeps – ensures that the acoustical signals are always audible to the wearer
- 8-channel digital signal processing
- AGC-I compression system 8 channels
- AGC-O output limitation 8/4

SIEMENS HEARING

Features of Pure 700/500 RIC S 108/45

- Receiver supplies 45 dB of gain with 108 dB peak output SPL

Features of Pure 700/500 RIC M 119/55

- Receiver supplies 55 dB of gain with 119 dB peak output SPL

Features of Pure 700/500 RIC P 122/65

- Receiver supplies 65 dB of gain with 121 dB peak output SPL

Features of Pure 700/500 CIC 113/35

- Receiver supplies 35 dB of gain with 113 dB peak output SPL
- Option of memory button

- Option of wireless connectivity
- Option of both memory button and wireless connectivity

Features of Pure 700/500 CIC 113/40

- Receiver supplies 40 dB of gain with 113dB peak output SPL
- Option of memory button
- Option of wireless connectivity
- Option of both memory button and wireless connectivity

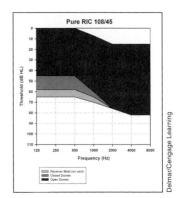

Fitting range for Pure® 700/500 RIC 108/45 for the open dome (dark gray), closed dome (dark and medium gray areas), and receiver mold with no vent (all shaded areas)

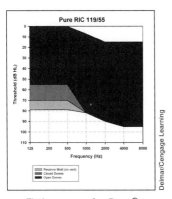

Fitting range for Pure® 700/500 RIC 119/55 for the open dome (dark gray), closed dome (dark and medium gray areas), and receiver mold with no vent (all shaded areas)

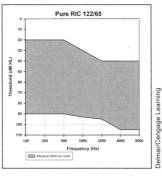

Fitting range for Pure® 700/500 RIC 112/65

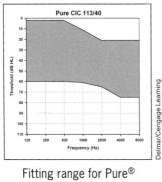

Fitting range for Pure® 700/500 CIC 113/40

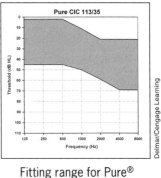

Fitting range for Pure® 700/500 CIC 113/35

Typical Specifications		Pure RIC 45dB receiver	Pure RIC 55dB receiver	Pure RIC 65dB receiver
Standard ANSI S3.22-1996				
Output sound pressure level	Max OSPL 90 (dB)	108	119	121
	HF-Average OSPL 90 (dB)	101	114	115
Full-on gain	Peak gain (dB)	45	55	65
	HF-Average full-on gain (dB)	35	46	54
Total harmonic distortion	500 Hz	1%	1%	1%
	800 Hz	1%	1%	1%
	1600 Hz	1%	2%	1%
Equivalent input noise (dB)		19	19	19
Telecoil sensitivity	HFA-SPLITS (dB)	n/a	n/a	n/a
Battery	Operating current (mA)	0.8	0.9	0.9
	Battery type	312 cell zinc-air	312 cell zinc-air	312 cell zinc-air
Compression characteristics – channel AGC-O (CK= –21 dB)	Attack (ms)	5	5	5
	Release (ms)	680	680	680

Delmar/Cengage Learning

Typical Specifications		Pure CIC 35dB receiver	Pure CIC 40dB receiver
Standard ANSI S3.22-1996			
Output sound pressure level	Max OSPL 90 (dB)	113	113
	HF-Average OSPL 90 (dB)	109	109
Full-on gain	Peak gain (dB)	35	40
	HF-Average full-on gain (dB)	30	35
Total harmonic distortion	500 Hz	<8%	<8%
	800 Hz	<8%	<8%
	1600 Hz	<8%	<8%
Equivalent input noise (dB)		<28	<28
Telecoil sensitivity	HFA-SPLITS (dB)	n/a	n/a
Battery	Operating current (mA)	<120	<120
	Battery type	10	10

continues

SIEMENS HEARING

continued

Typical Specifications		Pure CIC 35dB receiver	Pure CIC 40dB receiver
Compression characteristics – channel AGC-O (CK= –21 dB)	Attack (ms)	5	5
	Release (ms)	680	680

Delmar/Cengage Learning

PRODUCT 4: VIBE

Product Application

Vibe 500 RIC

Features of Vibe 500 RIC

- Hearing system for mild to moderate hearing losses
- Extremely lightweight
- Colored and patterned covers – up to 5 different covers come with purchase
- SoundSmoothing – effective transient noise suppression technology
- Data-logging – tracks information such as program use and wearing time for faster, more precise fine-tuning and better counseling
- FeedbackBlocker – automatically and quickly eliminates or reduces feedback noise without affecting sound quality
- 8-channel digital signal processing – provides for robust performance and flexibility to meet each individual's specific needs
- Vibe microphone – its unique positioning takes advantage of the natural contours of the outer ear and the way it collects and funnels sound into the ear canal
- In-the-crest fit – means it won't interfere with eyeglasses or other devices and keeps the ear canal open for comfort
- Single push-button control – combines cutting-edge technology with easy operation
- Speech and noise management – advanced technologies combine to automatically identify and reduce environmental background noise to a comfortable level while isolating and selectively enhancing speech
- Power-on delay – the power-on delay feature eliminates the possibility of feedback whistling while putting on the instruments

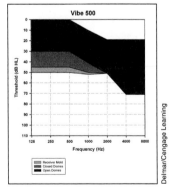

Fitting range for Vibe 500: open dome (dark gray), closed dome (medium and dark gray areas), and receiver mold (all shaded areas)

Options of Vibe 500 RIC

- 4 different receiver lengths for optimum fit
- Exchangeable covers in 19 different colors and patterns

Typical Specifications		Vibe 500 RIC
Standard ANSI S3.22-1996		
Output sound pressure level	Max OSPL 90 (dB)	108
	HF-Average OSPL 90 (dB)	100
Full-on gain	Peak gain (dB)	35
	HF-Average full-on gain (dB)	28
Total harmonic distortion	500 Hz	1%
	800 Hz	1%
	1600 Hz	1%
Equivalent input noise (dB)		16
Telecoil sensitivity	HFA-SPLITS (dB)	n/a
Battery	Operating current (mA)	0.8
	Battery type	10
Compression characteristics – channel AGC-O (CK= –21 dB)	Attack (ms)	5
	Release (ms)	500

Delmar/Cengage Learning

PRODUCT 5: EXPLORER

Product Application

Explorer 500 P BTE

Features of Explorer 500 P BTE

- Pediatric BTE for moderate to severe hearing losses
- Tamper-proof battery door
- Nanocoated housing
- Programmable end-stop volume control with clear markings and power-off functionality
- Programmable push button for program selection and power-off
- 8-channel AGC-I and AGC-O
- Feedback blocker
- Audibility-focused speech and noise management
- DAI with speech-activated FM
- High-performance directional microphone (static, automatic, and adaptive)
- SoundSmoothing
- eWindScreen – wind noise reduction system
- T-coil – manual and automatic

SIEMENS HEARING

- Optional visual status indicator
- Tek-ready
- Up to 5 individual hearing programs for microphone, audio shoe, telecoil, and/or Bluetooth
- Alerting tones for low battery voltage and program change
- Compatible with ConnexxLink (wireless programming)

Options of Explorer 500 P BTE

- 16 colors, including transparent colors, light pink, and light blue
- Optional visual status indicator LED

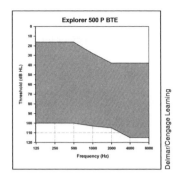

Fitting range for Explorer 500 P BTE

Typical Specifications		Explorer 500 P BTE
Standard ANSI S3.22-1996		
Output sound pressure level	Max OSPL 90 (dB)	136
	HF-Average OSPL 90 (dB)	129
Full-on gain	Peak gain (dB)	73
	HF-Average full-on gain (dB)	65
Total harmonic distortion	500 Hz	4%
	800 Hz	2%
	1600 Hz	1%
Equivalent input noise (dB)		15
Telecoil sensitivity	HFA-SPLITS (dB) (left/right)	111/114
Battery	Operating current (mA) (with LED/without LED)	1.8/1.4
	Battery type	13
Compression characteristics – channel AGC-O (CK= –21 dB)	Attack (ms)	5
	Release (ms)	550

Delmar/Cengage Learning

PRODUCT 6: CENTRA

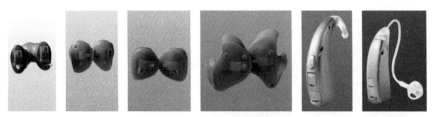

CENTRA Hearing Aid family including CENTRA CIC through CENTRA Life BTE
Compliments of Siemens Hearing Instruments, Inc.

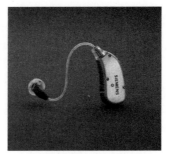

CENTRA Active BTE
Compliments of Siemens
Hearing Instruments, Inc.

Product Application

CENTRA Active BTE
CENTRA Life BTE
CENTRA P BTE
CENTRA HP BTE
CENTRA SP BTE
CENTRA S BTE
CENTRA S-VC BTE
CENTRA ITE
CENTRA ITC/HS
CENTRA MC
CENTRA CIC

Features of CENTRA Active BTE

- Digital 16-channel amplifier with 8 compression channels
- Appropriate for mild to moderate hearing losses
- Receiver-in-canal (RIC) hearing system
  - Rechargeable batteries
  - Ergonomically shaped receiver unit designed for optimum placement in the ear canal
  - Nanocoated housing – repels water and prevents moisture damage
  - Water-resistant domes with integrated C-Guard™ wax protection system available in various open and closed sizes
  - Clip-on replacement microphone covers protect microphones from moisture and debris
- e2e wireless – binaural synchronization system
- SoundSmoothing – suppresses transient sounds to reduce fatigue
- DataLearning – Siemens's proprietary data-logging system that automatically fine-tunes volume settings
- eWindScreen – wind noise reduction system
- Automatic and multichannel adaptive directional microphone system

SIEMENS
HEARING

- Automatic and adaptive feedback cancellation
- Automatic situation detection with music detection – changes settings depending on listening situation
- Adaptive noise reduction and adaptive speech enhancement – noise reduction algorithms that work either when there is noise alone or when there is speech in noise, respectively
- Connexx fitting software
- Battery compartment with ON/OFF switch
- Up to 3 hearing programs (only with ePocket™)
- Alerting tones for low battery voltage

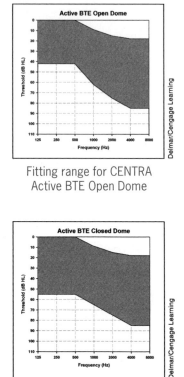

Fitting range for CENTRA Active BTE Open Dome

Options for CENTRA Active BTE

- Colors: beige, brown, gray, granite, silver, black, pearl white, sandy brown, golden blond, chestnut, charcoal
- Intelligent charger that charges up to 2 instruments (both instruments work all day and evening on a single charge)
- Size 13 rechargeable or standard batteries
- ePocket remote control option for discreet and easy adjustment

Fitting range for CENTRA Active BTE Closed Dome

Features of CENTRA Life BTE

- Digital 16-channel amplifier with 8 fully adjustable compression channels
- Appropriate for mild to moderate hearing losses
- Programmable BTE instrument
  - SoundSmoothing – suppresses transient sounds to reduce fatigue
  - DataLearning – Siemens's proprietary data-logging system that automatically fine-tunes volume settings
  - e2e wireless – binaural synchronization system
- Automatic and multichannel adaptive directional microphone system
- Automatic and adaptive feedback cancellation
- Automatic situation detection with music detection – changes settings depending on listening situation
- Adaptive noise reduction and adaptive speech enhancement – noise reduction algorithms that work either when there is noise alone or when there is speech in noise, respectively
- eWindScreen – wind noise reduction system
- Nanocoated housing – repels water and prevents moisture damage

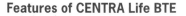

- Connexx fitting software
- Battery compartment with ON/OFF switch
- Up to 3 hearing programs (only with ePocket)
- Alerting tones for low battery voltage

Options for CENTRA Life BTE

- Colors: beige, brown, gray, granite, silver, black, and transparent; translucent fun colors: purple, green, blue, orange, and pink
- Life Fitting Set including LifeTubes, LifeTips, and other fitting accessories, with refill packages available
- ePocket – bidirectional remote control with readout function, program change, and volume adjustment
- Standard earhook

Features of CENTRA P BTE, CENTRA HP BTE, and CENTRA SP BTE

- Digital 16-channel amplifier with 8 fully adjustable compression channels
- CENTRA P BTE for moderate to severe hearing losses
- CENTRA HP BTE for moderate to profound hearing losses
- CENTRA SP BTE for severe to profound hearing losses
- Programmable BTE instruments
  - SoundSmoothing – suppresses transient sounds to reduce fatigue
  - DataLearning – Siemens's proprietary data-logging system that automatically fine-tunes volume settings
  - e2e wireless – binaural synchronization system
- Automatic and multichannel adaptive directional microphone system
- Automatic and adaptive feedback cancellation
- Automatic situation detection with music detection – changes settings depending on listening situation
- Adaptive noise reduction and adaptive speech enhancement – noise reduction algorithms that work either when there is noise alone or when there is speech in noise, respectively
- eWindScreen – wind noise reduction system

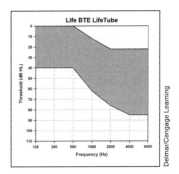

Fitting range for CENTRA Life BTE with LifeTube

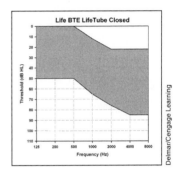

Fitting range for CENTRA Life BTE with LifeTube Closed

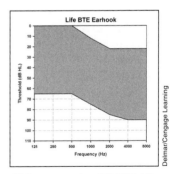

Fitting range for CENTRA Life BTE Earhook

- Nanocoated housing – repels water and prevents moisture damage
- Connexx fitting software
- Audio input compatibility with FM systems
- Telecoil with AutoPhone – automatically switches to telecoil
- Volume control with learning function
- Battery compartment with lock and ON/OFF switch
- Push button for program selection with alerting tones for program change
- Up to 4 individual hearing programs for microphone, audio input, and telecoil mode
- Alerting tones for low battery voltage
- Programmable ON/OFF function for push button

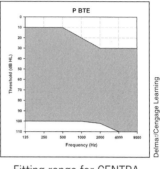

Fitting range for CENTRA P BTE

Options for CENTRA P BTE, CENTRA HP BTE, and CENTRA SP BTE

- Colors: beige, brown, gray, granite, silver, black, and transparent; translucent fun colors: purple, green, blue, orange, and pink
- ePocket – bidirectional remote control with readout function, program change, and volume adjustment
- Audio input boot
- Small earhook
- Materials to support pediatric fittings (use and care kit, storybooks, and more)

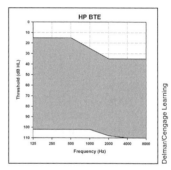

Fitting range for CENTRA HP BTE

Features of CENTRA S BTE and CENTRA S-VC BTE

- Digital 16-channel amplifier with 8 fully adjustable compression channels
- Appropriate for mild to moderate hearing losses
- Programmable BTE instruments
  - SoundSmoothing – suppresses transient sounds to reduce fatigue
  - DataLearning – Siemens's proprietary data-logging system that automatically fine-tunes volume settings
  - e2e wireless – binaural synchronization system

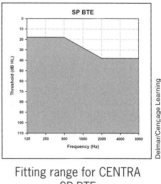

Fitting range for CENTRA SP BTE

- Automatic and multichannel adaptive directional microphone system
- Automatic and adaptive feedback cancellation
- Automatic situation detection with music detection – changes settings depending on listening situation
- Adaptive noise reduction and adaptive speech enhancement – noise reduction algorithms that work either when there is noise alone or when there is speech in noise, respectively
- eWindScreen – wind noise reduction system
- Connexx fitting software
- Volume control with learning function (S-VC only)
- Audio input compatibility with FM systems
- Telecoil with AutoPhone – automatically switches to telecoil
- Battery compartment with lock and ON/OFF switch
- Push button for program selection with alerting tones for program change (S only)
- Up to 4 individual hearing programs for microphone, audio shoe, and telecoil mode
- Alerting tones for low battery voltage
- Programmable ON/OFF function for push button

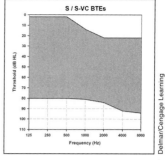

Fitting range for CENTRA S S-VC BTE

Options for CENTRA S BTE and CENTRA S-VC BTE

- Colors: beige, brown, gray, granite, silver, black, and transparent; translucent fun colors: purple, green, blue, orange, and pink
- ePocket – bidirectional remote control with readout function, program change, and volume adjustment
- Audio input boot
- Small earhook
- Materials to support pediatric fittings (use and care kit, storybooks, and more)

Features of CENTRA ITE, CENTRA ITC/HS, CENTRA MC, and CENTRA CIC

- Digital 16-channel amplifier with 8 fully programmable compression handles
- Appropriate for mild to severe hearing losses

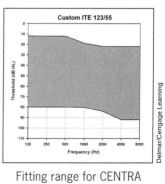

Fitting range for CENTRA ITE 123/55

SIEMENS HEARING

- SoundSmoothing technology – suppresses transient sounds to reduce fatigue
- DataLearning (with volume control or ePocket only) – Siemens's proprietary data-logging system that automatically fine-tunes volume settings
- e2e wireless – binaural synchronization system
- Automatic and adaptive feedback cancellation
- Automatic situation detection including music detection – changes settings depending on listening situation
- Adaptive noise reduction and adaptive speech enhancement – noise reduction algorithms that work either when there is noise alone or when there is speech in noise, respectively
- Connexx fitting software
- Power-on delay
- Alerting tones for low battery voltage

Options for CENTRA ITE, CENTRA ITC/HS, CENTRA MC, and CENTRA CIC

- Automatic and multichannel adaptive directional microphone system (except CENTRA MC and CIC models)
- Volume control with learning function and optional alerting tones for volume changes and volume limits (CENTRA CIC – only with ePocket)
- Telecoil (except CENTRA CIC)
- AutoPhone function – automatically switches to telecoil (except CENTRA MC and CIC models)
- Push button for program selection with programmable tones for memory change (CENTRA CIC – only with ePocket)
- Programmable ON/OFF function for push button
- C-Guard wax protection system
- ePocket – bidirectional remote control with readout function, program change, and volume adjustment

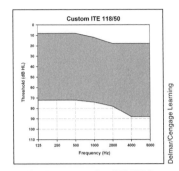

Fitting range for CENTRA ITE 118/50

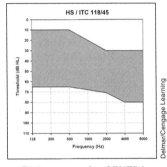

Fitting range for CENTRA ITC/HS 118/45

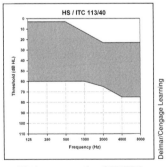

Fitting range for CENTRA ITC/HS 113/40

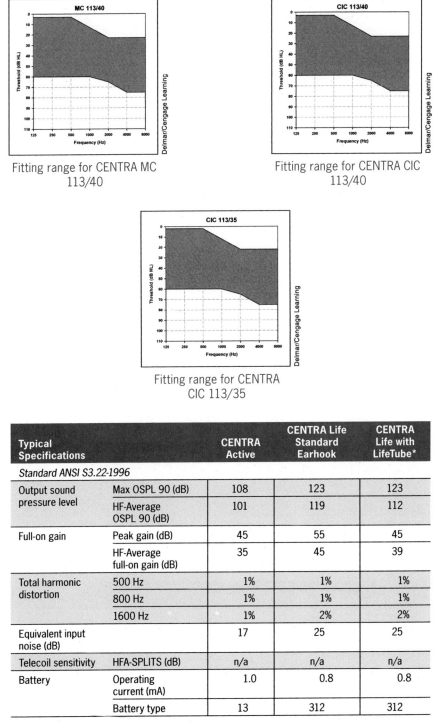

Fitting range for CENTRA MC
113/40

Fitting range for CENTRA CIC
113/40

Fitting range for CENTRA
CIC 113/35

Typical Specifications		CENTRA Active	CENTRA Life Standard Earhook	CENTRA Life with LifeTube*
Standard ANSI S3.22-1996				
Output sound pressure level	Max OSPL 90 (dB)	108	123	123
	HF-Average OSPL 90 (dB)	101	119	112
Full-on gain	Peak gain (dB)	45	55	45
	HF-Average full-on gain (dB)	35	45	39
Total harmonic distortion	500 Hz	1%	1%	1%
	800 Hz	1%	1%	1%
	1600 Hz	1%	2%	2%
Equivalent input noise (dB)		17	25	25
Telecoil sensitivity	HFA-SPLITS (dB)	n/a	n/a	n/a
Battery	Operating current (mA)	1.0	0.8	0.8
	Battery type	13	312	312

continues

continued

Typical Specifications		CENTRA Active	CENTRA Life Standard Earhook	CENTRA Life with LifeTube*
Compression characteristics – channel AGC-O (CK= –21 dB)	Attack (ms)	4	4	4
	Release (ms)	100	100	100

*measured with LifeTube

Delmar/Cengage Learning

Typical Specifications		CENTRA P BTE	CENTRA HP BTE	CENTRA SP BTE
Standard ANSI S3.22-1996				
Output sound pressure level	Max OSPL 90 (dB)	131	136	139
	HF-Average OSPL 90 (dB)	126	129	132
Full-on gain	Peak gain (dB)	70	75	80
	HF-Average full-on gain (dB)	63	67	73
Total harmonic distortion	500 Hz	4%	4%	5%
	800 Hz	4%	2%	2%
	1600 Hz	3%	1%	1%
Equivalent input noise (dB)		<16	11	26
Telecoil sensitivity	HFA-SPLITS (dB)	107.5	110	113
Battery	Operating current (mA)	1.6	1.4	2
	Battery type	13	13	675
Compression characteristics – channel AGC-O (CK= –21 dB)	Attack (ms)	4	5	8
	Release (ms)	100	100	100

Delmar/Cengage Learning

Typical Specifications		CENTRA PBTE	CENTRA HP BTE
Standard ANSI S3.22-1996			
Output sound pressure level	Max OSPL 90 (dB)	123	123
	HF-Average OSPL 90 (dB)	121	121
Full-on gain	Peak gain (dB)	55	55
	HF-Average full-on gain (dB)	52	52

continues

continued

Typical Specifications		CENTRA PBTE	CENTRA HP BTE
Total harmonic distortion	500 Hz	4%	4%
	800 Hz	3%	3%
	1600 Hz	1%	1%
Equivalent input noise (dB)		18	18
Telecoil sensitivity	HFA-SPLITS (dB)	102.5	102.5
Battery	Operating current (mA)	1.2	1.2
	Battery type	13	13
Compression characteristics – channel AGC-O (CK= −21 dB)	Attack (ms)	4	4
	Release (ms)	100	100

Delmar/Cengage Learning

Typical Specifications		CENTRA ITE		CENTRA HS ITC/HS		CENTRA MC		CENTRA CIC
Matrix		123/ 55	118/ 50	118/ 45	113/ 40	113/ 40	113/ 40	113/ 35
Standard ANSI S3.22-1996								
Output sound pressure level	Max OSPL 90 (dB)	118	116	114	109	109	110	109
Average gain	Average gain (dB)	49	44	38	35	34	36	31
Battery	Operating current (mA)	1.1	1.1	1.1	0.9	0.9	0.9	0.9
	Battery type	312	312	312	312	10	10	10

Delmar/Cengage Learning

PRODUCT 7: ARTIS 2

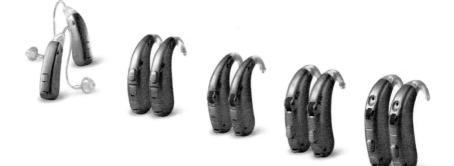

ARTIS 2 BTE series
Compliments of Siemens Hearing Instruments, Inc.

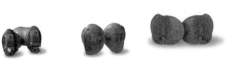

ARTIS 2 custom series including CIC, MC, ITC/HS, and ITE
Compliments of Siemens Hearing Instruments, Inc.

Product Application

ARTIS 2 S BTE	ARTIS 2 ITE
ARTIS 2 S VC BTE	ARTIS 2 ITC/HS
ARTIS 2 P BTE	ARTIS 2 MC
ARTIS 2 SP BTE	ARTIS 2 CIC
ARTIS 2 Life BTE	

FEATURES OF ARTIS 2 S BTE, ARTIS 2 S VC BTE, ARTIS 2 P BTE, AND ARTIS 2 SP BTE

- Fully digital and programmable 12-channel BTE instrument
- ARTIS 2 S BTE and ARTIS 2 S VC BTE recommended for mild to moderate hearing losses
- ARTIS 2 P BTE recommended for moderate to severe hearing losses
- ARTIS 2 SP BTE recommended for severe to profound hearing losses
- e2e wireless – binaural synchronization system
- DataLearning – Siemens's proprietary data-logging system that automatically fine-tunes volume settings
- Automatic and multichannel adaptive directional microphone system
- Automatic and adaptive feedback cancellation
- Automatic situation detection including music detection – changes settings depending on listening situation
- Adaptive noise reduction and adaptive speech enhancement in 12 channels – noise reduction algorithms that work either when there is noise alone or when there is speech in noise, respectively
- eWindScreen – wind noise reduction system
- 4 individual hearing programs for microphone, audio shoe, and/or telecoil (only with ePocket for ARTIS 2 S VC BTE)
- AutoPhone – automatically switches to telecoil
- Audio input
- Volume control
- Battery compartment with lock and ON/OFF switch
- Alerting tones for low battery voltage
- Nanocoated housing – repels water and prevents moisture damage

Options for ARTIS 2 S BTE, ARTIS 2 S VC BTE, ARTIS 2 P BTE, and ARTIS 2 SP BTE

- Colors: beige, brown, gray, granite, silver, black, pearl white, light pink, and light blue; translucent fun colors: purple, green, blue, orange, and pink
- ePocket remote control
- Audio input boot
- Small earhook

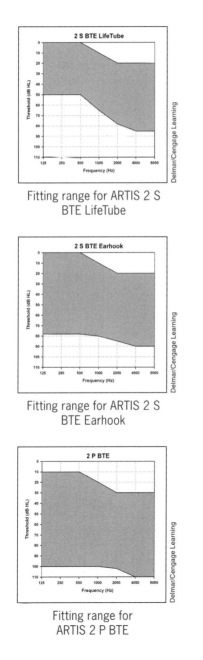

Fitting range for ARTIS 2 S BTE LifeTube

Fitting range for ARTIS 2 S BTE LifeTube Closed

Fitting range for ARTIS 2 S BTE Earhook

Fitting range for ARTIS 2 S VC BTE

Fitting range for ARTIS 2 P BTE

Fitting range for ARTIS 2 SP BTE

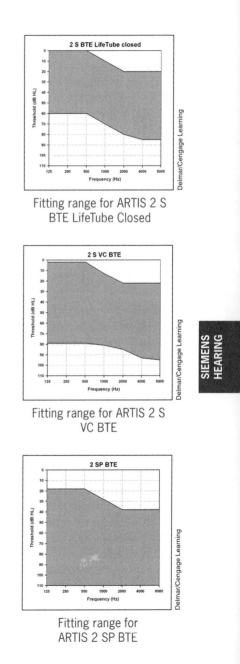

SIEMENS HEARING

Features of ARTIS 2 Life BTE

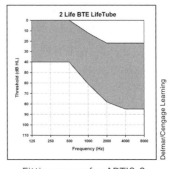

Fitting range for ARTIS 2
Life BTE LifeTube

- Fully digital and programmable 12-channel BTE instrument
- For mild to moderate hearing losses, ski-slope hearing loss, and first-time wearers
- Very thin and inconspicuous LifeTube for right and left sides
- e2e wireless – binaural synchronization system
- DataLearning – Siemens's proprietary data-logging system that automatically fine-tunes volume settings
- Automatic and multichannel adaptive directional microphone system
- Automatic and adaptive feedback cancellation
- Automatic situation detection including music detection – changes settings depending on listening situation
- Adaptive noise reduction and adaptive speech enhancement in 12 channels – noise reduction algorithms that work either when there is noise alone or when there is speech in noise, respectively
- eWindScreen – wind noise reduction system
- 4 individual hearing programs with optional ePocket
- Battery compartment with ON/OFF function
- Alerting tones for low battery voltage
- Nanocoated housing – repels water and prevents moisture damage

Options for ARTIS 2 Life BTE

- Colors: beige, brown, gray, granite, silver, black, pearl white, light pink, and light blue; translucent fun colors: purple, green, blue, orange, and pink
- ePocket bidirectional remote control with readout function
- Life Fitting Set including LifeTubes, LifeTips, and other fitting accessories
- Standard earhook

Features of ARTIS 2 Custom: ARTIS 2 ITE, ARTIS 2 ITC/HS, ARTIS 2 MC, and ARTIS 2 CIC

- Programmable 12-channel custom instruments
  - e2e wireless – binaural synchronization system
  - DataLearning – Siemens's proprietary data-logging system that automatically fine-tunes volume settings
- Automatic and adaptive feedback cancellation
- Automatic situation detection including music detection – changes settings depending on listening situation
- Adaptive noise reduction and speech enhancement in 12 channels – noise reduction algorithms that work either when there is noise alone or when there is speech in noise, respectively

- eWindScreen – wind noise reduction system on directional models
- Up to 4 programs
- Alerting tones for low battery voltage

Options of ARTIS 2 Custom: ARTIS 2 ITE, ARTIS 2 ITC/HS, ARTIS 2 MC, and ARTIS 2 CIC

- Automatic and multichannel adaptive directional microphone system (except ARTIS 2 CIC)
- Volume control with optional alert tones for volume changes and volume limits (except ARTIS 2 CIC)
- AutoPhone function – automatically switches to telecoil (except ARTIS 2 CIC)
- Push button for program selection with alert tones for program change (ARTIS 2 CIC – only with optional ePocket)
- Programmable ON/OFF function for push button
- C-Guard wax protection system
- ePocket – bidirectional remote control with readout function, program change, and volume adjustment

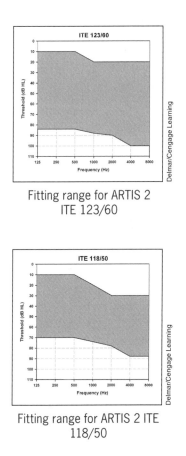

Fitting range for ARTIS 2
ITE 123/60

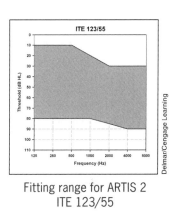

Fitting range for ARTIS 2
ITE 123/55

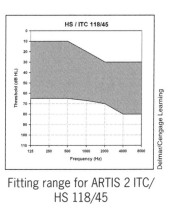

Fitting range for ARTIS 2 ITE
118/50

Fitting range for ARTIS 2 ITC/
HS 118/45

SIEMENS
HEARING

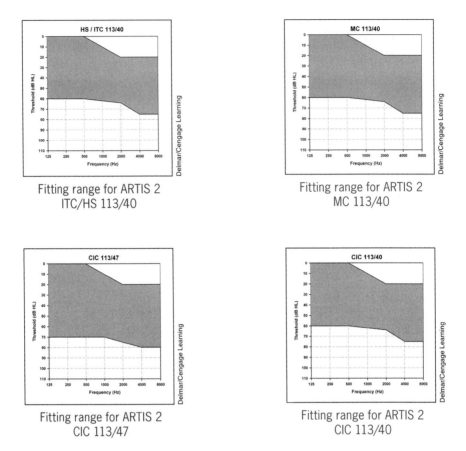

Fitting range for ARTIS 2
ITC/HS 113/40

Fitting range for ARTIS 2
MC 113/40

Fitting range for ARTIS 2
CIC 113/47

Fitting range for ARTIS 2
CIC 113/40

Typical Specifications		ARTIS 2 S BTE Standard Earhook	ARTIS 2 S BTE LifeTube*	ARTIS 2 S VC BTE Standard Earhook	ARTIS 2 S VC BTE LifeTube*
Standard ANSI S3.22-1996					
Output sound pressure level	Max OSPL 90 (dB)	123	123	123	123
	HF-Average OSPL 90 (dB)	122	114	122	114
Full-on gain	Peak gain (dB)	55	55	55	55
	HF-Average full-on gain (dB)	52	43	52	43
Total harmonic distortion	500 Hz	4%	4%	4%	4%
	800 Hz	3%	3%	3%	3%
	1600 Hz	1%	1%	1%	1%
Equivalent input noise (dB)		18	18	18	18

continues

continued

Typical Specifications		ARTIS 2 S BTE Standard Earhook	ARTIS 2 S BTE LifeTube*	ARTIS 2 S VC BTE Standard Earhook	ARTIS 2 S VC BTE LifeTube*
Telecoil sensitivity	HFA-SPLITS (dB)	106.5	97.5	106.5	97.5
Battery	Operating current (mA)	1.2	1.2	1.2	1.2
	Battery type	13	13	13	13
Compression characteristics – channel AGC-O (CK= −21 dB)	Attack (ms)	4	4	4	4
	Release (ms)	100	100	100	100

*measured with LifeTube2

Delmar/Cengage Learning

Typical Specifications		ARTIS 2 P BTE	ARTIS 2 SP BTE	ARTIS 2 Life BTE Standard Earhook	ARTIS 2 Life BTE LifeTube*
Standard ANSI S3.22-1996					
Output sound pressure level	Max OSPL 90 (dB)	131	138	123	123
	HF-Average OSPL 90 (dB)	126	132	120	112
Full-on gain	Peak gain (dB)	70	80	55	45
	HF-Average full-on gain (dB)	61	73	46	39
Total harmonic distortion	500 Hz	2%	5%	1%	1%
	800 Hz	1%	2%	1%	1%
	1600 Hz	1%	1%	2%	2%
Equivalent input noise (dB)		<16	26	25	25
Telecoil sensitivity	HFA-SPLITS (dB)	108	109.5	n/a	n/a
Battery	Operating current (mA)	1.0	2.0	0.8	0.8
	Battery type	13	675	312	312
Compression characteristics – channel AGC-O (CK= −21 dB)	Attack (ms)	5	8	5	5
	Release (ms)	100	100	100	100

*measured with LifeTube

Delmar/Cengage Learning

SIEMENS HEARING

Typical Specifications		ARTIS 2 ITE			ARTIS 2 ITC/HS		ARTIS 2 MC		ARTIS 2 CIC	
Matrix		118/ 50	123/ 55	123/ 60	113/ 40	118/ 45	113/ 40	113/ 47	113/ 40	113/ 47
Standard ANSI S3.22-1996										
Output sound pressure level	Max OSPL 90 (dB)	118/ 50	123/ 55	123/ 60	113/ 40	118/ 45	113/ 40	113/ 47	113/ 40	113/ 47
Average gain	Average gain (dB)	115/ 45	118/ 50	118/ 53	110/ 35	114/ 39	110/ 35	109/ 42	110/ 30	110/ 43
Battery	Operating current (mA)	1.0	1.0	1.0	0.9	1.0	0.9	0.9	0.9	0.9
	Battery type	13/ 312	13/ 312	13/ 312	312/ 10	312/ 10	10	10	10	10

Delmar/Cengage Learning

PRODUCT 8: CIELO 2

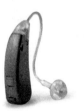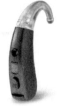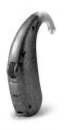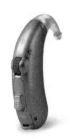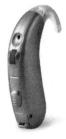

CIELO 2 BTE series
Compliments of Siemens Hearing Instruments, Inc.

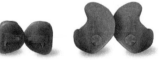

CIELO 2 custom series including ITE, ITC/HS, MC and CIC
Compliments of Siemens Hearing Instruments, Inc.

Product Application

CIELO 2 BTE   CIELO 2 ITE
CIELO 2 S BTE   CIELO 2 ITC/HS
CIELO 2 P BTE   CIELO 2 MC
CIELO 2 SP BTE   CIELO 2 CIC
CIELO 2 Life BTE

Features of CIELO 2 BTE

- Programmable BTE instrument with optional ePocket
- Appropriate for mild to moderate hearing losses
- Data-logging
- Automatic and adaptive directional microphone system
- Automatic and adaptive feedback cancellation
- Automatic situation detection including music detection – changes settings depending on listening situation
- Adaptive noise reduction and speech enhancement in 6 channels – noise reduction algorithms that work either when there is noise alone or when there is speech in noise, respectively
- Wind noise reduction
- 4 individual hearing programs for microphone, audio input, and/or telecoil (only available with ePocket)
- Alerting tones for low battery
- AutoPhone – automatically switches to telecoil
- Audio input
- Volume control
- Battery compartment with lock and ON/OFF switch
- Nanocoated housing – repels water and prevents moisture damage

Options of CIELO 2 BTE

- Colors: beige, brown, gray, granite, silver, black, pearl white, light pink, and light blue; translucent fun colors: purple, green, blue, orange, and pink
- Small earhook
- Audio input boot
- Materials and accessories to support pediatric fittings

Features of CIELO 2 S BTE

- Programmable BTE instrument with optional ePocket
- Data-logging

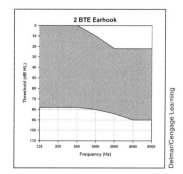

Fitting range for CIELO 2 BTE Earhook

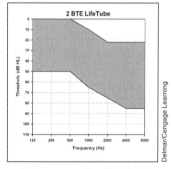

Fitting range for CIELO 2 BTE LifeTube

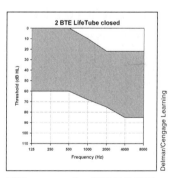

Fitting range for CIELO 2 BTE LifeTube Closed

SIEMENS HEARING

- Fully digital 6-channel amplifier
- Automatic and adaptive directional microphone system
- Automatic and adaptive feedback cancellation
- Automatic situation detection including music detection – changes settings depending on listening situation
- Adaptive noise reduction and speech enhancement in 6 channels – noise reduction algorithms that work either when there is noise alone or when there is speech in noise, respectively
- Wind noise reduction
- 4 individual hearing programs for microphone and/or telecoil
- AutoPhone – automatically switches to telecoil
- Battery compartment with lock and ON/ OFF switch
- Push button for program selection with alert tones for program change
- Alert tones for low battery
- Nanocoated housing – repels water and prevents moisture damage

Options of CIELO 2 S BTE

- Colors: beige, brown, gray, granite, silver, black, pearl white, light pink, and light blue; translucent fun colors: purple, green, blue, orange, and pink
- Small earhook

Features of CIELO 2 P BTE and CIELO 2 SP BTE

- Programmable BTE instrument with optional ePocket
- Fully digital 6-channel amplifier
- CIELO 2 P BTE recommended for moderate to severe hearing losses
- CIELO 2 SP BTE recommended for severe to profound hearing losses
- Data-logging
- Automatic and adaptive directional microphone system
- Automatic and adaptive feedback cancellation

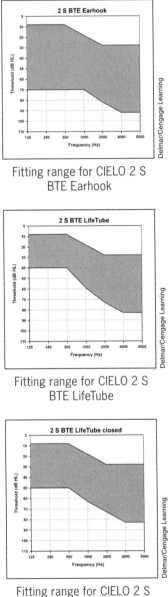

Fitting range for CIELO 2 S BTE Earhook

Fitting range for CIELO 2 S BTE LifeTube

Fitting range for CIELO 2 S LifeTube Closed

Delmar/Cengage Learning

- Automatic situation detection including music detection – changes settings depending on listening situation
- Adaptive noise reduction and speech enhancement in 6 channels – noise reduction algorithms that work either when there is noise alone or when there is speech in noise, respectively
- Wind noise reduction
- 4 individual hearing programs for microphone, audio shoe, and/or telecoil
- Nanocoated housing – repels water and prevents moisture damage
- AutoPhone – automatically switches to telecoil
- Audio input
- Volume control
- Battery compartment with lock and ON/OFF switch
- Push button for program selection with alert tones for program change
- Alert tones for low battery

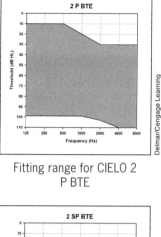

Fitting range for CIELO 2 P BTE

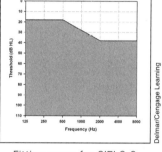

Fitting range for CIELO 2 SP BTE

Options of CIELO 2 P BTE and CIELO 2 SP BTE

- Colors: beige, brown, gray, granite, silver, black, pearl white, light pink, and light blue; translucent fun colors: purple, green, blue, orange, and pink
- Small earhook
- Audio input boot
- Materials and accessories to support pediatric fittings

Features of CIELO 2 Life BTE

- Programmable BTE instrument with optional ePocket
- Fully digital 6-channel amplifier
- Data logging
- Automatic and adaptive directional microphone system
- Automatic and adaptive feedback cancellation
- Automatic situation detection including music detection – changes settings depending on listening situation
- Adaptive noise reduction and speech enhancement in 6 channels – noise reduction algorithms that work either when there is noise alone or when there is speech in noise, respectively
- Wind noise reduction

- 3 individual hearing programs available with optional ePocket
- Alert tones for low battery
- Battery compartment with ON/OFF function
- Nanocoated housing – repels water and prevents moisture damage

Options of CIELO 2 Life BTE

- Colors: beige, brown, gray, granite, silver, black, pearl white, light pink, and light blue; translucent fun colors: purple, green, blue, orange, and pink
- Life Fitting Set including LifeTubes, Life-Tips, and other fitting accessories
- Small earhook

Features of CIELO 2 Custom: CIELO 2 ITE, CIELO 2 ITC/HS, CIELO 2 MC, and CIELO 2 CIC

- Programmable custom instrument with ePocket remote control and data-logging technology
- Appropriate for mild to moderate hearing losses
- Automatic situation detection including music detection – changes settings depending on listening situation
- Automatic and adaptive feedback cancellation
- Adaptive noise reduction and speech enhancement in 6 channels – noise reduction algorithms that work either when there is noise alone or when there is speech in noise, respectively
- Wind noise reduction
- Up to 4 programs
- Alerting tones for low battery voltage

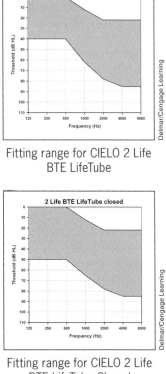

Fitting range for CIELO 2 Life BTE LifeTube

Fitting range for CIELO 2 Life BTE LifeTube Closed

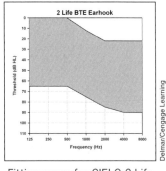

Fitting range for CIELO 2 Life BTE Earhook

Options for CIELO 2 Custom: CIELO 2 ITE, CIELO 2 ITC/HS, CIELO 2 MC, and CIELO 2 CIC

- Automatic and adaptive directional microphone (except CIELO 2 CIC)
- Volume control with optional alerting tones for volume changes and volume limits (CIELO 2 CIC – only with optional ePocket)
- AutoPhone – automatically switches to telecoil (except CIELO 2 CIC)

- Push button for program selection with alert tones for program change (CIELO 2 CIC – only with optional ePocket)
- Programmable ON/OFF function for push button
- ePocket – bidirectional remote control with readout function, program change, and volume adjustment

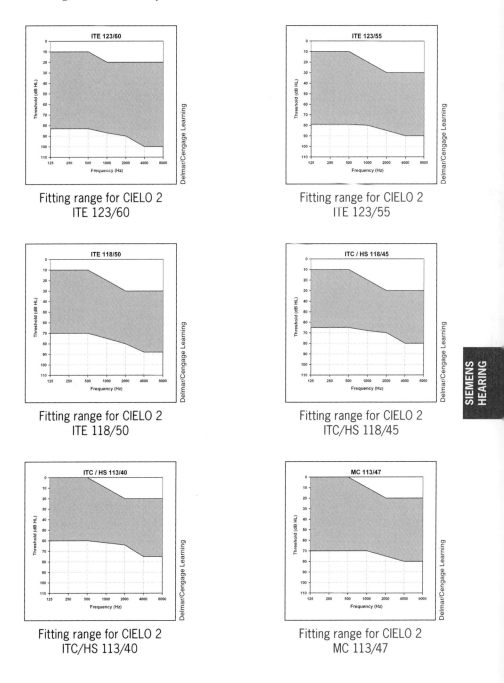

Fitting range for CIELO 2
ITE 123/60

Fitting range for CIELO 2
ITE 123/55

Fitting range for CIELO 2
ITE 118/50

Fitting range for CIELO 2
ITC/HS 118/45

Fitting range for CIELO 2
ITC/HS 113/40

Fitting range for CIELO 2
MC 113/47

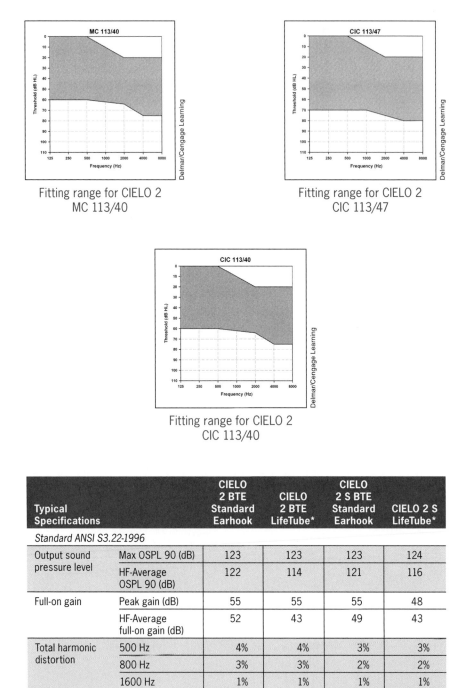

Fitting range for CIELO 2
MC 113/40

Fitting range for CIELO 2
CIC 113/47

Fitting range for CIELO 2
CIC 113/40

Typical Specifications		CIELO 2 BTE Standard Earhook	CIELO 2 BTE LifeTube*	CIELO 2 S BTE Standard Earhook	CIELO 2 S LifeTube*
Standard ANSI S3.22-1996					
Output sound pressure level	Max OSPL 90 (dB)	123	123	123	124
	HF-Average OSPL 90 (dB)	122	114	121	116
Full-on gain	Peak gain (dB)	55	55	55	48
	HF-Average full-on gain (dB)	52	43	49	43
Total harmonic distortion	500 Hz	4%	4%	3%	3%
	800 Hz	3%	3%	2%	2%
	1600 Hz	1%	1%	1%	1%
Equivalent input noise (dB)		18	18	16	16

continues

continued

Typical Specifications		CIELO 2 BTE Standard Earhook	CIELO 2 BTE LifeTube*	CIELO 2 S BTE Standard Earhook	CIELO 2 S LifeTube*
Telecoil sensitivity	HFA-SPLITS (dB)	106.5	97.5	102	96.5
Battery	Operating current (mA)	1.2	1.2	1.0	1.0
	Battery type	13	13	13	13
Compression characteristics – channel AGC-O (CK= –21 dB)	Attack (ms)	4	4	4	4
	Release (ms)	100	100	100	100

*measured with LifeTube2

Delmar/Cengage Learning

Typical Specifications		CIELO 2 P BTE	CIELO 2 SP BTE	CIELO 2 Life BTE Standard Earhook	CIELO 2 Life BTE LifeTube*
Standard ANSI S3.22-1996					
Output sound pressure level	Max OSPL 90 (dB)	131	138	123	123
	HF-Average OSPL 90 (dB)	126	132	120	112
Full-on gain	Peak gain (dB)	70	80	55	45
	HF-Average full-on gain (dB)	61	73	46	39
Total harmonic distortion	500 Hz	2%	5%	1%	1%
	800 Hz	1%	2%	1%	1%
	1600 Hz	1%	1%	2%	2%
Equivalent input noise (dB)		16	26	25	25
Telecoil sensitivity	HFA-SPLITS (dB)	107.5	109.5	n/a	n/a
Battery	Operating current (mA)	1.0	2.0	0.8	0.8
	Battery type	13	675	312	312
Compression characteristics – channel AGC-O (CK= –21 dB)	Attack (ms)	5	8	4	4
	Release (ms)	100	100	100	100

*measured with LifeTube

Delmar/Cengage Learning

Typical Specifications		CIELO 2 ITE		CIELO 2 ITC/HS			CIELO 2 MC		CIELO 2 CIC	
Matrix		123/ 600	123/ 55	118/ 50	118/ 45	113/ 40	113/ 47	113/ 40	113/ 47	113/ 40
Standard ANSI S3.22-1996										
Output sound pressure level	Max OSPL 90 (dB)	123	123	118	118	113	113	113	113	113
Average gain	Average gain (dB)	60	55	50	45	40	47	40	47	40
Battery	Operating current (mA)	n/a	n/a	n/a	n/a	n/a	n/a	n/a	n/a	n/a
	Battery type	13/ 312	13/ 312	13/ 312	312/ 10	312/ 10	10	10	10	10

PRODUCT 9: NITRO

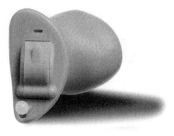

Nitro CIC
Compliments of Siemens Hearing
Instruments, Inc.

Product Application

Nitro CIC

Features of Nitro CIC

- Fully digital, 6-channel CIC instruments
- Appropriate for severe to profound hearing losses
- Adaptive noise reduction and speech enhancement in 6 channels
- Data-logging
- Automatic situation detection including music detection
- Up to 3 programs
- Alert tone for low battery

Options of Nitro CIC

- Push button for program selection with alert tones for program change
- Programmable ON/OFF function for push button
- C-Guard wax guard
  - Nitro CIC 118/55 matrix only

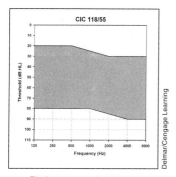

Fitting range for Nitro
CIC 118/50

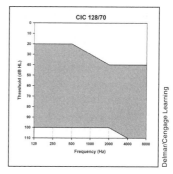

Fitting range for Nitro
CIC 128/70

Typical Specifications		Nitro CIC	
Matrix		118/50	128/70
Standard ANSI S3.22-2000			
Output sound pressure level	Max OSPL 90 (dB)	119	127
Average gain	Average gain (dB)	35	63
Battery	Operating current (mA)	0.9	1.0
	Battery type	10	10

Delmar/Cengage Learning

PRODUCT 10: INTUIS

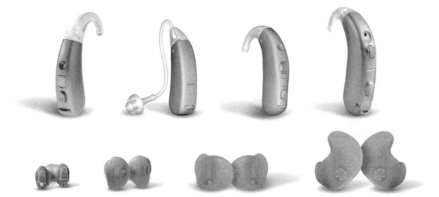

INTUIS family product line from BTE through CIC
Compliments of Siemens Hearing Instruments, Inc.

Product Application

INTUIS Life BTE   INTUIS ITE/Power ITE
INTUIS Dir BTE   INTUIS ITC/HS
INTUIS S Dir BTE   INTUIS MC
INTUIS SP Dir BTE   INTUIS CIC/Power CIC

Features of INTUIS Life BTE

- Fully digital, programmable 4-channel BTE instrument
- Appropriate for mild to moderate hearing losses, ski-slope hearing losses, and first-time wearers
- Very thin and inconspicuous LifeTube for right and left sides
- High-speed automatic feedback cancellation
- 4 adjustable compression channels with configurable crossover frequency
- Adaptive noise reduction – noise reduction algorithm to reduce steady-state noise
- Battery compartment with ON/OFF function
- Alerting tones for low battery power
- Nanocoated housing – repels water and prevents moisture damage
- Connexx fitting software

Options for INTUIS Life BTE

- Colors: beige, brown, gray, granite, silver, black, and transparent; translucent fun colors: purple, green, blue, orange, and pink
- Life Fitting Set
- Refill sets for Life Fitting Set
- Standard earhook

Features of INTUIS Dir BTE

- Fully digital, programmable 4-channel BTE instrument
- TwinMic directional microphone system
- Feedback cancellation
- 4 adjustable compression channels with configurable crossover frequency
- 4 individual hearing programs for microphone, audio input, and/or telecoil
- Programmable volume control
- Compatible with FM systems
- Battery compartment with ON/OFF function
- Push button for program selection with alert tones for program change
- ON/OFF function for push button
- Alerting tones for low battery
- Professional and efficient fitting with the workflow-oriented Connexx software

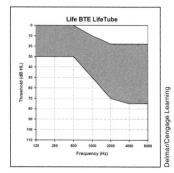

Fitting range for INTUIS Life BTE LifeTube

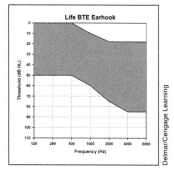

Fitting range for INTUIS Life BTE Earhook

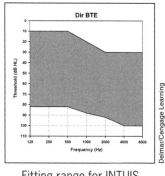

Fitting range for INTUIS Dir BTE

Options for INTUIS Dir BTE

- Colors: beige, brown, gray, granite, silver, black, pearl white, light pink, light blue, and transparent; translucent fun colors: purple, green, blue, orange, and pink
- Small earhook
- Audio input boot
- Volume control cover
- Materials to support pediatric fittings (use and care kit, storybooks, and more)

Features of INTUIS S Dir BTE

- Fully digital programmable 4-channel BTE instrument
- TwinMic directional microphone system
- Feedback cancellation
- 4 adjustable compression channels with configurable crossover frequency
- 4 individual hearing programs for microphone and telecoil
- Adaptive noise reduction – noise reduction algorithm to reduce steady-state noise
- Push button for program selection with alert tones for program change
- Nanocoated housing – repels water and prevents moisture damage
- Alert tones for low battery
- Connexx fitting software

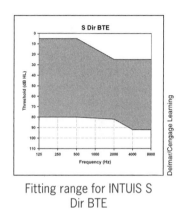

Fitting range for INTUIS S Dir BTE

Options for INTUIS S Dir BTE

- Colors: beige, brown, gray, granite, silver, black, pearl white, and transparent; translucent colors: purple, green, blue, orange, and pink
- Small earhook

Features of INTUIS SP Dir BTE

- Fully digital programmable 4-channel BTE instrument
- TwinMic directional microphone system
- Feedback cancellation
- Adaptive noise reduction in 4 channels – noise reduction algorithm to reduce steady-state noise
- 4 adjustable compression channels with configurable crossover frequency
- 4 individual hearing programs for microphone, telecoil, and audio input
- Nanocoated housing – repels water and prevents moisture damage
- Telecoil
- Audio input and FM compatibility

- Volume control
- Battery compartment with ON/OFF function
- Push button for program selection with alert tones for program change
- Alert tones for low battery voltage
- Connexx fitting software

Options for INTUIS SP Dir BTE

- Colors: beige, brown, gray, granite, silver, black, pearl white, light pink, light blue, and transparent; translucent colors: purple, green, blue, orange, and pink
- Small earhook
- Audio input boot
- Materials and accessories to support pediatric fittings

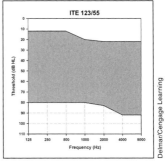

Fitting range for INTUIS SP Dir BTE

Features of INTUIS ITE/Power ITE, INTUIS ITC/HS, INTUIS MC, and INTUIS CIC/Power CIC

- Fully digital 4-channel amplifier
- Programmable custom instruments in all models from CIC to ITE
- 4 adjustable compression channels with one configurable crossover frequency
- Up to 4 individual hearing programs for microphone and/or telecoil
- Automatic feedback cancellation
- Connexx fitting software
- Alert tones for low battery voltage

Fitting range for INTUIS ITE 123/55

Options for INTUIS ITE/Power ITE, INTUIS ITC/HS, INTUIS MC, and INTUIS CIC/Power CIC

- Directional microphone system (except INTUIS CIC/Power CIC)
- Programmable telecoil with AutoPhone – automatically switches to telecoil (except INTUIS CIC/Power CIC)
- Programmable volume control (except INTUIS CIC/Power CIC)
- Push button for multiple memories and programmable ON/OFF function
- C-Guard wax protection system

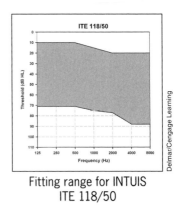

Fitting range for INTUIS ITE 118/50

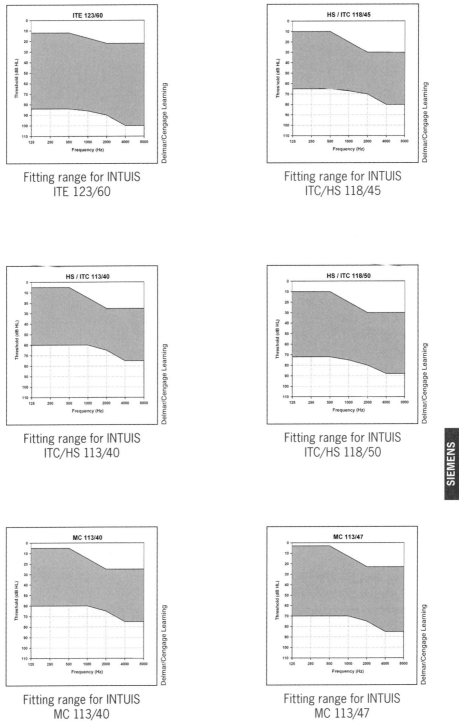

Fitting range for INTUIS
ITE 123/60

Fitting range for INTUIS
ITC/HS 118/45

Fitting range for INTUIS
ITC/HS 113/40

Fitting range for INTUIS
ITC/HS 118/50

Fitting range for INTUIS
MC 113/40

Fitting range for INTUIS
MC 113/47

SIEMENS
HEARING

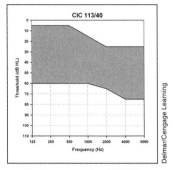

Fitting range for INTUIS
CIC 113/40

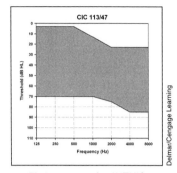

Fitting range for INTUIS
CIC 113/47

Typical Specifications		INTUIS Life Standard Earhook	INTUIS Life with LifeTube*
Standard ANSI S3.22-1996			
Output sound pressure level	Max OSPL 90 (dB)	117	115
	HF-Average OSPL 90 (dB)	114	105
Full-on gain	Peak gain (dB)	45	35
	HF-Average full-on gain (dB)	35	28
Total harmonic distortion	500 Hz	1%	1%
	800 Hz	1%	1%
	1600 Hz	1%	1%
Equivalent input noise (dB)		13	13
Telecoil sensitivity	HFA-SPLITS (dB)	n/a	n/a
Battery	Operating current (mA)	0.5	0.5
	Battery type	312	312
Compression characteristics – channel AGC-O (CK= –21 dB)	Attack (ms)	3	3
	Release (ms)	95	95

*measured with LifeTube
Delmar/Cengage Learning

Typical Specifications		INTUIS Dir BTE	INTUIS S Dir BTE	INTUIS SP Dir BTE
Standard ANSI S3.22-1996				
Output sound pressure level	Max OSPL 90 (dB)	130	124	138
	HF-Average OSPL 90 (dB)	125	122	131

continues

continued

Typical Specifications		INTUIS Dir BTE	INTUIS S Dir BTE	INTUIS SP Dir BTE
Full-on gain	Peak gain (dB)	60	55	80
	HF-Average full-on gain (dB)	55	51	72
Total harmonic distortion	500 Hz	4%	3%	3%
	800 Hz	4%	2%	2%
	1600 Hz	1%	1%	1%
Equivalent input noise (dB)		20	19	15
Telecoil sensitivity	HFA-SPLITS (dB)	105.5	103	112.5
Battery	Operating current (mA)	0.8	0.8	1.6
	Battery type	13	13	675
Compression characteristics – channel AGC-O (CK= −21 dB)	Attack (ms)	3	5	3
	Release (ms)	95	95	100

Delmar/Cengage Learning

Typical Specifications		INTUIS ITE			INTUIS ITC/HS			INTUIS MC		INTUIS CIC	
Matrix		118/50	123/55	123/60	113/40	118/45	118/50	113/40	113/47	113/40	113/47
Standard ANSI S3.22-1996											
Output sound pressure level	Max OSPL 90 (dB)	115	119	118	108	114	115	108	109	110	109
Average gain	Average gain (dB)	44	47	53	34	38	44	34	42	42	42
Battery	Operating current (mA)	0.6	0.6	0.6	0.6	0.6	0.6	0.6	0.6	0.6	0.6
	Battery type	13	13	13	312	312	312	10	10	10	10

Delmar/Cengage Learning

SIEMENS HEARING

CHAPTER NINE

Sonic Innovations

GET IN TOUCH WITH SONIC!

World Headquarters
Sonic Innovations
2795 East Cottonwood Pkwy, Suite 660
Salt Lake City, UT 84121
Phone: 1 (888) 678-4327 (consumers)
Phone: 1 (888) 423-7834 (HA professionals)
E-mail: directmail@sonici.com
Web site: http://sonici.com

> *To improve the quality of life of the hearing impaired*
> — Sonic Innovations vision (Sonic, 2008c)

The majority of companies and brands comprising the hearing industry can be traced back many decades, especially the major players. Sonic Innovations (hereafter Sonic) is the clear outlier in this generalization. 2008 marked Sonic's tenth anniversary, as celebrated by the launch of two new hearing aids, the Velocity miniBTE and the ion 400 (Global Markets Direct, 2008b). To be complete, however, Sonic originated as Sonix in 1991 and changed their name to Sonic Innovations in 1997 (Life Sciences Analytics, 2008). Sonic was founded and have maintained their headquarters in Salt Lake City, Utah. Their growth, however, has led them to have distribution partners in more than 25 countries (Sonic, 2008a, 2008b, 2008d). Some of Sonic's milestones are as follows (Global Markets Direct, 2008b; Life Sciences Analytics, 2008):

1991: Sonix founded
1997: Name changed to Sonic Innovations

2000: The NATURA digital hearing aid won Sonic a gold award in the
       2000 Medical Design Excellence Awards competition
2000: Entered the NASDAQ market
2002: Acquired two Canadian hearing aid companies: Sentech Systems
       and Orsonique
2002: Launched the Adesso
2003: Acquired the hearing aid distribution company Sanomed Handels-
       gesellschaft mbH
2004: Acquired Tympani, Inc.
2005: Launched a high-end digital hearing aid, the Innova
2006: Launched their first open-fit hearing aid, the Ion
2007: Launched a high-end digital hearing aid, the Velocity
2007: Sold Tympany, Inc. to a privately held company, Tympany Holdings,
       LLC
2008: Launched the Velocity miniBTE and the ion400
2009: Sonic's new, smaller, and more powerful hearing instrument
       introduced, the Touch

Transitions in any industry often provide the opportunity for new players to enter the market. The mid- to late 1990s were marked by the transition to fully digital hearing aids. Rather than having to maintain analog devices while spending heavy research and development dollars on digital devices, Sonic could simply jump directly into the fully digital hearing aid world. As a result of this timing and a pattern of good business decisions, Sonic is the only publicly traded hearing aid company in the United States. The exception to this pattern would be the purchase of Tympany, Inc., the manufacturer of an automated hearing evaluation system called the Otogram, in 2004. This single product cost them almost $15 million in losses over 2005 and 2006 (Life Sciences Analytics, 2008). Despite this relative hiccup, Sonic is quickly becoming a significant entity in the industry. As such, they may become a target for an acquisition in the upcoming years (Zable & Anand, 2008).

Philanthropy

For several months in 2008, Sonic donated $50 to the Armed Forces Foundation for every purchase of a Velocity hearing aid. The fund was intended to help veterans in several ways to improve their quality of life, with hearing loss (if applicable), educational expenses, or emergency funds (Sonic, 2008b).

In May 2008, Sonic collaborated with the America Speech-Language-Hearing Association's "Better Hearing Month" to provide free hearing screenings in over 40 clinics in 10 states in the United States (Sonic, 2008d).

SONIC
INNOVATIONS

PRODUCT INFORMATION

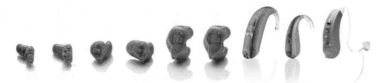

Sonic Innovations family product line
Courtesy of Sonic Innovations, Inc.

PRODUCT 1: TOUCH™

Product Application

Touch™ 24 BTE
Touch™ 12 BTE
Touch™ 6 BTE

Features of Touch 24 BTE

- 24 SonicSound™ channels – independent processing channels each with its own compression ratio and adaptive gain
- 9 fitting handles
- Speech enhancement – a proprietary algorithm designed to enhance speech understanding and improve listening comfort
- Best Fit Fast Fitting Rationale
- Superior Phase Canceling – proprietary algorithm using acoustic cancelation to minimize feedback
- User Control Retrain – an option in feedback management allowing algorithm to adapt to new conditions
- Superior Expansion – applies expansion below compression knee point
- Superior Digital Noise Reduction– helps speech understanding in noise
- Superior Wind Noise Reduction – detects noise and provides part of decision to determine state of directionality
- Superior Fixed Directionality
- Superior Automatic Directionality – automatically switches on directionality depending on listening conditions
- Superior Adaptive Directionality
- Superior Multi-Channel Adaptive Directionality

Options of Touch 24 BTE

- Superior Automatic Program
- 4 Manual Programs
- Data Logging
- 12 Environments
- Voice Alerts
- Program Selection Indicators

- Low Battery Indicators
- Comfort Delay Indicators

Features of Touch 12 BTE

- 12 SonicSound™ channels – independent processing channels each with its own compression ratio and adaptive gain
- 9 fitting handles
- Speech enhancement – a proprietary algorithm designed to enhance speech understanding and improve listening comfort
- Best Fit Fast Fitting Rationale
- Superior Phase Canceling – proprietary algorithm using acoustic cancelation to minimize feedback
- User Control Retrain – an option in feedback management allowing algorithm to adapt to new conditions
- Superior Expansion – applies expansion below compression knee point
- Good Digital Noise Reduction – helps speech understanding in noise
- Superior Wind Noise Reduction – detects noise and provides part of decision to determine state of directionality
- Good Fixed Directionality
- Superior Automatic Directionality – automatically switches on directionality depending on listening conditions
- Good Adaptive Directionality
- Good Multi-Channel Adaptive Directionality

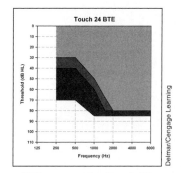

Fitting range for Touch 24 BTE open dome (light gray), tulip dome (light gray and medium gray), and closed dome (all shaded areas)

Options of Touch 12 BTE

- Good Automatic Program
- 3 Manual Programs
- Data Logging
- 10 Environments
- Program Selection Indicators
- Low Battery Indicators
- Comfort Delay Indicators

Features of Touch 6 BTE

- 6 SonicSound™ channels – independent processing channels each with its own compression ratio and adaptive gain
- 6 fitting handles
- Speech enhancement – a proprietary algorithm designed to enhance speech understanding and improve listening comfort

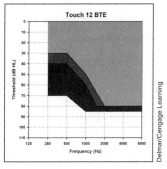

Fitting range for Touch 12 BTE open dome (light gray), tulip dome (light gray and medium gray), and closed dome (all shaded areas)

- Best Fit Fast Fitting Rationale
- Superior Phase Canceling – proprietary algorithm using acoustic cancelation to minimize feedback
- User Control Retrain – an option in feedback management allowing algorithm to adapt to new conditions
- Basic Expansion – applies expansion below compression knee point
- Good Digital Noise Reduction – helps speech understanding in noise
- Superior Wind Noise Reduction – detects noise and provides part of decision to determine state of directionality
- Good Fixed Directionality
- Superior Automatic Directionality – automatically switches on directionality depending on listening conditions
- Basic Adaptive Directionality
- Basic Multi-Channel Adaptive Directionality

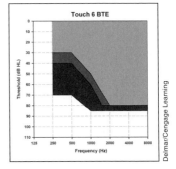

Fitting range for Touch 6 BTE open dome (light gray), tulip dome (light gray and medium gray), and closed dome (all shaded areas)

Options of Touch 6 BTE

- Good Automatic Program
- 2 Manual Programs
- Data Logging
- 8 Environments
- Program Selection Indicators
- Low Battery Indicators
- Comfort Delay Indicators

Typical Specifications		Touch 24 BTE	Touch 12 BTE	Touch 6 BTE
Standard ANSI S3.22-2003				
Output sound pressure level	Max OSPL 90 (dB SPL)	109	109	109
	HFAOSPL 90 (dB SPL)	108	108	108
Full-on gain (50 dB SPL input)	Peak gain (dB)	48	48	48
	HFA (dB)	47	47	47
Total harmonic distortion	500 Hz	0.6%	0.6%	0.6%
	800 Hz	0.7%	0.7%	0.7%
	1600 Hz	0.7%	0.7%	0.7%
Equivalent input noise (dB SPL)		25	25	25

continues

continued

Typical Specifications		Touch 24 BTE	Touch 12 BTE	Touch 6 BTE
Telecoil sensitivity	HFA SPLITS (dB SPL)	n/a	n/a	n/a
Battery	Operating current (mA)	1.1	1.1	1.1
	Battery type	10	10	10

Delmar/Cengage Learning

PRODUCT 2: ION

Product Application

ion 400 BTE
ion 200 BTE
ion BTE

Features of ion 400 BTE

- 24 channels
- 4 listening programs
- Auto-Morphic™ Switching – automatically switches between omnidirectional and directional mode
- Focused Null Steering – adapts among polar patterns based on the angle of arrival of the loudest input signal
- DIRECTIONAL*focus*™ – adaptive manipulation of gain based on location of noise
- Adaptive and fixed feedback cancellation
- iNR™ – uses signal-to-noise ratio and input level of noise to calculate level of noise reduction
- 8 environment-based programs
- Voice alerts
- Data logging
- Memory switch
- Integrated ON/OFF in battery door

Options of ion 400 BTE

- Up to 4 configurable program memories
- SmartTones™ – intelligently alerts the user
- 9 different color options

Features of ion 200 BTE

- 16 channels
- 4 listening programs
- DIRECTIONAL*focus* – adaptive manipulation of gain based on location of noise

- Adaptive and fixed feedback cancellation
- EXPRESSfit® – finds frequencies where feedback occurs and adjust gain levels to prevent feedback
- Hybrid noise reduction – attenuates low-input and high-input noise independently
- 7 environment-based programs
- Memory switch
- Integrated ON/OFF in battery door

Options of ion 200 BTE

- Up to 4 configurable program memories
- SmartTones – intelligently alerts the user
- 9 different color options

Features of ion BTE

- 16 channels
- 3 listening programs
- DIRECTIONAL*focus* – adaptive manipulation of gain based on location of noise
- Fixed feedback cancellation
- Automatic or fixed noise reduction programs
- Memory switch
- Integrated ON/OFF in Battery Door

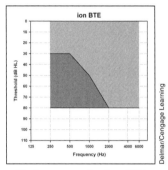

Options of ion BTE

- Up to 3 configurable program memories
- SmartTones – intelligently alerts the user
- 5 different color options

Fitting range for ion BTE with thin tube (light gray) or traditional ear hook (dark gray)

Typical Specifications		ion 400 BTE Open	ion 400 BTE Ear Hook
Standard ANSI S3.22-1996			
Output sound pressure level	Max OSPL 90 (dB SPL)	115	119
	HFAOSPL 90 (dB SPL)	109	116
Full-on gain (50 dB SPL input)	Peak gain (dB)	35	51
	HFA (dB)	35	48
Total harmonic distortion	500 Hz	1%	3.6%
	800 Hz	1%	1.5%
	1600 Hz	1%	1%
Equivalent input noise (dB SPL)		32	32
Telecoil sensitivity	HFA SPLITS (dB SPL)	n/a	n/a
Battery	Operating current (mA)	1.3	1.3
	Battery type	10	10

Typical Specifications		ion 200 BTE Open	ion 200 BTE Ear Hook
Standard ANSI S3.22-1996			
Output sound pressure level	Max OSPL 90 (dB SPL)	113	121
	HFAOSPL 90 (dB SPL)	108	115
Full-on gain (50 dB SPL input)	Peak gain (dB)	38	53
	HFA (dB)	35	49
Total harmonic distortion	500 Hz	3%	4%
	800 Hz	2%	2%
	1600 Hz	1%	1%
Equivalent input noise (dB SPL)		32	32
Telecoil sensitivity	HFA SPLITS (dB SPL)	n/a	n/a
Battery	Operating current (mA)	1.0	1.0
	Battery type	10	10

Delmar/Cengage Learning

Typical Specifications		ion BTE Open	ion BTE Ear Hook
Standard ANSI S3.22-1996			
Output sound pressure level	Max OSPL 90 (dB SPL)	115	114
	HFAOSPL 90 (dB SPL)	108	108
Full-on gain (50 dB SPL input)	Peak gain (dB)	39	36
	HFA (dB)	35	35
Total harmonic distortion	500 Hz	3%	2.5%
	800 Hz	2%	1.5%
	1600 Hz	1%	1%
Equivalent input noise (dB SPL)		32	32
Telecoil sensitivity	HFA SPLITS (dB SPL)	n/a	n/a
Battery	Operating current (mA)	1.0	1.0
	Battery type	10	10

Delmar/Cengage Learning

PRODUCT 3: VELOCITY SERIES 24, 12, 6, 4

Product Application

Velocity 24 BTE
Velocity 24 miniBTE
Velocity 24 ITE
Velocity 24 ITE-P

Velocity 24 HS
Velocity 24 ITC
Velocity 24 MC
Velocity 24 CIC

Features of Velocity 24 BTE, miniBTE, ITE, ITE-P, HS, ITC, MC, and CIC

- Overdrive System™ – set of algorithms that help to seamlessly react to any environment
- SonicSound™ – digital signal processing that preserves the natural sound quality provided by the cochlea
- iNR Noise Reduction – calculates optimal level of noise reduction
- DIRECTIONAL*focus* – predetermined focus area to provide maximum amplification and also to adapt gain when sounds "move out of focus"
- FLEXI*focus*™ – provides additional level of adaptation to DIRECTIONAL*focus*
- Focused Null Steering – uses the angle of arrival estimate from DIRECTIONAL*focus* to guide polar pattern selection
- Auto-Morphic Switching – continuously changes between omni and directional modes
- Adaptive feedback canceller – maintains stable system gain by monitoring and adjusting for subtle changes in the feedback path
- Situational feedback control – quickly eliminates feedback introduced by sudden changes in the environment
- Symmetric attack and release times
- Environment-based programming – common listening scenarios that configure the fitting parameters for each unique environment
- 24 compression channels
- 9 fitting handles
- Speech enhancement – a proprietary algorithm designed to enhance speech understanding and improve listening comfort
- Superior feedback cancellation
- Superior automatic directionality
- Superior adaptive directionality
- Superior fixed directionality
- Superior digital noise reduction – helps speech understanding in noise
- Superior universal program
- 4 listening programs
- Voice alerts
- Data logging
- Bluetooth capabilities

Product Application

Velocity 12 BTE
Velocity 12 miniBTE
Velocity 12 ITE
Velocity 12 ITE-P
Velocity 12 HS
Velocity 12 ITC
Velocity 12 MC
Velocity 12 CIC

Features of Velocity 12 BTE, miniBTE, ITE, ITE-P, HS, ITC, MC, and CIC

- Overdrive System – set of algorithms that help to seamlessly react to any environment
- SonicSound – digital signal processing that preserves the natural sound quality provided by the cochlea
- iNR Noise Reduction – calculates optimal level of noise reduction
- DIRECTIONAL*focus* – predetermined focus area to provide maximum amplification and also to adapt gain when sounds "move out of focus"
- Auto-Morphic Switching – continuously changes between omni and directional modes
- FLEXI*focus* – provides additional level of adaptation to DIRECTIONAL*focus*
- Focused Null Steering – uses the angle of arrival estimate from DIREC-TIONAL*focus* to guide polar pattern selection
- Adaptive feedback canceller – maintains stable system gain by monitoring and adjusting for subtle changes in the feedback path
- Situational feedback control – quickly eliminates feedback introduced by sudden changes in the environment
- Symmetric attack and release times
- Environment-based programming – common listening scenarios that configure the fitting parameters for each unique environment
- 12 compression channels
- 9 fitting handles
- Speech enhancement – a proprietary algorithm designed to enhance speech understanding and improve listening comfort
- Superior feedback cancellation
- Superior automatic directionality
- Good adaptive directionality
- Basic fixed directionality
- Good digital noise reduction – helps speech understanding in noise
- Good universal program
- 3 listening programs
- Data logging
- Bluetooth capabilities

Product Application

Velocity 6 BTE
Velocity 6 miniBTE
Velocity 6 ITE
Velocity 6 ITE-P
Velocity 6 HS
Velocity 6 ITC
Velocity 6 MC
Velocity 6 CIC

Features of Velocity 6 BTE, miniBTE, ITE, ITE-P, HS, ITC, MC, and CIC

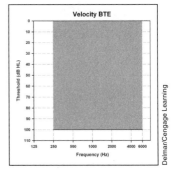

Fitting range for Velocity BTE

- Overdrive System – set of algorithms that help to seamlessly react to any environment
- SonicSound – digital signal processing that preserves the natural sound quality provided by the cochlea
- iNR Noise Reduction – calculates optimal level of noise reduction
- DIRECTIONAL*focus* – predetermined focus area to provide maximum amplification and also to adapt gain when sounds "move out of focus"
- FLEXI*focus* – provides additional level of adaptation to DIRECTIONAL*focus*
- Focused Null Steering – uses the angle of arrival estimate from DIRECTIONAL*focus* to guide polar pattern selection
- Auto-Morphic Switching – continuously changes between omni and directional modes
- Adaptive feedback canceller – maintains stable system gain by monitoring and adjusting for subtle changes in the feedback path
- Situational feedback control – quickly eliminates feedback introduced by sudden changes in the environment
- Symmetric attack and release times
- Environment-based programming – common listening scenarios that configure the fitting parameters for each unique environment
- 6 compression channels
- 6 fitting handles
- Speech enhancement – a proprietary algorithm designed to enhance speech understanding and improve listening comfort
- Superior feedback cancellation
- Superior automatic directionality
- Basic adaptive directionality
- Basic fixed directionality
- Good digital noise reduction – helps speech understanding in noise
- Good universal program
- 2+ listening programs
- Data logging
- Bluetooth capabilities

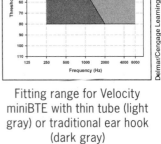

Fitting range for Velocity miniBTE with thin tube (light gray) or traditional ear hook (dark gray)

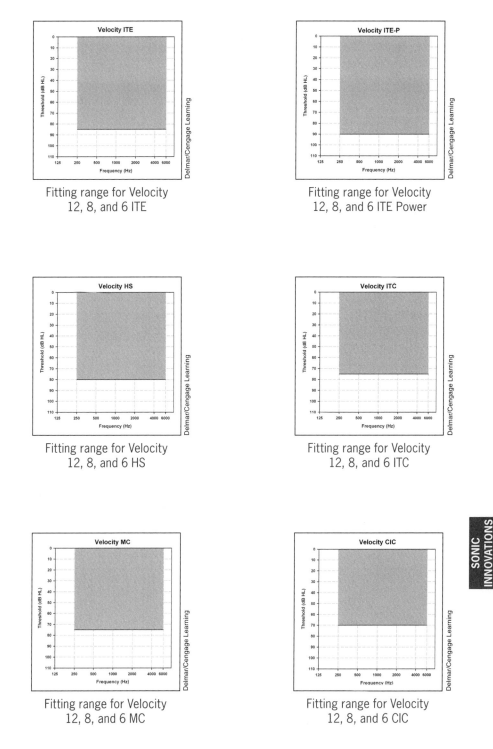

Fitting range for Velocity
12, 8, and 6 ITE

Fitting range for Velocity
12, 8, and 6 ITE Power

Fitting range for Velocity
12, 8, and 6 HS

Fitting range for Velocity
12, 8, and 6 ITC

Fitting range for Velocity
12, 8, and 6 MC

Fitting range for Velocity
12, 8, and 6 CIC

Product Application

Velocity 4 BTE
Velocity 4 Open BTE
Velocity 4 ITE
Velocity 4 ITE-P
Velocity 4 HS
Velocity 4 ITC
Velocity 4 MC
Velocity 4 CIC

Features of Velocity 4 BTE, Open BTE, ITE, ITE-P, HS, ITC, MC, and CIC

- Overdrive System – sct of algorithms that help to seamlessly react to any environment
- SonicSound – digital signal processing that preserves the natural sound quality provided by the cochlea
- iNR Noise Reduction – calculates optimal level of noise reduction
- DIRECTIONAL*focus* – predetermined focus area to provide maximum amplification and also to adapt gain when sounds "move out of focus"
- FLEXI*focus* – provides additional level of adaptation to DIRECTIONAL*focus*
- Focused Null Steering – uses the angle of arrival estimate from DIRECTIONAL*focus* to guide polar pattern selection
- Auto-Morphic Switching – continuously changes between omni and directional modes
- Adaptive feedback canceller – maintains stable system gain by monitoring and adjusting for subtle changes in the feedback path
- Situational feedback control – quickly eliminates feedback introduced by sudden changes in the environment
- Symmetric attack and release times
- Environment-based programming – common listening scenarios that configure the fitting parameters for each unique environment
- 4 compression channels
- 4 fitting handles
- Speech enhancement – a proprietary algorithm designed to enhance speech understanding and improve listening comfort
- Basic feedback cancellation
- Basic fixed directionality
- Basic digital noise reduction – helps speech understanding in noise
- 2+ listening programs
- Bluetooth capabilities

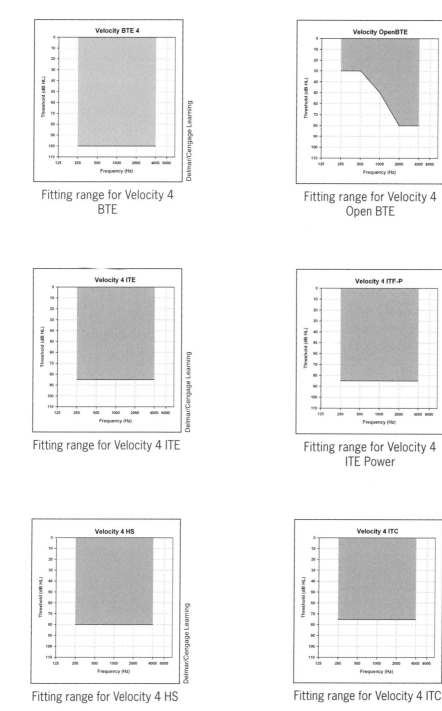

Fitting range for Velocity 4
BTE

Fitting range for Velocity 4
Open BTE

Fitting range for Velocity 4 ITE

Fitting range for Velocity 4
ITE Power

Fitting range for Velocity 4 HS

Fitting range for Velocity 4 ITC

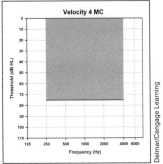

Fitting range for Velocity 4 MC

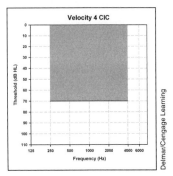

Fitting range for Velocity 4 CIC

Options of Velocity 24 BTE, Velocity 12 BTE, Velocity 6 BTE, and Velocity 4 BTE

- Program button
- Programmable telecoil
- Auto telephone (NA w/V4)
- Volume control
- Directionality
- sonicBLU-compatible
- DIA-compatible
- Tamper-resistant door
- Integrated ON/OFF in battery door
- Direct audio input capability

Options of Velocity 24 miniBTE, Velocity 12 miniBTE, and Velocity 6 miniBTE

- Memory switch
- Program button
- Programmable telecoil
- Auto telephone (NA w/V4)
- Volume control
- Directionality
- sonicBLU-compatible
- DIA-compatible
- Thin tube fitting
- Tamper-resistant door
- Integrated ON/OFF in battery door
- Direct audio input capability

Options of Velocity 4 Open BTE

- Program button
- Directionality
- Thin tube fitting

Options of Velocity 24 ITE, Velocity 24 ITC, Velocity 24 HS, Velocity 12 ITE, Velocity 12 ITC, Velocity 12 HS, Velocity 6 ITE, Velocity 6 ITC, Velocity 6 HS, Velocity 4 ITE, Velocity 4 ITC, and Velocity 4 HS

- Program button
- Programmable telecoil
- Auto telephone (NA w/V4)
- Volume control
- Directionality
- sonicBLU-compatible
- Memory switch

Options of Velocity 24 CIC, Velocity 24 MC, Velocity 12 CIC, Velocity 12 MC, Velocity 6 CIC, Velocity 6 MC, Velocity 4 CIC, and Velocity 4 MC

- Program button

Typical Specifications		Velocity BTE	Velocity BTE Open	Velocity miniBTE Open Fit	Velocity miniBTE Ear Hook
Standard ANSI S3.22-1996					
Output sound pressure level	Max OSPL 90 (dB SPL)	130	111	114	120
	HFAOSPL 90 (dB SPL)	124	108	109	116
Full-on gain (50 dB SPL input)	Peak gain (dB)	63	39	36	52
	HFA (dB)	60	35	35	50
Total harmonic distortion	500 Hz	4%	2.5%	1%	3%
	800 Hz	2%	1.5%	1%	1%
	1600 Hz	1%	1%	1%	1%
Equivalent input noise (dB SPL)		29	29	29	29
Telecoil sensitivity	HFA SPLITS (dB SPL)	108	n/a	n/a	n/a
Battery	Operating current (mA)	1.5	1.0	1.4	1.4
	Battery type	13	13	13	13

Delmar/Cengage Learning

Typical Specifications		Velocity ITE	Velocity ITE-P	Velocity ITC
Standard ANSI S3.22-1996				
Output sound pressure level	Max OSPL 90 (dB SPL)	117	120	111
	HFAOSPL 90 (dB SPL)	111	115	106
Full-on gain (50 dB SPL input)	Peak gain (dB)	48	52	38
	HFA (dB)	45	50	36

continues

continued

Typical Specifications		Velocity ITE	Velocity ITE-P	Velocity ITC
Total harmonic distortion	500 Hz	2%	3%	2%
	800 Hz	1%	2%	1%
	1600 Hz	1%	1%	1%
Equivalent input noise (dB SPL)		29	29	29
Telecoil sensitivity	HFA SPLITS (dB SPL)	95	99	88
Battery	Operating current (mA)	1.3	1.4	1.2
	Battery type	312 or 13	13	10 or 312

Delmar/Cengage Learning

Typical Specifications		Velocity CIC	Velocity MC	Velocity HS
Standard ANSI S3.22-1996				
Output sound pressure level	Max OSPL 90 (dB SPL)	111	111	117
	HFAOSPL 90 (dB SPL)	106	106	111
Full-on gain (50 dB SPL input)	Peak gain (dB)	31	36	43
	HFA (dB)	30	34	40
Total harmonic distortion	500 Hz	2%	2%	2%
	800 Hz	1%	1%	1%
	1600 Hz	1%	1%	1%
Equivalent input noise (dB SPL)		32	32	32
Telecoil sensitivity	HFA SPLITS (dB SPL)	n/a	n/a	n/a
Battery	Operating current (mA)	1.2	1.2	1.3
	Battery type	10	10	312

Delmar/Cengage Learning

PRODUCT 4: BALANCE

Product Application

balance BTE
balance microBTE
balance ITE
balance ITE-P
balance HS
balance ITC
balance MC
balance CIC

Features of balance BTE and balance microBTE

- Environment-based programming – common listening scenarios that configure the fitting parameters for each unique environment
- Adaptive directionality using DIRECTIONAL*focus*

- 16 channels
- 9 programming handles
- 7 different presets
- Hybrid noise reduction – both low and high input noise are attenuated to an appropriate amount
- S.M.A.R.T.™ technology – feedback management
- Feedback canceller – fixed or adaptive

Options of balance BTE and balance microBTE

- 4 listening programs
- Memory switch
- Directionality
- Integrated ON/OFF in battery door
- Volume control with ON/OFF (BTE only)
- Direct audio input capability (BTE only)

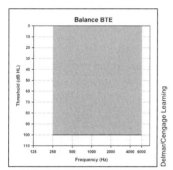

Fitting range for balance BTE

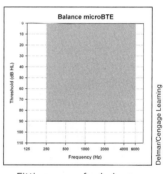

Fitting range for balance microBTE

Features of balance ITE, balance ITE-P, balance HS, and balance ITC

- Environment-based programming – common listening scenarios that configure the fitting parameters for each unique environment
- Adaptive directionality using DIRECTIONAL*focus*
- 16 channels
- 9 programming handles
- 7 different presets
- Hybrid noise reduction – both low and high input noise are attenuated to an appropriate amount
- S.M.A.R.T. technology – feedback management
- Feedback canceller – fixed or adaptive

Options of balance ITE, balance ITE-P, balance HS, and balance ITC

- 4 listening programs
- Memory switch
- Directionality
- ON/OFF switch
- Volume control with ON/OFF (BTE only)
- Programmable telecoil

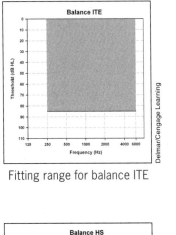

Fitting range for balance ITE

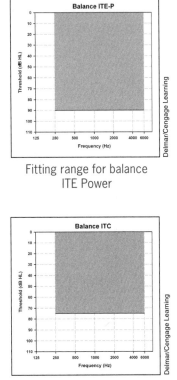

Fitting range for balance
ITE Power

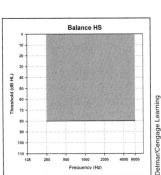

Fitting range for balance HS

Fitting range for balance ITC

Features of balance MC and balance CIC

- Environment-based programming – common listening scenarios that configure the fitting parameters for each unique environment
- Adaptive directionality using DIRECTIONAL*focus*
- 16 channels
- 9 programming handles
- 7 different presets
- Hybrid noise reduction – both low and high input noise are attenuated to an appropriate amount
- S.M.A.R.T. technology – feedback management
- Feedback canceller – fixed or adaptive

Options of balance MC and balance CIC

* 4 listening programs
* Memory switch

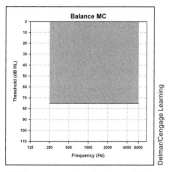

Fitting range for balance MC

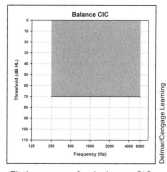

Fitting range for balance CIC

Typical Specifications		balance BTE	balance microBTE
Standard ANSI S3.22-1996			
Output sound pressure level	Max OSPL 90 (dB SPL)	121	130
	HFAOSPL 90 (dB SPL)	114	123
Full-on gain (50 dB SPL input)	Peak gain (dB)	53	63
	HFA (dB)	50	60
Total harmonic distortion	500 Hz	4%	3%
	800 Hz	2%	2%
	1600 Hz	1%	1%
Equivalent input noise (dB SPL)		23	23
Telecoil sensitivity	HFA SPLITS (dB SPL)	106	n/a
Battery	Operating current (mA)	1.0	1.05
	Battery type	13	10

Delmar/Cengage Learning

Typical Specifications		balance ITE	balance ITE-P
Standard ANSI S3.22-1996			
Output sound pressure level	Max OSPL 90 (dB SPL)	117	120
	HFAOSPL 90 (dB SPL)	111	115
Full-on gain (50 dB SPL input)	Peak gain (dB)	48	52
	HFA (dB)	45	50
Total harmonic distortion	500 Hz	3%	3%
	800 Hz	2%	2%
	1600 Hz	1%	1%

continues

continued

Typical Specifications		balance ITE	balance ITE-P
Equivalent input noise (dB SPL)		23	23
Telecoil sensitivity	HFA SPLITS (dB SPL)	94	97
Battery	Operating current (mA)	.89	.95
	Battery type	312	13

Delmar/Cengage Learning

Typical Specifications		balance HS	balance ITC	balance CIC
Standard ANSI S3.22-1996				
Output sound pressure level	Max OSPL 90 (dB SPL)	117	111	111
	HFAOSPL 90 (dB SPL)	111	106	106
Full-on gain (50 dB SPL input)	Peak gain (dB)	43	38	31
	HFA (dB)	40	36	30
Total harmonic distortion	500 Hz	3%	2%	2%
	800 Hz	2%	1%	1%
	1600 Hz	1%	1%	1%
Equivalent input noise (dB SPL)		23	23	23
Telecoil sensitivity	HFA SPLITS (dB SPL)	95	90	n/a
Battery	Operating current (mA)	0.89	0.89	0.88
	Battery type	312	10	10

Delmar/Cengage Learning

PRODUCT 5: APPLAUSE

Product application

applause BTE
applause ITE
applause ITE-P
applause HS
applause ITC
applause CIC
applause MC

Features of applause BTE

- Digital signal processing
- Personalized noise reduction

- DIRECTIONAL*focus* – predetermined focus area to provide maximum amplification and also to adapt gain when sounds "move out of focus"

Options of applause BTE

- Memory switch
- Directionality
- Programmable telecoil
- Integrated ON/OFF battery door
- Volume control with ON/OFF
- Direct audio input capability

Features of applause ITE, applause ITE-P, applause HS, and applause ITC

- Digital signal processing
- Personalized noise reduction
- DIRECTIONAL*focus* – predetermined focus area to provide maximum amplification and also to adapt gain when sounds "move out of focus"

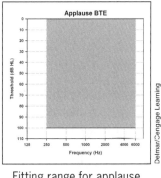

Fitting range for applause BTE

Options of applause ITE, applause ITE-P, applause HS, and applause ITC

- Memory switch
- Directionality
- Programmable telecoil
- ON/OFF switch
- Volume control with ON/OFF

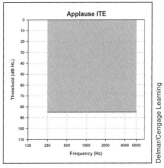

Fitting range for applause ITE

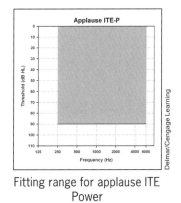

Fitting range for applause ITE Power

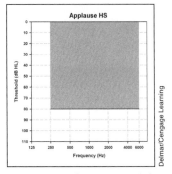

Fitting range for applause HS

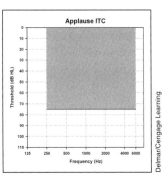

Fitting range for applause ITC

Features of applause CIC and applause MC

- Digital signal processing
- Personalized noise reduction
- DIRECTIONAL*focus* – predetermined focus area to provide maximum amplification and also to adapt gain when sounds "move out of focus"

Options of applause CIC and applause MC

- Memory switch

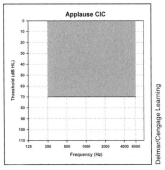

Fitting range for applause CIC

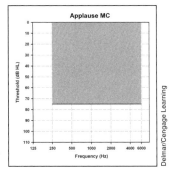

Fitting range for applause MC

Typical Specifications		applause BTE	applause ITE	applause ITE-P
Standard ANSI S3.22-1996				
Output sound pressure level	Max OSPL 90 (dB SPL)	130	117	120
	HFAOSPL 90 (dB SPL)	123	111	115
Full-on gain (50 dB SPL input)	Peak gain (dB)	63	48	52
	HFA (dB)	60	45	50

continues

continued

Typical Specifications		applause BTE	applause ITE	applause ITE-P
Total harmonic distortion	500 Hz	4%	3%	3%
	800 Hz	2%	2%	2%
	1600 Hz	1%	1%	1%
Equivalent input noise (dB SPL)		<23	<23	<23
Telecoil sensitivity	HFA SPLITS (dB SPL)	106	94	97
Battery	Operating current (mA)	1.05	0.89	0.95
	Battery type	13	312	13

Delmar/Cengage Learning

Typical Specifications		applause HS	applause ITC
Standard ANSI S3.22-1996			
Output sound pressure level	Max OSPL 90 (dB SPL)	117	111
	HFAOSPL 90 (dB SPL)	111	106
Full-on gain (50 dB SPL input)	Peak gain (dB)	43	38
	HFA (dB)	40	36
Total harmonic distortion	500 Hz	3%	2%
	800 Hz	2%	1%
	1600 Hz	1%	1%
Equivalent input noise (dB SPL)		<23	<23
Telecoil sensitivity	HFA SPLITS (dB SPL)	95	90
Battery	Operating current (mA)	0.89	0.89
	Battery type	312	10

Delmar/Cengage Learning

Typical Specifications		applause CIC	applause MC
Standard ANSI S3.22-1996			
Output sound pressure level	Max OSPL 90 (dB SPL)	111	111
	HFAOSPL 90 (dB SPL)	106	106
Full-on gain (50 dB SPL input)	Peak gain (dB)	31	36
	HFA (dB)	30	34
Total harmonic distortion	500 Hz	2%	2%
	800 Hz	1%	1%
	1600 Hz	1%	1%
Equivalent input noise (dB SPL)		<23	<23
Telecoil sensitivity	HFA SPLITS (dB SPL)	n/a	n/a
Battery	Operating current (mA)	0.88	0.89
	Battery type	10	10

Delmar/Cengage Learning

PRODUCT 6: NATURA PRO

Product Application

Natura Pro BTE
Natura Pro ITE
Natura Pro ITE-P
Natura Pro HS
Natura Pro ITC
Natura Pro CIC
Natura Pro MC

Features of Natura Pro BTE

- Digital signal processing (third-generation)
- S.M.A.R.T. technology – very fast-acting compression with 4 expansion settings
- Noise reduction – 4 fixed settings (high, medium, low, off)
- 3 optional directionality patterns
- Feedback canceller
- Gain adjuster
- 4 fixed expansion levels
- SmartTones – intelligently alert the user
- 3 memory settings

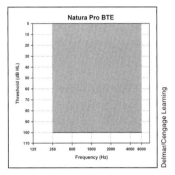

Fitting range for Natura
Pro BTE

Options of Natura Pro BTE

- Memory switch
- Directionality
- Programmable telecoil
- Integrated ON/OFF battery door
- Volume control with ON/OFF
- Direct audio input capability

Features of Natura Pro ITE, ITE-P, HS, and ITC

- Digital signal processing (third-generation)
- S.M.A.R.T. technology – very fast-acting compression with 4 expansion settings
- Noise reduction – 4 fixed settings (high, medium, low, off)
- 3 optional directionality patterns
- Feedback canceller
- Gain adjuster
- 4 fixed expansion levels
- SmartTones – intelligently alert the user
- 3 memory settings

Options of Natura Pro ITE, ITE-P, HS, and ITC

- Memory switch
- Directionality
- Programmable telecoil
- ON/OFF switch
- Volume control with ON/OFF

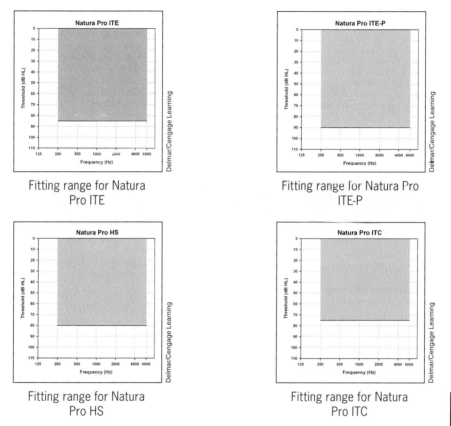

Fitting range for Natura Pro ITE

Fitting range for Natura Pro ITE-P

Fitting range for Natura Pro HS

Fitting range for Natura Pro ITC

Features of Natura Pro CIC and Natura Pro MC

- Digital signal processing (third-generation)
- S.M.A.R.T. technology – very fast-acting compression with 4 expansion settings
- Noise reduction – 4 fixed settings (high, medium, low, off)
- 3 optional directionality patterns
- Feedback canceller
- Gain adjuster
- 4 fixed expansion levels
- SmartTones – intelligently alert the user
- 2 or 3 memory settings

Options of Natura Pro CIC, Natura Pro MC

• Memory switch

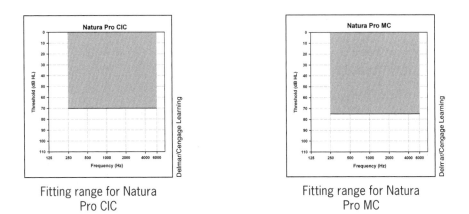

Fitting range for Natura
Pro CIC

Fitting range for Natura
Pro MC

Typical Specifications		Natura Pro BTE	Natura Pro ITE	Natura Pro ITE-P
Standard ANSI S3.22-1996				
Output sound pressure level	Max OSPL 90 (dB SPL)	130	117	120
	HFAOSPL 90 (dB SPL)	123	111	115
Full-on gain (50 dB SPL input)	Peak gain (dB)	63	48	52
	HFA (dB)	60	45	50
Total harmonic distortion	500 Hz	3%	3%	3%
	800 Hz	2%	2%	2%
	1600 Hz	1%	1%	1%
Equivalent input noise (dB SPL)		<23	<23	<23
Telecoil sensitivity	HFA SPLITS (dB SPL)	106	94	97
Battery	Operating current (mA)	1.05	0.89	0.95
	Battery type	13	312	13

Delmar/Cengage Learning

Typical Specifications		Natura Pro HS	Natura Pro ITC
Standard ANSI S3.22-1996			
Output sound pressure level	Max OSPL 90 (dB SPL)	117	111
	HFAOSPL 90 (dB SPL)	111	106
Full-on gain (50 dB SPL input)	Peak gain (dB)	43	38
	HFA (dB)	40	36
Total harmonic distortion	500 Hz	3%	2%
	800 Hz	2%	1%
	1600 Hz	1%	1%

continues

continued

Typical Specifications		Natura Pro HS	Natura Pro ITC
Equivalent input noise (dB SPL)		<23	<23
Telecoil sensitivity	HFA SPLITS (dB SPL)	95	90
Battery	Operating current (mA)	0.89	0.89
	Battery type	312	10

Delmar/Cengage Learning

Typical Specifications		Natura Pro CIC	Natura Pro MC
Standard ANSI S3.22-1996			
Output sound pressure level	Max OSPL 90 (dB SPL)	111	111
	HFAOSPL 90 (dB SPL)	106	106
Full-on gain (50 dB SPL input)	Peak gain (dB)	31	36
	HFA (dB)	30	34
Total harmonic distortion	500 Hz	2%	2%
	800 Hz	1%	1%
	1600 Hz	1%	1%
Equivalent input noise (dB SPL)		<23	<23
Telecoil sensitivity	HFA SPLITS (dB SPL)	n/a	n/a
Battery	Operating current (mA)	0.88	0.89
	Battery type	10	10

Delmar/Cengage Learning

PRODUCT 7: NATURA 2 SE

Product Application

Natura 2 SE BTE
Natura 2 SE ITE
Natura 2 SE ITE-P
Natura 2 SE HS
Natura 2 SE ITC
Natura 2 SE ITC-P
Natura 2 SE CIC
Natura 2 SE MC

Features of Natura 2 SE BTE

- Digital signal processing (second-generation)
- Dynamic speech enhancement – a proprietary algorithm designed to enhance speech understanding and improve listening comfort
- Noise reduction fixed or 3 levels
- Conventional directionality
- Feedback manager

- 2 memory settings
- 4 fixed expansion levels
- Standard alerting tones

Options of Natura 2 SE BTE

- Program 1/Program 2 switch
- Directional/omnidirectional switch
- ON/OFF switch
- Programmable telecoil
- Direct audio input

Features of Natura 2 SE ITE and Natura 2 SE ITE-P

- Digital signal processing (second-generation)
- Dynamic speech enhancement – a proprietary algorithm designed to enhance speech understanding and improve listening comfort
- Noise reduction fixed or 3 levels
- Conventional directionality
- Feedback manager
- 2 memory settings
- 4 fixed expansion levels
- Standard alerting tones

Options of Natura 2 SE ITE and Natura 2 SE ITE-P

- Program 1/Program 2 switch
- Directional/omnidirectional switch (ITE only)
- Directional/telecoil/omnidirectional (ITE only)
- Programmable telecoil
- ON/OFF switch

Features of Natura 2 SE HS, Natura 2 SE ITC, and Natura 2 SE ITC-P

- Digital signal processing (second-generation)
- Dynamic speech enhancement – a proprietary algorithm designed to enhance speech understanding and improve listening comfort
- Noise reduction fixed or 3 levels
- Conventional directionality

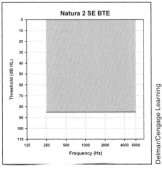

Fitting range for Natura 2 SE BTE

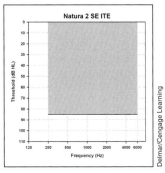

Fitting range for Natura 2 SE ITE

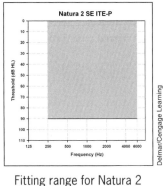

Fitting range for Natura 2 SE ITE Power

- Feedback manager
- 2 memory settings
- 4 fixed expansion levels
- Standard alerting tones

Options of Natura 2 SE HS, Natura 2 SE ITC, and Natura 2 SE ITC-P

- Program 1/Program 2 switch
- Directional/omnidirectional switch (HS and ITC only)
- Programmable telecoil
- ON/OFF switch
- Volume control

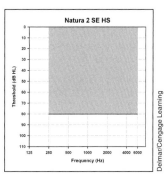

Fitting range for Natura 2 SE HS

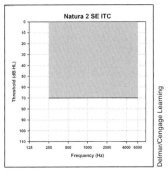

Fitting range for Natura 2 SE ITC

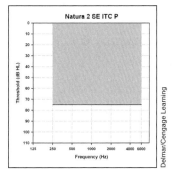

Fitting range for Natura 2 SE ITC Power

Features of Natura 2 SE CIC and Natura 2 SE MC

- Digital signal processing (second-generation)
- Dynamic speech enhancement – a proprietary algorithm designed to enhance speech understanding and improve listening comfort
- Noise reduction fixed or 3 levels
- Conventional directionality
- Feedback manager
- 2 memory settings
- 4 fixed expansion levels
- Standard alerting tones

Options of Natura 2 SE MC

- Program 1/Program 2 switch

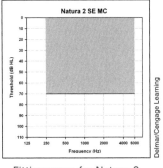

Fitting range for Natura 2
SE MC

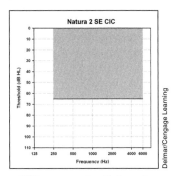

Fitting range for Natura 2
SE CIC

Typical Specifications		Natura 2 SE BTE	Natura 2 SE ITE	Natura 2 SE ITE-P
Standard ANSI S3.22-1996				
Output sound pressure level	Max OSPL 90 (dB SPL)	119	116	118
	HFAOSPL 90 (dB SPL)	114	111	115
Full-on gain (50 dB SPL input)	Peak gain (dB)	54	47	53
	HFA (dB)	52	45	49
Total harmonic distortion	500 Hz	4%	2.5%	3%
	800 Hz	2%	1.5%	2%
	1600 Hz	1%	1%	1%
Equivalent input noise (dB SPL)		<23	<23	<23
Telecoil sensitivity	HFA SPLITS (dB SPL)	96	92	96
Battery	Operating current (mA)	1.5	1.4	1.4
	Battery type	13	312	13

Delmar/Cengage Learning

Typical Specifications		Natura 2 SE HS	Natura 2 SE ITC	Natura 2 SE ITC-P
Standard ANSI S3.22-1996				
Output sound pressure level	Max OSPL 90 (dB SPL)	113	106	113
	HFAOSPL 90 (dB SPL)	108	102	108
Full-on gain (50 dB SPL input)	Peak gain (dB)	46	39	43
	HFA (dB)	44	36	40
Total harmonic distortion	500 Hz	2.5%	2%	2%
	800 Hz	1.5%	1%	1%
	1600 Hz	1%	1%	1%
Equivalent input noise (dB SPL)		<23	<23	<23

continues

continued

Typical Specifications		Natura 2 SE HS	Natura 2 SE ITC	Natura 2 SE ITC-P
Telecoil sensitivity	HFA SPLITS (dB SPL)	92	86	92
Battery	Operating current (mA)	1.4	0.96	1.4
	Battery type	312	13	312

Delmar/Cengage Learning

Typical Specifications		Natura 2 SE CIC	Natura 2 SE MC
Standard ANSI S3.22-1996			
Output sound pressure level	Max OSPL 90 (dB SPL)	106	106
	HFAOSPL 90 (dB SPL)	102	102
Full-on gain (50 dB SPL input)	Peak gain (dB)	32	39
	HFA (dB)	28	36
Total harmonic distortion	500 Hz	2%	2%
	800 Hz	1%	1%
	1600 Hz	1%	1%
Equivalent input noise (dB SPL)		<23	<23
Telecoil sensitivity	HFA SPLITS (dB SPL)	n/a	n/a
Battery	Operating current (mA)	0.8	0.96
	Battery type	10	10

Delmar/Cengage Learning

PRODUCT 8: TRIBUTE

Product Application

Tribute BTE
Tribute ITE
Tribute ITE-P
Tribute HS
Tribute ITC
Tribute CIC
Tribute MC

Features of Tribute BTE

- 9-channel DSP
- Memory switch (2 programs)
- Programmable telecoil
- Switchable directionality

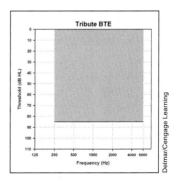

Fitting range for Tribute BTE

Options of Tribute BTE

- Telecoil
- Directional/omni switch
- Direct audio input

Features of Tribute ITE and Tribute ITE-P

- 9-channel DSP
- Memory switch (2 programs)
- Programmable telecoil
- Volume control
- Switchable directionality

Options of Tribute ITE and Tribute ITE-P

- Program 1/Program 2 switch
- Directional/omni switch (ITE only)
- Directional/telecoil/omni (ITE only)
- ON/OFF switch

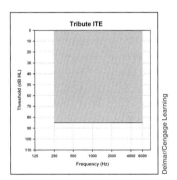

Fitting range for Tribute ITE

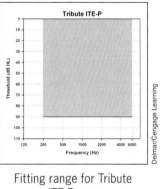

Fitting range for Tribute
ITE Power

Features of Tribute HS, Tribute ITC, Tribute CIC, and Tribute MC

- 9-channel DSP
- Memory switch (2 programs)
- Programmable telecoil
- Volume control
- Switchable directionality

Options of Tribute HS and Tribute ITC

- Telecoil
- Directional/omni switch
- Volume control

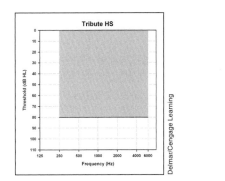

Fitting range for Tribute HS

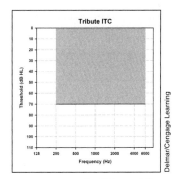

Fitting range for Tribute ITC

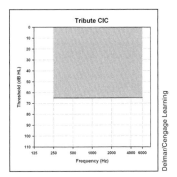

Fitting range for Tribute CIC

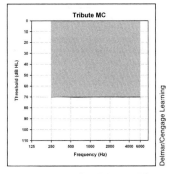

Fitting range for Tribute MC

Typical Specifications		Tribute BTE	Tribute ITE	Tribute ITE-P
Standard ANSI S3.22-1996				
Output sound pressure level	Max OSPL 90 (dB SPL)	119	116	118
	HFAOSPL 90 (dB SPL)	114	111	115
Full-on gain (50 dB SPL input)	Peak gain (dB)	54	47	53
	HFA (dB)	52	45	49
Total harmonic distortion	500 Hz	4%	2.5%	3%
	800 Hz	2%	1.5%	2%
	1600 Hz	1%	1%	1%
Equivalent input noise (dB SPL)		<23	<23	<23
Telecoil sensitivity	HFA SPLITS (dB SPL)	96	92	96
Battery	Operating current (mA)	1.5	1.4	1.4
	Battery type	13	312	13

Delmar/Cengage Learning

Typical Specifications		Tribute HS	Tribute ITC
Standard ANSI S3.22-1996			
Output sound pressure level	Max OSPL 90 (dB SPL)	113	106
	HFAOSPL 90 (dB SPL)	108	102
Full-on gain (50 dB SPL input)	Peak gain (dB)	46	39
	HFA (dB)	44	36
Total harmonic distortion	500 Hz	2.5%	2%
	800 Hz	1.5%	1%
	1600 Hz	1%	1%
Equivalent input noise (dB SPL)		<23	<23
Telecoil sensitivity	HFA SPLITS (dB SPL)	92	86
Battery	Operating current (mA)	1.4	0.96
	Battery type	312	13

Delmar/Cengage Learning

Typical Specifications		Tribute CIC	Tribute MC
Standard ANSI S3.22-1996			
Output sound pressure level	Max OSPL 90 (dB SPL)	106	106
	HFAOSPL 90 (dB SPL)	102	102
Full-on gain (50 dB SPL input)	Peak gain (dB)	32	32
	HFA (dB)	28	28
Total harmonic distortion	500 Hz	2%	2%
	800 Hz	1%	1%
	1600 Hz	1%	1%
Equivalent input noise (dB SPL)		<23	<23
Telecoil sensitivity	HFA SPLITS (dB SPL)	n/a	n/a
Battery	Operating current (mA)	0.8	0.8
	Battery type	10	10

Delmar/Cengage Learning

CHAPTER TEN

Starkey Laboratories

STARKEY LABORATORIES: HELPING PEOPLE EVERYWHERE

World Headquarters
Starkey Laboratories, Inc.
World Headquarters
6700 Washington Ave. S
Eden Prairie, MN 55344
Phone: 1 (800) 328-8602
Web site: http://www.starkey.com

Contrary to popular notions, Bill Austin was not the founder of Starkey Laboratories (Eden Prairie, MN; http://www.starkey.com). But it would be foolhardy not to credit Bill Austin for making Starkey what it is today: the third-largest business in hearing instrument market share worldwide, holding 13 percent of the market (Gretler, 2004). In fact, it is one of the few businesses to have grown to such worldwide prominence and yet remain privately held. Starkey's secret to success has been its staunch orientation to the end user. Starkey has consistently maintained a high level of service and has led the industry in these arenas. Since the new millennium, Starkey Laboratories has caught up in its technology.

Bill Austin entered the hearing aid scene in 1967 when, frustrated with the relatively poor repair quality for hearing instruments, he founded Professional Hearing Aid Service, a hearing instrument repair company for any brand. Aside from high-quality repairs, the hallmark of the business was flat-charge repairs. Starkey Laboratories, a small ear mold company, was founded by Harold Starkey. Looking to expand his company, Bill Austin acquired Starkey Laboratories (hereafter Starkey) in 1971. Bill carried his high value for service into his new venture of hearing instrument manufacturing and sales. Within 2 years, Starkey began offering both a 1-year unconditional warranty, which put Starkey on the map as a major competitor, as well as a 90-day trial period on particular models, an industry first (Starkey, 2006c). In keeping with this service-first idea, the Starkey Fund was created in 1978 to help people without resources to receive hearing assistance. Eventually, the Starkey Fund grew into the Starkey Hearing Foundation, which annually provides over 20,000 hearing instruments to those in need (Starkey, 2006d).

In 1976, Starkey began expanding worldwide by opening a facility in Manchester, England, and the company opened four more facilities within the next five years. Currently, Starkey employs over 3,500 people in 22 facilities to enable the business to operate in over 100 markets (Starkey, 2006c, 2007, 2009a).

As far as product innovation is concerned, Starkey's early major initiatives are as follows:

1983: The industry's first ITC hearing instrument is introduced (CE-5)

1993: Starkey's first CIC introduced (Tympanette)

1996: First custom programmable instrument introduced (Sequel Custom Programmable)

1999: Acquired Micro-Tech

1999: First digital hearing instruments entered the market (Cetera and Aries)

2006: Destiny line is introduced; subsequently expanded to include open-fit and receiver-in-the-canal styles

2008: Starkey Zōn wins multiple design awards (Klemme, 2008a, 2008b)

2009: Introduces new device line with Drive Architecture (S Series) (Starkey, 2009)

Philanthropy

Starkey has, I dare say, the most active and comprehensive philanthropic programs in the industry. As a personal example, in 1999, Starkey loaned me an audiometer and a tympanometer to take to Indonesia to do hearing screenings. Though my trip was just a survey trip at the time, they made two things clear to me: (a) that they would provide free hearing instruments and batteries to those in need based on my findings and (b) that they would only do so if I could provide Starkey a plan to provide batteries on an ongoing basis. It is this kind of thoughtful planning that is required for philanthropic programs to be successful.

The Starkey Hearing Foundation, an incorporated charitable organization, receives private donations to provide hearing instruments to the needy around the world. As previously stated, the Starkey Hearing Foundation provides over 20,000 hearing instruments per year and has provided over 32,000 hearing instruments to African countries, over 37,000 to Asian countries, over 34,000 to Caribbean and Central American countries, over 25,000 to Europe and the Middle East, over 77,000 to Mexico, over 26,000 to South America, and over 100,000 to the United States through April 2009. It has accomplished this by doing over 150 missions per year (Starkey Hearing Foundation, 2009; Starkey, 2007; Starkey Hearing Foundation, 2006c).

The Starkey Hearing Foundation's Hear Now program is the foundation's domestic program that provides hearing instruments to those who cannot afford them. Part of its program works on the donation of used hearing instruments that can be "recycled" and then donated to an appropriate recipient (Starkey Hearing Foundation, 2006b).

Warranty

Every Starkey hearing instrument carries a 1-year warranty, called the Worry-Free Warranty. Certain models carry a 2-year warranty. This covers mechanical problems due to defect or fitting problems. With this is a one-time replacement in the rare situation the hearing instrument is lost or totally destroyed. For a fee, extended warrantees can be purchased (Starkey, 2006b).

If a patient owns a Starkey device currently under the standard warranty, he or she can purchase the Worry-Free Extended Warranty. This add-on extends the coverage to internal component failure, accidental damage, or remakes due to fitting issues (Starkey, 2006b).

Starkey also offers three warranty packages for any brand of hearing instruments: Worry-Free Repair Warranty; Worry-Free Loss and Damage Warranty; and Worry-Free Deluxe Loss, Damage, and Repair Warranty. The hearing instrument must be in proper working condition at the time of warranty purchase. Pricing can vary, as the warrantees are sold through hearing professionals (Starkey, 2006b).

Worry-Free Repair Warranty

This warranty covers if the hearing aid "breaks down" due to an internal component. Think of it as similar to power-train warranty on a car (Starkey, 2006b).

Worry-Free Loss and Damage Warranty

This warranty replaces any brand of hearing instrument with a Starkey equivalent device in the event of loss, theft, or if it is completely destroyed (Starkey, 2006b).

Worry-Free Deluxe Loss, Damage, and Repair Warranty

This warranty combines the coverage of the Worry-Free Repair Warranty and the Worry-Free Loss and Damage Warranty. Therefore, breakdowns, loss, and theft are covered as described above (Starkey, 2006b).

PRODUCT INFORMATION

PRODUCT 1: S SERIES™ SERIES 11, 9, 7, AND 5

Product Application

S Series 11 RIC BTE
S Series 11 RIC BTE Absolute Power
S Series 11 ITE
S Series 11 HS
S Series 11 ITC
S Series 11 CIC
S Series 9 RIC BTE
S Series 9 RIC BTE Absolute Power
S Series 9 ITE
S Series 9 HS
S Series 9 ITC
S Series 9 CIC
S Series 7 RIC BTE
S Series 7 RIC BTE Absolute Power
S Series 7 ITE
S Series 7 HS
S Series 7 ITC
S Series 7 CIC
S Series 5 RIC BTE
S Series 5 RIC BTE Absolute Power
S Series 5 ITE
S Series 5 HS
S Series 5 ITC
S Series 5 CIC

Features of S Series 11 RIC BTE, S Series 11 ITE, S Series 11 HS, S Series 11 ITC, and S Series 11 CIC

- Optimal high-resolution sound imaging
- Frequency shaping in all 16 channels and 16 bands
- PureWave Feedback Eliminator – proprietary feedback management system
- Acoustic Scene Analyzer – an algorithm designed to implement appropriate combination of processing strategies depending on listening environment
- AudioScape – adjusts program settings according to listening conditions
- Comfort Control – a tool to assist clinician in adjusting instrument to patient preferences
- InVision Directionality – proprietary directional microphone system
- Live Real Ear Measurement – a real-ear measurement system integrated into the instrument
- T^2 (Touch-Tone) – allows the patient to use a cell phone or touch-tone phone to switch modes or adjust volume

- Automatic Telephone Solutions – automatically detects telephone use and adjusts the frequency response
- Auto Path – an automatic fitting routine designed to streamline the fitting process
- Live 3D Speech Mapping – verifies instrument output using speech as an input in a visually clear manner
- Live Speech Mapping – verifies instrument output using speech as an input

Options of S Series 11 RIC BTE, S Series 11 ITE, S Series 11 HS, S Series 11 ITC, and S Series 11 CIC

- Self-Check – allows a diagnostic check of the microphone, circuit, and receiver
- Appointment Reminders – to remind patients of follow up appointments and maintenance checks
- Leisure Listening Memories – settings for various music genres
- Voice Indicators – alerts patient on status of battery, memory and telephone modes
- Tonal Indicators – unique tones for memory, low battery, etc.
- Verify Comfort
- In-Situ Audiometry
- Data Logging

Features of S Series 9 RIC BTE, S Series 9 ITE, S Series 9 HS, S Series 9 ITC, and S Series 9 CIC

- High-resolution sound imaging
- Frequency shaping in 12 channels and 12 bands
- PureWave Feedback Eliminator – proprietary feedback management system
- Acoustic Scene Analyzer – an algorithm designed to implement appropriate combination of processing strategies depending on listening environment
- AudioScape – adjusts program settings according to listening conditions
- InVision Directionality – proprietary directional microphone system
- Live Real Ear Measurement – a real-ear measurement system integrated into the instrument
- T^2 (Touch-Tone) – allows the patient to use a cell phone or touch-tone phone to switch modes or adjust volume
- Automatic Telephone Solutions – automatically detects telephone use and adjusts the frequency response
- Auto Path – an automatic fitting routine designed to streamline the fitting process
- Live Speech Mapping – verifies instrument output using speech as an input

Options of S Series 9 RIC BTE, S Series 9 ITE, S Series 9 HS, S Series 9 ITC, and S Series 9 CIC

- Tonal Indicators – unique tones for memory, low battery, etc.
- Verify Comfort

- In-Situ Audiometry
- Data Logging

Features of S Series 7 RIC BTE, S Series 7 ITE, S Series 7 HS, S Series 7 ITC, and S Series 7 CIC

- Frequency shaping in 8 channels and 8 bands
- PureWave Feedback Eliminator – proprietary feedback management system
- Acoustic Scene Analyzer – an algorithm designed to implement appropriate combination of processing strategies depending on listening environment
- AudioScape – adjusts program settings according to listening conditions
- InVision Directionality – proprietary directional microphone system
- Live Real Ear Measurement – a real-ear measurement system integrated into the instrument
- T^2 (Touch-Tone) – allows the patient to use a cell phone or touch-tone phone to switch modes or adjust volume
- Automatic Telephone Solutions – automatically detects telephone use and adjusts the frequency response
- Auto Path – an automatic fitting routine to help provide an accurate first fit
- Live Speech Mapping – verifies instrument output using speech as an input

Options of S Series 7 RIC BTE, S Series 7 ITE, S Series 7 HS, S Series 7 ITC, and S Series 7 CIC

- Tonal Indicators – unique tones for memory, low battery, etc.
- Verify Comfort
- In-Situ Audiometry
- Data Logging

Features of S Series 5 RIC BTE, S Series 5 ITE, S Series 5 HS, S Series 5 ITC, and S Series 5 CIC

- 6 channels
- 6 bands
- PureWave Feedback Eliminator – proprietary feedback management system
- Acoustic Scene Analyzer – an algorithm designed to implement appropriate combination of processing strategies depending on listening environment
- AudioScape – adjusts program settings according to listening conditions
- InVision Directionality – proprietary directional microphone system
- Live Real Ear Measurement – a real-ear measurement system integrated into the instrument

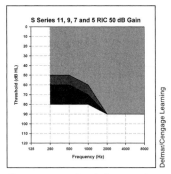

Fitting range for S Series 11, 9, 7 and 5 RIC 50 dB Gain open earbud (light gray), occluded earbud (gray) and custom earearmold (dark gray)

- T² (Touch-Tone) – allows the patient to use a cell phone or touch-tone phone to switch modes or adjust volume
- Automatic Telephone Solutions – automatically detects telephone use and adjusts the frequency response
- Auto Path – an automatic fitting routine to help provide an accurate first fit
- Live Speech Mapping – verifies instrument output using speech as an input

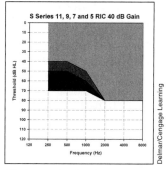

Fitting range for S Series 11, 9, 7 and 5 RIC 40 dB Gain open earbud (light gray), occluded earbud (gray) and custom earearmold (dark gray)

Options of S Series 5 RIC BTE, S Series 5 ITE, S Series 5 HS, S Series 5 ITC, and S Series 5 CIC

- Tonal Indicators – unique tones for memory, low battery, etc.
- Verify Comfort
- In-Situ Audiometry
- Data Logging

Features of S Series 11 RIC Absolute Power BTE

- Optimal high-resolution sound imaging
- Frequency shaping in all 16 channels and 16 bands
- PureWave Feedback Eliminator – proprietary feedback management system
- Acoustic Scene Analyzer – an algorithm designed to implement appropriate combination of processing strategies depending on listening environment
- AudioScape – adjusts program settings according to listening conditions
- Comfort Control – a tool to assist clinician in adjusting instrument to patient preferences
- InVision Directionality – proprietary directional microphone system
- T² (Touch-Tone) – allows the patient to use a cell phone or touch-tone phone to switch modes or adjust volume
- Automatic Telephone Solutions – automatically detects telephone use and adjusts the frequency response
- Auto Path – an automatic fitting routine to help provide an accurate first fit
- Live 3D Speech Mapping – verifies instrument output using speech as an input in a visually clear manner
- Live Speech Mapping – verifies instrument output using speech as an input

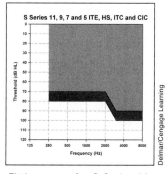

Fitting range for S Series 11, 9, 7 and 5 ITE, HS and ITC (light gray) and CIC (dark gray)

Options of S Series 11 RIC Absolute Power BTE

- Self-Check – allows a diagnostic check of the microphone, circuit, and receiver
- Appointment Reminders – to remind patients of follow up appointments and maintenance checks
- Leisure Listening Memories – settings for various music genres
- Voice Indicators – alerts patient on status of battery, memory and telephone modes
- Tonal Indicators – unique tones for memory, low battery, etc.
- Verify Comfort
- In-Situ Audiometry
- Data Logging

Features of S Series 9 RIC Absolute Power BTE

- High-resolution sound imaging
- Frequency shaping in all 12 channels and 12 bands
- PureWave Feedback Eliminator – proprietary feedback management system
- Acoustic Scene Analyzer – an algorithm designed to implement appropriate combination of processing strategies depending on listening environment
- AudioScape – adjusts program settings according to listening conditions
- InVision Directionality – proprietary directional microphone system
- T^2 (Touch-Tone) – allows the patient to use a cell phone or touch-tone phone to switch modes or adjust volume
- Automatic Telephone Solutions – automatically detects telephone use and adjusts the frequency response
- Auto Path – an automatic fitting routine to help provide an accurate first fit
- Live Speech Mapping – verifies instrument output using speech as an input

Options of S Series 9 RIC Absolute Power BTE

- Tonal Indicators – unique tones for memory, low battery, etc.
- Verify Comfort
- In-Situ Audiometry
- Data Logging

Features of S Series 7 RIC Absolute Power BTE

- Frequency shaping in all 8 channels and 8 bands
- PureWave Feedback Eliminator – proprietary feedback management system
- Acoustic Scene Analyzer – an algorithm designed to implement appropriate combination of processing strategies depending on listening environment
- AudioScape – adjusts program settings according to listening conditions
- InVision Directionality – proprietary directional microphone system
- T^2 (Touch-Tone) – allows the patient to use a cell phone or touch-tone phone to switch modes or adjust volume

- Automatic Telephone Solutions – automatically detects telephone use and adjusts the frequency response
- Auto Path – an automatic fitting routine to help provide an accurate first fit
- Live Speech Mapping – verifies instrument output using speech as an input

Options of S Series 7 RIC Absolute Power BTE

- Tonal Indicators – unique tones for memory, low battery, etc.
- Verify Comfort
- In-Situ Audiometry
- Data Logging

Features of S Series 5 RIC Absolute Power BTE

- 6 channels
- 6 bands
- PureWave Feedback Eliminator – proprietary feedback management system
- Acoustic Scene Analyzer – an algorithm designed to implement appropriate combination of processing strategies depending on listening environment
- AudioScape – adjusts program settings according to listening conditions
- InVision Directionality – proprietary directional microphone system
- T^2 (Touch-Tone) – allows the patient to use a cell phone or touch-tone phone to switch modes or adjust volume
- Automatic Telephone Solutions – automatically detects telephone use and adjusts the frequency response
- Auto Path – an automatic fitting routine to help provide an accurate first fit
- Live Speech Mapping – verifies instrument output using speech as an input

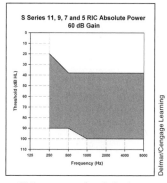

Fitting range for S Series 11, 9, 7 and 5 RIC Absolute Power 60 dB Gain with occluded earmold

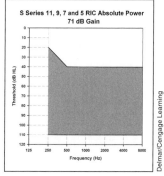

Fitting range for S Series 11, 9, 7 and 5 RIC Absolute Power 71 dB Gain with occluded earmold

Options of S Series 5 RIC Absolute Power BTE

- Tonal Indicators – unique tones for memory, low battery, etc.
- Verify Comfort
- In-Situ Audiometry
- Data Logging

Features of E Series 3 RIC BTE and E Series 3 RIC Absolute Power BTE

- Feedback Canceller – proprietary feedback cancellation algorithm
- Environmental Adaptation – Scans the environment and adapts appropriately to noise or quiet
- Dynamic Directionality
- Tonal Indicators – unique tones for memory, low battery, etc.
- 4 memories standard

Features of E Series 3 ITE, E Series 3 HS, E Series 3 ITC, E Series 3 CIC

- Feedback Canceller – proprietary feedback cancellation algorithm
- Environmental Adaptation – Scans the environment and adapts appropriately to noise or quiet
- Dynamic Directionality
- Tonal Indicators   unique tones for memory, low battery, etc.
- 1 memory standard

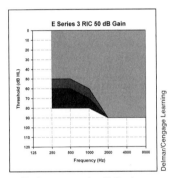

Fitting range for E Series 3 RIC 50 dB Gain open earbud (light gray), occluded earbud (gray) and custom earearmold (dark gray)

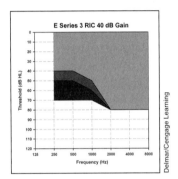

Fitting range for E Series 3 RIC 40 dB Gain open earbud (light gray), occluded earbud (gray) and custom earearmold (dark gray)

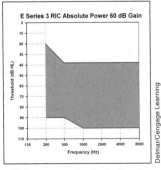

Fitting range for E Series 3 RIC Absolute Power 60 dB Gain with occluded earmold

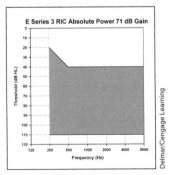

Fitting range for E Series 3 RIC Absolute Power 71 dB Gain with occluded earmold

Options of E Series 3 ITE, E Series 3 HS, E Series 3 ITC, E Series 3 CIC

• Induction Coil – unique tones for memory, low battery, etc.
• 4 memories optional

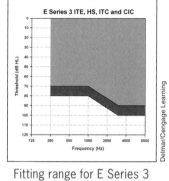

Fitting range for E Series 3
ITE, HS and ITC (light gray)
and CIC (dark gray)

Typical Specifications		S Series 11, 9, 7, and 5 RIC BTE 40 dB gain	S Series 11, 9, 7, and 5 RIC BTE 50 dB gain
Standard ANSI S3.22-2003			
Output sound pressure level	Max OSPL 90 (dB SPL)	110	115
	HF-average OSPL 90 (dB SPL)	102	108
Full-on gain	Peak gain (dB)	40	50
	HF-average full-on gain (dB)	31	44
Total harmonic distortion	500 Hz	<3%	<3%
	800 Hz	<3%	<3%
	1600 Hz	<3%	<3%
Equivalent input noise (dB SPL)		<25	<25
Telecoil sensitivity	HFA-SPLITS (dB SPL)	n/a	n/a
Battery	Operating current (mA)	1.2	1.3
	Battery type	312	312
Compression characteristics – channel AGC	Attack (ms)	20	20
	Release 0.1s (ms)	5-150	5-150
	Release 2.0s (ms)	5-150	5-150

Delmar/Cengage Learning

Typical Specifications		S Series 11, 9, 7, and 5 RIC Absolute Power BTE – 60 dB gain	S Series 11, 9, 7, and 5 RIC Absolute Power BTE – 71 dB gain
Standard ANSI S3.22-2003			
Output sound pressure level	Max OSPL 90 (dB SPL)	123	131
	HF-average OSPL 90 (dB SPL)	115	125
Full-on gain	Peak gain (dB)	60	71
	HF-average full-on gain (dB)	52	64
Total harmonic distortion	500 Hz	<3%	<3%
	800 Hz	<3%	<3%
	1600 Hz	<3%	<3%
Equivalent input noise (dB SPL)		<25	<25
Telecoil sensitivity	HFA-SPLITS (dB SPL)	n/a	n/a
Battery	Operating current (mA)	1.2	1.6
	Battery type	312	312
Compression characteristics – channel AGC	Attack (ms)	20	20
	Release 0.1s (ms)	5-150	5-150
	Release 2.0s (ms)	5-150	5-150

Delmar/Cengage Learning

Typical Specifications		S Series 11, 9, 7, and 5 ITE	S Series 11, 9, 7, and 5 HS/ITC	S Series 11, 9, 7, and 5 CIC
Standard ANSI S3.22-2003				
Output sound pressure level	Max OSPL 90 (dB SPL)	115-131	110-131	110-131
	HF-average OSPL 90 (dB SPL)	111-126	106-126	106-126
Full-on gain	Peak Gain (dB)	45-71	40-71	35-71
	HF-average full-on gain (dB)	41-65	36-65	31-65
Total harmonic distortion	500 Hz	<3%	<3%	<3%
	800 Hz	<3%	<3%	<3%
	1600 Hz	<3%	<3%	<3%
Equivalent input noise (dB SPL)		<28	<28	<28
Telecoil sensitivity	HFA-SPLITS (dB SPL)	94-109	89-109	n/a
Battery	Operating current (mA)	1.1-1.7	1.1-1.7	1.1-1.7
	Battery type	13, 312, 10	13, 312, 10	13, 312, 10

continues

continued

Typical Specifications		S Series 11, 9, 7, and 5 ITE	S Series 11, 9, 7, and 5 HS/ITC	S Series 11, 9, 7, and 5 CIC
Compression characteristics – channel AGC	Attack (ms)	20	20	20
	Release 0.1s (ms)	5-150	5-150	5-150
	Release 2.0s (ms)	5-150	5-150	5-150

Delmar/Cengage Learning

Typical Specifications		E Series 3 RIC BTE – 40 dB gain	E Series 3 RIC BTE – 50 dB gain
Standard ANSI S3.22-2003			
Output sound pressure level	Max OSPL 90 (dB SPL)	110	115
	HF-average OSPL 90 (dB SPL)	102	108
Full-on gain	Peak gain (dB)	40	50
	HF-average full-on gain (dB)	31	44
Total harmonic distortion	500 Hz	<3%	<3%
	800 Hz	<3%	<3%
	1600 Hz	<3%	<3%
Equivalent input noise (dB SPL)		<25	<25
Telecoil sensitivity	HFA-SPLITS (dB SPL)	n/a	n/a
Battery	Operating current (mA)	1.2	1.3
	Battery type	312	312
Compression characteristics – channel AGC	Attack (ms)	20	20
	Release 0.1s (ms)	5-150	5-150
	Release 2.0s (ms)	5-150	5-150

Delmar/Cengage Learning

Typical Specifications		E Series 3 RIC Absolute Power BTE – 60 dB gain	E Series 3 Absolute Power BTE – 71 dB gain
Standard ANSI S3.22-2003			
Output sound pressure level	Max OSPL 90 (dB SPL)	123	131
	HF-average OSPL 90 (dB SPL)	115	125
Full-on gain	Peak gain (dB)	60	71
	HF-average full-on gain (dB)	52	64

STARKEY LABORATORIES

continues

continued

Typical Specifications		E Series 3 RIC Absolute Power BTE – 60 dB gain	E Series 3 Absolute Power BTE – 71 dB gain
Total harmonic distortion	500 Hz	<3%	<3%
	800 Hz	<3%	<3%
	1600 Hz	<3%	<3%
Equivalent input noise (dB SPL)		<25	<25
Telecoil sensitivity	HFA-SPLITS (dB SPL)	n/a	n/a
Battery	Operating current (mA)	1.2	1.6
	Battery type	312	312
Compression characteristics – channel AGC	Attack (ms)	20	20
	Release 0.1s (ms)	5-150	5-150
	Release 2.0s (ms)	5-150	5-150

Delmar/Cengage Learning

Typical Specifications		E Series 3 ITE	E Series 3 HS/ITC	E Series 3 CIC
Standard ANSI S3.22-2003				
Output sound pressure level	Max OSPL 90 (dB SPL)	115-131	110-131	110-131
	HF-average OSPL 90 (dB SPL)	111-126	106-126	106-126
Full-on gain	Peak gain (dB)	45-71	40-71	35-71
	HF-average full-on gain (dB)	41-65	36-65	31-65
Total harmonic distortion	500 Hz	<3%	<3%	<3%
	800 Hz	<3%	<3%	<3%
	1600 Hz	<3%	<3%	<3%
Equivalent input noise (dB SPL)		<28	<28	<28
Telecoil sensitivity	HFA-SPLITS (dB SPL)	94-109	89-109	n/a
Battery	Operating current (mA)	1.1-1.7	1.1-1.7	1.1-1.7
	Battery type	13, 312, 10	13, 312, 10	13, 312, 10
Compression characteristics – channel AGC	Attack (ms)	20	20	20
	Release 0.1s (ms)	5-150	5-150	5-150
	Release 2.0s (ms)	5-150	5-150	5-150

Delmar/Cengage Learning

PRODUCT: DESTINY

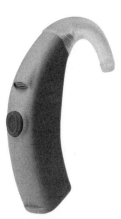

Destiny Mini BTE
Starkey Laboratories

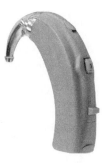

Destiny Power Plus BTE
Starkey Laboratories

Product Application

Destiny 1600 Mini BTE
Destiny 1200 Mini BTE
Destiny 800 Mini BTE
Destiny 400 Mini BTE
Destiny 1200 Power Plus

Features of Destiny 1600 Mini BTE

- Integrated real-ear measurement (IREM) – performs real-ear measurement and incorporates data immediately through Inspire OS 2.0
- Auto Path – initial fitting protocol designed to significantly shorten the fitting process
- Voice indicators – use speech to alert wearers of hearing aid status
- Self-check – a diagnostic check of the microphone, circuit, and receiver
- Patient reminder – provides an audible reminder for follow-up appointments
- Environmental adaptation including acoustic signature – auto-adjusts to various listening situations as well as for unwanted sounds (e.g., wind noise)
- Advanced data-logging – records the time spent in various listening situations
- 8 channels
- 12 bands
- 4 programs
- Active feedback intercept (off, adaptive [default], static) – proprietary feedback reduction system
- Automatic telephone response – automatically adjusts device for telephone use
- Induction coil – selectable as telecoil or autocoil (enable M/T)

- Adaptive indicator tones – unique tones for memory, low battery, volume, and the like
- Directional speech detector (DSD) – autoswitching to directional microphone system
- Power-on delay
- Audiometer – for frequency-specific in situ threshold and UCL measures
- Verify comfort – frequency-specific verification of the patient's dynamic range
- Direct audio input (DAI) – FM and Bluetooth
- Tamper-resistant battery door
- Programmed via Inspire OS software
- Acoustic signature – with acoustic signature, patients experience superior environmental management
- Intelligent environmental adaptation – identifies unique sound environments and adjusts to them instantly
- Auto Path fitting – leads professional through an automatic, binaural fitting protocol using real-ear data in less than 2 minutes

Features of Destiny 1200 Mini BTE

- Integrated real-ear measurement – performs real-ear measurement and incorporates data immediately through Inspire OS 2.0
- Auto Path fitting – leads professional through an automatic, binaural fitting protocol using real-ear data in less than 2 minutes
- Acoustic signature – superior environmental management
- Intelligent environmental adaptation – includes acoustic signature, a system that identifies unique sound environments and adjusts to them instantly
- Advanced data logging with acoustic signature linking
- 8 channels for sound adaptation
- 12 bands for precise fine-tuning
- Active feedback intercept with acoustic signature and DSD
- Adaptive indicator tones – available for memory selection, standby, volume control, low battery, telephone mode, and shutdown
- Directional speech detector – automatically adjusts to provide the optimal setting in quiet or noisy environments
- Automatic telephone response

Features of Destiny 800 Mini BTE

- Integrated real-ear measurement – performs real-ear measurement and incorporates data immediately through Inspire OS 2.0
- Auto Path fitting – leads professional through an automatic, binaural fitting protocol using real-ear data in less than 2 minutes
- Enhanced environmental adaptation – transitions seamlessly from one acoustic environment to the next
- 8 channels for sound adaptation
- 10 bands for enhanced fine-tuning

- Active feedback intercept with environmental adaptation
- Adaptive indicator tones – available for memory selection, standby, volume control, low battery, telephone mode, and shutdown
- Directional speech detector – automatically adjusts to provide the optimal setting in quiet or noisy environments
- Automatic telephone response

Features of Destiny 400 Mini BTE

- Integrated real-ear measurement – performs real-ear measurement and incorporates data immediately through Inspire OS 2.0
- Auto Path fitting – leads professional through an automatic, binaural fitting protocol using real-ear data in less than 2 minutes
- Environmental adaptation – transitions easily from one acoustic environment to the next
- 4 channels for sound adaptation
- 8 bands for fine-tuning
- Active feedback intercept with environmental adaptation
- Adaptive indicator tones – available for memory selection, standby, volume control, low battery, telephone mode, and shutdown
- Directional speech detector – automatically adjusts to provide the optimal setting in quiet or noisy environments
- Automatic telephone response

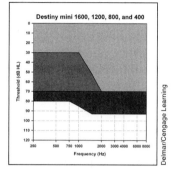

Fitting range for Destiny Mini 1600, 1200, 800, and 400 for thin tube open (light gray), thin tube occluded (light and medium gray), and standard earhook (all shaded areas)

Features of Destiny 1200 Power Plus BTE

- 8 channels for sound adaptation
- 12 bands for fine-tuning
- 4 memories
- WDRC
- Induction coil selectable as telecoil or autocoil (enable M/T)
- Automatic telephone response – automatically adjusts device for telephone use
- DAI – FM and Bluetooth
- Expanded dynamic range
- Active feedback intercept (off, adaptive [default], static) – proprietary feedback reduction system
- Environmental detection including acoustic signature – auto-adjusts to various listening situations as well as for unwanted sounds (e.g., wind noise)
- DSD – autoswitching to directional microphone system
- Indicator tones – memory, low battery, volume control, battery shutdown, telephone
- Data-logging – records the time spent in various listening situations

- Power-on delay
- Audiometer – for frequency-specific in situ threshold and UCL measures
- Verify comfort – for frequency-specific verification of the patient's dynamic range
- Volume control (can be disabled through software)
- Tamper-resistant battery door
- Programmed via Inspire OS Software

Options of Destiny 1200 Power Plus BTE

- CROS/BiCROS

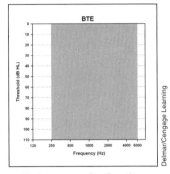

Fitting range for Destiny 1200 Power Plus BTE

Typical Specifications		Destiny 400, 800, 1200, and 1600 Mini BTE	Destiny 1200 Power Plus BTE
Standard ANSI S3.22-1996			
Output sound pressure level	Max OSPL 90 (dB SPL)	123	140
	HF-Average OSPL 90 (dB SPL)	117	134
Full-on gain	Peak gain (dB)	55	80
	HF-Average full-on gain (dB)	49	72
Total harmonic distortion	500 Hz	7%	1%
	800 Hz	3%	1%
	1600 Hz	3%	1%
Equivalent input noise (dB SPL)		28	30
Telecoil sensitivity	HFA-SPLITS (dB SPL)	n/a	114
Battery	Operating current (mA)	1.25-1.6	2.8
	Battery type	312	675
Compression Characteristics – Channel AGC	Attack (ms)	25	5
	Release 0.1s (ms)	55	20
	Release 2.0s (ms)	55	20

Delmar/Cengage Learning

CHAPTER ELEVEN

Unitron

UNITRON: KEEPING EVERYTHING CONNECTED

International Headquarters
Unitron Corporate Office
20 Beasley Dr
P.O. Box 9017
Kitchener, Ontario, Canada
N2G 4X1
Phone: 1 (877) 492-6244
Fax: 1 (519) 895-0108
E-mail: info@unitron.com
Web site: http://unitron.com

U.S. Headquarters
Unitron U.S.
2300 N Berkshire Ln
Suite A
Plymouth, MN 55441
Phone: 1 (800) 888-8882
Fax: 1 (763) 557-8828
E-mail: info@unitronhearing.com
Web site: http://www.unitron.com/us

We provide services to the professionals who serve people with hearing loss.
— Cameron Hay, president and CEO, Unitron (Dorich, 2005)

In 1965, a group consisting largely of hearing experts founded what was known at the time as Unitron Industries. As a new player in the industry, they focused their efforts on the development of hearing instruments and new technology (Dorich, 2005). Over time, they have become more people-oriented, committed to "purpose-driven innovation" to show their care for "people with hearing loss and the professionals who support them" (Unitron, 2009a). A large part of this shift came in 2001 when they changed their name to Unitron Hearing and underwent a time of introspection to reevaluate their branding and identity. As a result, they increased their research and development efforts and promoted a "customer-intimate behavior" (Dorich, 2005). In 2009, they reinvented their brand identity by including the "Connect" tagline after the Unitron name (Unitron, 2009c). These expanded research and development efforts have included a focus on signal processing, software development, and custom-made devices. The Passport is Unitron's most advanced hearing instrument to date (Unitron, 2009b). So now, over 40 years later, Unitron has grown to a point where it employs around 600 people serving 70 countries (Unitron, 2007).

Unitron has not been absent in the consolidation process that has marked the industry in recent years. Between 1999 and 2001, Unitron merged with Argosy Hearing Solutions and Lori Medical Labs (Unitron, 2007). These are currently a subsidiary of Sonova, yet maintain their own branding and sense of corporate culture. Cameron Hay, the CEO of Unitron, clearly states, "We are not Phonak Lite," as evidenced by its own sales, distribution, and research and development (Beck, 2005). Furthermore, Hay states that Unitron is a "strongly Canadian company," with the United States its largest geographic market (Beck, 2005).

Philanthropy

At the time of this writing, no information was available on Unitron's philanthropic activities.

Warranty

Unitron offers a 2-year warranty on Indigo, Conversa.NT, Conversa, Unison 6, Unison 3, and the WiFi Mic System. Other product lines, including the Unison Essential, Breeze, and other conventional hearing instruments, include a 1-year warranty. Additional years of coverage can be purchased during the warranty period. All Unitron hearing instruments also come with 1-year loss and damage coverage. A fee will be charged for the processing of a loss and damage claim. Additional years of loss and damage coverage can be purchased during this first year.

PRODUCT INFORMATION

PRODUCT 1: PASSPORT™

Product Application

Passport BTE
Passport BTE HP
Passport Moxi 13 CRT BTE
Passport Moxi 13 CRT BTE Power
Passport Moxi CRT BTE
Passport Moxi CRT BTE Power
Passport Moda 13 BTE
Passport Moda II BTE
Passport Shift CRT BTE
Passport Full Shell
Passport Full Shell Power

Passport Half Shell/Canal
Passport Half Shell/Canal Power
Passport Mini Canal/CIC
Passport CIC Power
Passport Fuse Crossover (open-fit CIC)

Features of Passport BTE and Passport BTE HP

- Smart focus – designed to provide patient with a method to enhance speech by allowing adjustments to microphone strategy, speech enhancement, noise reduction and gain
- Enhanced auto pro 4 – uses five parameters to adapt hearing aid to listening environment
- Enhanced feedback management system – proprietary feedback management reduction
- Self-learning – a learning algorithm that automatically learns volume and comfort – clarity preferences
- Learn now – learns patient's preferences for Smart focus and volume control
- Unifi wireless system with duo link – connects the two hearing instruments to ensure changes are made to both instruments
- 20 channels of signal processing
- Automatic program with 4 listening destinations, 3 manual, and 2 wireless streaming programs
- Speech enhancement LD – increases gain in each band where speech dominates over noise
- Noise reduction – reduces gain in bands with poor SNRs
- Anti-shock – reduces the level of impulse noises
- Data logging
- Easy DAI
- Easy-t – auto switching to t-coil program when phone is picked up
- Suitable for mild to severe hearing losses and can fit audiogram configurations ranging from reverse to precipitously sloping

Options of Passport BTE and Passport BTE HP

- Smart control – a remote control allowing patients to adjust their devices
- uDirect – a device worn around the neck acts as a wireless interface between the hearing aids and other Bluetooth-enabled devices. Devices include:
  - uPhone – activates streaming program when signal is received from Bluetooth-enabled cell phone and Bluetooth-enabled audio devices
  - uAudio – activates streaming program when signal is received from FM transmitters or wired audio inputs
- Multiple microphones – omnidirectional, fixed directional, and multiband adaptive directional
- Wireless programming with iCube

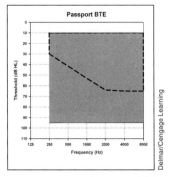

Fitting range for Passport BTE
(full shaded area) and slim
tube (dotted line and above)

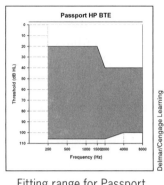

Fitting range for Passport
BTE HP

Features of Passport Moxi 13 CRT BTE and Passport Moxi 13 CRT BTE Power

- Smart focus – designed to provide patient with a method to enhance speech by allowing adjustments to microphone strategy, speech enhancement, noise reduction and gain
- Enhanced auto pro 4 – four programs each with adaptive parameters; includes automatic and smooth program changes
- Enhanced feedback management system – proprietary feedback management reduction
- Self-learning – can be configured to automatically learn volume and comfort – clarity preferences
- Learn now – learns patient's preferences for Smart focus and volume control
- uDirect – a device worn around the neck acts as a wireless interface between the hearing aids and other Bluetooth-enabled devices. Devices include:
  - uPhone – activates streaming program when signal is received from Bluetooth-enabled cell phone and Bluetooth-enabled audio devices
  - uAudio – activates streaming program when signal is received from FM transmitters or wired audio inputs
- 20 channels of signal processing
- Automatic program with 4 listening destinations and 3 manual
- Speech enhancement LD – increases gain in each band where speech dominates over noise
- Noise reduction – reduces gain in bands with poor SNRs

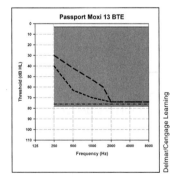

Fitting range for Passport Moxi 13 CRT BTE open dome (long dash and above), closed dome (short dash and above), and sleeve mold (all shaded region)

- Anti-shock reduces the level of impulse noises
- Data logging
- Easy-t – auto switching to t-coil program when phone is picked up
- Suitable for mild to severe hearing losses and can fit audiogram configurations ranging from reverse to precipitously sloping

Options of Passport Moxi 13 CRT and Passport Moxi 13 CRT BTE Power

- Smart control – allows patient to adjust the hearing aids using a remote control
- Multiple microphones – omnidirectional, fixed directional, and multiband adaptive directional
- Wireless programming with iCube
- Choice of 2 receivers

Features of Passport Moxi CRT BTE and Passport Moxi CRT BTE Power

- Smart focus – designed to provide patient with a method to enhance speech by allowing adjustments to microphone strategy, speech enhancement, noise reduction and gain
- Enhanced auto pro 4 – four programs each with adaptive parameters; includes automatic and smooth program changes
- Enhanced feedback management system – proprietary feedback management reduction
- Self-learning – can be configured to automatically learn volume and comfort – clarity preferences
- Learn now – learns patient's preferences for Smart focus and volume control
- 20 channels of signal processing
- Automatic program with 4 listening destinations and 3 manual
- Speech enhancement LD – increases gain in each band where speech dominates over noise
- Noise reduction – reduces gain in bands with poor SNRs
- Anti-shock reduces the level of impulse noises

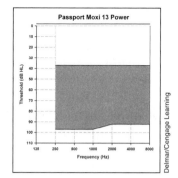

Fitting range for Passport Moxi 13 CRT BTE Power

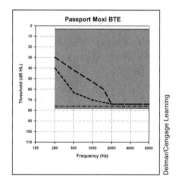

Fitting range for Passport Moxi CRT BTE open dome (long dash and above), closed dome (short dash and above), and sleeve mold (all shaded region)

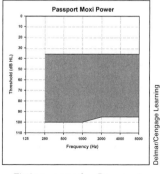

Fitting range for Passport Moxi CRT BTE Power

- Data logging
- Easy-t – auto switching to t-coil program when phone is picked up
- Passport Moxi and Passport Moxi Power are suitable for mild to severe hearing losses and can fit audiogram configurations ranging from reverse to precipitously sloping

Options of Passport Moxi CRT BTE and Passport Moxi CRT BTE Power

- Smart control – allows patient to adjust the hearing aids using a remote control
- Multiple microphones – omnidirectional, fixed directional, and multiband adaptive directional
- Choice of 2 receivers

Features of Passport Moda 13

- Smart focus – designed to provide patient with a method to enhance speech by allowing adjustments to microphone strategy, speech enhancement, noise reduction and gain
- Enhanced auto pro 4 – four programs each with adaptive parameters; includes automatic and smooth program changes
- Enhanced feedback management system – proprietary feedback management reduction
- Self-learning – a learning algorithm that automatically learns volume and comfort – clarity preferences
- Learn now – learns patient's preferences for Smart focus and volume control
- Unifi wireless system with duo link – connects the two hearing instruments to ensure changes are made to both instruments
- 20 channels of signal processing
- Automatic program with 4 listening destinations, 3 manual, and 2 wireless streaming programs
- Speech enhancement LD – increases gain in each band where speech dominates over noise
- Noise reduction – reduces gain in bands with poor SNRs
- Anti-shock reduces the level of impulse noises
- Data logging
- Easy DAI
- Easy-t – auto switching to t-coil program when phone is picked up
- Suitable for mild to moderately severe hearing losses and can fit audiogram configurations ranging from reverse to precipitously sloping

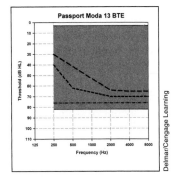

Fitting range for Passport Moda 13 Open dome (long dash and above), closed dome (short dash and above), and sleeve mold (all shaded region)

Options of Passport Moda 13

- Smart control – allows patient to adjust the hearing aids using a remote control
- uDirect – a device worn around the neck acts as a wireless interface between the hearing aids and other Bluetooth-enabled devices. Devices include:
  - uPhone – activates streaming program when signal is received from Bluetooth-enabled cell phone and Bluetooth-enabled audio devices
  - uAudio – activates streaming program when signal is received from FM transmitters or wired audio inputs
- Multiple microphones – omnidirectional, fixed directional, and multiband adaptive directional
- Wireless programming with iCube

Features of Passport Moda II

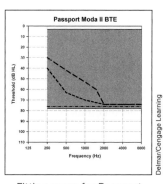

- Smart focus – designed to provide patient with a method to enhance speech by allowing adjustments to microphone strategy, speech enhancement, noise reduction and gain
- Enhanced auto pro 4 – four programs each with adaptive parameters; includes automatic and smooth program changes
- Enhanced feedback management system – proprietary feedback management reduction
- Self-learning – can be configured to automatically learn volume and comfort – clarity preferences
- Learn now – learns patient's preferences for Smart focus and volume control
- 20 channels of signal processing
- Automatic program with 4 listening destinations and 3 manual
- Speech enhancement LD – increases gain in each band where speech dominates over noise
- Noise reduction – reduces gain in bands with poor SNRs
- Anti-shock reduces the level of impulse noises
- Data logging
- Suitable for mild to moderately severe hearing losses and can fit audiogram configurations ranging from reverse to precipitously sloping

Fitting range for Passport Moda II open dome (long dash and above), closed dome (short dash and above), and sleeve mold (all shaded region)

Options of Passport Moda II

- Smart control – allows patient to adjust the hearing aids using a remote control
- Multiple microphones – omnidirectional, fixed directional, and multiband adaptive directional

Features of Passport Shift

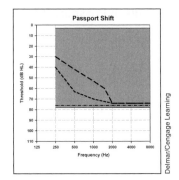

Fitting range for Passport Shift open dome (long dash and above), closed dome (short dash and above), and sleeve mold (all shaded region)

- Smart focus – designed to provide patient with a method to enhance speech by allowing adjustments to microphone strategy, speech enhancement, noise reduction and gain
- Enhanced auto pro 4 – four programs each with adaptive parameters; includes automatic and smooth program changes
- Enhanced feedback management system – proprietary feedback management reduction
- Self-learning – a learning algorithm that automatically learns volume and comfort – clarity preferences
- Learn now – learns patient's preferences for Smart focus and volume control
- 20 channels of signal processing
- Automatic +3 manual programs
- Speech enhancement LD – increases gain in each band where speech dominates over noise
- Noise reduction – reduces gain in bands with poor SNRs
- Anti-shock reduces the level of impulse noises
- Data logging
- Telecoil
- Suitable for mild to moderately severe hearing losses and can fit audiogram configurations ranging from reverse to precipitously sloping

Options of Passport Shift

- Smart control – allows patient to adjust the hearing aids using a remote control
- Multiple microphones – omnidirectional, fixed directional, and multiband adaptive directional

Features of Passport Full Shell, Passport Full Shell Power, Passport Half Shell/Canal, Passport Half Shell/Canal Power, Passport Mini Canal/CIC, Passport CIC Power

- Smart focus – designed to provide patient with a method to enhance speech by allowing adjustments to microphone strategy, speech enhancement, noise reduction and gain
- Enhanced auto pro 4 – four programs each with adaptive parameters; includes automatic and smooth program changes
- Enhanced feedback management system – proprietary feedback management reduction

- Self-learning – a learning algorithm that automatically learns volume and comfort – clarity preferences
- Learn now – learns patient's preferences for Smart focus and volume control
- uDirect – a device worn around the neck acts as a wireless interface between the hearing aids and other Bluetooth-enabled devices. Devices include:
  - uPhone – activates streaming program when signal is received from Bluetooth-enabled cell phone and Bluetooth-enabled audio devices
  - uAudio – activates streaming program when signal is received from FM transmitters or wired audio inputs
- 20 channels of signal processing
- Automatic program with 4 listening destinations, 3 manual, and 2 wireless streaming programs (where available)
- Speech enhancement LD – increases gain in each band where speech dominates over noise
- Noise reduction – reduces gain in bands with poor SNRs
- Anti-shock reduces the level of impulse noises
- Data logging
- Easy-t – auto switching to t-coil program when phone is picked up
- IntelliVent Technology
- Suitable for mild to severe hearing losses and can fit audiogram configurations ranging from reverse to precipitously sloping

Options of Passport Full Shell, Passport Full Shell Power, Passport Half Shell/Canal, Passport Half Shell/Canal Power, Passport Mini Canal/CIC, Passport CIC Power

- Smart control – allows patient to adjust the hearing aids using a remote control
- Multiple microphones – omnidirectional, fixed directional, and multiband adaptive directional
- Wireless programming with iCube

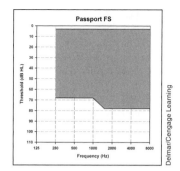

Fitting range for Passport Full Shell

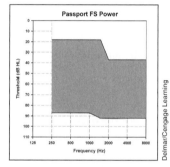

Fitting range for Passport Full Shell Power

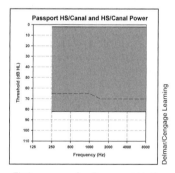

Fitting range for Passport Half Shell/Canal (dotted line and above) and Passport Half Shell/Canal Power (full shaded area)

Features of Passport Fuse Crossover Open-Fit CIC

- Smart focus – designed to provide patient with a method to enhance speech by allowing adjustments to microphone strategy, speech enhancement, noise reduction and gain
- Enhanced auto pro 4 – four programs each with adaptive parameters; includes automatic and smooth program changes
- Enhanced feedback management system – proprietary feedback management reduction
- Self-learning – a learning algorithm that automatically learns volume and comfort – clarity preferences
- Learn now – learns patient's preferences for Smart focus and volume control
- Articulation joint – flexes with the bend of the patient's ear canal
- Dual-flow vents – venting on both sides of the aid provide an open style fit to reduce the occlusion effect
- 20 channels of signal processing
- Automatic program with 4 listening destinations and 3 manual programs
- Speech enhancement LD – increases gain in each band where speech dominates over noise
- Omnidirectional microphone
- Noise reduction – reduces gain in bands with poor SNRs
- Anti-shock reduces the level of impulse noises
- My music™
- Wind noise manager
- Data logging
- Suitable for mild to moderately severe hearing losses and can fit audiogram configurations ranging from reverse to precipitously sloping

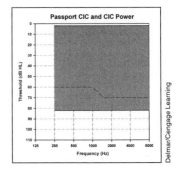

Fitting range for Passport Mini Canal/CIC and (dotted line and above) Passport CIC Power (full shaded area)

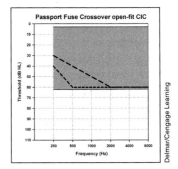

Fitting range for Passport Fuse crossover open-fit CIC open dome (long dash and above), closed dome (short dash and above), and power dome (all shaded region)

Options of Passport Fuse Crossover open-fit CIC

- Smart control – allows patient to adjust the hearing aids using a remote control
- Secure-fit tab-additional attachment to the body of the hearing aid to provide a more secure fit for patients with large ear canals

Typical Specifications		Passport (Slim tube)	Passport BTE	Passport (High power)
Standard ANSI S3.22-1996				
Output sound pressure level	Max OSPL 90 (dB SPL)	124	125	135
	HFA OSPL 90 (dB SPL)	108	122	128
Full-on gain (50 dB SPL input)	Peak gain (dB)	52	60	75
	HFA (dB)	38	52	68
Total harmonic distortion	500 Hz	1%	3%	2%
	800 Hz	1%	2%	2%
	1600 Hz	1%	1%	1%
Equivalent input noise (dB SPL)		26	19	19
Telecoil sensitivity	HFA SPLITS (dB SPL)	90	105	111
Battery	Operating current (mA)	1.2	1.3	2.2
	Battery type	13	13	13

Delmar/Cengage Learning

Typical Specifications		Passport Moxi 13 (xS receiver)	Passport Moxi 13 Power (xP receiver)	Passport Moxi (xS receiver)	Passport Moxi Power (xP receiver)
Standard ANSI S3.22-1996					
Output sound pressure level	Max OSPL 90 (dB SPL)	109	123	109	123
	HFA OSPL 90 (dB SPL)	104	118	104	118
Full-on gain (50 dB SPL input)	Peak gain (dB)	44	55	44	55
	HFA (dB)	36	47	36	47
Total harmonic distortion	500 Hz	1%	1.5%	1%	1.5%
	800 Hz	0.5%	1.3%	0.5%	1.3%
	1600 Hz	0.5%	0.5%	0.5%	0.5%
Equivalent input noise (dB SPL)		24	24	24	24
Telecoil sensitivity	HFA SPLITS (dB SPL)	87	101	87	101
Battery	Operating current (mA)	1.25	1.35	1.15	1.25
	Battery type	13	13	312	312

Delmar/Cengage Learning

Typical Specifications		Passport Moda 13	Passport Moda II	Passport Shift
Standard ANSI S3.22-1996				
Output sound pressure level	Max OSPL 90 (dB SPL)	124	117	109
	HFA OSPL 90 (dB SPL)	113	109	104
Full-on gain (50 dB SPL input)	Peak gain (dB)	53	45	44
	HFA (dB)	49	35	36
Total harmonic distortion	500 Hz	1.5%	1.5%	1%
	800 Hz	1.3%	1.3%	0.5%
	1600 Hz	1%	1%	0.5%
Equivalent input noise (dB SPL)		24	24	24
Telecoil sensitivity	HFA SPLITS (dB SPL)	96	92	87
Battery	Operating current (mA)	1.3	1.15	1.15
	Battery type	312	312	10A

Delmar/Cengage Learning

Typical Specifications		Passport Full Shell	Passport Full shell Power	Passport HS/Canal	Passport HS/Canal Power
Standard ANSI S3.22-1996					
Output sound pressure level	Max OSPL 90 (dB SPL)	115	112	113	117
	HFA OSPL 90 (dB SPL)	110	119	109	114
Full-on gain (50 dB SPL input)	Peak gain (dB)	50	60	48	55
	HFA (dB)	43	53	42	50
Total harmonic distortion	500 Hz	1%	1%	1%	1%
	800 Hz	0.5%	0.5%	0.5%	0.5%
	1600 Hz	0.5%	0.5%	0.5%	0.5%
Equivalent input noise (dB SPL)		20	20	20	21
Telecoil sensitivity	HFA SPLITS (dB SPL)	94	102	92	98
Battery	Operating current (mA)	1.1	1.1	1.1	1.1
	Battery type	13	13	312	312

Delmar/Cengage Learning

Typical Specifications		Passport MC/CIC	Passport MC/CIC Power	Passport Fuse Crossover open-fit CIC
Standard ANSI S3.22-1996				
Output sound pressure level	Max OSPL 90 (dB SPL)	112	116	109
	HFA OSPL 90 (dB SPL)	108	112	104
Full-on gain (50 dB SPL input)	Peak gain (dB)	40	55	40
	HFA (dB)	32	50	34
Total harmonic distortion	500 Hz	1%	1%	1%
	800 Hz	0.5%	0.5%	0.5%
	1600 Hz	0.5%	1.5%	0.5%
Equivalent input noise (dB SPL)		20	21	22
Telecoil sensitivity	HFA SPLITS (dB SPL)	n/a	n/a	n/a
Battery	Operating current (mA)	1.1	1.1	1.0
	Battery type	10A	10A	10A

Delmar/Cengage Learning

PRODUCT 2: LATITUDE™

Product Application

Latitude 16 BTE
Latitude 16 BTE HP
Latitude 16 Moxi 13 CRT BTE xS
Latitude 16 Moxi 13 CRT BTE Power xP
Latitude 16 Moxi 13 CRT BTE OptimumFit
Latitude 16 Moxi CRT BTE xS
Latitude 16 Moxi CRT BTE Power xP
Latitude 16 Moxi CRT BTE OptimumFit
Latitude 16 Moda 13 BTE
Latitude 16 Moda II BTE
Latitude 16 Shift CRT BTE
Latitude 16 Shift CRT BTE OptimumFit xS
Latitude 16 Full Shell
Latitude 16 Full Shell Power
Latitude 16 Half Shell/Canal
Latitude 16 Half Shell/Canal Power
Latitude 16 Mini Canal/CIC
Latitude 16 Mini Canal Power/CIC Power
Latitude 16 Fuse Crossover (open-fit CIC)

Features of Latitude 16 BTE and Latitude 16 BTE HP

- Smart focus – designed to provide patient with a method to enhance speech by allowing adjustments to microphone strategy, speech enhancement, noise reduction and gain
- Enhanced auto pro3™ – three programs each with adaptive parameters; includes automatic and smooth program changes
- Enhanced feedback management system – proprietary feedback management reduction
- Self-learning – a learning algorithm that automatically learns volume and comfort – clarity preferences
- Unifi wireless system with duoLink – connects the two hearing instruments to ensure changes are made to both instruments
- 16 channels of signal processing
- 16 bands
- Automatic program with 3 listening destinations, 3 manual, and 2 wireless streaming programs
- Speech enhancement LD – increases gain in each band where speech dominates over noise
- Noise reduction – reduces gain in bands with poor SNRs
- Anti-shock-reduces the level of impulse noises
- Data logging
- Easy DAI
- Easy-t – auto switching to t-coil program when phone is picked up
- Wind noise manager – reduces low-frequency gain during windy conditions
- Suitable for mild to severe hearing losses and can fit audiogram configurations ranging from reverse to precipitously sloping

Options of Latitude 16 BTE and Latitude 16 BTE HP

- Smart control – a remote control allowing patients to adjust their devices
- uDirect – a device worn around the neck acts as a wireless interface between the hearing aids and other Bluetooth-enabled devices. Devices include:
  - uPhone – activates streaming program when signal is received from Bluetooth-enabled cell phone and Bluetooth-enabled audio devices
  - uAudio – activates streaming program when signal is received from FM transmitters or wired audio inputs
- Duo link – program and/or volume adjustments made on one hearing instruments are automatically synchronized with the other
- Binaural phone – allows for binaural hearing while on a landline or mobile phone by automatically streams audio signal to the non-phone ear
- Multiple microphones – omnidirectional, fixed directional, and multiband adaptive directional
- My music
- Wireless programming with iCube

Features of Latitude 16 Moxi 13 CRT BTE xS, Latitude 16 Moxi 13 CRT BTE Power xP, and Latitude 16 Moxi 13 CRT BTE OptimumFit

- Smart focus – designed to provide patient with a method to enhance speech by allowing adjustments to microphone strategy, speech enhancement, noise reduction and gain
- Enhanced auto pro 3 – three programs each with adaptive parameters; includes automatic and smooth program changes
- Enhanced feedback management system – proprietary feedback management reduction
- Self-learning – a learning algorithm that automatically learns volume and comfort – clarity preferences
- Unifi wireless system with duoLink – connects the two hearing instruments to ensure changes are made to both instruments
- 16 channels of signal processing
- 16 bands
- Automatic program with 3 listening destinations, 3 manual, and 2 wireless streaming programs
- Speech enhancement LD – increases gain in each band where speech dominates over noise
- Noise reduction – reduces gain in bands with poor SNRs
- Wind noise manager – reduces low-frequency gain during windy conditions
- Anti-shock reduces the level of impulse noises
- Data logging
- Easy-t – auto switching to t-coil program when phone is picked up
- Telecoil
- Suitable for mild to severe hearing losses and can fit audiogram configurations ranging from reverse to precipitously sloping

Options of Latitude 16 Moxi 13 CRT BTE xS, Latitude 16 Moxi 13 CRT BTE Power xP, and Latitude 16 Moxi 13 CRT BTE OptimumFit

- Smart control – a remote control allowing patients to adjust their devices
- uDirect – a device worn around the neck acts as a wireless interface between the hearing aids and other Bluetooth-enabled devices. Devices include:
  - uPhone – activates streaming program when signal is received from Bluetooth-enabled cell phone and Bluetooth-enabled audio devices
  - uAudio – activates streaming program when signal is received from FM transmitters or wired audio inputs
- Duo link – program and/or volume adjustments made on one hearing instruments are automatically synchronized with the other
- Binaural phone – allows for binaural hearing while on a landline or mobile phone by automatically streams audio signal to the non-phone ear
- Multiple microphones – omnidirectional, fixed directional, and multiband adaptive directional

- My music – allows clinician to customize frequency response for music listening
- Wireless programming with iCube
- OptimumFit – with intelliVent technology
- Choice of 2 receivers

Features of Latitude 16 Moxi CRT BTE xS, Latitude 16 Moxi CRT BTE Power xP, and Latitude 16 Moxi CRT BTE OptimumFit

- Smart focus – designed to provide patient with a method to enhance speech by allowing adjustments to microphone strategy, speech enhancement, noise reduction and gain
- Enhanced auto pro 3 – three programs each with adaptive parameters; includes automatic and smooth program changes
- Enhanced feedback management system – proprietary feedback management reduction
- Self-learning – a learning algorithm that automatically learns volume and comfort – clarity preferences
- 16 channels of signal processing
- 16 bands
- Automatic program with 3 listening destinations, 3 manual, and 2 wireless streaming programs
- Speech enhancement LD – increases gain in each band where speech dominates over noise
- Noise reduction – reduces gain in bands with poor SNRs
- Anti-shock reduces the level of impulse noises
- Wind noise manager – reduces low-frequency gain during windy conditions
- Data logging
- Easy-t – auto switching to t-coil program when phone is picked up
- Telecoil
- Suitable for mild to severe hearing losses and can fit audiogram configurations ranging from reverse to precipitously sloping

Options of Latitude 16 Moxi CRT BTE xS, Latitude 16 Moxi CRT BTE Power xP, and Latitude 16 Moxi CRT BTE OptimumFit

- Smart control – a remote control allowing patients to adjust their devices
- Multiple microphones – omnidirectional, fixed directional, and multiband adaptive directional
- My music – allows clinician to customize frequency response for music listening
- OptimumFit with intelliVent technology
- Choice of 2 receivers

Features of Latitude 16 Moda 13 BTE

- Smart focus – designed to provide patient with a method to enhance speech by allowing adjustments to microphone strategy, speech enhancement, noise reduction and gain

- Enhanced auto pro 3 – three programs each with adaptive parameters; includes automatic and smooth program changes
- Enhanced feedback management system – proprietary feedback management reduction
- Self-learning – a learning algorithm that automatically learns volume and comfort – clarity preferences
- Unifi wireless system with duo link – connects the two hearing instruments to ensure changes are made to both instruments
- 16 channels of signal processing
- 16 bands
- Automatic program with 3 listening destinations, 3 manual, and 2 wireless streaming programs
- Speech enhancement LD – increases gain in each band where speech dominates over noise
- Noise reduction – reduces gain in bands with poor SNRs
- Anti-shock reduces the level of impulse noises
- Wind noise manager – reduces low-frequency gain during windy conditions
- Data logging
- Easy-t – auto switching to t-coil program when phone is picked up
- Telecoil
- Suitable for mild to moderately severe hearing losses and can fit audiogram configurations ranging from reverse to precipitously sloping

Options of Latitude 16 Moda 13 BTE

- Smart control – a remote control allowing patients to adjust their devices
- uDirect – a device worn around the neck acts as a wireless interface between the hearing aids and other Bluetooth-enabled devices. Devices include:
  - uPhone – activates streaming program when signal is received from Bluetooth-enabled cell phone and Bluetooth-enabled audio devices
  - uAudio – activates streaming program when signal is received from FM transmitters or wired audio inputs
- Duo link – program and/or volume adjustments made on one hearing instruments are automatically synchronized with the other
- Binaural phone – allows for binaural hearing while on a landline or mobile phone by automatically streams audio signal to the non-phone ear
- Multiple microphones – omnidirectional, fixed directional, and multiband adaptive directional
- My music – allows clinician to customize frequency response for music listening
- Wireless programming with iCube

Features of Latitude 16 Moda II BTE

- Smart focus – designed to provide patient with a method to enhance speech by allowing adjustments to microphone strategy, speech enhancement, noise reduction and gain

- Enhanced auto pro 3 – three programs each with adaptive parameters; includes automatic and smooth program changes
- Enhanced feedback management system – proprietary feedback management reduction
- Self-learning – a learning algorithm that automatically learns volume and comfort – clarity preferences
- 16 channels of signal processing
- 16 bands
- Automatic program with 3 listening destinations, 3 manual, and 2 wireless streaming programs
- Speech enhancement LD – increases gain in each band where speech dominates over noise
- Noise reduction – reduces gain in bands with poor SNRs
- Anti-shock reduces the level of impulse noises
- Wind noise manager – reduces low-frequency gain during windy conditions
- Data logging
- Telecoil
- Suitable for mild to moderately severe hearing losses and can fit audiogram configurations ranging from reverse to precipitously sloping

Options of Latitude 16 Moda II BTE

- Smart control – a remote control allowing patients to adjust their devices
- Multiple microphones – omnidirectional, fixed directional, and multiband adaptive directional
- My music – allows clinician to customize frequency response for music listening

Features of Latitude 16 Shift CRT BTE and Latitude 16 Shift CRT BTE OptimumFit xS

- Smart focus – designed to provide patient with a method to enhance speech by allowing adjustments to microphone strategy, speech enhancement, noise reduction and gain
- Enhanced auto pro 3 – three programs each with adaptive parameters; includes automatic and smooth program changes
- Enhanced feedback management system – proprietary feedback management reduction
- Self-learning – a learning algorithm that automatically learns volume and comfort – clarity preferences
- 16 channels of signal processing
- 16 bands
- Automatic program with 3 listening destinations, 3 manual, and 2 wireless streaming programs
- Speech enhancement LD – increases gain in each band where speech dominates over noise

- Noise reduction – reduces gain in bands with poor SNRs
- Anti-shock reduces the level of impulse noises
- Wind noise manager – reduces low-frequency gain during windy conditions
- Data logging
- Telecoil
- Suitable for mild to moderately severe hearing losses and can fit audiogram configurations ranging from reverse to precipitously sloping

Options of Latitude 16 Shift CRT BTE and Latitude 16 Shift CRT BTE OptimumFit xS

- Smart control – a remote control allowing patients to adjust their devices
- Multiple microphones – omnidirectional, fixed directional, and multiband adaptive directional
- My music – allows clinician to customize frequency response for music listening
- OptimumFit™ with intelliVent technology

Features of Latitude 16 Full Shell, Latitude 16 Full Shell Power, Latitude 16 Half Shell/Canal, Latitude 16 Half Shell/Canal Power, Latitude 16 Mini Canal/CIC, Latitude 16 Mini Canal Power/CIC Power

- Smart focus – designed to provide patient with a method to enhance speech by allowing adjustments to microphone strategy, speech enhancement, noise reduction and gain
- Enhanced auto pro 3 – three programs each with adaptive parameters; includes automatic and smooth program changes
- Enhanced feedback management system – proprietary feedback management reduction
- Self-learning – a learning algorithm that automatically learns volume and comfort – clarity preferences
- Unifi wireless system with duoLink – connects the two hearing instruments to ensure changes are made to both instruments
- 16 channels of signal processing
- 16 bands
- Automatic program with 3 listening destinations, 3 manual, and 2 wireless streaming programs
- Speech enhancement LD – increases gain in each band where speech dominates over noise
- Noise reduction – reduces gain in bands with poor SNRs
- Anti-shock reduces the level of impulse noises
- Wind noise manager – reduces low-frequency gain during windy conditions
- Data logging
- Easy DAI
- Suitable for mild to severe hearing losses and can fit audiogram configurations ranging from reverse to precipitously sloping

Options of Latitude 16 Full Shell, Latitude 16 Full Shell Power, Latitude 16 Half Shell/Canal, Latitude 16 Half Shell/Canal Power, Latitude 16 Mini Canal/CIC, Latitude 16 Mini Canal Power/CIC Power

- Smart control – a remote control allowing patients to adjust their devices
- uDirect – a device worn around the neck acts as a wireless interface between the hearing aids and other Bluetooth-enabled devices. Devices include:
  - uPhone – activates streaming program when signal is received from Bluetooth-enabled cell phone and Bluetooth-enabled audio devices
  - uAudio – activates streaming program when signal is received from FM transmitters or wired audio inputs
- Duo link – program and/or volume adjustments made on one hearing instruments are automatically synchronized with the other
- Binaural phone – allows for binaural hearing while on a landline or mobile phone by automatically streams audio signal to the non-phone ear
- Multiple microphones – omnidirectional, fixed directional, and multiband adaptive directional
- My music – allows clinician to customize frequency response for music listening
- Easy-t – auto switching to t-coil program when phone is picked up
- IntelliVent technology
- Wireless programming with iCube

Features of Latitude 16 Fuse Crossover Open-Fit CIC

- Smart focus – designed to provide patient with a method to enhance speech by allowing adjustments to microphone strategy, speech enhancement, noise reduction and gain
- Enhanced auto pro 3 – four programs each with adaptive parameters; includes automatic and smooth program changes
- Enhanced feedback management system – proprietary feedback management reduction
- Self-learning – a learning algorithm that automatically learns volume and comfort – clarity preferences
- Articulation joint- flexes with the bend of the patient's ear canal
- Dual-flow vents – venting on both sides of the aid provide an open style fit to reduce the occlusion effect
- 16 channels of signal processing
- Automatic program with 3 listening destinations and 3 manual programs
- Speech enhancement LD – increases gain in each band where speech dominates over noise
- Omnidirectional microphone
- Noise reduction – reduces gain in bands with poor SNRs
- Anti-shock reduces the level of impulse noises
- My music
- Wind noise manager

- Data logging
- Suitable for mild to moderately severe hearing losses and can fit audiogram configurations ranging from reverse to precipitously sloping

Options of Latitude 16 Fuse Crossover open-fit CIC

- Smart control – allows patient to adjust the hearing aids using a remote control
- Secure-fit tab- additional attachment to the body of the hearing aid to provide a more secure fit for patients with large ear canals

Product Application

    Latitude 8 BTE
    Latitude 8 BTE HP
    Latitude 8 Moxi 13 CRT BTE xS
    Latitude 8 Moxi 13 CRT BTE Power xP
    Latitude 8 Moxi 13 CRT BTE OptimumFit
    Latitude 8 Moxi CRT BTE xS
    Latitude 8 Moxi CRT BTE Power xP
    Latitude 8 Moxi CRT BTE OptimumFit
    Latitude 8 Moda 13 BTE
    Latitude 8 Moda II BTE
    Latitude 8 Shift CRT BTE
    Latitude 8 Shift CRT BTE OptimumFit xS
    Latitude 8 Full Shell
    Latitude 8 Full Shell Power
    Latitude 8 Half Shell/Canal
    Latitude 8 Half Shell/Canal Power
    Latitude 8 Mini Canal/CIC
    Latitude 8 Mini Canal Power/CIC Power
    Latitude 8 Fuse Crossover (open-fit CIC)

Features of Latitude 8 BTE and Latitude 8 BTE HP

- Speech enhancement LD – increases gain in each band where speech dominates over noise
- Auto pro 2 – allows patient smooth transitions between 2 programs
- Enhanced feedback management system – proprietary feedback management reduction
- Unifi wireless system with duoLink – connects the two hearing instruments to ensure changes are made to both instruments
- 8 channels of signal processing
- 8 bands
- Automatic program with 2 listening destinations, 3 manual, and 2 wireless streaming programs
- Noise reduction – reduces gain in bands with poor SNRs

- Anti-shock reduces the level of impulse noises
- Wind noise manager – reduces low-frequency gain during windy conditions
- Data logging
- Easy DAI
- Easy-t – auto switching to t-coil program when phone is picked up
- Suitable for mild to severe hearing losses and can fit audiogram configurations ranging from reverse to precipitously sloping

Options of Latitude 8 BTE and Latitude 8 BTE HP

- Smart control – a remote control allowing patients to adjust their devices
- uDirect – a device worn around the neck acts as a wireless interface between the hearing aids and other Bluetooth-enabled devices. Devices include:
  - uPhone – activates streaming program when signal is received from Bluetooth-enabled cell phone and Bluetooth-enabled audio devices
  - uAudio – activates streaming program when signal is received from FM transmitters or wired audio inputs
- Duo link – program and/or volume adjustments made on one hearing instruments are automatically synchronized with the other
- Multiple microphones – omnidirectional, fixed directional, and multiband adaptive directional
- My music – allows clinician to customize frequency response for music listening
- Wireless programming with iCube

Features of Latitude 8 Moxi 13 CRT BTE xS, Latitude 8 Moxi 13 CRT BTE Power xP, and Latitude 8 Moxi 13 CRT BTE OptimumFit

- Speech enhancement LD – increases gain in each band where speech dominates over noise
- Auto pro 2 – allows patient smooth transitions between 2 programs
- Enhanced feedback management system – proprietary feedback management reduction
- Unifi wireless system with duo link – connects the two hearing instruments to ensure changes are made to both instruments
- 8 channels of signal processing
- 8 bands
- Automatic program with 2 listening destinations, 3 manual, and 2 wireless streaming programs
- Noise reduction – reduces gain in bands with poor SNRs
- Anti-shock reduces the level of impulse noises
- Wind noise manager – reduces low-frequency gain during windy conditions
- Data logging
- Easy-t – auto switching to t-coil program when phone is picked up
- Telecoil
- Suitable for mild to severe hearing losses and can fit audiogram configurations ranging from reverse to precipitously sloping

Options of Latitude 8 Moxi 13 CRT BTE xS, Latitude 8 Moxi 13 CRT BTE Power xP, and Latitude 8 Moxi 13 CRT BTE OptimumFit

- Smart control – a remote control allowing patients to adjust their devices
- uDirect – a device worn around the neck acts as a wireless interface between the hearing aids and other Bluetooth-enabled devices. Devices include:
  - uPhone – activates streaming program when signal is received from Bluetooth-enabled cell phone and Bluetooth-enabled audio devices
  - uAudio – activates streaming program when signal is received from FM transmitters or wired audio inputs
- Duo link – program and/or volume adjustments made on one hearing instruments are automatically synchronized with the other
- Multiple microphones – omnidirectional, fixed directional, and multiband adaptive directional
- My music – allows clinician to customize frequency response for music listening
- Wireless programming with iCube
- OptimunFit with IntelliVent technology
- Choice of 2 receivers

Features of Latitude 8 Moxi CRT BTE xS, Latitude 8 Moxi CRT BTE Power xP, and Latitude 8 Moxi CRT BTE OptimumFit

- Speech enhancement LD – increases gain in each band where speech dominates over noise
- Auto pro 2 – allows patient smooth transitions between 2 programs
- Enhanced feedback management system – proprietary feedback management reduction
- 8 channels of signal processing
- 8 bands
- Automatic program with 2 listening destinations, 3 manual, and 2 wireless streaming programs
- Noise reduction – reduces gain in bands with poor SNRs
- Anti-shock reduces the level of impulse noises
- Wind noise manager – reduces low-frequency gain during windy conditions
- Data logging
- Easy-t – auto switching to t-coil program when phone is picked up
- Telecoil
- Suitable for mild to severe hearing losses and can fit audiogram configurations ranging from reverse to precipitously sloping

Options of Latitude 8 Moxi CRT BTE xS, Latitude 8 Moxi CRT BTE Power xP, and Latitude 8 Moxi CRT BTE OptimumFit

- Smart control – a remote control allowing patients to adjust their devices
- Multiple microphones – omnidirectional, fixed directional, and multiband adaptive directional

- My music – allows clinician to customize frequency response for music listening
- OptimunFit with IntelliVent technology
- Choice of 2 receivers

Features of Latitude 8 Moda 13 BTE

- Speech enhancement LD – increases gain in each band where speech dominates over noise
- Auto pro 2 – allows patient smooth transitions between 2 programs
- Enhanced feedback management system – proprietary feedback management reduction
- Unifi wireless system with duo link – connects the two hearing instruments to ensure changes are made to both instruments
- 8 channels of signal processing
- 8 bands
- Automatic program with 2 listening destinations, 3 manual, and 2 wireless streaming programs
- Noise reduction – reduces gain in bands with poor SNRs
- Anti-shock reduces the level of impulse noises
- Wind noise manager – reduces low-frequency gain during windy conditions
- Data logging
- Easy-t – auto switching to t-coil program when phone is picked up
- Telecoil
- Suitable for mild to moderately severe hearing losses and can fit audiogram configurations ranging from reverse to precipitously sloping

Options of Latitude 8 Moda 13 BTE

- Smart control – a remote control allowing patients to adjust their devices
- uDirect – a device worn around the neck acts as a wireless interface between the hearing aids and other Bluetooth-enabled devices. Devices include:
  - uPhone – activates streaming program when signal is received from Bluetooth-enabled cell phone and Bluetooth-enabled audio devices
  - uAudio – activates streaming program when signal is received from FM transmitters or wired audio inputs
- Duo link – program and/or volume adjustments made on one hearing instruments are automatically synchronized with the other
- Multiple microphones – omnidirectional, fixed directional, and multiband adaptive directional
- My music – allows clinician to customize frequency response for music listening
- Wireless programming with iCube

Features of Latitude 8 Moda II BTE

- Speech enhancement LD – increases gain in each band where speech dominates over noise
- Auto pro 2 – allows patient smooth transitions between 2 programs

- Enhanced feedback management system – proprietary feedback management reduction
- 8 channels of signal processing
- 8 bands
- Automatic program with 2 listening destinations, 3 manual, and 2 wireless streaming programs
- Noise reduction – reduces gain in bands with poor SNRs
- Anti-shock reduces the level of impulse noises
- Wind noise manager – reduces low-frequency gain during windy conditions
- Data logging
- Telecoil
- Suitable for mild to moderately severe hearing losses and can fit audiogram configurations ranging from reverse to precipitously sloping

Options of Latitude 8 Moda II BTE

- Smart control – a remote control allowing patients to adjust their devices
- Multiple microphones – omnidirectional, fixed directional, and multiband adaptive directional
- My music – allows clinician to customize frequency response for music listening

Features of Latitude 8 Shift CRT BTE and Latitude 8 Shift CRT BTE OptimumFit xS

- Speech enhancement LD – increases gain in each band where speech dominates over noise
- Auto pro 2 – allows patient smooth transitions between 2 programs
- Enhanced Feedback Management System – proprietary feedback management reduction
- 8 channels of signal processing
- 8 bands
- Automatic program with 2 listening destinations, 3 manual, and 2 wireless streaming programs
- Noise reduction – reduces gain in bands with poor SNRs
- Anti-shock reduces the level of impulse noises
- Wind noise manager – reduces low-frequency gain during windy conditions
- Data logging
- Telecoil
- Suitable for mild to moderately severe hearing losses and can fit audiogram configurations ranging from reverse to precipitously sloping

Options of Latitude 8 Shift CRT BTE and Latitude 8 Shift CRT BTE OptimumFit xS

- Smart control – a remote control allowing patients to adjust their devices
- Multiple microphones – omnidirectional, fixed directional, and multiband adaptive directional

- My music – allows clinician to customize frequency response for music listening
- OptimunFit xS with IntelliVent technology

Features of Latitude 8 Full Shell, Latitude 8 Full Shell Power, Latitude 8 Half Shell/Canal, Latitude 8 Half Shell/Canal Power, Latitude 8 Mini Canal/CIC, and Latitude 8 Mini Canal Power/CIC Power

- Speech enhancement LD – increases gain in each band where speech dominates over noise
- Auto pro 2 – allows patient smooth transitions between 2 programs
- Enhanced feedback management system – proprietary feedback management reduction
- Unifi wireless system with duo link – connects the two hearing instruments to ensure changes are made to both instruments
- 8 channels of signal processing
- 8 bands
- Automatic program with 2 listening destinations, 3 manual, and 2 wireless streaming programs
- Noise reduction – reduces gain in bands with poor SNRs
- Anti-shock reduces the level of impulse noises
- Wind noise manager – reduces low-frequency gain during windy conditions
- Data logging
- Suitable for mild to severe hearing losses and can fit audiogram configurations ranging from reverse to precipitously sloping

Options of Latitude 8 Full Shell, Latitude 8 Full Shell Power, Latitude 8 Half Shell/Canal, Latitude 8 Half Shell/Canal Power, Latitude 8 Mini Canal/CIC, and Latitude 8 Mini Canal Power/CIC Power

- Smart control – a remote control allowing patients to adjust their devices
- uDirect – a device worn around the neck acts as a wireless interface between the hearing aids and other Bluetooth-enabled devices. Devices include:
  - uPhone – activates streaming program when signal is received from Bluetooth-enabled cell phone and Bluetooth-enabled audio devices
  - uAudio – activates streaming program when signal is received from FM transmitters or wired audio inputs
- Duo link – program and/or volume adjustments made on one hearing instruments are automatically synchronized with the other
- Multiple microphones – omnidirectional, fixed directional, and multiband adaptive directional
- My music – allows clinician to customize frequency response for music listening
- Easy-t – auto switching to t-coil program when phone is picked up
- IntelliVent technology
- Wireless programming with iCube

Features of Latitude 8 Fuse Crossover open-fit CIC

- Speech enhancement LD – increases gain in each band where speech dominates over noise
- Enhanced auto pro 2 – four programs each with adaptive parameters; includes automatic and smooth program changes
- Enhanced feedback management system – proprietary feedback management reduction
- Articulation joint-flexes with the bend of the patient's ear canal
- Dual-flow vents-venting on both sides of the aid provide an open style fit to reduce the occlusion effect
- 8 channels of signal processing
- Automatic program with 2 listening destinations and 3 manual programs
- Omnidirectional microphone
- Noise reduction – reduces gain in bands with poor SNRs
- Anti-shock reduces the level of impulse noises
- My music
- Wind noise manager
- Data logging
- Suitable for mild to moderately severe hearing losses and can fit audiogram configurations ranging from reverse to precipitously sloping

Options of Latitude 8 Fuse Crossover Open-Fit CIC

- Smart control – allows patient to adjust the hearing aids using a remote control
- Secure-fit tab-additional attachment to the body of the hearing aid to provide a more secure fit for patients with large ear canals

Product Application

Latitude 4 BTE
Latitude 4 BTE HP
Latitude 4 Moxi 13 CRT BTE xS
Latitude 4 Moxi 13 CRT BTE Power xP
Latitude 4 Moxi 13 CRT BTE OptimumFit
Latitude 4 Moxi CRT BTE xS
Latitude 4 Moxi CRT BTE Power xP
Latitude 4 Moxi CRT BTE OptimumFit
Latitude 4 Moda 13 BTE
Latitude 4 Moda II BTE
Latitude 4 Shift CRT BTE
Latitude 4 Shift CRT BTE OptimumFit xS
Latitude 4 Full Shell
Latitude 4 Full Shell Power
Latitude 4 Half Shell/Canal
Latitude 4 Half Shell/Canal Power
Latitude 4 Mini Canal/CIC
Latitude 4 Mini Canal/CIC Power

Features of Latitude 4 BTE and Latitude 4 BTE HP

- Speech enhancement LD – increases gain in each band where speech dominates over noise
- Enhanced feedback management system – proprietary feedback management reduction
- Unifi wireless system with duo link – connects the two hearing instruments to ensure changes are made to both instruments
- 4 channels of signal processing
- 8 bands
- 4 manual + 2 wireless streaming programs
- Noise reduction – reduces gain in bands with poor SNRs
- Anti-shock reduces the level of impulse noises
- Wind noise manager – reduces low-frequency gain during windy conditions
- Data logging
- Easy-t – auto switching to t-coil program when phone is picked up
- Suitable for mild to severe hearing losses and can fit audiogram configurations ranging from reverse to precipitously sloping

Options of Latitude 4 BTE and Latitude 4 BTE HP

- Smart control – a remote control allowing patients to adjust their devices
- uDirect – a device worn around the neck acts as a wireless interface between the hearing aids and other Bluetooth-enabled devices. Devices include:
  - uPhone – activates streaming program when signal is received from Bluetooth-enabled cell phone and Bluetooth-enabled audio devices
  - uAudio – activates streaming program when signal is received from FM transmitters or wired audio inputs
- Duo link – program and/or volume adjustments made on one hearing instruments are automatically synchronized with the other
- Multiple microphones – omnidirectional, fixed directional, and multiband adaptive directional
- Wireless programming with iCube

Features of Latitude 4 Moxi 13 CRT BTE xS, Latitude 4 Moxi 13 CRT BTE Power xP, and Latitude 4 Moxi 13 CRT BTE OptimumFit

- Speech enhancement LD – increases gain in each band where speech dominates over noise
- Enhanced feedback management system – proprietary feedback management reduction
- Unifi wireless system with duo link – connects the two hearing instruments to ensure changes are made to both instruments
- 4 channels of signal processing
- 8 bands
- 4 manual + 2 wireless streaming programs

- Noise reduction – reduces gain in bands with poor SNRs
- Anti-shock reduces the level of impulse noises
- Wind noise manager – reduces low-frequency gain during windy conditions
- Data logging
- Easy-t – auto switching to t-coil program when phone is picked up
- Telecoil
- Suitable for mild to severe hearing losses and can fit audiogram configurations ranging from reverse to precipitously sloping

Options of Latitude 4 Moxi 13 CRT BTE xS, Latitude 4 Moxi 13 CRT BTE Power xP, and Latitude 4 Moxi 13 CRT BTE OptimumFit

- Smart control – a remote control allowing patients to adjust their devices
- uDirect – a device worn around the neck acts as a wireless interface between the hearing aids and other Bluetooth-enabled devices. Devices include:
  - uPhone – activates streaming program when signal is received from Bluetooth-enabled cell phone and Bluetooth-enabled audio devices
  - uAudio – activates streaming program when signal is received from FM transmitters or wired audio inputs
- Duo link – program and/or volume adjustments made on one hearing instruments are automatically synchronized with the other
- Multiple microphones – omnidirectional, fixed directional, and multiband adaptive directional
- Wireless programming with iCube
- OptimunFit with IntelliVent technology
- Choice of 2 receivers

Features of Latitude 4 Moxi CRT BTE xS, Latitude 4 Moxi CRT BTE Power xP, and Latitude 4 Moxi CRT BTE OptimumFit

- Speech enhancement LD – increases gain in each band where speech dominates over noise
- Enhanced feedback management system – proprietary feedback management reduction
- 4 channels of signal processing
- 8 bands
- 4 manual programs
- Noise reduction – reduces gain in bands with poor SNRs
- Anti-shock reduces the level of impulse noises
- Wind noise manager – reduces low-frequency gain during windy conditions
- Data logging
- Easy-t – auto switching to t-coil program when phone is picked up
- Telecoil
- Suitable for mild to severe hearing losses and can fit audiogram configurations ranging from reverse to precipitously sloping

Options of Latitude 4 Moxi CRT BTE xS, Latitude 4 Moxi CRT BTE Power xP, and Latitude 4 Moxi CRT BTE OptimumFit

- Smart control – a remote control allowing patients to adjust their devices
- Multiple microphones – omnidirectional, fixed directional, and multiband adaptive directional
- OptimunFit with IntelliVent technology
- Choice of 2 receivers

Features of Latitude 4 Moda 13 BTE

- Speech enhancement LD – increases gain in each band where speech dominates over noise
- Enhanced feedback management system – proprietary feedback management reduction
- Unifi wireless system with duoLink – connects the two hearing instruments to ensure changes are made to both instruments
- 4 channels of signal processing
- 8 bands
- 4 manual + 2 wireless streaming programs
- Noise reduction – reduces gain in bands with poor SNRs
- Anti-shock reduces the level of impulse noises
- Wind noise manager – reduces low-frequency gain during windy conditions
- Data logging
- Easy-t – auto switching to t-coil program when phone is picked up
- Telecoil
- Suitable for mild to moderately severe hearing losses and can fit audiogram configurations ranging from reverse to precipitously sloping

Options of Latitude 4 Moda 13 BTE

- Smart control – a remote control allowing patients to adjust their devices
- uDirect – a device worn around the neck acts as a wireless interface between the hearing aids and other Bluetooth-enabled devices. Devices include:
  - uPhone – activates streaming program when signal is received from Bluetooth-enabled cell phone and Bluetooth-enabled audio devices
  - uAudio – activates streaming program when signal is received from FM transmitters or wired audio inputs
- Duo link – program and/or volume adjustments made on one hearing instruments are automatically synchronized with the other
- Multiple microphones – omnidirectional, fixed directional, and multiband adaptive directional
- Wireless programming with iCube

Features of Latitude 4 Moda II BTE

- Speech enhancement LD – increases gain in each band where speech dominates over noise
- Enhanced feedback management system – proprietary feedback management reduction

- 4 channels of signal processing
- 8 bands
- 4 manual programs
- Noise reduction – reduces gain in bands with poor SNRs
- Anti-shock reduces the level of impulse noises
- Wind noise manager – reduces low-frequency gain during windy conditions
- Data logging
- Telecoil
- Suitable for mild to moderately severe hearing losses and can fit audiogram configurations ranging from reverse to precipitously sloping

Options of Latitude 4 Moda II BTE

- Smart control – a remote control allowing patients to adjust their devices
- Multiple microphones – omnidirectional, fixed directional, and multiband adaptive directional

Features of Latitude 4 Shift CRT BTE and Latitude 4 Shift CRT BTE OptimumFit xS

- Speech enhancement LD – increases gain in each band where speech dominates over noise
- Enhanced feedback management system – proprietary feedback management reduction
- 4 channels of signal processing
- 8 bands
- 4 manual programs
- Noise reduction – reduces gain in bands with poor SNRs
- Anti-shock reduces the level of impulse noises
- Wind noise manager – reduces low-frequency gain during windy conditions
- Data logging
- Telecoil
- Suitable for mild to moderately severe hearing losses and can fit audiogram configurations ranging from reverse to precipitously sloping

Options of Latitude 4 Shift CRT BTE and Latitude 4 Shift CRT BTE OptimumFit xS

- Smart control – a remote control allowing patients to adjust their devices
- Multiple microphones – omnidirectional, fixed directional, and multiband adaptive directional
- OptimunFit xS with IntelliVent technology

Features of Latitude 4 Full Shell, Latitude 4 Full Shell Power, Latitude 4 Half Shell/Canal, Latitude 4 Half Shell/Canal Power, Latitude 4 Mini Canal/CIC, and Latitude 4 Mini Canal Power/CIC Power

- Speech enhancement LD – increases gain in each band where speech dominates over noise
- Enhanced feedback management system – proprietary feedback management reduction

UNITRON

- Unifi wireless system with duo link – connects the two hearing instruments to ensure changes are made to both instruments
- 4 channels of signal processing
- 8 bands
- 4 manual + 2 wireless streaming programs (where available)
- Noise reduction – reduces gain in bands with poor SNRs
- Anti-shock reduces the level of impulse noises
- Wind noise manager – reduces low-frequency gain during windy conditions
- Data logging
- Suitable for mild to severe hearing losses and can fit audiogram configurations ranging from reverse to precipitously sloping

Options of Latitude 4 Full Shell, Latitude 4 Full Shell Power, Latitude 4 Half Shell/Canal, Latitude 4 Half Shell/Canal Power, Latitude 4 Mini Canal/CIC, and Latitude 4 Mini Canal Power/CIC Power

- Smart control – a remote control allowing patients to adjust their devices
- uDirect – a device worn around the neck acts as a wireless interface between the hearing aids and other Bluetooth-enabled devices. Devices include:
  - uPhone – activates streaming program when signal is received from Bluetooth-enabled cell phone and Bluetooth-enabled audio devices
  - uAudio – activates streaming program when signal is received from FM transmitters or wired audio inputs
- Duo link – program and/or volume adjustments made on one hearing instruments are automatically synchronized with the other
- Multiple microphones – omnidirectional, fixed directional, and multiband adaptive directional
- Easy-t – auto switching to t-coil program when phone is picked up
- IntelliVent technology
- Wireless programming with iCube

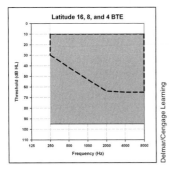

Fitting range for Latitude 16, 8, and 4 BTE (full shaded area) and slim tube (dotted line and above)

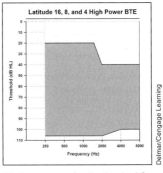

Fitting range for Latitude 16, 8, and 4 High Power BTE

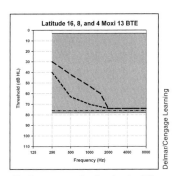

Fitting range for Latitude 16, 8, and 4 Moxi 13 BTE open dome (long dash and above), crosed dome (short dash and above), and sleeve mold (all shaded region)

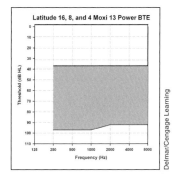

Fitting range for Latitude 16, 8, and 4 Moxi 13 Power BTE

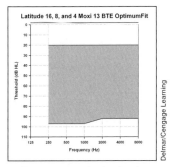

Fitting range for Latitude 16, 8, and 4 Moxi 13 BTE OptimumFit

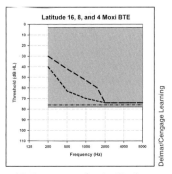

Fitting range for Latitude 16, 8, and 4 Moxi BTE open dome (long dash and above), closed dome (short dash and above), and sleeve mold (all shaded region)

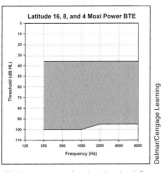

Fitting range for Latitude 16, 8, and 4 Moxi Power BTE

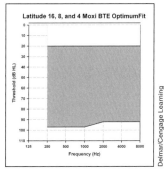

Fitting range for Latitude 16, 8, and 4 Moxi BTE OptimumFit

UNITRON

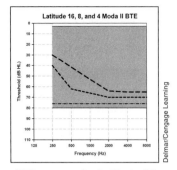

Fitting range for Latitude 16, 8, and 4 Moda 13 BTE open dome (long dash and above), closed dome (short dash and above), and sleeve mold (all shaded region)

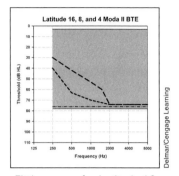

Fitting range for Latitude 16, 8, and 4 Moda II BTE open dome (long dash and above), closed dome (short dash and above), and sleeve mold (all shaded region)

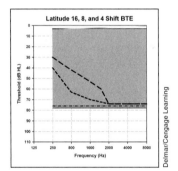

Fitting range for Latitude 16, 8, and 4 Shift BTE open dome (long dash and above), closed dome (short dash and above), and sleeve mold (all shaded region)

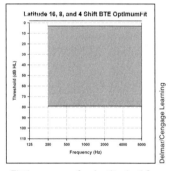

Fitting range for Latitude 16, 8, and 4 Shift BTE OptimumFit

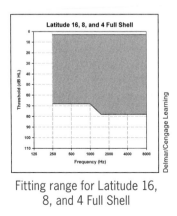

Fitting range for Latitude 16, 8, and 4 Full Shell

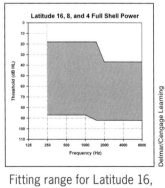

Fitting range for Latitude 16, 8, and 4 Full Shell Power

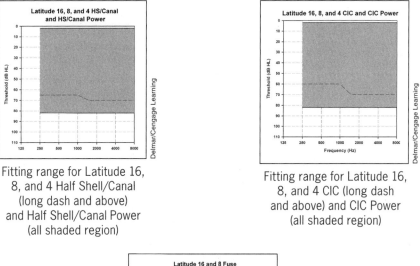

Fitting range for Latitude 16,
8, and 4 Half Shell/Canal
(long dash and above)
and Half Shell/Canal Power
(all shaded region)

Fitting range for Latitude 16,
8, and 4 CIC (long dash
and above) and CIC Power
(all shaded region)

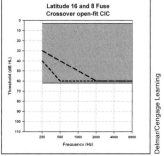

Fitting range for Latitude Fuse
crossover open-fit CIC open
dome (long dash and above),
closed dome (short dash and
above), and power dome
(all shaded region)

Typical Specifications		Latitude 16, 8, and 4 BTE (Slim tube)	Latitude 16, 8, and 4 BTE	Latitude 16, 8, and 4 BTE (High power)
Standard ANSI S3.22-1996				
Output sound pressure level	Max OSPL 90 (dB SPL)	124	125	135
	HFA OSPL 90 (dB SPL)	108	122	128
Full-on gain (50 dB SPL input)	Peak gain (dB)	52	60	75
	HFA (dB)	38	52	68
Total harmonic distortion	500 Hz	1%	3%	2%
	800 Hz	1%	2%	2%
	1600 Hz	1%	1%	1%

UNITRON

continues

continued

Typical Specifications		Latitude 16, 8, and 4 BTE (Slim tube)	Latitude 16, 8, and 4 BTE	Latitude 16, 8, and 4 BTE (High power)
Equivalent input noise (dB SPL)		26	19	19
Telecoil sensitivity	HFA SPLITS (dB SPL)	90	105	111
Battery	Operating current (mA)	1.2	1.3	2.2
	Battery type	13	13	13

Delmar/Cengage Learning

Typical Specifications		Latitude 16, 8, and 4 Moxi 13 (xS)	Latitude 16, 8, and 4 Moxi 13 Power (xP)
Standard ANSI S3.22-1996			
Output sound pressure level	Max OSPL 90 (dB SPL)	109	123
	HFA OSPL 90 (dB SPL)	104	118
Full-on gain (50 dB SPL input)	Peak gain (dB)	44	55
	HFA (dB)	36	47
Total harmonic distortion	500 Hz	1%	1.5%
	800 Hz	0.5%	1.3%
	1600 Hz	0.5%	0.5%
Equivalent input noise (dB SPL)		24	24
Telecoil sensitivity	HFA SPLITS (dB SPL)	87	101
Battery	Operating current (mA)	1.25	1.35
	Battery type	13	13

Delmar/Cengage Learning

Typical Specifications		Latitude 16, 8, and 4 Moxi (xS)	Latitude 16, 8, and 4 Moxi Power (xP)
Standard ANSI S3.22-1996			
Output sound pressure level	Max OSPL 90 (dB SPL)	109	123
	HFA OSPL 90 (dB SPL)	104	118
Full-on gain (50 dB SPL input)	Peak gain (dB)	44	55
	HFA (dB)	36	47
Total harmonic distortion	500 Hz	1%	1.5%
	800 Hz	0.5%	1.3%
	1600 Hz	0.5%	0.5%

continues

continued

Typical Specifications		Latitude 16, 8, and 4 Moxi (xS)	Latitude 16, 8, and 4 Moxi Power (xP)
Equivalent input noise (dB SPL)		24	24
Telecoil sensitivity	HFA SPLITS (dB SPL)	87	101
Battery	Operating current (mA)	1.25	1.35
	Battery type	13	13

Delmar/Cengage Learning

Typical Specifications		Latitude 16, 8, and 4 Moda 13	Latitude 16, 8, and 4 Moda II	Latitude 16, 8, and 4 Shift
Standard ANSI S3.22-1996				
Output sound pressure level	Max OSPL 90 (dB SPL)	124	117	109
	HFA OSPL 90 (dB SPL)	113	109	104
Full-on gain (50 dB SPL input)	Peak gain (dB)	53	45	44
	HFA (dB)	49	35	36
Total harmonic distortion	500 Hz	1.5%	1.5%	1%
	800 Hz	1.3%	1.3%	0.5%
	1600 Hz	1%	1%	0.5%
Equivalent input noise (dB SPL)		24	24	24
Telecoil sensitivity	HFA SPLITS (dB SPL)	96	92	87
Battery	Operating current (mA)	1.3	1.15	1.15
	Battery type	312	312	10A

Delmar/Cengage Learning

Typical Specifications		Latitude 16, 8, and 4 Full Shell	Latitude 16, 8, and 4 Full shell Power	Latitude 16, 8, and 4 HS/Canal	Latitude 16, 8, and 4 HS/Canal Power
Standard ANSI S3.22-1996					
Output sound pressure level	Max OSPL 90 (dB SPL)	115	112	113	117
	HFA OSPL 90 (dB SPL)	110	119	109	114
Full-on gain (50 dB SPL input)	Peak gain (dB)	50	60	48	55
	HFA (dB)	43	53	42	50
Total harmonic distortion	500 Hz	1%	1%	1%	1%
	800 Hz	0.5%	0.5%	0.5%	0.5%
	1600 Hz	0.5%	0.5%	0.5%	0.5%

UNITRON

continues

continued

Typical Specifications		Latitude 16, 8, and 4 Full Shell	Latitude 16, 8, and 4 Full shell Power	Latitude 16, 8, and 4 HS/Canal	Latitude 16, 8, and 4 HS/Canal Power
Equivalent input noise (dB SPL)		20	20	20	21
Telecoil sensitivity	HFA SPLITS (dB SPL)	94	102	92	98
Battery	Operating current (mA)	1.1	1.1	1.1	1.1
	Battery type	13	13	312	312

Delmar/Cengage Learning

Typical Specifications		Latitude 16, 8, and 4 MC/CIC	Latitude 16, 8, and 4 MC/ CIC Power	Latitude 16 and 8 Fuse Crossover open-fit CIC
Standard ANSI S3.22-1996				
Output sound pressure level	Max OSPL 90 (dB SPL)	112	116	109
	HFA OSPL 90 (dB SPL)	108	112	104
Full-on gain (50 dB SPL input)	Peak gain (dB)	40	55	40
	HFA (dB)	32	50	34
Total harmonic distortion	500 Hz	1%	1%	1%
	800 Hz	0.5%	0.5%	0.5%
	1600 Hz	0.5%	1.5%	0.5%
Equivalent input noise (dB SPL)		20	21	22
Telecoil sensitivity	HFA SPLITS (dB SPL)	n/a	n/a	n/a
Battery	Operating current (mA)	1.1	1.1	1
	Battery type	10A	10A	10A

Delmar/Cengage Learning

PRODUCT 3: YUU

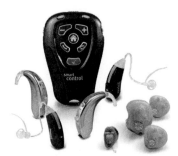

Yuu family
Courtesy of Unitron

Product Application

Yuu BTE (with or without VC)	Yuu Full-Shell Power
Yuu P BTE	Yuu Full-Shell
Yuu HP BTE	Yuu Half-Shell/Canal
Yuu Moxi CRT BTE	Yuu Mini Canal/CIC
Yuu Moda II BTE	

Features of Yuu BTE, Yuu P BTE, and Yuu HP BTE

- autoPro™ 4 – 4 programs, each with adaptive parameters; includes automatic and smooth program changes
- 3 additional manual programs
- Comfort – clarity balance – allows users to adjust adaptive features of noise reduction and speech enhancement
- AntiShock™ – reduces the level of impulse noises
- Speech Enhancement LD™ – increases gain in each band where speech dominates over noise
- 20 channels of signal processing
- Multiband adaptive directional microphone system
- Noise reduction – reduces gain in bands with poor SNRs
- Data logging
- Self-learning – can be configured to automatically learn volume and comfort – clarity preferences in autoPro4
- myMusic™ – allows the frequency response to be shaped to increase music enjoyment
- onBoard™ – a button that can be configured as a volume control or program button
- Easy-t – auto switching to t-coil program when phone is picked up
- Digital volume control with beep notifications
- Easy-DAI – automatically switches to DAI program when signal from external source is detected
- Low-battery warning
- Start-up delay
- ON/OFF by opening or closing the battery door

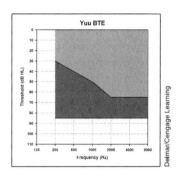

Fitting range for Yuu BTE with slim tube/open dome (light gray) or traditional earhook (all shaded regions)

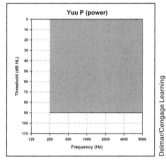

Fitting range for Yuu P BTE

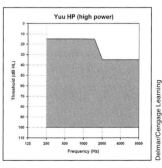

Fitting range for Yuu HP BTE

UNITRON

- Programmed using NOAH-compatible U:fit™ or Standalone U:fit fitting software
- Suitable for fitting mild to severe hearing losses and can fit audiogram configurations that range from reverse to precipitously sloping

Options of Yuu BTE, Yuu P BTE, and Yuu HP BTE

- SmartControl™ – a remote control allowing patients to adjust their devices
- Tamper-resistant volume control
- Tamper-resistant battery door
- Filtered earhook
- Slim tube coupling for instant open fittings (Yuu BTE only)
- Choice of shell colors
- Direct audio input battery door unit

Features of Yuu Moxi CRT BTE

- Canal receiver technology (CRT)
- autoPro4 – 4 programs, each with adaptive parameters; includes automatic and smooth program changes
- 3 additional manual programs
- Comfort – clarity balance – allows users to adjust adaptive features of noise reduction and speech enhancement
- AntiShock – reduces the level of impulse noises
- Speech Enhancement LD – increases gain in each band where speech dominates over noise
- 20 channels of signal processing
- Multiband adaptive directional microphone system
- Noise reduction – reduces gain in bands with poor SNRs
- Data logging
- Self-learning – can be configured to automatically learn volume and comfort – clarity preferences in autoPro4
- myMusic – allows the frequency response to be shaped to increase music enjoyment
- onBoard – a button that can be configured as a volume control or program button
- Easy-t – auto switching to t-coil program when phone is picked up
- Digital volume control with beep notifications

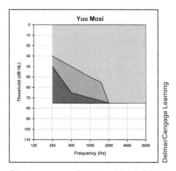

Fitting range for Yuu Moxi CRT BTE with open dome (light gray), closed dome (medium and light gray), and sleeve mold (all shaded regions)

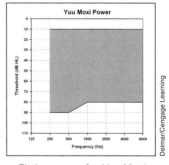

Fitting range for Yuu Moxi CRT P BTE

- Low-battery warning
- Start-up delay
- ON/OFF by opening or closing the battery door
- Can be programmed using NOAH-compatible U:fit and Standalone U:fit fitting software v1.3 or higher
- Choice of 2 receivers
- Suitable for mild to moderately severe hearing losses and can fit audiogram configurations ranging from reverse to precipitously sloping

Options of Yuu Moxi CRT BTE

- Remote control with volume control, comfort – clarity balance, LearnNow, program change button, and more
- Wide variety of coupling and venting options
- Choice of shell colors

Features of Yuu Moda II BTE

- autoPro4 – 4 programs, each with adaptive parameters; includes automatic and smooth program changes
- 3 additional manual programs
- Comfort – clarity balance – allows users to adjust adaptive features of noise reduction and speech enhancement
- AntiShock – reduces the level of impulse noises
- Speech Enhancement LD – increases gain in each band where speech dominates over noise
- 20 channels of signal processing
- Multiband adaptive directional microphone system
- Noise reduction – reduces gain in bands with poor SNRs
- Data logging
- Self-learning – can be configured to automatically learn volume and comfort – clarity preferences in autoPro4
- myMusic – allows the frequency response to be shaped to increase music enjoyment
- onBoard – a button that can be configured as a volume control or program button
- Digital volume control with beep notifications
- Telecoil (T) or microphone/telecoil (MT) can be set as 1 of the 3 programs
- Low-battery warning
- Start-up delay
- ON/OFF by opening or closing the battery door

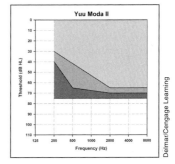

Fitting range for Yuu Moda II BTE with open dome (light gray), closed dome (medium and light gray), and sleeve mold (all shaded regions)

UNITRON

- Can be programmed using NOAH-compatible U:fit and Standalone U:fit fitting software v1.3 or higher
- Suitable for fitting mild to moderately severe hearing losses and can fit audiogram configurations ranging from reverse to precipitously sloping

Options of Yuu Moda II BTE

- Remote control with volume control, comfort – clarity balance, LearnNow, program change button, and more
- Slim tube coupling for open fittings
- Filtered/unfiltered earhooks
- Choice of shell colors

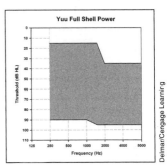

Fitting range for Yuu Full-Shell Power

Features of Yuu Full-Shell Power, Yuu Full-Shell, Yuu Half-Shell/Canal, and Yuu Mini Canal/CIC

- autoPro4 – 4 programs, each with adaptive parameters; includes automatic and smooth program changes
- 3 additional manual programs
- Comfort – clarity balance – allows users to adjust adaptive features of noise reduction and speech enhancement
- AntiShock – reduces the level of impulse noises
- Speech Enhancement LD – increases gain in each band where speech dominates over noise
- 20 channels of signal processing
- Multiband adaptive directional microphone system
- Noise reduction – reduces gain in bands with poor SNRs
- Data logging

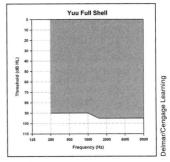

Fitting range for Yuu Full-Shell

- Self-learning – can be configured to auto-matically learn volume and comfort – clarity preferences in autoPro4
- myMusic – allows the frequency response to be shaped to increase music enjoyment
- onBoard – a button that can be configured as a volume control or program button
- Digital volume control with beep notifications
- Low-battery warning
- Start-up delay
- ON/OFF by opening or closing the battery door
- Can be programmed using NOAH-compatible U:fit and Standalone U:fit fitting software v1.3 or higher
- Suitable for fitting mild to severe hearing losses and can fit audiogram configurations ranging from reverse to precipitously sloping

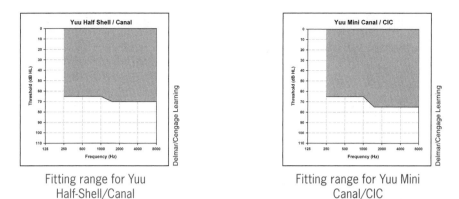

Fitting range for Yuu
Half-Shell/Canal

Fitting range for Yuu Mini
Canal/CIC

Options of Yuu Full-Shell Power, Yuu Full-Shell, Yuu Half-Shell/Canal, and Yuu Mini Canal/CIC

- Remote control with volume control, comfort – clarity balance, LearnNow, program change button, and more
- Telecoil (T) or microphone/telecoil (MT) can be set as 1 of the 3 programs
- Easy-t – auto switching to t-coil program when phone is picked up

Typical Specifications		Yuu Slim Tube (Optional)	Yuu BTE	Yuu P (Power) BTE	Yuu HP (High-Power)
Standard ANSI S3.22-1996					
Output sound pressure level	Max OSPL 90 (dB SPL)	124	125	130	135
	HFA OSPL 90 (dB SPL)	10	122	125	128
Full-on gain (50 dB SPL input)	Peak gain (dB)	54	60	70	75
	HFA (dB)	38	52	59	65
Total harmonic distortion	500 Hz	1%	4%	1%	2%
	800 Hz	1%	2%	1%	2%
	1600 Hz	1%	1%	1%	1%
Equivalent input noise (dB SPL)		25	20	20	20
Telecoil sensitivity	HFA SPLITS (dB SPL)	89	104	108	111
Battery	Operating current (mA)	1.1	1.2	1.7	2.2
	Battery type	13	13	13	13

Note: Measurement data obtained with hearing aid set to omni mode with all adaptive features disabled.
Delmar/Cengage Learning

UNITRON

Typical Specifications		Yuu Moxi BTE (xS Receiver)	Yuu Moxi Power BTE (xP Receiver)	Yuu Moda II BTE
Standard ANSI S3.22-1996				
Output sound pressure level	Max OSPL 90 (dB SPL)	109	123	118
	HFA OSPL 90 (dB SPL)	105	118	109
Full-on gain (50 dB SPL input)	Peak gain (dB)	44	55	45
	HFA (dB)	36	47	36
Total harmonic distortion	500 Hz	1%	1.5%	1.5%
	800 Hz	0.5%	1.3%	1.3%
	1600 Hz	0.5%	0.5%	0.5%
Equivalent input noise (dB SPL)		24	24	24
Telecoil sensitivity	HFA SPLITS (dB SPL)	89	102	94
Battery	Operating current (mA)	1.15	1.25	1.25
	Battery type	312	312	312

Note: Measurement data obtained with hearing aid set to linear, omni mode with all adaptive features disabled.
Delmar/Cengage Learning

Typical Specifications		Yuu Full-Shell Power	Yuu Full-Shell	Yuu Canal/ Half-Shell	Yuu CIC/Mini Canal
Standard ANSI S3.22-1996					
Output sound pressure level	Max OSPL 90 (dB SPL)	122	115	113	112
	HFA OSPL 90 (dB SPL)	119	110	109	108
Full-on gain (50 dB SPL input)	Peak gain (dB)	60	50	48	40
	HFA (dB)	53	43	42	32
Total harmonic distortion	500 Hz	1.0%	1.0%	1.5%	1%
	800 Hz	0.5%	0.5%	1.5%	0.5%
	1600 Hz	0.5%	0.5%	1.0%	0.5%
Equivalent input noise (dB SPL)		22	22	22	22
Telecoil sensitivity	HFA SPLITS (dB SPL)	102	94	92	92
Battery	Operating current (mA)	1.1	1.1	1.1	1.1
	Battery type	13	13	312	10

Delmar/Cengage Learning

PRODUCT 4: NEXT SERIES 16, 8, 4, AND ESSENTIAL

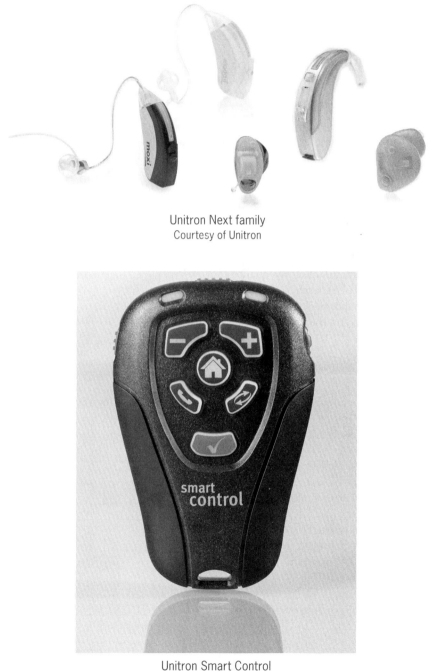

Unitron Next family
Courtesy of Unitron

Unitron Smart Control
Courtesy of Unitron

Product Application

Next 16 BTE	Next 16 Mini Canal/CIC
Next 16 BTE P	Next 16 CIC P
Next 16 BTE HP	Next 16 Moda II BTE
Next 16 FS P	Next 16 Moxi (xS)
Next 16 FS	Next 16 Moxi P (xP)
Next 16 HS/Canal	Next 16 Moxi Optimum Fit

Features of Next 16 BTE, Next 16 BTE P, and Next 16 BTE HP

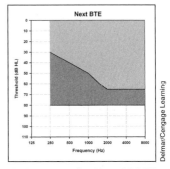

Fitting range for Next 16 BTE with slim tube/open dome (light gray) or traditional earhook (all shaded regions)

- autoPro3 – offers faster detection and response of the 3 listening destinations and the ability to adjust comfort and clarity in all destinations
- Feedback management
- Comfort – clarity balance – gives client control of adaptive features
- AntiShock – instantaneously reduces the level of impulse noises such as a door slam while maintaining the quality and intelligibility of speech
- Speech enhancement – emphasizes speech signals based on the input level
- 16 channels
- Adaptive directional microphone
- Noise reduction, wind noise manager
- Data logging
- myMusic – enhances the music listening experience by bringing out the rich, full tones of music
- onBoard – control is easily configured as a volume control with reduced dexterity
- Automatic switching to telephone program
- Ideal-volume indicator provides a beep notification when preferred gain is reached on the volume control
- 3 additional manual programs
- Easy-DAI – automatic switching to a dedicated DAI program
- Low-battery warning
- Start-up delay
- ON/OFF by opening or closing battery door
- Programmed by NOAH-compatible U:fit and Standalone U:fit software 1.4 or higher
- Choice of processing strategy – WDRC or Linear Limiting
- 13 size battery

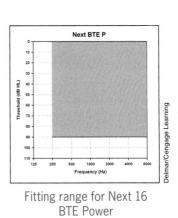

Fitting range for Next 16 BTE Power

Options of Next 16 BTE, Next 16 BTE P, and Next 16 BTE HP

- Remote control with volume control, comfort – clarity balance, program change button, and more
- Tamper-resistant volume control
- Tamper-resistant battery door
- Filtered earhook
- Slim tube coupling for instant open fittings (Next 16 BTE only)
- Choice of shell colors
- Direct audio input unit

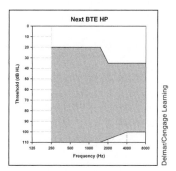

Fitting range for Next 16 BTE High-Power

Features of Next 16 Moda II BTE

- autoPro3 – offers faster detection and response of the 3 listening destinations and the ability to adjust comfort and clarity in all destinations
- Feedback management
- Comfort – clarity balance – gives client control of adaptive features
- AntiShock – instantaneously reduces the level of impulse noises such as a door slam while maintaining the quality and intelligibility of speech
- Speech enhancement – emphasizes speech signals based on the input level
- 16 channels
- Adaptive directional microphone
- Noise reduction, wind noise manager
- Data logging

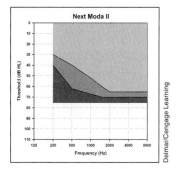

Fitting range for Next 16 Moda II BTE with open dome (light gray), closed dome (medium and light gray), and sleeve mold (all shaded regions)

- myMusic – enhances the music listening experience by bringing out the rich, full tones of music
- onBoard – control is easily configured as a volume control with reduced dexterity
- 3 additional manual programs
- Ideal-volume indicator provides a beep notification when preferred gain is reached on the volume control
- Low-battery warning
- Start-up delay
- ON/OFF by opening or closing battery door
- Programmed by NOAH-compatible U:fit and Standalone U:fit software 1.4 or higher
- Choice of processing strategy – WDRC or Linear Limiting
- 312 size battery

Options of Next 16 Moda II BTE

- Remote control with volume control, comfort – clarity balance, program change button, and more
- Telecoil (T) or microphone/telecoil (MT) option can be set as 1 of the 3 manual programs
- Choice of coupling and venting options
- Earhook

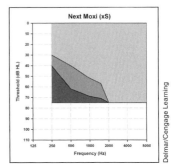

Fitting range for Next 16 Moxi (xS) with open dome (light gray), closed dome (medium and light gray), and sleeve mold (all shaded regions)

Features of Next 16 Moxi (xS), Next 16 Moxi P (xP), and Next 16 Moxi Optimum Fit

- autoPro3 – offers faster detection and response of the 3 listening destinations and the ability to adjust comfort and clarity in all destinations
- Feedback management
- Comfort – clarity balance – gives client control of adaptive features
- AntiShock – instantaneously reduces the level of impulse noises such as a door slam while maintaining the quality and intelligibility of speech
- Speech enhancement – emphasizes speech signals based on the input level
- 16 channels
- Adaptive directional microphone
- Noise reduction, wind noise manager
- Data logging
- myMusic – enhances the music listening experience by bringing out the rich, full tones of music
- onBoard – control is easily configured as a volume control with reduced dexterity
- Automatic switching to telephone program
- 3 additional manual programs
- Ideal-volume indicator provides a beep notification when preferred gain is reached on the volume control
- Low-battery warning
- Start-up delay
- ON/OFF by opening or closing battery door
- Programmed by NOAH-compatible U:fit and Standalone U:fit software 1.4 or higher

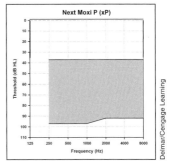

Fitting range for Next 16 Moxi (xP)

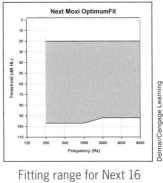

Fitting range for Next 16 Optimum Fit

- Choice of processing strategy – WDRC or Linear Limiting
- Choice of receivers
- 312 size battery

Options of Next 16 Moxi (xS), Next 16 Moxi P (xP), and Next 16 Moxi Optimum Fit

- Remote control with volume control, comfort – clarity balance, program change button, and more
- Choice of coupling and venting options

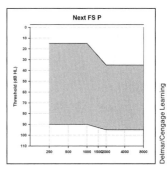

Features of Next 16 FS P, Next 16 FS, Next 16 HS/Canal, Next 16 Mini Canal/ CIC, and Next 16 CIC P

- autoPro3 – offers faster detection and response of the 3 listening destinations and the ability to adjust comfort and clarity in all destinations
- Feedback management
- Comfort – clarity balance – gives client control of adaptive features
- AntiShock – instantaneously reduces the level of impulse noises such as a door slam while maintaining the quality and intelligibility of speech
- Speech enhancement – emphasizes speech signals based on the input level
- 16 channels
- Adaptive directional microphone
- Noise reduction, wind noise manager
- Data logging
- myMusic – enhances the music listening experience by bringing out the rich, full tones of music
- onBoard – control is easily configured as a volume control with reduced dexterity
- Automatic switching to telephone program
- Ideal-volume indicator provides a beep notification when preferred gain is reached on the volume control
- 3 additional manual programs
- Low-battery warning
- Start-up delay
- ON/OFF by opening or closing battery door

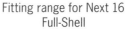

Fitting range for Next 16 Full-Shell Power

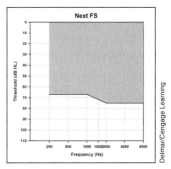

Fitting range for Next 16 Full-Shell

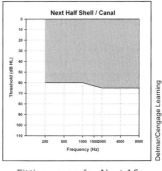

Fitting range for Next 16 Half-Shell/Canal

- Programmed by NOAH-compatible U:fit and Standalone U:fit software 1.4 or higher
- Choice of processing strategy – WDRC or Linear Limiting

Options of Next 16 FS P, Next 16 FS, Next 16 HS/Canal, Next 16 Mini Canal/CIC, and Next 16 CIC P

- Remote control with volume control, comfort – clarity balance, program change button, and more
- Telecoil (T) or microphone/telecoil (MT) option can be set as 1 of the 3 manual programs in canal to full-shell styles

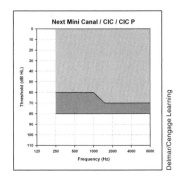

Fitting range for Next 16 Mini Canal/CIC/CIC Power Mini Canal/CIC (light gray) and CIC P (all shaded regions)

Typical Specifications		Next 16 Slim Tube (Optional)	Next 16 BTE	Next 16 BTE P	Next 16 BTE HP
Standard ANSI S3.22-1996					
Output sound pressure level	Max OSPL 90 (dB SPL)	124	125	130	135
	HFA OSPL 90 (dB SPL)	108	122	125	128
Full-on gain (50 dB SPL input)	Peak gain (dB)	53	60	70	75
	HFA (dB)	37	52	60	65
Total harmonic distortion	500 Hz	1%	4%	1%	2%
	800 Hz	1%	2%	1%	2%
	1600 Hz	1%	1%	1%	1%
Equivalent input noise (dB SPL)		28	20	20	20
Telecoil sensitivity	HFA SPLITS (dB SPL)	89	104	108	111
Battery	Operating current (mA)	1.1	1.2	1.7	2.2
	Battery type	13	13	13	13

Delmar/Cengage Learning

Typical Specifications		Next 16 Moda II BTE	Next 16 Moxi (xS)	Next 16 Moxi P (xP)
Standard ANSI S3.22-1996				
Output sound pressure level	Max OSPL 90 (dB SPL)	118	109	123
	HFA OSPL 90 (dB SPL)	109	105	118
Full-on gain (50 dB SPL input)	Peak gain (dB)	45	44	55
	HFA (dB)	36	36	47

continues

continued

Typical Specifications		Next 16 Moda II BTE	Next 16 Moxi (xS)	Next 16 Moxi P (xP)
Total harmonic distortion	500 Hz	1.5%	1%	1.5%
	800 Hz	1.3%	0.5%	1.3%
	1600 Hz	0.5%	0.5%	0.5%
Equivalent input noise (dB SPL)		19	24	24
Telecoil sensitivity	HFA SPLITS (dB SPL)	94	89	102
Battery	Operating current (mA)	1.25	1.15	1.25
	Battery type	312	312	312

Delmar/Cengage Learning

Typical Specifications		Next 16 CIC/Mini Canal	Next 16 CIC P	Next 16 Canal/HS	Next 16 FS	Next 16 FS P
Standard ANSI S3.22-1996						
Output sound pressure level	Max OSPL 90 (dB SPL)	112	116	113	115	122
	HFA OSPL 90 (dB SPL)	108	112	109	110	119
Full-on gain (50 dB SPL input)	Peak gain (dB)	40	55	48	50	60
	HFA (dB)	32	50	42	43	53
Total harmonic distortion	500 Hz	1%	1%	1.5%	1%	1%
	800 Hz	0.5%	0.5%	1.5%	0.5%	0.5%
	1600 Hz	0.5%	1%	1%	0.5%	0.5%
Equivalent input noise (dB SPL)		22	22	22	22	22
Telecoil sensitivity	HFA SPLITS (dB SPL)	92	N/A	92	94	102
Battery	Operating current (mA)	1.1	1.1	1.1	1.1	1.1
	Battery type	10	10	312	13	13

Delmar/Cengage Learning

Product Application

Next 8 BTE	Next 8 Mini Canal/CIC
Next 8 BTE P	Next 8 CIC P
Next 8 BTE HP	Next 8 Moda II BTE
Next 8 FS P	Next 8 Moxi (xS)
Next 8 FS	Next 8 Moxi P (xP)
Next 8 HS/Canal	Next 8 Moxi Optimum Fit

Features of Next 8 BTE, Next 8 BTE P, and Next 8 BTE HP

- autoPro2 – analyzes the input signal and quickly adapts to 1 of 2 distinct destinations; within each destination, the adaptive features can be customized for optimal listening and comfort
- Feedback management
- Comfort – clarity balance – gives client control of adaptive features
- AntiShock – instantaneously reduces the level of impulse noises such as a door slam while maintaining the quality and intelligibility of speech
- Speech enhancement – emphasizes speech signals based on the input level
- 8 channels
- Adaptive directional microphone
- Noise reduction, wind noise manager
- Data logging
- myMusic – enhances the music listening experience by bringing out the rich, full tones of music
- onBoard – control is easily configured as a volume control with reduced dexterity
- Automatic switching to telephone program
- Ideal-volume indicator provides a beep notification when preferred gain is reached on the volume control
- Digital volume control lever for easy control with reduced dexterity
- 3 additional manual programs
- Easy-DAI – automatic switching to a dedicated DAI program
- Low-battery warning
- Start-up delay
- ON/OFF by opening or closing battery door
- Programmed by NOAH-compatible U:fit and Standalone U:fit software 1.4 or higher
- Choice of processing strategy – WDRC or Linear Limiting
- 13 size battery

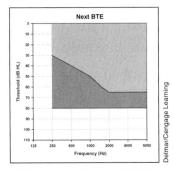

Fitting range for Next 8 BTE with slim tube/open dome (light gray) or traditional earhook (all shaded regions)

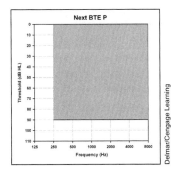
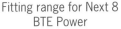

Fitting range for Next 8 BTE Power

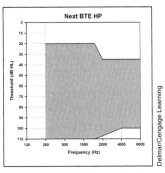

Fitting range for Next 8 BTE High-Power

Options of Next 8 BTE, Next 8 BTE P, and Next 8 BTE HP

- Remote control with volume control, comfort – clarity balance, program change button, and more
- Tamper-resistant volume control
- Tamper-resistant battery door
- Filtered earhook
- Slim tube coupling for instant open fittings (Next 8 BTE only)
- Choice of shell colors
- Direct audio input unit

Features of Next 8 Moda II BTE

- autoPro2 – analyzes the input signal and quickly adapts to 1 of 2 distinct destinations; within each destination, the adaptive features can be customized for optimal listening and comfort
- Feedback management
- AntiShock – instantaneously reduces the level of impulse noises such as a door slam while maintaining the quality and intelligibility of speech
- Speech enhancement – emphasizes speech signals based on the input level
- 8 channels
- Adaptive directional microphone
- Noise reduction, wind noise manager
- Data logging

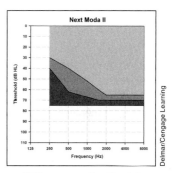

Fitting range for Next 8 Moda II BTE with open dome (light gray), closed dome (medium and light gray), and sleeve mold (all shaded regions)

- myMusic – enhances the music listening experience by bringing out the rich, full tones of music
- onBoard – control is easily configured as a volume control with reduced dexterity
- 3 additional manual programs
- Ideal-volume indicator provides a beep notification when preferred gain is reached on the volume control
- Low-battery warning
- Start-up delay
- ON/OFF by opening or closing battery door
- Programmed by NOAH-compatible U:fit and Standalone U:fit software 1.4 or higher
- Choice of processing strategy – WDRC or Linear Limiting
- 312 size battery

Options of Next 8 Moda II BTE

- Remote control with volume control, comfort – clarity balance, program change button, and more
- Telecoil (T) or microphone/telecoil (MT) option can be set as 1 of the 3 manual programs
- Choice of coupling and venting options
- Earhook

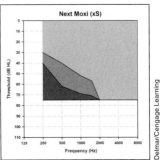

Fitting range for Next 8 Moxi (xS) with open dome (light gray), closed dome (medium and light gray), and sleeve mold (all shaded regions)

Features of Next 8 Moxi (xS), Next 8 Moxi P (xP), and Next 8 Moxi Optimum Fit

- autoPro2 – analyzes the input signal and quickly adapts to 1 of 2 distinct destinations; within each destination, the adaptive features can be customized for optimal listening and comfort
- Feedback management
- AntiShock – instantaneously reduces the level of impulse noises such as a door slam while maintaining the quality and intelligibility of speech
- Speech enhancement – emphasizes speech signals based on the input level
- 8 channels
- Adaptive directional microphone
- Noise reduction, wind noise manager
- Data logging
- myMusic – enhances the music listening experience by bringing out the rich, full tones of music
- onBoard – control is easily configured as a volume control with reduced dexterity
- Automatic switching to telephone program
- 3 additional manual programs
- Ideal-volume indicator provides a beep notification when preferred gain is reached on the volume control
- Low-battery warning
- Start-up delay
- ON/OFF by opening or closing battery door
- Programmed by NOAH-compatible U:fit and Standalone U:fit software 1.4 or higher
- Choice of processing strategy – WDRC or Linear Limiting

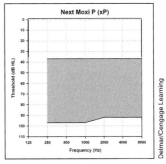
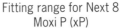

Fitting range for Next 8 Moxi P (xP)

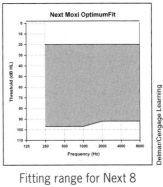

Fitting range for Next 8 Optimum Fit

- Choice of receivers
- 312 size battery

Options of Next 8 Moxi (xS), Next 8 Moxi P (xP), and Next 8 Moxi Optimum Fit

- Remote control with volume control, comfort – clarity balance, program change button, and more
- Choice of coupling and venting options

Features of Next 8 FS P, Next 8 FS, Next 8 HS/Canal, Next 8 Mini Canal/CIC, and Next 8 CIC P

- autoPro2 – analyzes the input signal and quickly adapts to 1 of 2 distinct destinations; within each destination, the adaptive features can be customized for optimal listening and comfort
- Feedback management
- Comfort – clarity balance – gives client control of adaptive features
- AntiShock – instantaneously reduces the level of impulse noises such as a door slam while maintaining the quality and intelligibility of speech
- Speech enhancement – emphasizes speech signals based on the input level
- 8 channels
- Adaptive directional microphone
- Noise reduction, wind noise manager
- Data logging
- myMusic – enhances the music listening experience by bringing out the rich, full tones of music
- onBoard – control is easily configured as a volume control with reduced dexterity
- Automatic switching to telephone program
- Ideal-volume indicator provides a beep notification when preferred gain is reached on the volume control
- 3 additional manual programs
- Low-battery warning
- Start-up delay
- ON/OFF by opening or closing battery door

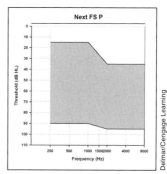

Fitting range for Next 8 Full-Shell Power

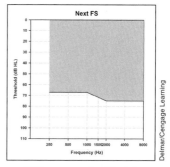

Fitting range for Next 8 Full-Shell

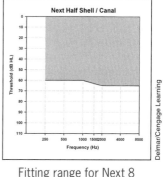

Fitting range for Next 8 Half-Shell/Canal

- Programmed by NOAH-compatible U:fit and Standalone U:fit software 1.4 or higher
- Choice of processing strategy – WDRC or Linear Limiting

Options of Next 8 FS P, Next 8 FS, Next 8 HS/Canal, Next 8 Mini Canal/CIC, and Next 8 CIC P

- Remote control with volume control, comfort – clarity balance, program change button, and more
- Telecoil (T) or microphone/telecoil (MT) option can be set as 1 of the 3 manual programs in canal to full-shell styles

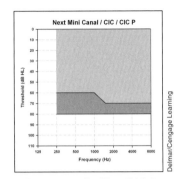

Fitting range for Next 8 Mini Canal/CIC/CIC Power Mini Canal/CIC (light gray) and CIC P (all shaded regions)

Typical Specifications		Next 8 Slim Tube (Optional)	Next 8 BTE	Next 8 BTE P	Next 8 BTE HP
Standard ANSI S3.22-1996					
Output sound pressure level	Max OSPL 90 (dB SPL)	124	125	130	135
	HFA OSPL 90 (dB SPL)	108	122	125	128
Full-on gain (50 dB SPL input)	Peak gain (dB)	53	60	70	75
	HFA (dB)	37	52	60	65
Total harmonic distortion	500 Hz	1%	4%	1%	2%
	800 Hz	1%	2%	1%	2%
	1600 Hz	1%	1%	1%	1%
Equivalent input noise (dB SPL)		28	20	20	20
Telecoil sensitivity	HFA SPLITS (dB SPL)	89	104	108	111
Battery	Operating current (mA)	1.1	1.2	1.7	2.2
	Battery type	13	13	13	13

Delmar/Cengage Learning

Typical Specifications		Next 8 Moda II BTE	Next 8 Moxi (xS)	Next 8 Moxi P (xP)
Standard ANSI S3.22-1996				
Output sound pressure level	Max OSPL 90 (dB SPL)	118	109	123
	HFA OSPL 90 (dB SPL)	109	105	118
Full-on gain (50 dB SPL input)	Peak gain (dB)	45	44	55
	HFA (dB)	36	36	47

continues

continued

Typical Specifications		Next 8 Moda II BTE	Next 8 Moxi (xS)	Next 8 Moxi P (xP)
Total harmonic distortion	500 Hz	1.5%	1%	1.5%
	800 Hz	1.3%	0.5%	1.3%
	1600 Hz	0.5%	0.5%	0.5%
Equivalent input noise (dB SPL)		24	24	24
Telecoil sensitivity	HFA SPLITS (dB SPL)	94	89	102
Battery	Operating current (mA)	1.25	1.15	1.25
	Battery type	312	312	312

Delmar/Cengage Learning

Typical Specifications		Next 8 CIC/Mini Canal	Next 8 CIC P	Next 8 Canal/HS	Next 8 FS	Next 8 FS P
Standard ANSI S3.22-1996						
Output sound pressure level	Max OSPL 90 (dB SPL)	112	116	113	115	122
	HFA OSPL 90 (dB SPL)	108	112	109	110	119
Full-on gain (50 dB SPL input)	Peak gain (dB)	40	55	48	50	60
	HFA (dB)	32	50	42	43	53
Total harmonic distortion	500 Hz	1%	1%	1.5%	1%	1%
	800 Hz	0.5%	0.5%	1.5%	0.5%	0.5%
	1600 Hz	0.5%	1%	1%	0.5%	0.5%
Equivalent input noise (dB SPL)		22	22	22	22	22
Telecoil sensitivity	HFA SPLITS (dB SPL)	92	N/A	92	94	102
Battery	Operating current (mA)	1.1	1.1	1.1	1.1	1.1
	Battery type	10	10	312	13	13

Delmar/Cengage Learning

Product Application

Next 4 BTE
Next 4 BTE P
Next 4 BTE HP
Next 4 FS P
Next 4 FS
Next 4 HS/Canal

Next 4 Mini Canal/CIC
Next 4 CIC P
Next 4 Moda II BTE
Next 4 Moxi (xS)
Next 4 Moxi P (xP)
Next 4 Optimum Fit

UNITRON

Features of Next 4 BTE, Next 4 BTE P, and Next 4 BTE HP

- Up to 4 manual programs provide customization for individual needs and preferences
- Feedback management
- AntiShock – instantaneously reduces the level of impulse noises such as a door slam while maintaining the quality and intelligibility of speech
- Speech enhancement – emphasizes speech signals based on the input level
- 4 channels, 8 bands provide flexible and accurate frequency shaping
- Fixed directional microphone
- Noise reduction, wind noise manager
- Data logging
- onBoard – control is easily configured as a volume control with reduced dexterity
- Automatic switching to telephone program
- Ideal-volume indicator provides a beep notification when preferred gain is reached on the volume control
- Digital volume control lever for easy control with reduced dexterity
- Low-battery warning
- Start-up delay
- ON/OFF by opening or closing battery door
- Programmed by NOAH-compatible U:fit and Standalone U:fit software 1.4 or higher
- Choice of processing strategy – WDRC or Linear Limiting
- 13 size battery

Options of Next 4 BTE, Next 4 BTE P, and Next 4 BTE HP

- Remote control with volume control, program change button, and more
- Tamper-resistant volume control
- Tamper-resistant battery door
- Filtered earhook
- Slim tube coupling for instant open fittings (Next 4 BTE only)
- Choice of shell colors
- Direct audio input unit

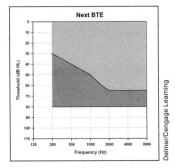

Fitting range for Next 4 BTE with slim tube/open dome (light gray) or traditional earhook (all shaded regions)

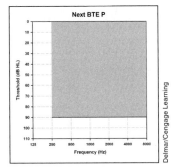

Fitting range for Next 4 BTE Power

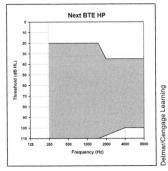

Fitting range for Next 4 BTE High-Power

Features of Next 4 Moda II BTE

- Up to 4 manual programs provide customization for individual needs and preferences
- Feedback management
- AntiShock – instantaneously reduces the level of impulse noises such as a door slam while maintaining the quality and intelligibility of speech
- Speech enhancement – emphasizes speech signals based on the input level
- 4 channels, 8 bands provide flexible and accurate frequency shaping
- Fixed directional microphone
- Noise reduction, wind noise manager
- Data logging
- onBoard – control is easily configured as a volume control with reduced dexterity
- Ideal-volume indicator provides a beep notification when preferred gain is reached on the volume control
- Low-battery warning
- Start-up delay
- ON/OFF by opening or closing battery door
- Programmed by NOAH-compatible U:fit and Standalone U:fit software 1.4 or higher
- Choice of processing strategy – WDRC or Linear Limiting
- 312 size battery

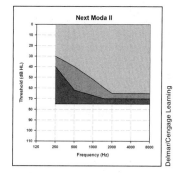

Fitting range for Next 4 Moda II BTE with open dome (light gray), closed dome (medium and light gray), and sleeve mold (all shaded regions)

Options of Next 4 Moda II BTE

- Remote control with volume control, program change button, and more
- Telecoil (T) or microphone/telecoil (MT) option can be set as 1 of the 4 manual programs
- Choice of coupling and venting options
- Earhook

Features of Next 4 Moxi (xS), Next 4 Moxi P (xP), and Next 4 Moxi Optimum Fit

- Up to 4 manual programs provide customization for individual needs and preferences
- Feedback management
- AntiShock – instantaneously reduces the level of impulse noises such as a door slam while maintaining the quality and intelligibility of speech
- Speech enhancement – emphasizes speech signals based on the input level
- 4 channels, 8 bands provide flexible and accurate frequency shaping
- Fixed directional microphone

- Noise reduction, wind noise manager
- Data logging
- onBoard – control is easily configured as a volume control with reduced dexterity
- Automatic switching to telephone program
- Ideal-volume indicator provides a beep notification when preferred gain is reached on the volume control
- Low-battery warning
- Start-up delay
- ON/OFF by opening or closing battery door
- Programmed by NOAH-compatible U:fit and Standalone U:fit software 1.4 or higher
- Choice of processing strategy – WDRC or Linear Limiting
- Choice of receivers
- 312 size battery

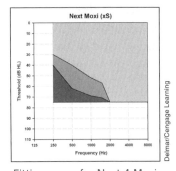

Fitting range for Next 4 Moxi (xS) with open dome (light gray), closed dome (medium and light gray), and sleeve mold (all shaded regions)

Options of Next 4 Moxi (xS), Next 4 Moxi P (xP), and Next 4 Moxi Optimum Fit

- Remote control with volume control, program change button, and more
- Choice of coupling and venting options

Features of Next 4 FS P, Next 4 FS, Next 4 HS/Canal, Next 4 Mini Canal/CIC, and Next 4 CIC P

- Up to 4 manual programs provide customization for individual needs and preferences
- Feedback management
- AntiShock – instantaneously reduces the level of impulse noises such as a door slam while maintaining the quality and intelligibility of speech
- Speech enhancement – emphasizes speech signals based on the input level
- 4 channels, 8 bands provide flexible and accurate frequency shaping
- Fixed directional microphone
- Noise reduction, wind noise manager
- Data logging
- onBoard – control is easily configured as a volume control with reduced dexterity
- Automatic switching to telephone program

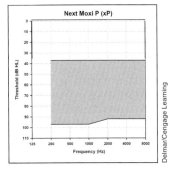

Fitting range for Next 4 Moxi P (xP)

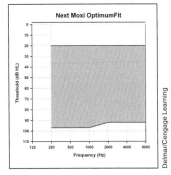

Fitting range for Next 4 Moxi Optimum Fit

- Ideal-volume indicator provides a beep notification when preferred gain is reached on the volume control
- Low-battery warning
- Start-up delay
- ON/OFF by opening or closing battery door
- Programmed by NOAH-compatible U:fit and Standalone U:fit software 1.4 or higher
- Choice of processing strategy – WDRC or Linear Limiting

Options of Next 4 FS P, Next 4 FS, Next 4 HS/Canal, Next 4 Mini Canal/CIC, and Next 4 CIC P

- Remote control with volume control, program change button, and more
- Telecoil (T) or microphone/telecoil (MT) option can be set as 1 of the 3 manual programs in canal to full-shell styles

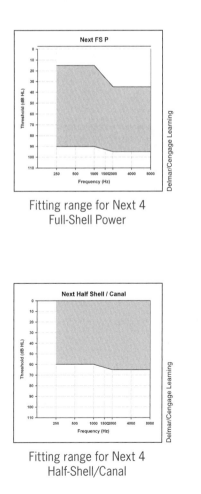

Fitting range for Next 4
Full-Shell Power

Fitting range for Next 4
Half-Shell/Canal

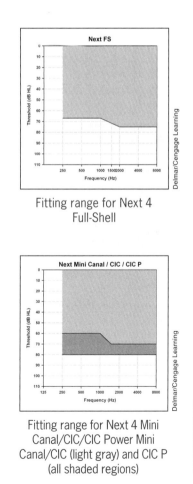

Fitting range for Next 4
Full-Shell

Fitting range for Next 4 Mini
Canal/CIC/CIC Power Mini
Canal/CIC (light gray) and CIC P
(all shaded regions)

Typical Specifications		Next 4 Slim Tube (Optional)	Next 4 BTE	Next 4 BTE P	Next 4 BTE HP
Standard ANSI S3.22-1996					
Output sound pressure level	Max OSPL 90 (dB SPL)	124	125	130	135
	HFA OSPL 90 (dB SPL)	108	122	125	128
Full-on gain (50 dB SPL input)	Peak gain (dB)	53	60	70	75
	HFA (dB)	37	52	60	65
Total harmonic distortion	500 Hz	1%	4%	1%	2%
	800 Hz	1%	2%	1%	2%
	1600 Hz	1%	1%	1%	1%
Equivalent input noise (dB SPL)		28	20	20	20
Telecoil sensitivity	HFA SPLITS (dB SPL)	89	104	108	111
Battery	Operating current (mA)	1.1	1.2	1.7	2.2
	Battery type	13	13	13	13

Delmar/Cengage Learning

Typical Specifications		Next 4 Moda II BTE	Next 4 Moxi (xS)	Next 4 Moxi P (xP)
Standard ANSI S3.22-1996				
Output sound pressure level	Max OSPL 90 (dB SPL)	118	109	123
	HFA OSPL 90 (dB SPL)	109	105	118
Full-on gain (50 dB SPL input)	Peak gain (dB)	45	44	55
	HFA (dB)	36	36	47
Total harmonic distortion	500 Hz	1.5%	1%	1.5%
	800 Hz	1.3%	0.5%	1.3%
	1600 Hz	0.5%	0.5%	0.5%
Equivalent input noise (dB SPL)		24	24	24
Telecoil sensitivity	HFA SPLITS (dB SPL)	94	89	102
Battery	Operating current (mA)	1.25	1.15	1.25
	Battery type	312	312	312

Delmar/Cengage Learning

Typical Specifications		Next 4 CIC/Mini Canal	Next 4 CIC P	Next 4 Canal/HS	Next 4 FS	Next 4 FS P
Standard ANSI S3.22-1996						
Output sound pressure level	Max OSPL 90 (dB SPL)	112	116	113	115	122
	HFA OSPL 90 (dB SPL)	108	112	109	110	119
Full-on gain (50 dB SPL input)	Peak gain (dB)	40	55	48	50	60
	HFA (dB)	32	50	42	43	53
Total harmonic distortion	500 Hz	1%	1%	1.5%	1%	1%
	800 Hz	0.5%	0.5%	1.5%	0.5%	0.5%
	1600 Hz	0.5%	1%	1%	0.5%	0.5%
Equivalent input noise (dB SPL)		22	22	22	22	22
Telecoil sensitivity	HFA SPLITS (dB SPL)	92	N/A	92	94	102
Battery	Operating current (mA)	1.1	1.1	1.1	1.1	1.1
	Battery type	10	10	312	13	13

Delmar/Cengage Learning

Product Application

Next Essential BTE
Next Essential BTE HP
Next Essential FS P
Next Essential FS

Next Essential HS/Canal
Next Essential Mini Canal/CIC
Next Essential CIC P
Next Essential Moda II BTE

Features of Next Essential BTE and Next Essential BTE HP

- 2 manual programs provide customization for individual needs and preferences
- Feedback management
- AntiShock – instantaneously reduces the level of impulse noises such as a door slam while maintaining the quality and intelligibility of speech
- 4 channels, 8 bands provide flexible and accurate frequency shaping
- Fixed directional microphone
- Noise reduction – reduces gain in bands with poor SNRs

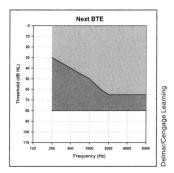

Fitting range for Next Essential BTE with slim tube/ open dome (light gray) or traditional earhook (all shaded regions)

- Data logging
- Automatic switching to telephone program
- Ideal-volume indicator provides a beep notification when preferred gain is reached on the volume control
- Digital volume control lever for easy control with reduced dexterity
- Low-battery warning
- Start-up delay
- ON/OFF by opening or closing battery door
- Programmed by NOAH-compatible U:fit and Standalone U:fit software 1.4 or higher
- Choice of processing strategy – WDRC or Linear Limiting
- 13 size battery

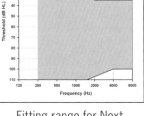

Fitting range for Next Essential BTE High-Power

Options of Next Essential BTE and Next Essential BTE HP

- Tamper-resistant volume control
- Tamper-resistant battery door
- Filtered earhook
- Slim tube coupling for instant open fittings (Next Essential BTE only)
- Choice of shell colors
- Direct audio input unit

Features of Next Essential Moda II BTE

- 2 manual programs provide customization for individual needs and preferences
- Feedback management
- AntiShock – instantaneously reduces the level of impulse noises such as a door slam while maintaining the quality and intelligibility of speech
- 4 channels, 8 bands provide flexible and accurate frequency shaping
- Fixed directional microphone
- Noise reduction – reduces gain in bands with poor SNRs
- Data logging
- Low-battery warning
- Start-up delay
- ON/OFF by opening or closing battery door
- Programmed by NOAH-compatible U:fit and Standalone U:fit software 1.4 or higher

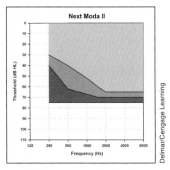

Fitting range for Next Essential Moda II BTE with open dome (light gray), closed dome (medium and light gray), and sleeve mold (all shaded regions)

- Choice of processing strategy – WDRC or Linear Limiting
- 312 size battery

Options of Next Essential Moda II BTE

- Telecoil (T) or microphone/telecoil (MT) option can be set as 1 of 2 manual programs
- Choice of coupling and venting options
- Earhook

Features of Next Essential FS P, Next Essential FS, Next Essential HS/Canal, Next Essential Mini Canal/CIC, and Next Essential CIC P

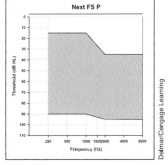

Fitting range for Next Essential Full-Shell Power

- 2 manual programs provide customization for individual needs and preferences
- Feedback management
- AntiShock – instantaneously reduces the level of impulse noises such as a door slam while maintaining the quality and intelligibility of speech
- 4 channels, 8 bands provide flexible and accurate frequency shaping
- Fixed directional microphone
- Noise reduction – reduces gain in bands with poor SNRs
- Data logging
- Automatic switching to telephone program
- Ideal-volume indicator provides a beep notification when preferred gain is reached on the volume control
- Low-battery warning
- Start-up delay
- ON/OFF by opening or closing battery door
- Programmed by NOAH-compatible U:fit and Standalone U:fit software 1.4 or higher
- Choice of processing strategy – WDRC or Linear Limiting

Options of Next Essential FS P, Next Essential FS, Next Essential HS/Canal, Next Essential Mini Canal/CIC, and Next Essential CIC P

- Telecoil (T) or microphone/telecoil (MT) option can be set as 1 of the 3 manual programs in canal to full-shell styles

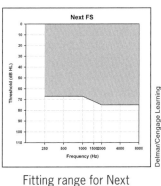

Fitting range for Next Essential Full-Shell

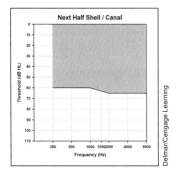

Fitting range for Next
Essential Half-Shell/Canal

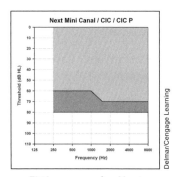

Fitting range for Next
Essential Mini Canal/CIC/
CIC Power Mini Canal/CIC
(light gray) and CIC P
(all shaded regions)

Typical Specifications		Next Essential Slim Tube (Optional)	Next Essential BTE	Next Essential BTE HP
Standard ANSI S3.22-1996				
Output sound pressure level	Max OSPL 90 (dB SPL)	124	125	135
	HFA OSPL 90 (dB SPL)	108	122	128
Full-on gain (50 dB SPL input)	Peak gain (dB)	53	60	75
	HFA (dB)	37	52	65
Total harmonic distortion	500 Hz	1%	4%	2%
	800 Hz	1%	2%	2%
	1600 Hz	1%	1%	1%
Equivalent input noise (dB SPL)		28	20	20
Telecoil sensitivity	HFA SPLITS (dB SPL)	89	104	111
Battery	Operating current (mA)	1.1	1.2	2.2
	Battery type	13	13	13

Delmar/Cengage Learning

Typical Specifications		Next Essential Moda II BTE
Standard ANSI S3.22-1996		
Output sound pressure level	Max OSPL 90 (dB SPL)	118
	HFA OSPL 90 (dB SPL)	109
Full-on gain (50 dB SPL input)	Peak gain (dB)	45
	HFA (dB)	36
Total harmonic distortion	500 Hz	1.5%
	800 Hz	1.3%
	1600 Hz	0.5%
Equivalent input noise (dB SPL)		24
Telecoil sensitivity	HFA SPLITS (dB SPL)	94
Battery	Operating current (mA)	1.25
	Battery type	312

Delmar/Cengage Learning

Typical Specifications		Next Essential CIC/Mini Canal	Next Essential CIC P	Next Essential Canal/HS	Next Essential FS	Next Essential FS P
Standard ANSI S3.22-1996						
Output sound pressure level	Max OSPL 90 (dB SPL)	112	116	113	115	122
	HFA OSPL 90 (dB SPL)	108	112	109	110	119
Full-on gain (50 dB SPL input)	Peak gain (dB)	40	55	48	50	60
	HFA (dB)	32	50	42	43	53
Total harmonic distortion	500 Hz	1%	1%	1.5%	1%	1%
	800 Hz	0.5%	0.5%	1.5%	0.5%	0.5%
	1600 Hz	0.5%	1%	1%	0.5%	0.5%
Equivalent input noise (dB SPL)		22	22	22	22	22
Telecoil sensitivity	HFA SPLITS (dB SPL)	92	N/A	92	94	102
Battery	Operating current (mA)	1.1	1.1	1.1	1.1	1.1
	Battery type	10	10	312	13	13

Delmar/Cengage Learning

PRODUCT 5: 360

Product Application

360 + Power BTE

360 e Power BTE

Features of 360 + Power BTE

- Range of loss severe to profound
- 8 channels
- 8 bands
- WDRC Linear Limiting processing
- autoPro2 – analyzes the input signal and quickly adapts to 1 of 2 distinct destinations; within each destination, the adaptive features can be customized for optimal listening and comfort
- Up to 3 manual listening programs
- onBoard control (VC or program control)
- Directional microphone system – multiband adaptive directional
- AntiShock – instantaneously reduces the level of impulse noises such as a door slam while maintaining the quality and intelligibility of speech
- Speech Enhancement
- Phase canceller enhanced
- Advanced data logging
- myMusic – enhances the music listening experience by bringing out the rich, full tones of music
- Noise reduction – reduces gain in bands with poor SNRs
- Bass enhancer
- Wind noise manager
- Easy-t – auto switching to t-coil program when phone is picked up
- Telecoil
- Easy-DAI – automatic switching to a dedicated DAI program
- Program beep indicator
- Low-battery warning
- FM-compatible

Options of 360 + Power BTE

- Smart Control – a remote control allowing patients to adjust their devices
- Mini earhook
- Tamper-proof volume control cover and battery door
- Kids' club – an information kit with resources and special tools to assist children and their parents/caregivers to make the most of their hearing instruments

Features of 360 e Power BTE

- Range of loss severe to profound
- 4 channels
- 8 bands

- WDRC Linear Limiting processing
- Up to 2 manual listening programs – plus 1 program for telephone or DAI
- Directional microphone system – omnidirectional
- AntiShock – instantaneously reduces the level of impulse noises such as a door slam while maintaining the quality and intelligibility of speech
- Phase canceller enhanced
- Data logging
- Noise reduction – reduces gain in bands with poor SNRs
- Easy-t – auto switching to t-coil program when phone is picked up
- Telecoil
- Program beep indicator
- Low-battery warning
- FM-compatible

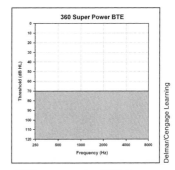

Fitting range for 360 Super Power BTE

Options of 360 e Power BTE

- Mini earhook
- Tamper-proof volume control cover and battery door
- Kids' club – an information kit with resources and special tools to assist children and their parents/caregivers to make the most of their hearing instruments

Typical Specifications		360 e Power BTE and 360 + Power BTE
Standard ANSI S3.22-1996		
Output sound pressure level	Max OSPL 90 (dB SPL)	141
	HFA OSPL 90 (dB SPL)	138
Full-on gain (50 dB SPL input)	Peak gain (dB)	82
	HFA (dB)	72
Total harmonic distortion	500 Hz	3%
	800 Hz	2%
	1600 Hz	1%
Equivalent input noise (dB SPL)		19
Telecoil sensitivity	HFA SPLITS (dB SPL)	116
Battery	Operating current (mA)	2.0
	Battery type	675

Delmar/Cengage Learning

PRODUCT 6: INDIGO

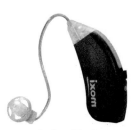

Indigo Moxi
Courtesy of Unitron

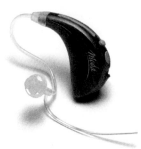

Indigo Moda BTE
Courtesy of Unitron

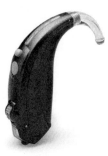

Indigo BTE
Courtesy of Unitron

Indigo Full-Shell
Courtesy of Unitron

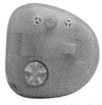

Indigo Half-Shell
Courtesy of Unitron

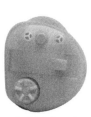

Indigo Canal
Courtesy of Unitron

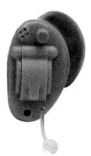

Indigo CIC
Courtesy of Unitron

Product Application

Indigo Moxi BTE	Indigo Moda BTE
Indigo Moxi Power BTE	Indigo Full-Shell Power
Indigo BTE	Indigo Full-Shell
Indigo M (No VC) BTE	Indigo Half-Shell/Canal
Indigo P BTE	Indigo Mini Canal/CIC

Features of Indigo Moxi BTE and Indigo Moxi Power BTE

- Canal receiver technology
- autoPro4 – 4 programs, each with adaptive parameters; includes automatic and smooth program changes
- 3 additional manual programs
- Multiband adaptive directional microphone system
- AntiShock – reduces the level of impulse noises
- Speech Enhancement LD – increases gain in each band where speech dominates over noise
- Phase canceller for feedback cancellation

- myMusic – allows the frequency response to be shaped to increase music enjoyment
- Noise reduction – reduces gain in bands with poor SNRs
- Wind noise manager
- Data logging
- 16 channels of signal processing
- Low-battery warning
- Start-up delay
- ON/OFF by opening or closing battery door
- Programmed using NOAH-compatible U:fit and Standalone U:fit fitting software
- Easy-t – auto switching to t-coil program when phone is picked up
- Choice of 2 receivers
- Suitable for fitting mild to severe hearing losses and can fit audiogram configurations ranging from reverse to precipitously sloping

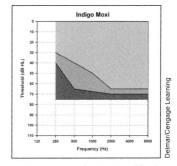

Fitting range for Indigo Moxi BTE with open dome (light gray), closed dome (medium gray and light gray), and sleeve mold/power dome (all shaded regions)

Options of Indigo Moxi BTE and Indigo Moxi Power BTE

- onBoard – a button that can be configured as a volume control or program button
- Coupling options for instant fittings
- Choice of shell colors

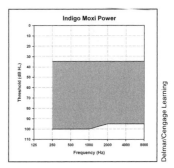

Fitting range for Indigo Moxi Power BTE

Features of Indigo BTE, Indigo M (No VC) BTE, and Indigo P BTE

- autoPro4 – 4 programs, each with adaptive parameters; includes automatic and smooth program changes
- Multiband adaptive directional microphone system
- Noise reduction – reduces gain in bands with poor SNRs
- Phase canceller for feedback cancellation
- Wind noise manager
- myMusic – allows the frequency response to be shaped to increase music enjoyment
- Speech Enhancement LD – increases gain in each band where speech dominates over noise
- AntiShock – reduces the level of impulse noises
- 16 channels of signal processing

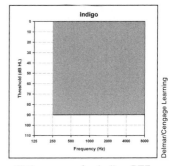

Fitting range for Indigo BTE

- Dynamic range-mapping functions
- 3 additional manual programs
- Volume indicator with beep notification
- Data logging
- Easy-t – auto switching to t-coil program when phone is picked up
- Low-battery warning
- Start-up delay
- ON/OFF by opening or closing the battery door
- Programmed using NOAH-compatible U:fit and Standalone U:fit fitting software
- Suitable for fitting mild to profound hearing losses and can fit audiogram configurations ranging from reverse to precipitously sloping

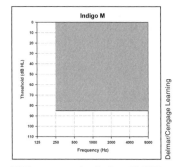

Fitting range for Indigo M BTE

Options of Indigo BTE, Indigo M (No VC) BTE, and Indigo P BTE

- Tamper-resistant volume control
- Tamper-resistant battery door
- Filtered earhook
- onBoard – a button that can be configured as a volume control or program button (Indigo M (No VC) BTE only)
- Slim tube coupling for instant open fittings (Indigo M (No VC) BTE only)
- Choice of shell colors
- Direct audio input battery door unit

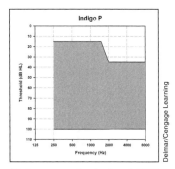

Fitting range for Indigo P BTE

Features of Indigo Moda BTE

- autoPro4 – 4 programs, each with adaptive parameters; includes automatic and smooth program changes
- Multiband adaptive directional microphone system
- Noise reduction – reduces gain in bands with poor SNRs
- myMusic – allows the frequency response to be shaped to increase music enjoyment
- Speech Enhancement LD – increases gain in each band where speech dominates over noise
- AntiShock – reduces the level of impulse noises
- Phase canceller for feedback cancellation
- Wind noise manager
- 16 channels of signal processing
- 3 additional manual programs

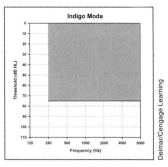

Fitting range for Indigo Moda BTE

- Data logging
- Easy-t – auto switching to t-coil program when phone is picked up
- Low-battery warning
- Start-up delay
- ON/OFF by opening or closing the battery door
- Programmed using NOAH-compatible U:fit and Standalone U:fit fitting software
- Suitable for fitting mild to moderately severe hearing losses and can fit audiogram configurations ranging from revere to precipitously sloping

Options of Indigo Moda BTE

- onBoard – a button that can be configured as a volume control or program button
- Slim tube coupling for open fittings
- Filtered earhook
- Choice of shell colors

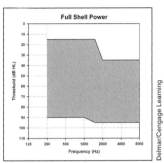

Fitting range for Indigo
Full-Shell Power

Features of Indigo Full-Shell Power, Indigo Full-Shell, Indigo Half-Shell/Canal, and Indigo Mini Canal/CIC

- autoPro4 – 4 programs, each with adaptive parameters; includes automatic and smooth program changes
- Multiband adaptive directional microphone system (excludes Indigo Mini Canal/CIC)
- myMusic – allows the frequency response to be shaped to increase music enjoyment
- Speech Enhancement LD – increases gain in each band where speech dominates over noise
- AntiShock – reduces the level of impulse noises
- Noise reduction – reduces gain in bands with poor SNRs
- Phase canceller for feedback cancellation
- Wind noise manager
- 16 channels of signal processing
- 3 additional manual programs
- Volume indicator with beep notification
- Data logging
- Low-battery warning
- Start-up delay
- ON/OFF by closing or opening the battery door or manual volume control (if present)

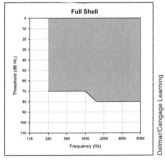

Fitting range for Indigo
Full-Shell

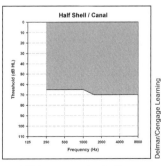

Fitting range for Indigo
Half-Shell/Canal

UNITRON

- Programmed using NOAH-compatible U:fit and Standalone U:fit fitting software
- Suitable for fitting mild to severe hearing losses and can fit audiogram configurations ranging from reverse to precipitously sloping

Options of Indigo Full-Shell Power, Indigo Full-Shell, Indigo Half-Shell/Canal, and Indigo Mini Canal/CIC

- onBoard – a button that can be configured as a volume control or program button telecoil (T) or microphone/telecoil (MT) option can be set as 1 of the 3 manual programs (excludes Indigo Mini Canal/CIC)
- Easy-t – auto switching to t-coil program when phone is picked up

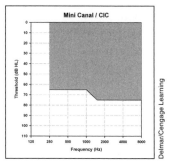

Fitting range for Indigo Mini Canal/CIC

Typical Specifications		Indigo Moxi BTE (xS Receiver)	Indigo Moxi Power BTE (xP Receiver)
Standard ANSI S3.22-1996			
Output sound pressure level	Max OSPL 90 (dB SPL)	109	123
	HFA OSPL 90 (dB SPL)	105	118
Full-on gain (50 dB SPL input)	Peak gain (dB)	44	55
	HFA (dB)	36	46
Total harmonic distortion	500 Hz	1%	1.5%
	800 Hz	0.5%	1.3%
	1600 Hz	0.5%	0.5%
Equivalent input noise (dB SPL)		19	19
Telecoil sensitivity	HFA SPLITS (dB SPL)	90	102
Battery	Operating current (mA)	1.0	1.1
	Battery type	312	312

Note: Measurement data obtained with hearing aid set to linear, omni mode with all adaptive features disabled.
Delmar/Cengage Learning

Typical Specifications		Indigo M (No VC) Slim Tube (Optional)	Indigo M (No VC)	Indigo	Indigo P (Power)
Standard ANSI S3.22-1996					
Output sound pressure level	Max OSPL 90 (dB SPL)	122	125	125	131
	HFA OSPL 90 (dB SPL)	107	119	118	124
Full-on gain (50 dB SPL input)	Peak gain (dB)	51	55	60	70
	HFA (dB)	36	50	56	63

continues

continued

Typical Specifications		Indigo M (No VC) Slim Tube (Optional)	Indigo M (No VC)	Indigo	Indigo P (Power)
Total harmonic distortion	500 Hz	1%	1%	1%	2%
	800 Hz	1%	1%	1%	1%
	1600 Hz	1%	1%	1%	1%
Equivalent input noise (dB SPL)		24	<20	<20	<20
Telecoil sensitivity	HFA SPLITS (dB SPL)	91	103	103	109
Battery	Operating current (mA)	1.1	1.1	1.1	1.2
	Battery type	13	13	13	13

Note: Measurement data obtained with hearing aid set to linear, omni mode with all adaptive features disabled.
Delmar/Cengage Learning

Typical Specifications		Indigo Moda Slim Tube (Optional)	Indigo Moda Unfiltered Earhook (Standard)
Standard ANSI S3.22-1996			
Output sound pressure level	Max OSPL 90 (dB SPL)	117	125
	HFA OSPL 90 (dB SPL)	102	117
Full-on gain (50 dB SPL input)	Peak gain (dB)	43	47
	HFA (dB)	31	43
Total harmonic distortion	500 Hz	2%	1%
	800 Hz	1%	1%
	1600 Hz	1%	1%
Equivalent input noise (dB SPL)		23	15
Telecoil sensitivity	HFA SPLITS (dB SPL)	86	101
Battery	Operating current (mA)	1.1	1.1
	Battery type	10	10

Note: Measurement data obtained with hearing aid set to linear, omni mode with all adaptive features disabled.
Delmar/Cengage Learning

Typical Specifications		Indigo Full-Shell Power	Indigo Full-Shell	Indigo Canal/ Half-Shell	Indigo CIC/Mini Canal
Standard ANSI S3.22-2003					
Output sound pressure level	Max OSPL 90 (dB SPL)	122	115	113	112
	HFA OSPL 90 (dB SPL)	119	110	109	108
Full-on gain (50 dB SPL input)	Peak gain (dB)	60	50	48	40
	HFA (dB)	53	42	41	33

continues

continued

Typical Specifications		Indigo Full-Shell Power	Indigo Full-Shell	Indigo Canal/ Half-Shell	Indigo CIC/Mini Canal
Total harmonic distortion	500 Hz	<5%	<5%	<5%	<5%
	800 Hz	<4%	<4%	<4%	<4%
	1600 Hz	<4%	<4%	<4%	<4%
Equivalent input noise (dB SPL)		22	22	22	22
Telecoil sensitivity	HFA SPLITS (dB SPL)	102	94	92	91
Battery	Operating current (mA)	1.1	1.1	1.1	1.0
	Battery type	13	13	312	10

Note: Measurement data obtained with hearing aid set to omni mode with all adaptive features disabled.
Delmar/Cengage Learning

PRODUCT 7: ELEMENT SERIES 16, 8, AND 4

Product Application

Element 16 Moxi BTE
Element 16 Moxi Power BTE
Element 16 M (No VC) BTE
Element 16 BTE
Element 16 P BTE

Element 16 Moda BTE
Element 16 Full-Shell Power
Element 16 Full-Shell
Element 16 Half-Shell/Canal
Element 16 Mini Canal/CIC

Features of Element 16 Moxi BTE and Element 16 Moxi Power BTE

- Canal receiver technology
- autoPro2 – a program that automatically adapts to the listening environment
- 3 additional manual programs
- Adaptive directional microphone system
- Noise reduction – reduces gain in bands with poor SNRs
- Speech Enhancement LD – increases gain in each band where speech dominates over noise
- AntiShock – reduces the level of impulse noises
- Phase canceller for feedback cancellation
- onBoard – a button that can be configured as a volume control or program button

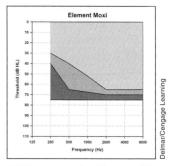

Fitting range for Element 16 Moxi BTE with open dome (light gray), closed dome (medium and light gray), and sleeve mold/power dome (all shaded regions)

- Wind noise manager
- 16 channels of signal processing
- Choice of 2 processing strategies – WDRC and Linear Limiting
- Data logging
- Low-battery warning
- Start-up delay
- ON/OFF by opening or closing the battery door
- Programmed using NOAH-compatible U:fit and Standalone U:fit fitting software
- Easy-t – auto switching to t-coil program when phone is picked up
- Suitable for fitting mild to severe hearing losses and can fit audiogram configurations ranging from reverse to precipitously sloping

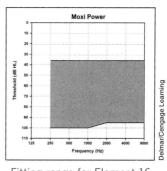

Fitting range for Element 16 Moxi Power BTE

Options of Element 16 Moxi BTE and Element 16 Moxi Power BTE

- Coupling options for instant fittings
- Choice of shell colors

Features of Element 16 M (No VC) BTE, Element 16 BTE, and Element 16 P BTE

- autoPro2 – a program that automatically adapts to the listening environment
- Adaptive directional microphone system
- Noise reduction – reduces gain in bands with poor SNRs
- Speech Enhancement LD – increases gain in each band where speech dominates over noise
- AntiShock – reduces the level of impulse noises
- Phase canceller for feedback cancellation
- Wind noise manager
- 16 channels of signal processing
- Choice of 2 processing strategies – WDRC and Linear Limiting
- 3 additional manual programs
- Volume indicator with beep notification (excludes Element 16 M (No VC) BTE)
- Data logging
- Easy-t – auto switching to t-coil program when phone is picked up

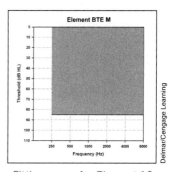

Fitting range for Element 16 M BTE

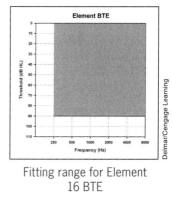

Fitting range for Element 16 BTE

UNITRON

- Low-battery warning
- Start-up delay
- ON/OFF by opening or closing the battery door
- Programmed using NOAH-compatible U:fit and Standalone U:fit fitting software
- Suitable for fitting mild to severe hearing losses and can fit audiogram configurations ranging from reverse to precipitously sloping

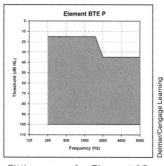

Fitting range for Element 16 P BTE

Options of Element 16 M (No VC) BTE, Element 16 BTE, and Element 16 P BTE

- Tamper-resistant volume control
- Tamper-resistant battery door
- Filtered earhook
- Slim tube coupling for instant open fittings (Element 16 M (No VC) BTE)
- Choice of shell colors
- Direct audio input battery door unit

Features of Element 16 Moda BTE

- autoPro2 – a program that automatically adapts to the listening environment
- Adaptive directional microphone system
- Noise reduction – reduces gain in bands with poor SNRs
- Speech Enhancement LD – increases gain in each band where speech dominates over noise
- AntiShock – reduces the level of impulse noises
- Phase canceller for feedback cancellation
- Wind noise manager
- 16 channels of signal processing
- Choice of 2 processing strategies – WDRC and Linear Limiting
- 3 additional manual programs
- Data logging
- Easy-t – auto switching to t-coil program when phone is picked up
- Low-battery warning
- Start-up delay
- ON/OFF by opening or closing the battery door

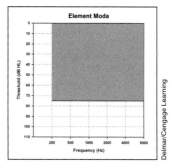

Fitting range for Element 16 Moda BTE

- Programmed using NOAH-compatible U:fit and Standalone U:fit fitting software
- Suitable for fitting mild to moderately severe hearing losses and can fit audiogram configurations ranging from reverse to precipitously sloping

Features of Element 16 Full-Shell Power, Element 16 Full-Shell, Element 16 Half-Shell/Canal, and Element 16 Mini Canal/CIC

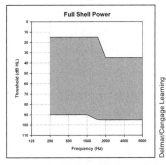
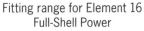

Fitting range for Element 16 Full-Shell Power

- autoPro2 – a program that automatically adapts to the listening environment
- Adaptive directional microphone system (excludes Element 16 Mini Canal/CIC)
- Noise reduction – reduces gain in bands with poor SNRs
- Speech Enhancement LD – increases gain in each band where speech dominates over noise
- AntiShock – reduces the level of impulse noises
- Phase canceller for feedback cancellation
- Wind noise manager
- 16 channels of signal processing
- Choice of 2 processing strategies – WDRC and Linear Limiting
- 3 additional manual programs
- Volume indicator with beep notification
- Data logging
- Low-battery warning
- Start-up delay
- ON/OFF by opening or closing the battery door or by rotating the manual VC
- Programmed using NOAH-compatible U:fit and Standalone U:fit fitting software
- Suitable for fitting mild to severe hearing losses and can fit audiogram configurations ranging from reverse to precipitously sloping

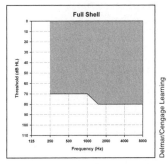

Fitting range for Element 16 Full-Shell

Options of Element 16 Full-Shell Power, Element 16 Full-Shell, Element 16 Half-Shell/Canal, and Element 16 Mini Canal/CIC

- Telecoil (T) or microphone/telecoil (MT) option can be set as 1 of the 3 manual programs (excludes Element 16 Mini Canal/CIC)
- Easy-t – auto switching to t-coil program when phone is picked up

UNITRON

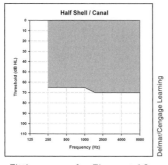

Fitting range for Element 16
Half-Shell/Canal

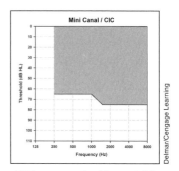

Fitting range for Element 16
Mini Canal/CIC

Typical Specifications		Element 16 Moxi BTE	Element 16 Moxi Power BTE
Standard ANSI S3.22-1996			
Output sound pressure level	Max OSPL 90 (dB SPL)	109	123
	HFA OSPL 90 (dB SPL)	105	118
Full-on gain (50 dB SPL input)	Peak gain (dB)	44	55
	HFA (dB)	36	46
Total harmonic distortion	500 Hz	1%	1.5%
	800 Hz	0.5%	1.3%
	1600 Hz	0.5%	0.5%
Equivalent input noise (dB SPL)		19	19
Telecoil sensitivity	HFA SPLITS (dB SPL)	90	102
Battery	Operating current (mA)	1.0	1.1
	Battery type	312	312

Note: Measurement data obtained with hearing aid set to linear, omni mode with all adaptive features disabled.
Delmar/Cengage Learning

Typical Specifications		Element 16 M (No VC) Slim Tube (Optional)	Element 16 M (No VC)	Element 16	Element 16 P (Power)
Standard ANSI S3.22-1996					
Output sound pressure level	Max OSPL 90 (dB SPL)	122	125	125	131
	HFA OSPL 90 (dB SPL)	107	119	118	124
Full-on gain (50 dB SPL input)	Peak gain (dB)	51	55	60	70
	HFA (dB)	36	50	56	63

continues

continued

Typical Specifications		Element 16 M (No VC) Slim Tube (Optional)	Element 16 M (No VC)	Element 16	Element 16 P (Power)
Total harmonic distortion	500 Hz	1%	1%	1%	2%
	800 Hz	1%	1%	1%	1%
	1600 Hz	1%	1%	1%	1%
Equivalent input noise (dB SPL)		24	<20	<20	<20
Telecoil sensitivity	HFA SPLITS (dB SPL)	91	103	103	109
Battery	Operating current (mA)	1.1	1.1	1.1	1.2
	Battery type	13	13	13	13

Delmar/Cengage Learning

Typical Specifications		Element 16 Moda Slim Tube (Optional)	Element Moda Unfiltered Earhook (Standard)
Standard ANSI S3.22-1996			
Output sound pressure level	Max OSPL 90 (dB SPL)	117	125
	HFA OSPL 90 (dB SPL)	102	117
Full-on gain (50 dB SPL input)	Peak gain (dB)	43	47
	HFA (dB)	31	43
Total harmonic distortion	500 Hz	2%	1%
	800 Hz	1%	1%
	1600 Hz	1%	1%
Equivalent input noise (dB SPL)		23	15
Telecoil sensitivity	HFA SPLITS (dB SPL)	86	101
Battery	Operating current (mA)	1.1	1.1
	Battery type	10	10

Delmar/Cengage Learning

Typical Specifications		Element 16 Full-Shell Power	Element 16 Full-Shell	Element 16 Canal/ Half-Shell	Element 16 CIC/Mini Canal
Standard ANSI S3.22-2003					
Output sound pressure level	Max OSPL 90 (dB SPL)	122	115	113	112
	HFA OSPL 90 (dB SPL)	119	110	109	108
Full-on gain (50 dB SPL input)	Peak gain (dB)	60	50	48	40
	HFA (dB)	53	42	41	33

continues

UNITRON

continued

Typical Specifications		Element 16 Full-Shell Power	Element 16 Full-Shell	Element 16 Canal/ Half-Shell	Element 16 CIC/Mini Canal
Total harmonic distortion	500 Hz	1.0%	1.0%	1.5%	1.0%
	800 Hz	0.5%	0.5%	1.5%	0.5%
	1600 Hz	0.5%	0.5%	1.5%	0.5%
Equivalent input noise (dB SPL)		22	22	22	22
Telecoil sensitivity	HFA SPLITS (dB SPL)	102	94	92	91
Battery	Operating current (mA)	1.1	1.1	1.1	1.0
	Battery type	13	13	312	10

Note: Measurement data obtained with hearing aid set to linear, omni mode with all adaptive features disabled.

Product Application

Element 8 Moxi BTE

Element 8 Moxi Power BTE

Element 8 M (No VC) BTE

Element 8 BTE

Element 8 P BTE

Element 8 Moda BTE

Element 8 Full-Shell Power

Element 8 Full-Shell

Element 8 Half-Shell/Canal

Element 8 Mini Canal/CIC

Features of Element 8 Moxi BTE and Element 8 Moxi Power BTE

- Canal receiver technology
- autoMic™ – automatically switches between omni and directional mode
- 3 additional manual programs
- Adaptive directional microphone system
- Noise reduction – reduces gain in bands with poor SNRs
- Speech enhancement
- AntiShock – reduces the level of impulse noises
- Phase canceller for feedback cancellation
- onBoard – a button that can be configured as a volume control or program button
- Wind noise manager
- 8 channels of signal processing
- Choice of 2 processing strategies – WDRC and Linear Limiting
- Data logging
- Low-battery warning
- Start-up delay

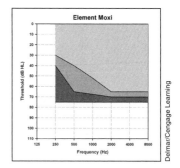

Fitting range for Element 8 Moxi BTE with open dome (light gray), closed dome (medium and light gray), and sleeve mold/power dome (all shaded regions)

- ON/OFF by opening or closing the battery door
- Programmed using NOAH-compatible U:fit and Standalone U:fit fitting software
- Suitable for fitting mild to severe hearing losses and can fit audiogram configurations ranging from reverse to precipitously sloping
- Easy-t – auto switching to t-coil program when phone is picked up
- Choice of 2 receivers

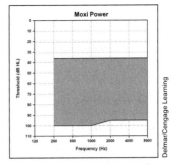

Fitting range for Element 8 Moxi Power BTE

Options of Element 8 Moxi BTE and Element 8 Moxi Power BTE

- Coupling options for instant fittings
- Choice of shell colors

Features of Element 8 M (No VC) BTE, Element 8 BTE, and Element 8 P BTE

- autoMic – automatically switches between omni and directional mode
- Adaptive directional microphone system
- Noise reduction – reduces gain in bands with poor SNRs
- Speech enhancement
- AntiShock – reduces the level of impulse noises
- Phase canceller for feedback cancellation
- Wind noise manager
- 8 channels of signal processing
- Choice of 2 processing strategies – WDRC and Linear Limiting
- 3 additional manual programs
- Volume indicator with beep notification (excludes Element 8 M (No VC) BTE)
- Data logging
- Easy-t – auto switching to t-coil program when phone is picked up
- Low-battery warning
- Start-up delay
- ON/OFF by opening or closing the battery door
- Programmed using NOAH-compatible U:fit and Standalone U:fit fitting software
- Suitable for fitting mild to severe hearing losses and can fit audiogram configurations ranging from reverse to precipitously sloping

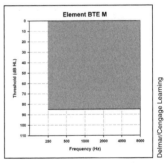

Fitting range for Element 8 M BTE

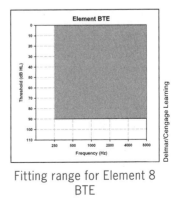

Fitting range for Element 8 BTE

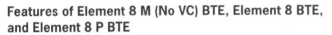

UNITRON

Options of Element 8 M (No VC) BTE, Element 8 BTE, and Element 8 P BTE

- Tamper-resistant volume control
- Tamper-resistant battery door
- Filtered earhook
- Slim tube coupling for instant open fittings (Element 8 M BTE (No VC) only)
- Choice of shell colors
- Direct audio input battery door unit

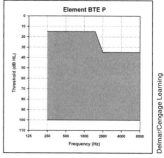

Fitting range for Element 8 P BTE

Features of Element 8 Moda BTE

- autoMic – automatically switches between omni and directional mode
- Adaptive directional microphone system
- Noise reduction – reduces gain in bands with poor SNRs
- Speech enhancement in each of the 8 bands
- AntiShock – reduces the level of impulse noises
- Phase canceller for feedback cancellation
- Wind noise manager
- 8 channels of signal processing
- Choice of 2 processing strategies – WDRC and Linear Limiting
- 3 additional manual programs
- Data logging
- Easy-t – auto switching to t-coil program when phone is picked up
- Low-battery warning
- Start-up delay
- ON/OFF by opening or closing the battery door
- Programmed using NOAH-compatible U:fit and Standalone U:fit fitting software
- Suitable for fitting mild to moderately severe hearing losses and can fit audiogram configurations ranging from reverse to precipitously sloping

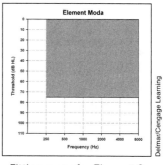

Fitting range for Element 8 Moda BTE

Options of Element 8 Moda BTE

- Slim tube coupling for open fittings
- Filtered earhooks
- Choice of shell colors

Features of Element 8 Full-Shell Power, Element 8 Full-Shell, Element 8 Half-Shell/Canal, and Element 8 Mini Canal/CIC

- autoMic – automatically switches between omni and directional mode
- Adaptive directional microphone system (excludes Element 8 Mini Canal/CIC)

- Noise reduction – reduces gain in bands with poor SNRs
- Speech enhancement
- AntiShock – reduces the level of impulse noises
- Phase canceller for feedback cancellation
- Wind noise manager
- 8 channels of signal processing
- Choice of 2 processing strategies – WDRC and Linear Limiting
- 3 additional manual programs
- Volume indicator with beep notification
- Data logging
- Low-battery warning
- Start-up delay
- ON/OFF by opening or closing the battery door
- Programmed using NOAH-compatible U:fit and Standalone U:fit fitting software
- Suitable for fitting mild to severe hearing losses and can fit audiogram configurations ranging from reverse to precipitously sloping

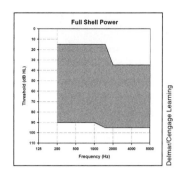

Fitting range for Element 8
Full-Shell Power

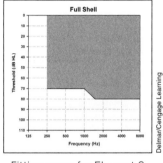

Fitting range for Element 8
Full-Shell

Options of Element 8 Full-Shell Power, Element 8 Full-Shell, Element 8 Half-Shell/Canal, and Element 8 Mini Canal/CIC

- Telecoil (T) or microphone/telecoil (MT) option can be set as 1 of the 3 manual programs (excludes Element 8 Mini Canal/CIC)
- Easy-t – auto switching to t-coil program when phone is picked up

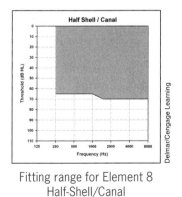

Fitting range for Element 8
Half-Shell/Canal

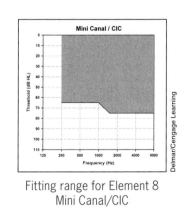

Fitting range for Element 8
Mini Canal/CIC

UNITRON

Typical Specifications		Element 8 Moxi BTE	Element 8 Moxi Power BTE
Standard ANSI S3.22-1996			
Output sound pressure level	Max OSPL 90 (dB SPL)	109	123
	HFA OSPL 90 (dB SPL)	105	118
Full-on gain (50 dB SPL input)	Peak gain (dB)	44	55
	HFA (dB)	36	46
Total harmonic distortion	500 Hz	1%	1.5%
	800 Hz	0.5%	1.3%
	1600 Hz	0.5%	0.5%
Equivalent input noise (dB SPL)		19	19
Telecoil sensitivity	HFA SPLITS (dB SPL)	90	102
Battery	Operating current (mA)	1.0	1.1
	Battery type	312	312

Note: Measurement data obtained with hearing aid set to linear, omni mode with all adaptive features disabled.
Delmar/Cengage Learning

Typical Specifications		Element 8 M (No VC) Slim Tube (Optional)	Element 8 (No VC)	Element 8	Element 8 P (Power)
Standard ANSI S3.22-1996					
Output sound pressure level	Max OSPL 90 (dB SPL)	122	125	125	131
	HFA OSPL 90 (dB SPL)	107	119	118	124
Full-on gain (50 dB SPL input)	Peak gain (dB)	51	55	60	70
	HFA (dB)	36	50	56	63
Total harmonic distortion	500 Hz	1%	1%	1%	2%
	800 Hz	1%	1%	1%	1%
	1600 Hz	1%	1%	1%	1%
Equivalent input noise (dB SPL)		24	<20	<20	<20
Telecoil sensitivity	HFA SPLITS (dB SPL)	91	103	103	109
Battery	Operating current (mA)	1.1	1.1	1.1	1.2
	Battery type	13	13	13	13

Note: Measurement data obtained with hearing aid set to linear, omni mode with all adaptive features disabled.
Delmar/Cengage Learning

Typical Specifications		Element 8 Moda Slim Tube (Optional)	Element 8 Moda Unfiltered Earhook (Standard)
Standard ANSI S3.22-1996			
Output sound pressure level	Max OSPL 90 (dB SPL)	117	125
	HFA OSPL 90 (dB SPL)	102	117
Full-on gain (50 dB SPL input)	Peak gain (dB)	43	47
	HFA (dB)	31	43
Total harmonic distortion	500 Hz	2%	1%
	800 Hz	1%	1%
	1600 Hz	1%	1%
Equivalent input noise (dB SPL)		23	15
Telecoil sensitivity	HFA SPLITS (dB SPL)	86	101
Battery	Operating current (mA)	1.1	1.1
	Battery type	10	10

Note: Measurement data obtained with hearing aid set to linear, omni mode with all adaptive features disabled.
Delmar/Cengage Learning

Typical Specifications		Element 8 Full-Shell Power	Element 8 Full-Shell	Element 8 Canal/ Half-Shell	Element 8 CIC/Mini Canal
Standard ANSI S3.22-2003					
Output sound pressure level	Max OSPL 90 (dB SPL)	122	115	113	112
	HFA OSPL 90 (dB SPL)	119	110	109	108
Full-on gain (50 dB SPL input)	Peak gain (dB)	60	50	48	40
	HFA (dB)	53	42	41	33
Total harmonic distortion	500 Hz	1.0%	1.0%	1.5%	1.0%
	800 Hz	0.5%	0.5%	1.5%	0.5%
	1600 Hz	0.5%	0.5%	1.5%	0.5%
Equivalent input noise (dB SPL)		22	22	22	22
Telecoil sensitivity	HFA SPLITS (dB SPL)	102	94	92	91
Battery	Operating current (mA)	1.1	1.1	1.1	1.0
	Battery type	13	13	312	10

Note: Measurement data obtained with hearing aid set to linear, omni mode with all adaptive features disabled.
Delmar/Cengage Learning

Product Application

Element 4 Moxi BTE

Element 4 Moxi Power BTE

Element 4 M (No VC) BTE

Element 4 BTE

Element 4 P BTE

Element 4 Moda BTE

Element 4 Full-Shell Power

Element 4 Full-Shell

Element 4 Half-Shell/Canal

Element 4 Mini Canal/CIC

Features of Element 4 Moxi BTE and Element 4 Moxi Power BTE

- Canal receiver technology
- Choice of 3 manual programs
- Fixed directional microphone system
- Noise reduction – reduces gain in bands with poor SNRs
- AntiShock – reduces the level of impulse noises
- Phase canceller for feedback cancellation
- onBoard – a button that can be configured as a volume control or program button
- Wind noise manager
- 4 channels, 8 bands
- Choice of 2 processing strategies – WDRC and Linear Limiting
- Data logging
- Low-battery warning
- Start-up delay
- ON/OFF by opening or closing the battery door
- Programmed using NOAH-compatible U:fit and Standalone U:fit fitting software
- Suitable for fitting mild to severe hearing losses and can fit audiogram configurations ranging from reverse to precipitously sloping
- Easy-t – auto switching to t-coil program when phone is picked up
- Choice of 2 receivers

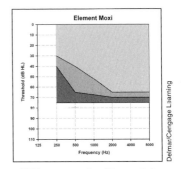

Fitting range for Element 4 Moxi BTE with open dome (light gray), closed dome (medium and light gray), and sleeve mold/power dome (all shaded regions)

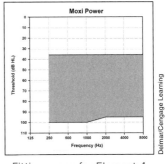

Fitting range for Element 4 Moxi Power BTE

Options of Element 4 Moxi BTE and Element 4 Moxi Power BTE

- Coupling options for instant fittings
- Choice of shell colors

Features of Element 4 M (No VC) BTE, Element 4 BTE, Element 4 P BTE, and Element 4 Moda BTE

- Choice of 3 manual programs
- Fixed directional microphone system

- Noise reduction – reduces gain in bands with poor SNRs
- AntiShock – reduces the level of impulse noises
- Phase canceller for feedback cancellation
- Wind noise manager
- 4 channels, 8 bands
- Choice of 2 processing strategies – WDRC and Linear Limiting
- Volume indicator with beep notification (excludes Element 4 Moda BTE and Element 4 M (No VC) BTE)
- Data logging
- Easy-t – auto switching to t-coil program when phone is picked up
- Low-battery warning
- Start-up delay
- ON/OFF by opening or closing the battery door
- Programmed using NOAH-compatible U:fit and Standalone U:fit fitting software
- Element 4 – suitable for fitting mild to severe hearing losses and can fit audiogram configurations ranging from reverse to precipitously sloping
- Element 4 Moda – suitable for fitting mild to moderately severe hearing losses and can fit audiogram configurations ranging from reverse to precipitously sloping

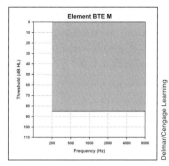

Fitting range for Element 4 M BTE

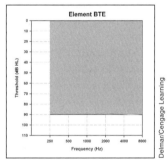

Fitting range for Element 4 BTE

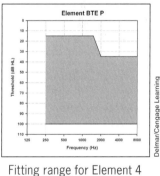

Fitting range for Element 4 P BTE

Options of Element 4 M (No VC) BTE, Element 4 BTE, Element 4 P BTE, and Element 4 Moda BTE

- Tamper-resistant volume control (excludes Element 4 Moda BTE)
- Tamper-resistant battery door (excludes Element 4 Moda BTE)
- Filtered earhook
- Slim tube coupling for open fittings (Element 4 Moda BTE and Element 4 M (No VC) BTE only)
- Choice of shell colors
- Direct audio input battery door unit (excludes Element 4 Moda BTE)

UNITRON

Features of Element 4 Full-Shell Power, Element 4 Full-Shell, Element 4 Half-Shell/Canal, and Element 4 Mini Canal/CIC

- Choice of 3 manual programs
- Fixed directional microphone system (excludes Element 4 Mini Canal/CIC)
- Noise reduction – reduces gain in bands with poor SNRs
- AntiShock – reduces the level of impulse noises
- Phase canceller for feedback cancellation
- Wind noise manager
- 4 channels, 8 bands
- Choice of 2 processing strategies – WDRC and Linear Limiting
- Volume indicator with beep notification
- Data logging
- Low-battery warning
- Start-up delay
- ON/OFF by opening or closing the battery door or by rotating the manual VC
- Programmed using NOAH-compatible U:fit and Standalone U:fit fitting software
- Suitable for fitting mild to severe hearing losses and can fit audiogram configurations ranging from revere to precipitously sloping

Options of Element 4 Full-Shell Power, Element 4 Full-Shell, Element 4 Half-Shell/Canal, and Element 4 Mini Canal/CIC

- Telecoil (T) or microphone/telecoil (MT) option can be set as 1 of the 3 manual programs (excludes Element 4 Mini Canal/CIC)
- Easy-t – auto switching to t-coil program when phone is picked up

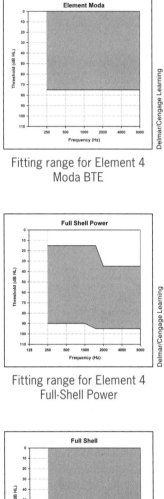

Fitting range for Element 4 Moda BTE

Fitting range for Element 4 Full-Shell Power

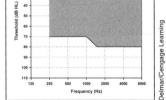

Fitting range for Element 4 Full-Shell

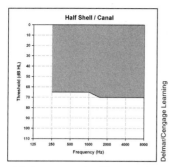

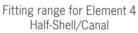

Fitting range for Element 4
Half-Shell/Canal

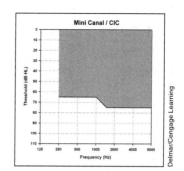

Fitting range for Element 4
Mini Canal/CIC

Typical Specifications		Element 4 Moxi BTE	Element 4 Moxi Power BTE
Standard ANSI S3.22-1996			
Output sound pressure level	Max OSPL 90 (dB SPL)	109	123
	HFA OSPL 90 (dB SPL)	105	118
Full-on gain (50 dB SPL input)	Peak gain (dB)	44	55
	HFA (dB)	36	46
Total harmonic distortion	500 Hz	1%	1.5%
	800 Hz	0.5%	1.3%
	1600 Hz	0.5%	0.5%
Equivalent input noise (dB SPL)		19	19
Telecoil sensitivity	HFA SPLITS (dB SPL)	90	102
Battery	Operating current (mA)	1.0	1.1
	Battery type	312	312

Note: Measurement data obtained with hearing aid set to linear, omni mode with all adaptive feature disabled.
Delmar/Cengage Learning

Typical Specifications		Element 4 M (No VC) Slim Tube (Optional)	Element 4M (No VC)	Element 4	Element 4 P (Power)
Standard ANSI S3.22-1996					
Output sound pressure level	Max OSPL 90 (dB SPL)	122	125	125	131
	HFA OSPL 90 (dB SPL)	107	119	118	124
Full-on gain (50 dB SPL input)	Peak gain (dB)	51	55	60	70
	HFA (dB)	36	50	56	63

continues

UNITRON

continued

Typical Specifications		Element 4 M (No VC) Slim Tube (Optional)	Element 4M (No VC)	Element 4	Element 4 P (Power)
Total harmonic distortion	500 Hz	1%	1%	1%	2%
	800 Hz	1%	1%	1%	1%
	1600 Hz	1%	1%	1%	1%
Equivalent input noise (dB SPL)		24	<20	<20	<20
Telecoil sensitivity	HFA SPLITS (dB SPL)	91	103	103	109
Battery	Operating current (mA)	1.1	1.1	1.1	1.2
	Battery type	13	13	13	13

Note: Measurement data obtained with hearing aid set to linear, omni mode with all adaptive features disabled.
Delmar/Cengage Learning

Typical Specifications		Element 4Moda Slim Tube (Optional)	Element 4 Moda Unfiltered Earhook (Standard)
Standard ANSI S3.22-1996			
Output sound pressure level	Max OSPL 90 (dB SPL)	117	125
	HFA OSPL 90 (dB SPL)	102	117
Full-on gain (50 dB SPL input)	Peak gain (dB)	43	47
	HFA (dB)	31	43
Total harmonic distortion	500 Hz	2%	1%
	800 Hz	1%	1%
	1600 Hz	1%	1%
Equivalent input noise (dB SPL)		23	15
Telecoil sensitivity	HFA SPLITS (dB SPL)	86	101
Battery	Operating current (mA)	1.1	1.1
	Battery type	10	10

Note: Measurement data obtained with hearing aid set to linear, omni mode with all adaptive features disabled.
Delmar/Cengage Learning

Typical Specifications		Element 4 Full-Shell Power	Element 4 Full-Shell	Element 4 Canal/ Half-Shell	Element 4 CIC/Mini Canal
Standard ANSI S3.22-2003					
Output sound pressure level	Max OSPL 90 (dB SPL)	122	115	113	112
	HFA OSPL 90 (dB SPL)	119	110	109	108
Full-on gain (50 dB SPL input)	Peak gain (dB)	60	50	48	40
	HFA (dB)	53	42	41	33

continues

continued

Typical Specifications		Element 4 Full-Shell Power	Element 4 Full-Shell	Element 4 Canal/ Half-Shell	Element 4 CIC/Mini Canal
Total harmonic distortion	500 Hz	1.0%	1.0%	1.5%	1.0%
	800 Hz	0.5%	0.5%	1.5%	0.5%
	1600 Hz	0.5%	0.5%	1.5%	0.5%
Equivalent input noise (dB SPL)		22	22	22	22
Telecoil sensitivity	HFA SPLITS (dB SPL)	102	94	92	91
Battery	Operating current (mA)	1.1	1.1	1.1	1.0
	Battery type	13	13	312	10

Note: Measurement data obtained with hearing aid set to linear, omni mode with all adaptive features disabled.

Delmar/Cengage Learning

PRODUCT 8: CONVERSA.NT

Product Application

Conversa.NT BTE
Conversa.NT Full-Shell
Conversa.NT Half-Shell
Conversa.NT Canal
Conversa.NT M (No VC) BTE

Conversa.NT P BTE
Conversa.NT Moda BTE
Conversa.NT Mini Canal
Conversa.NT CIC

Features of Conversa.NT BTE, Conversa.NT M (No VC) BTE, Conversa. NT P BTE, and Conversa.NT Moda BTE

- Speech enhancement with 3 choices of settings: off, moderate, maximum
- autoMic – automatically switches between omni and directional mode
- Adaptive beamformer directional microphone system
- Real-time feedback canceller for noise cancellation
- Intelligent noise reduction with 4 choices of settings: off, mild, moderate, maximum
- Wind noise manager
- 16 channels of signal processing
- Dynamic range mapping across 16 channels
- Up to 3 programs
- Telecoil (T) or microphone/telecoil (MT) option can be set in any of the 3 programs
- Wearers choose program through program button; audible beeps confirm selection
- Ideal volume indicator provides beep notification when correct gain is reached on the volume control
- Manual volume control can be disabled through Unifit™

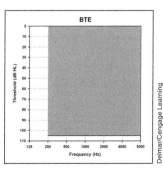

Fitting range for Conversa. NT BTE

- ON/OFF feature through the battery door
- Start-up mute
- Low-battery warning
- Direct audio input – MLx-compatible
- Can be programmed using NOAH-compatible Unifit software or Standalone Unifit
- Conversa.NT BTE – suitable for fitting mild to profound hearing losses and can fit audiogram configurations ranging from reverse to precipitously sloping
- Conversa.NT Moda BTE – suitable for fitting mild to moderately severe hearing losses and can fit audiogram configurations ranging from reverse to precipitously sloping

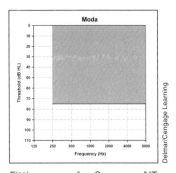

Fitting range for Conversa.NT Moda BTE

Options of Conversa.NT BTE, Conversa.NT M (No VC) BTE, and Conversa.NT P BTE

- WiFi Mic digital wireless CROS/BiCROS system
- Slim tube coupling for instant open fittings (Conversa.NT M (No VC) BTE)
- Tamper-resistant volume control
- Tamper-resistant battery door
- Filtered earhook
- Choice of shell colors
- Direct audio input battery door unit

Options of Conversa.NT Moda BTE

- Slim tube coupling for instant open fittings
- Unfiltered earhooks
- Choice of shell colors

Features of Conversa.NT Full-Shell, Conversa.NT Half-Shell, Conversa. NT Canal, Conversa.NT Mini Canal, and Conversa.NT CIC

- Speech enhancement with 3 choices of settings: off, moderate, maximum
- autoMic – automatically switches between omni and directional mode
- Adaptive beamformer directional microphone system
- Real-time feedback canceller for noise cancellation
- Intelligent noise reduction with 4 choices of settings: off, mild, moderate, maximum
- Wind noise manager
- 16 channels of signal processing
- Dynamic range mapping across 16 channels
- Up to 3 programs
- Wearers choose program through program button; audible beeps confirm selection

- Ideal volume indicator provides beep notification when correct gain is reached on the volume control
- Manual volume control can be disabled through Unifit
- Start-up mute
- Low-battery warning
- Can be programmed using NOAH-compatible Unifit software or Standalone Unifit
- Suitable for fitting mild to severe hearing losses and can fit audiogram configurations ranging from reverse to precipitously sloping

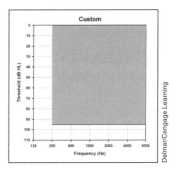

Fitting range for Conversa.NT Custom

Options of Conversa.NT Full-Shell, Conversa.NT Half-Shell, Conversa.NT Canal, Conversa.NT Mini Canal, and Conversa.NT CIC

- Telecoil (T) or microphone/telecoil (MT) option can be set in any of the 3 programs (excludes Conversa.NT Mini Canal and Conversa.NT CIC)
- Easy-t – auto switching to t-coil program when phone is picked up
- Directional microphone (excludes Conversa.NT Mini Canal and Conversa.NT CIC)

Typical Specifications		Conversa. NT M (No VC) Slim Tube	Conversa. NT M (No VC)	Conversa. NT	Conversa. NT P (Power)
Standard ANSI S3.22-1996					
Output sound pressure level	Max OSPL 90 (dB SPL)	112	130	127	135
	HFA OSPL 90 (dB SPL)	105*	123	119	127
Full-on gain	Peak gain (dB)	38	55	60	70
	HFA (dB)	32*	50	54	63
Total harmonic distortion	500 Hz	<5%	<5%	<5%	<7%
	800 Hz	<5%	<3%	<5%	<5%
	1600 Hz	<5%	<3%	<5%	<5%
Equivalent input noise (dB SPL)		23	15	15	15
Telecoil sensitivity	HFA SPLITS (dB SPL)	87*	105	100	108
Battery	Operating current (mA)	1.3	1.3	1.1	1.4
	Battery type	13	13	13	13
Fast time constant	Attack (ms)	<40	<40	<40	<40
	Release (ms)	100	100	100	100

continues

UNITRON

continued

Typical Specifications		Conversa. NT M (No VC) Slim Tube	Conversa. NT M (No VC)	Conversa. NT	Conversa. NT P (Power)
Slow time constant	Attack (ms)	250	250	250	250
	Release (ms)	300	300	300	300
Compression ratio	Wide dynamic range compression	4:1 to 1:1	4:1 to 1:1	4:1 to 1:1	4:1 to 1:1
	Compression limiting	20:1	20:1	20:1	20:1

*SPA frequencies: 1600, 2500, and 4000 Hz
Note: Technical data generated with quiet mode expansion on.
Delmar/Cengage Learning

Typical Specifications		Conversa.NT Moda Filtered Earhook	Conversa.NT Moda Filtered Earhook	Conversa.NT Moda Slim Tube Coupling
Standard ANSI S3.22-1996				
Output sound pressure level	Max OSPL 90 (dB SPL)	117	124	108
	HFA OSPL 90 (dB SPL)	114	116	100*
Full-on gain	Peak gain (dB)	40	47	38
	HFA (dB)	38	40	30*
Total harmonic distortion	500 Hz	5%	5%	5%
	800 Hz	4%	4%	4%
	1600 Hz	4%	4%	4%
Equivalent input noise (dB SPL)		15	15	23
Telecoil sensitivity	HFA SPLITS (dB SPL)	87*	105	100
Battery	Operating current (mA)	1.3	1.3	1.1
	Battery type	10	10	10
Fast time constant	Attack (ms)	<40	<40	<40
	Release (ms)	100	100	100
Slow time constant	Attack (ms)	250	250	250
	Release (ms)	300	300	300
Compression ratio	Wide dynamic range compression	4:1 to 1:1	4:1 to 1:1	4:1 to 1:1
	Compression limiting	20:1	20:1	20:1

*SPA frequencies: 1600, 2500, and 4000 Hz
Note: Technical data generated with quiet mode expansion on.
Delmar/Cengage Learning

Typical Specifications		Conversa. NT Full-Shell Power	Conversa. NT Full-Shell	Conversa. NT Canal Half-Shell	Conversa. NT Mini Canal	Conversa. NT CIC
Standard ANSI S3.22-1996						
Output sound pressure level	Max OSPL 90 (dB SPL)	125	118	115	112	112
	HFA OSPL 90 (dB SPL)	120	113	110	109	109
Full-on gain	Peak gain (dB)	60	50	45	45	40
	HFA (dB)	52	43	37	36	32
Total harmonic distortion	500 Hz	5%	5%	5%	5%	5%
	800 Hz	7%	4%	4%	4%	4%
	1600 Hz	4%	4%	4%	4%	4%
Equivalent input noise (dB SPL)		20	20	21	19	20
Telecoil sensitivity	HFA SPLITS (dB SPL)	103	96	92	92	n/a
Battery	Operating current (mA)	1.2	1.0	1.0	1.0	1.0
	Battery type	13	13/312	312	10	10
Fast time constant	Attack (ms)	40	40	40	40	40
	Release (ms)	100	100	100	100	100
Slow time constant	Attack (ms)	200	200	200	200	200
	Release (ms)	300	300	300	300	300
Compression ratio	Wide dynamic range compression	4:1 to 1:1	4:1 to 1:1	4:1 to 1:1	4:1 to 1:1	4:1 to 1:1
	Compression limiting	20:1	20:1	20:1	20:1	20:1

Note: Technical data generated with quiet mode expansion on.

Delmar/Cengage Learning

PRODUCT 9: UNISON SERIES 6, 3, AND ESSENTIAL

Product Application

Unison 6 M (No VC) BTE

Unison 6 BTE

Unison 6 P BTE

Unison 6 HP BTE

Unison 6 Moda BTE

Unison 6 Full-Shell Power

Unison 6 Full-Shell

Unison 6 Canal/Half-Shell

Unison 6 Mini Canal

Unison 6 CIC

Features of Unison 6 M (No VC) BTE, Unison 6 BTE, Unison 6 P BTE, and Unison 6 HP BTE

- 6 channels with 6 bands
- 4 processing choices to tailor to client needs

UNITRON

- Digital wide dynamic range compression (Digital WDRC[6])
- ASP noise suppression for automatic low-frequency attenuation
- Adaptive compression (AGCi)
- Linear with output compression limiting (AGCo)
- Adaptive feedback canceller addresses feedback in everyday listening situations
- Multiband feedback manager at time of fitting via Unifit software
- Intelligent noise reduction analyzes input on 3 dimensions and automatically reduces noise signals; choice of off, mild, moderate, maximum

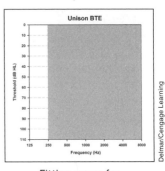

Fitting range for
Unison 6 BTE

- Selective dual-microphone directionality for improved signal-to-noise ratio, AI–DI = 5.0
- Multichannel quiet mode expansion reduces gain for very soft inputs, yet preserves moderately soft inputs such as speech for more pure, natural sound
- Intelligent power management responds to environmental inputs more efficiently to maximize battery life
- Choice of moderate-gain, power, or high-power versions
- Up to 3 programs allow customization for different listening environments
- Telecoil (T) mode or microphone/telecoil (MT) mode can be set as 1 of the 3 independent programs
- Wearers choose program through push button; audible beep confirms selection
- Ideal volume indicator provides beep notification when correct gain is reached on the volume control
- Manual volume control can be disabled through Unifit
- OFF position in volume control on high power
- Start-up mute
- Low-battery warning
- Direct audio input – MLx-compatible
- Can be programmed using NOAH-compatible Unifit software or Standalone Unifit
- Suitable for fitting mild to profound hearing losses and can fit audiogram configurations ranging from reverse to precipitously sloping

Options of Unison 6 M (No VC) BTE, Unison 6 BTE, Unison 6 P BTE, and Unison 6 HP BTE

- WiFi Mic digital wireless CROS/BiCROS system available with moderate and power versions
- Slim tube coupling for instant open fittings (Unison 6 M (No VC) BTE)
- Tamper-resistant battery door and volume control

- Filtered earhook
- Choice of shell colors
- Direct audio input battery door unit

Features of Unison 6 Moda BTE

- 6 channels with 6 bands
- 4 processing choices to tailor to client needs
  - Digital WDRC
  - ASP noise suppression for automatic low-frequency attenuation
  - Adaptive compression (AGCi)
  - Linear with output compression limiting (AGCo)
- Adaptive feedback canceller addresses feedback in everyday listening situations
- Multiband feedback manager at time of fitting via Unifit software
- Intelligent noise reduction analyzes input on 3 dimensions and automatically reduces noise signals; choice of off, mild, moderate, maximum
- Multichannel quiet mode expansion reduces gain for very soft inputs, yet preserves moderately soft inputs such as speech for more pure, natural sound
- Intelligent power management responds to environmental inputs more efficiently to maximize battery life
- Up to 3 programs allow customization for different listening environments
- Telecoil (T) mode or microphone/telecoil (MT) mode can be set as 1 of the 3 independent programs
- Wearers choose program through push button; audible beep confirms selection
- Selectable dual-microphone directionality for improved signal-to-noise ratio, AI–DI = 5.0 dB
- Start-up mute
- Low-battery warning
- Filtered earhook
- Can be programmed using NOAH-compatible Unifit software or Standalone Unifit
- Suitable for fitting mild to moderately severe hearing losses and can fit audiogram configurations from reverse to precipitously sloping

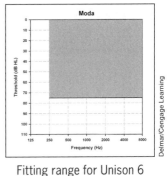

Fitting range for Unison 6 Moda BTE

Delmar/Cengage Learning

Options of Unison 6 Moda BTE

- Slim tube coupling for instant open fittings
- Unfiltered earhook
- Choice of shell colors

UNITRON

Features of Unison 6 Full-Shell, Unison 6 Full-Shell Power, Unison 6 Canal/Half-Shell, Unison 6 Mini Canal, and Unison 6 CIC

- 6 channels with 6 bands
- 4 processing choices to tailor to client needs
  - Digital WDRC[6]
  - ASP noise suppression for automatic low-frequency attenuation
  - Adaptive compression (AGCi)
  - Linear with output compression limiting (AGCo)

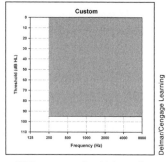

Fitting range for Unison 6 Custom

- Adaptive feedback canceller addresses feedback in everyday listening situations
- Multiband feedback manager at time of fitting via Unifit software
- Intelligent noise reduction analyzes input on 3 dimensions and automatically reduces noise signals; choice of off, mild, moderate, maximum
- Multichannel quiet mode expansion reduces gain for very soft inputs, yet preserves moderately soft inputs such as speech for more pure, natural sound
- Intelligent power management responds to environmental inputs more efficiently to maximize battery life
- Up to 3 programs allow customization for different listening environments
- Wearers choose program through push button; audible beep confirms selection
- Start-up mute
- Low-battery warning
- Manual volume control can be disabled through Unifit
- Ideal volume indicator provides beep notification when correct gain is reached on the volume control
- Can be programmed using NOAH-compatible Unifit or Standalone Unifit
- Suitable for fitting mild to severe hearing losses and can fit audiogram configurations ranging from reverse to precipitously sloping

Options of Unison 6 Full-Shell, Unison 6 Full-Shell Power, Unison 6 Canal/Half-Shell, Unison 6 Mini Canal, and Unison 6 CIC

- Selectable dual-microphone directionality for improved signal-to-noise ratio, AI–DI = 5.9 dB (Unison 6 Full-Shell, Unison 6 Half-Shell, and Unison 6 Canal only)
- Telecoil (T) mode or microphone/telecoil (MT) mode can be set as 1 of the 3 independent programs (Unison 6 Full-Shell, Unison 6 Half-Shell, and Unison 6 Canal only)
- Easy t-coil for automatic telecoil operation

Typical Specifications		Unison 6 M (No VC) Slim Tube (Optional)	Unison 6 M (No VC) (Standard)	Unison 6	Unison 6 P	Unison 6 HP
Standard ANSI S3.22-1996						
Output sound pressure level	Max OSPL 90 (dB SPL)	112	130	127	135	138
	HFA OSPL 90 (dB SPL)	105	123	117	125	130
Full-on gain	Peak gain (dB)	38	55	60	70	76
	HFA (dB)	32	50	54	63	70
Total harmonic distortion	500 Hz	<5%	<5%	<5%	<7%	<5%
	800 Hz	<5%	<5%	<5%	<5%	<5%
	1600 Hz	<5%	<5%	<5%	<5%	<5%
Equivalent input noise (dB SPL)		23	15	15	15	15
Telecoil sensitivity	HFA SPLITS (dB SPL)	87	105	100	108	112
Battery	Operating current (mA)	1.3	1.3	1.1	1.2	1.4
	Battery type	13	13	13	13	675
Fast time constant	Attack (ms)	<40	<40	<40	<40	<40
	Release (ms)	100	100	50	50	50
Slow time constant	Attack (ms)	250	250	250	250	250
	Release (ms)	300	300	300	300	300
Compression ratio	Wide dynamic range compression	4:1 to 1:1	4:1 to 1:1	4:1 to 1:1	4:1 to 1:1	4:1 to 1:1
	AGCi	6:1	6:1	6:1	6:1	6:1
	AGCo	20:1	20:1	20:1	20:1	20:1

Note: Technical data generated with quiet mode expansion on.

Delmar/Cengage Learning

Typical Specifications		Unison 6 Moda Filtered Earhook	Unison 6 Moda Unfiltered Earhook	Unison 6 Slim Tube Coupling
Standard ANSI S3.22-1996				
Output sound pressure level	Max OSPL 90 (dB SPL)	117	124	108
	HFA OSPL 90 (dB SPL)	114	116	100*
Full-on gain	Peak gain (dB)	40	47	38
	HFA (dB)	38	40	30*

continues

UNITRON

continued

Typical Specifications		Unison 6 Moda Filtered Earhook	Unison 6 Moda Unfiltered Earhook	Unison 6 Slim Tube Coupling
Total harmonic distortion	500 Hz	5%	5%	5%
	800 Hz	4%	4%	4%
	1600 Hz	4%	4%	4%
Equivalent input noise (dB SPL)		15	15	23
Telecoil sensitivity	HFA SPLITS (dB SPL)	96	99	83*
Battery	Operating current (mA)	1.1	1.1	1.1
	Battery type	10	10	10
Fast time constant	Attack (ms)	<40	<40	<40
	Release (ms)	100	100	100
Slow time constant	Attack (ms)	250	250	250
	Release (ms)	300	300	300
Compression ratio	Wide dynamic range compression	4:1 to 1:1	4:1 to 1:1	4:1 to 1:1
	AGCi	6:1	6:1	6:1
	AGCo	20:1	20:1	20:1

*SPA frequencies: 1600, 2500, and 4000 Hz

Note: Technical data generated with quiet mode expansion on.

Delmar/Cengage Learning

Typical Specifications		Unison 6 Full-Shell Power	Unison 6 Full-Shell	Unison 6 Canal Half-Shell	Unison 6 Mini Canal	Unison 6 CIC
Standard ANSI S3.22-1996						
Output sound pressure level	Max OSPL 90 (dB SPL)	125	118	115	112	112
	HFA OSPL 90 (dB SPL)	120	113	110	109	109
Full-on gain	Peak gain (dB)	60	50	45	45	40
	HFA (dB)	52	43	37	36	32
Total harmonic distortion	500 Hz	5%	5%	5%	5%	5%
	800 Hz	7%	4%	4%	4%	4%
	1600 Hz	4%	4%	4%	4%	4%
Equivalent input noise (dB SPL)		20	20	21	19	20
Telecoil sensitivity	HFA SPLITS (dB SPL)	103	95	93	92	n/a

continues

continued

Typical Specifications		Unison 6 Full-Shell Power	Unison 6 Full-Shell	Unison 6 Canal Half-Shell	Unison 6 Mini Canal	Unison 6 CIC
Battery	Operating current (mA)	1.2	1.0	1.0	1.0	1.0
	Battery type	13	13/312	312	10	10
Fast time constant	Attack (ms)	40	40	40	40	40
	Release (ms)	100	100	100	100	100
Slow time constant	Attack (ms)	200	200	200	200	200
	Release (ms)	300	300	300	300	300
Compression ratio	Wide dynamic range compression	4:1 to 1:1	4:1 to 1:1	4:1 to 1:1	4:1 to 1:1	4:1 to 1:1
	AGCi	6:1	6:1	6:1	6:1	6:1
	AGCo	20:1	20:1	20:1	20:1	20:1

Delmar/Cengage Learning

Product Application

Unison 3 DM (No VC) BTE	Unison 3 D Moda BTE
Unison 3 BTE	Unison 3 Full-Shell Power
Unison 3D BTE	Unison 3 Full-Shell
Unison 3P BTE	Unison 3 Canal/Half-Shell
Unison 3P D BTE	Unison 3 Mini Canal
Unison 3 HP BTE	Unison 3 CIC
Unison 3 HP D BTE	

Features of Unison 3 DM (No VC) BTE, Unison 3 BTE, Unison 3D BTE, Unison 3P BTE, Unison 3P D BTE, Unison 3 HP BTE, and Unison 3 HP D BTE

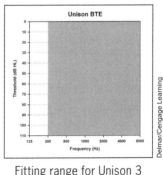

Fitting range for Unison 3 BTE

- 3 channels and 6 bands
- 2 processing choices to tailor to client needs: Digital WDRC[3] and Linear with output compression limiting (AGCo)
- Adaptive feedback canceller addresses feedback in everyday listening situations
- Multiband feedback manager at time of fitting via Unifit software
- Multichannel quiet mode expansion reduces gain for very soft inputs, yet preserves moderately soft inputs such as speech for more pure, natural sound
- Intelligent power management responds to environmental inputs more efficiently to maximize battery life
- Choice of moderate-gain, power, or high-power versions

UNITRON

- Up to 3 programs allow customization for different listening environments
- Telecoil (T) mode or microphone/telecoil (MT) mode can be set as 1 of the 3 independent programs
- Wearers choose program through push button; audible beep confirms selection
- Ideal volume indicator provides beep notification when correct gain is reached on the volume control
- Manual volume control can be disabled through Unifit
- OFF position in volume control on high power
- Start-up mute
- Low-battery warning
- Direct audio input – MLx-compatible
- Can be programmed using NOAH-compatible Unifit software or Standalone Unifit
- Suitable for fitting mild to profound hearing losses and can fit audiogram configurations ranging from reverse to precipitously sloping

Options of Unison 3 DM (No VC) BTE, Unison 3 BTE, Unison 3D BTE, Unison 3P BTE, Unison 3P D BTE, Unison 3 HP BTE, and Unison 3 HP D BTE

- Unison 3 DM BTE, Unison 3 D BTE, Unison 3P D BTE, and Unison 3HP D BTE with selectable dual-microphone directionality for improved signal-to-noise ratio, AI–DI = 5.0 dB
- Slim tube coupling for instant open fitting (Unison 3 DM (No VC) BTE)
- WiFi Mic digital wireless CROS/BiCROS system available with moderate and power versions
- Tamper-resistant battery door and volume control
- Filtered earhook
- Choice of shell colors
- Direct audio input battery door unit

Features of Unison 3 D Moda BTE

- 3 channels and 6 bands
- 2 processing choices to tailor to client needs: Digital WDRC[3] and Linear with output compression limiting (AGCo)
- Adaptive feedback canceller addresses feedback in every day listening situations
- Multiband feedback manager at time of fitting via Unifit software
- Multichannel quiet mode expansion reduces gain for very soft inputs, yet preserves moderately soft inputs such as speech for more pure, natural sound

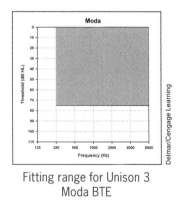

Fitting range for Unison 3 Moda BTE

- Intelligent power management responds to environmental inputs more efficiently to maximize battery life
- Up to 3 programs allow customization for different listening environments
- Telecoil (T) mode or microphone/telecoil (MT) mode can be set as 1 of the 3 independent programs
- Wearers choose program through push button; audible beep confirms selection
- Selectable dual-microphone directionality for improved signal-to-noise ratio, AI–DI = 5.0 dB
- Start-up mute
- Low-battery warning
- Filtered earhook
- Can be programmed using NOAH-compatible Unifit software or Standalone software
- Suitable for mild to moderately severe hearing losses and can fit audiogram configurations ranging from reverse to precipitously sloping

Options of Unison 3 D Moda BTE

- Slim tube coupling for instant open fittings
- Unfiltered earhook
- Choice of shell colors

Features of Unison 3 Full-Shell Power, Unison 3 Full-Shell, Unison 3 Canal/ Half-Shell, Unison 3 Mini Canal, and Unison 3 CIC

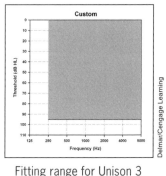

Fitting range for Unison 3 Custom

- 3 channels and 6 bands
- 2 processing choices to tailor to client needs: Digital WDRC[3] and Linear with output compression limiting (AGCo)
- Adaptive feedback canceller addresses feedback in everyday listening situations
- Multiband feedback manager at time of fitting via Unifit software
- Multichannel quiet mode expansion reduces gain for very soft inputs, yet preserves moderately soft inputs such as speech for more pure, natural sound
- Up to 3 programs allow customization for different listening environments
- Wearers choose program through push button; audible beep confirms selection
- Start-up mute
- Low-battery warning
- Manual volume control can be disabled through Unifit
- Ideal volume indicator provides beep notification when correct gain is reached on the volume control

- Can be programmed using NOAH-compatible Unifit or Standalone Unifit
- Suitable for fitting mild to severe hearing losses and can fit audiogram configurations ranging from reverse to precipitously sloping

Options of Unison 3 Full-Shell Power, Unison 3 Full-Shell, Unison 3 Canal/Half-Shell, Unison 3 Mini Canal, and Unison 3 CIC

- Selectable dual-microphone directionality for improved signal-to-noise ratio, AI–DI = 5.9 dB (Unison 3 Full-Shell, Unison 3 Half-Shell, and Unison 3 Canal only)
- Telecoil (T) mode or microphone/telecoil (MT) mode can be set as 1 of the 3 independent programs (Unison 3 Full-Shell, Unison 3 Half-Shell, and Unison 3 Canal only)
- Easy t-coil for automatic telecoil operation

Typical Specifications		Unison 3 DM (No VC) Slim Tube (Optional)	Unison 3 DM (No VC) Unfiltered (Standard)	Unison 3 & 3D
Standard ANSI S3.22-1996				
Output sound pressure level	Max OSPL 90 (dB SPL)	112	130	127
	HFA OSPL 90 (dB SPL)	105*	123	117
Full-on gain	Peak gain (dB)	38	55	60
	HFA (dB)	32*	50	54
Total harmonic distortion	500 Hz	<5%	<5%	<5%
	800 Hz	<5%	<5%	<5%
	1600 Hz	<5%	<5%	<5%
Equivalent input noise (dB SPL)		23	15	15
Telecoil sensitivity	HFA SPLITS (dB SPL)	87*	105	100
Battery	Operating current (mA)	1.3	1.3	1.1
	Battery type	13	13	13
Fast time constant	Attack (ms)	<40	<40	<40
	Release (ms)	100	100	100
Slow time constant	Attack (ms)	250	250	250
	Release (ms)	300	300	300
Compression ratio	Wide dynamic range compression	4:1 to 1:1	4:1 to 1:1	4:1 to 1:1
	AGCo	20:1	20:1	20:1

*SPA frequencies: 1600, 2500, and 4000 Hz

Delmar/Cengage Learning

Typical Specifications		Unison 3P and 3P D	Unison 3 HP	Unison 3 HP D
Standard ANSI S3.22-1996				
Output sound pressure level	Max OSPL 90 (dB SPL)	135	138	138
	HFA OSPL 90 (dB SPL)	125	130	130
Full-on gain	Peak gain (dB)	70	76	76
	HFA (dB)	63	68	70
Total harmonic distortion	500 Hz	<7%	<5%	<5%
	800 Hz	<5%	<5%	<5%
	1600 Hz	<5%	<5%	<5%
Equivalent input noise (dB SPL)		15	15	15
Telecoil sensitivity	HFA SPLITS (dB SPL)	108	112	112
Battery	Operating current (mA)	1.2	1.4	1.4
	Battery type	13	675	675
Fast time constant	Attack (ms)	<40	<40	<40
	Release (ms)	100	50	50
Slow time constant	Attack (ms)	250	250	250
	Release (ms)	300	300	300
Compression ratio	Wide dynamic range compression	4:1 to 1:1	4:1 to 1:1	4:1 to 1:1
	AGCo	20:1	20:1	20:1

Delmar/Cengage Learning

Typical Specifications		Unison 3 Moda Filtered Earhook	Unison 3 Moda Unfiltered Earhook	Unison 3 Slim Tube Coupling
Standard ANSI S3.22-1996				
Output sound pressure level	Max OSPL 90 (dB SPL)	117	124	108
	HFA OSPL 90 (dB SPL)	114	116	100*
Full-on gain	Peak gain (dB)	40	47	38
	HFA (dB)	38	40	30*
Total harmonic distortion	500 Hz	5%	5%	5%
	800 Hz	4%	4%	4%
	1600 Hz	4%	4%	4%
Equivalent input noise (dB SPL)		15	15	23

continues

UNITRON

continued

Typical Specifications		Unison 3 Moda Filtered Earhook	Unison 3 Moda Unfiltered Earhook	Unison 3 Slim Tube Coupling
Telecoil sensitivity	HFA SPLITS (dB SPL)	96	99	83*
Battery	Operating current (mA)	1.1	1.1	1.1
	Battery type	10	10	10
Fast time constant	Attack (ms)	<40	<40	<40
	Release (ms)	100	100	100
Slow time constant	Attack (ms)	250	250	250
	Release (ms)	300	300	300
Compression ratio	Wide dynamic range compression	4:1 to 1:1	4:1 to 1:1	4:1 to 1:1
	AGCo	20:1	20:1	20:1

*SPA frequencies: 1600, 2500, and 4000 Hz

Note: Technical data generated with quiet mode expansion on.

Delmar/Cengage Learning

Typical Specifications		Unison 3 Full-Shell Power	Unison 3 Full-Shell	Unison 3 Canal Half-Shell	Unison 3 Mini Canal	Unison 3 CIC
Standard ANSI S3.22-1996						
Output sound pressure level	Max OSPL 90 (dB SPL)	125	118	115	112	112
	HFA OSPL 90 (dB SPL)	120	113	110	109	109
Full-on gain	Peak gain (dB)	60	50	45	45	40
	HFA (dB)	52	43	37	36	32
Total harmonic distortion	500 Hz	5%	5%	5%	5%	5%
	800 Hz	7%	4%	4%	4%	4%
	1600 Hz	4%	4%	4%	4%	4%
Equivalent input noise (dB SPL)		20	20	21	19	20
Telecoil sensitivity	HFA SPLITS (dB SPL)	103	95	93	92	n/a
Battery	Operating current (mA)	1.2	1.0	1.0	1.0	1.0
	Battery type	13	13/312	312	10	10
Fast time constant	Attack (ms)	40	40	40	40	40
	Release (ms)	100	100	100	100	100

continues

continued

Typical Specifications		Unison 3 Full-Shell Power	Unison 3 Full-Shell	Unison 3 Canal Half-Shell	Unison 3 Mini Canal	Unison 3 CIC
Slow time constant	Attack (ms)	200	200	200	200	200
	Release (ms)	300	300	300	300	300
Compression ratio	Wide dynamic range compression	4:1 to 1:1	4:1 to 1:1	4:1 to 1:1	4:1 to 1:1	4:1 to 1:1
	AGCo	20:1	20:1	20:1	20:1	20:1

Delmar/Cengage Learning

Product Application

Unison Essential BTE

Unison Essential P BTE

Unison Essential HP BTE

Unison Essential Full-Shell Power

Unison Essential Full-Shell

Unison Essential Canal/Half-Shell

Unison Essential Mini Canal

Unison Essential CIC

Features of Unison Essential BTE, Unison Essential P BTE, and Unison Essential HP BTE

- 3 channels and 6 bands
- Digital WDRC[3]
- Multiband feedback manager at time of fitting via Unifit software
- Multiband quiet mode expansion reduces gain for very soft inputs, yet preserves moderately soft inputs such as speech for more pure, natural sound
- Intelligent power management responds to environmental inputs more efficiently to maximize battery life
- Choice of moderate-gain, power, or high-power versions
- 1 program + telecoil program
- Telecoil (T) mode or microphone/telecoil (MT) mode fixed in telecoil program
- Wearers choose program through push button; audible beep confirms selection
- Ideal volume indicator provides beep notification when correct gain is reached on the volume control
- Manual volume control can be disabled through Unifit
- OFF position in volume control on high power
- Low-battery warning
- Direct audio input – MLx-compatible

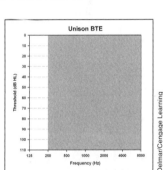

Fitting range for Unison Essential BTE

- Can be programmed using NOAH-compatible Unifit software or Standalone Unifit
- Suitable for fitting mild to profound hearing losses and can fit audiogram configurations ranging from reverse to precipitously sloping

Options of Unison Essential BTE, Unison Essential P BTE, and Unison Essential HP BTE

- Tamper-resistant battery door
- Tamper-resistant volume control
- Filtered earhook
- Choice of shell colors
- Direct audio input battery door unit

Features of Unison Essential Full-Shell Power, Unison Essential Full-Shell, Unison Essential Canal/Half-Shell, Unison Essential Mini Canal, and Unison Essential CIC

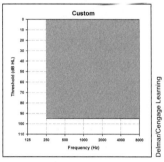

Fitting range for Unison Essential Custom

- 3 channels and 6 bands
- Digital WDRC[3]
- Multiband feedback manager at time of fitting via Unifit software
- Intelligent power management responds to environmental inputs more efficiently to maximize battery life
- Multiband quiet mode expansion reduces gain for very soft inputs, yet preserves moderately soft inputs such as speech for more pure, natural sound
- 1 program + optional telecoil program
- Wearers choose telecoil program through push button; audible beep confirms selection
- Low-battery warning
- Manual volume control can be disabled in Unifit
- Ideal volume indicator provides beep notification when correct gain is reached on the volume control
- Can be programmed using NOAH-compatible Unifit software or Standalone Unifit
- Suitable for fitting mild to severe hearing losses and can fit audiogram configurations ranging from reverse to precipitously sloping

Options of Unison Essential Full-Shell Power, Unison Essential Full-Shell, Unison Essential Canal/Half-Shell, Unison Essential Mini Canal, and Unison Essential CIC

- Telecoil (T) mode or microphone/telecoil (MT) mode fixed in additional telecoil program (Unison Essential Full-Shell, Unison Essential Half-Shell, and Unison Essential Canal only)
- Easy t-coil for automatic telecoil operation

Typical Specifications		Unison Essential	Unison Essential P	Unison Essential HP
Standard ANSI S3.22-1996				
Output sound pressure level	Max OSPL 90 (dB SPL)	127	135	138
	HFA OSPL 90 (dB SPL)	117	125	130
Full-on gain	Peak gain (dB)	60	70	76
	HFA (dB)	54	63	68
Total harmonic distortion	500 Hz	<5%	<7%	<5%
	800 Hz	<5%	<5%	<5%
	1600 Hz	<5%	<5%	<5%
Equivalent input noise (dB SPL)		15	15	15
Telecoil sensitivity	HFA SPLITS (dB SPL)	100	108	112
Battery	Operating current (mA)	1.1	1.2	1.4
	Battery type	13	13	675
Fast time constant	Attack (ms)	<40	<40	<40
	Release (ms)	100	100	50
Slow time constant	Attack (ms)	250	250	250
	Release (ms)	300	300	300
Compression ratio	Wide dynamic range compression	4:1 to 1:1	4:1 to 1:1	4:1 to 1:1

Delmar/Cengage Learning

Typical Specifications		Unison Essential Full-Shell Power	Unison Essential Full-Shell	Unison Essential Canal Half-Shell	Unison Essential Mini Canal	Unison Essential CIC
Standard ANSI S3.22-1996						
Output sound pressure level	Max OSPL 90 (dB SPL)	125	118	115	112	112
	HFA OSPL 90 (dB SPL)	120	113	110	109	109
Full-on gain	Peak gain (dB)	60	50	45	45	40
	HFA (dB)	52	43	37	36	32
Total harmonic distortion	500 Hz	5%	5%	5%	5%	5%
	800 Hz	7%	4%	4%	4%	4%
	1600 Hz	4%	4%	4%	4%	4%
Equivalent input noise (dB SPL)		20	20	21	19	20

UNITRON

continues

continued

Typical Specifications		Unison Essential Full-Shell Power	Unison Essential Full-Shell	Unison Essential Canal Half-Shell	Unison Essential Mini Canal	Unison Essential CIC
Telecoil sensitivity	HFA SPLITS (dB SPL)	103	95	93	92	n/a
Battery	Operating current (mA)	1.2	1.0	1.0	1.0	1.0
	Battery type	13	13/312	312	10	10
Fast time constant	Attack (ms)	40	40	40	40	40
	Release (ms)	100	100	100	100	100
Slow time constant	Attack (ms)	200	200	200	200	200
	Release (ms)	300	300	300	300	300
Compression ratio	Wide dynamic range compression	4:1 to 1:1	4:1 to 1:1	4:1 to 1:1	4:1 to 1:1	4:1 to 1:1

Delmar/Cengage Learning

PRODUCT 10: BREEZE

Product Application

> Breeze Mini BTE
> Breeze Custom AGCo (Full-Shell Power, Full-Shell, Canal Power, Canal Half-Shell, and CIC)
> Breeze Custom Linear (Full-Shell Power, Full-Shell, Canal Power, Canal Half-Shell, and CIC)
> Breeze Custom WDRC (Full-Shell, Canal Half-Shell, and CIC)

Features of Breeze Mini BTE

- Digital sound processing for clear, comfortable sound
- 2-channel WDRC
- 3 controls provide fitting flexibility:
  - L – low-channel gain (green)
  - F – crossover frequency (white)
  - P – maximum power output (blue)
- Controls continuously adjustable in steps for precise adjustment
- Set F control counterclockwise for 4000 Hz position
- Quiet mode expansion for improved sound quality in quiet environments and reduced circuit noise
- Power management system provides optimized battery door
- Low-battery warning

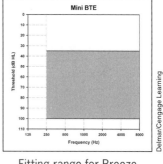

Fitting range for Breeze Mini BTE

Delmar/Cengage Learning

- Volume control – numbered 1 (low) to 4 (high)
- M–T–O switch – 3 positions: microphone–telecoil–OFF
- Direct audio input – MLx-compatible
- Unfiltered earhook
- Suitable for fitting moderate to severe hearing losses and can fit audiogram configurations ranging from flat to steeply sloping

Options of Breeze Mini BTE

- Tamper-resistant volume control
- Tamper-resistant battery door
- Filtered earhook
- Choice of shell colors

Features of Breeze Custom AGCo

- Digital sound processing for clear, comfortable sound
- Output compression limiting
- 4 controls provide fitting flexibility:
  - Low-cut (green dot)
  - High-cut (black dot)
  - Maximum power output (blue dot)
  - Gain (red dot)
- Controls continuously adjustable in steps for precise adjustment
- Set trimmers counterclockwise for maximum amplification

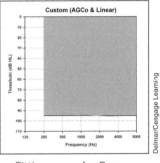

Fitting range for Breeze Custom AGCo

- Quiet mode expansion for improved sound quality in quiet environment and reduced circuit noise
- Power management system provides optimized battery life
- Low-battery warning
- Contoured matte faceplate provides attractive cosmetics
- Screw-set volume control (red arrow) (CIC only)
- Suitable for mild to severe hearing losses and can fit audiogram configurations ranging from reverse to sloping

Options of Breeze Custom AGCo

- Optional telecoil, accessible through push-button switch (canal, half-shell, and full-shell only)
- Optional dual-microphone directionality for improved signal-to-noise ratio, selectable by push button; AI–DI = 5.1 dB (canal, half-shell, and full-shell only)
- Manual volume control (canal, half-shell, and full-shell only)
- Screw-set volume control (red arrow) (canal, half-shell, and full-shell only)
- Power option (canal and full-shell only)

Features of Breeze Custom Linear

- Digital sound processing for clear, comfortable sound
- 4 controls provide fitting flexibility:
  - Low-cut (green dot)
  - High-cut (black dot)
  - Maximum power output (blue dot)
  - Gain (red dot)
- Controls continuously adjustable in steps for precise adjustment
- Set trimmers counterclockwise for maximum amplification
- Quiet mode expansion for improved sound quality in quiet environment and reduced circuit noise
- Power management system provides optimized battery life
- Low-battery warning
- Contoured matte faceplate provides attractive cosmetics
- Screw-set volume control (red arrow) (CIC only)
- Suitable for mild to severe hearing losses and can fit audiogram configurations ranging from reverse to sloping

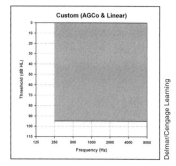

Fitting range for Breeze Custom Linear

Options of Breeze Custom Linear

- Optional telecoil, accessible through push-button switch (canal, half-shell, and full-shell only)
- Optional dual-microphone directionality for improved signal-to-noise ratio, selectable by push button; AI–DI = 5.1 dB (canal, half-shell, and full-shell only)
- Screw-set volume control (red arrow) (canal, half-shell, and full-shell only)
- Power option (canal and full-shell only)

Features of Breeze Custom WDRC

- Digital sound processing for clear, comfortable sound
- 2-channel WDRC
- Choice of 5 controls provide fitting flexibility:
  - Low-channel gain (green dot)
  - High-channel gain (black dot)
  - Crossover frequency (white dot)
  - Maximum power output (blue dot)
  - Threshold knee-point (orange dot)

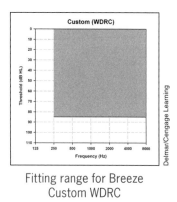

Fitting range for Breeze Custom WDRC

- Controls continuously adjustable in steps for precise adjustment
- Set F counterclockwise for 4000 Hz position, other trimmers counterclockwise for maximum amplification
- Quiet mode expansion for improved sound quality in quiet environments and reduced circuit noise
- Power management system provides optimized battery door
- Low-battery warning
- Contoured matte faceplate provides attractive cosmetics
- Manual volume control (canal, half-shell, and full-shell only)
- Screw-set volume control (red arrow) (CIC only)
- Suitable for mild to severe hearing losses and can fit audiogram configurations ranging from reverse to sloping

Options of Breeze Custom WDRC

- Optional telecoil, accessible through push-button switch (canal, half-shell, and full-shell only)
- Optional dual-microphone directionality for improved signal-to-noise ratio, selectable by push button; AI–DI = 5.1 dB (canal, half-shell, and full-shell only)
- Screw-set volume control (red arrow) (canal, half-shell, and full-shell only)

Typical Specifications		Breeze Mini BTE
Standard ANSI S3.22-1996		
Output sound pressure level	Max OSPL 90 (dB SPL)	130
	HFA OSPL 90 (dB SPL)	124
Full-on gain	Peak gain (dB)	65
	HFA (dB)	60
Total harmonic distortion	500 Hz	<3%
	800 Hz	<3%
	1600 Hz	<3%
Equivalent input noise (dB SPL)		20
Telecoil sensitivity	HFA SPLITS (dB SPL)	106
Battery	Operating current (mA)	1.3
	Battery type	13
	Attack (ms)	<40
	Release (ms)	100
Compression ratio	Wide dynamic range compression	2.9:1 to 1:1

Delmar/Cengage Learning

UNITRON

Typical Specifications		Breeze AGCo Full-Shell Power	Breeze AGCo Full-Shell	Breeze AGCo Canal Power	Breeze AGCo Canal Half-Shell	Breeze AGCo CIC
Standard ANSI						
Output sound pressure level	Max OSPL 90 (dB SPL)	123	117	115	112	112
	HFA OSPL 90 (dB SPL)	116	112	109	107	105
Full-on gain	Peak gain (dB)	50–60	35–55	50	35–45	20–40
	HFA (dB)	44–54	27–47	40–44	27–37	12–32
Total harmonic distortion	500 Hz	5%	5%	5%	5%	5%
	800 Hz	3%	3%	3%	3%	3%
	1600 Hz	3%	3%	3%	3%	3%
Equivalent input noise (dB SPL)		22	20	20	20	19–31
Telecoil sensitivity	HFA SPLITS (dB SPL)	103	90–97	95	91	n/a
Battery	Operating current (mA)	1.1	1.0	1.0	0.9–1.0	0.9
	Battery type	13	13	312	312	10
	Attack (ms)	<10	<10	<10	<10	<10
	Release (ms)	100	100	100	100	100
Compression ratio	AGCo	∞:1	∞:1	∞:1	∞:1	∞:1

Delmar/Cengage Learning

Typical Specifications		Breeze Linear Full-Shell Power	Breeze Linear Full-Shell	Breeze Linear Canal Power	Breeze Linear Canal Half-Shell	Breeze Linear CIC
Standard ANSI S3.22-1996						
Output sound pressure level	Max OSPL 90 (dB SPL)	123	117	115	112	112
	HFA OSPL 90 (dB SPL)	116	112	109	107	105
Full-on gain	Peak gain (dB)	50–60	35–55	50	35–45	20–40
	HFA (dB)	44–54	27–47	40–44	27–37	12–32
Total harmonic distortion	500 Hz	5%	5%	5%	5%	5%
	800 Hz	3%	3%	3%	3%	3%
	1600 Hz	3%	3%	3%	3%	3%
Equivalent input noise (dB SPL)		22	20	20	20	19–31
Telecoil sensitivity	HFA SPLITS (dB SPL)	103	90–97	95	91	n/a
Battery	Operating current (mA)	1.1	1.0	1.0	0.9–1.0	0.9
	Battery type	13	13	312	312	10

Delmar/Cengage Learning

Typical Specifications		Breeze WDRC Full-Shell	Breeze WDRC Canal Half-Shell	Breeze WDRC CIC
Standard ANSI S3.22-1996				
Output sound pressure level	Max OSPL 90 (dB SPL)	96–116	100–110	85–105
	HFA OSPL 90 (dB SPL)	91–110	94–104	78–99
Full-on gain	Peak gain (dB)	35–55	35–45	20–40
	HFA (dB)	28–48	29–39	13–35
Total harmonic distortion	500 Hz	5%	5%	5%
	800 Hz	3%	3%	3%
	1600 Hz	3%	3%	3%
Equivalent input noise (dB SPL)		18–26	22–25	23–37
Telecoil sensitivity	HFA SPLITS (dB SPL)	71–90	74–84	n/a
Battery	Operating current (mA)	0.9	0.8	0.85
	Battery type	13	312	10
	Attack (ms)	70	70	70
	Release (ms)	400	400	400
Compression ratio	WDRC	2.9:1 to 1:1	2.9:1 to 1:1	2.9:1 to 1:1

Delmar/Cengage Learning

PRODUCT 11: AGC-O (CONVENTIONAL)

Product Application

AGC-O Power Full-Shell

AGC-O Full-Shell

AGC-O Canal

AGC-O Half-Shell

AGC-O Mini Canal

AGC-O CIC

Features of AGC-O Power Full-Shell

- Output compression limiting (10:1 ratio) to prevent loudness discomfort
- Standard potentiometers – active low-frequency and output
- Microphone windscreen
- 2-year repair/1-year loss and damage warranty
- Pink color
- Volume control
- Select-A-Vent
- Wax spring

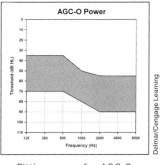

Fitting range for AGC-O Power Full-Shell

Options of AGC-O Power Full-Shell

- Optional potentiometers – high-frequency and gain
- High-power telecoil

UNITRON

- Extended warranty
- Stacked or screw-set volume control
- Colors – pink, tan, cocoa, or brown
- ON/OFF toggle switch
- Belled canal

Features of AGC-O Full-Shell, AGC-O Canal, AGC-O Half-Shell, AGC-O Mini Canal, and AGC-O CIC

- Output compression limiting (10:1 ratio) to prevent loudness discomfort
- Standard potentiometers – compression threshold and active low-frequency
- Microphone windscreen
- 2-year repair/1-year loss and damage warranty
- Pink color (cocoa standard for CIC)
- Volume control
- Select-A-Vent
- Wax spring

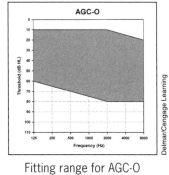

Fitting range for AGC-O Custom

Options of AGC-O Full-Shell, AGC-O Canal, AGC-O Half-Shell, AGC-O Mini Canal, and AGC-O CIC

- Optional potentiometers – high-frequency and gain
- High-power telecoil (AGC-O Full-Shell and AGC-O Canal only)
- Directional microphone
- Extended warranty
- Stacked or screw-set volume control
- Colors – pink, tan, cocoa, or brown
- ON/OFF toggle switch
- Belled canal

Typical Specifications		AGC-O Power Full-Shell	AGC-O Full-Shell, AGC-O Half-Shell, AGC-O Canal	AGC-O Mini Canal & AGC-O CIC
Standard ANSI S3.22-1996				
Output sound pressure level	Max OSPL 90 (dB SPL)	120	115	105
	HFA OSPL 90 (dB SPL)	118	109	102
Full-on gain	Peak gain (dB)	60	50	45
	HFA (dB)	51	45	40

continues

continued

Typical Specifications		AGC-O Power Full-Shell	AGC-O Full-Shell, AGC-O Half-Shell, AGC-O Canal	AGC-O Mini Canal & AGC-O CIC
Total harmonic distortion	800 Hz	<5%	<3%	<3%
	1250 Hz	<5%	<3%	<3%
	2000 Hz	<5%	<3%	<3%
Equivalent input noise (dB SPL)		<24	<24	<24
Telecoil sensitivity	HFA SPLITS (dB SPL)	103	90	n/a
Battery	Operating current (mA)	0.95	0.95	0.5
	Battery type	13	13/312	10
	Attack (ms)	11	2	2
	Release (ms)	86	207	225

Delmar/Cengage Learning

PRODUCT 12: ENHANCED LINEAR (CONVENTIONAL)

Product Application

Enhanced Linear Power Full-Shell
Enhanced Linear Full-Shell
Enhanced Linear Half-Shell
Enhanced Linear Canal
Enhanced Linear Mini Canal
Enhanced Linear CIC

Features of Enhanced Linear Power Full-Shell, Enhanced Linear Full-Shell, Enhanced Linear Half-Shell, Enhanced Linear Canal, Enhanced Linear Mini Canal, and Enhanced Linear CIC

- Linear with Class D Response
- Standard potentiometers – active low-frequency
- Microphone windscreen
- 2-year repair/1-year loss and damage warranty
- Pink color (cocoa standard for CIC)
- Volume control
- Wax spring

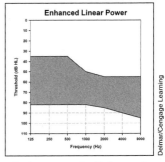

Fitting range for Enhanced Linear Power Full-Shell

Options of Enhanced Linear Power Full-Shell, Enhanced Linear Full-Shell, Enhanced Linear Half-Shell, Enhanced Linear Canal, Enhanced Linear Mini Canal, and Enhanced Linear CIC

- Optional potentiometers – high-frequency and gain
- High-power telecoil (excludes Enhanced Linear Mini Canal and Enhanced Linear CIC)
- Directional microphone (excludes Enhanced Linear Power Full-Shell)
- Extended warranty
- Stacked or screw-set volume control
- Colors – pink, tan, cocoa, or brown
- ON/OFF toggle switch
- Belled canal

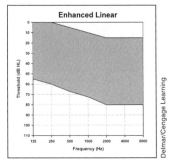

Fitting range for Enhanced Linear Custom

Typical Specifications		Enhanced Linear Power Full-Shell	Enhanced Linear Full-Shell, Enhanced Linear Half-Shell, and Enhanced Linear Canal	Enhanced Linear Mini Canal and Enhanced Linear CIC
Standard ANSI S3.22-1996				
Output sound pressure level	Max OSPL 90 (dB SPL)	125	117	112
	HFA OSPL 90 (dB SPL)	122	115	110
Full-on gain	Peak gain (dB)	60	50	45
	HFA (dB)	52	45	40
Total harmonic distortion	800 Hz	<5%	<3%	<3%
	1250 Hz	<5%	<3%	<3%
	2000 Hz	<5%	<3%	<3%
Equivalent input noise (dB SPL)		<23	<20	<20
Telecoil sensitivity	HFA SPLITS (dB SPL)	103	95	n/a
Battery	Operating current (mA)	0.95	0.95	0.5
	Battery type	13	13/312	10

Delmar/Cengage Learning

PRODUCT 13: US 80 CONVENTIONAL

Product Application

US 80 PP BTE
US 80 PPL BTE

Features of US 80 PP BTE and US 80 PPL BTE

- 4 controls provide full fitting flexibility:
  - L – low-cut tone
  - H – active high-cut
  - P – power
  - G – gain
- Controls continuously adjustable with end stops
- Adjustable gain control provides high-to-super power gain
- Powerful CI receiver for more distortion-free power
- Advanced AVM™ microphone with lower sensitivity to vibration helps reduce feedback problems
- Powerful push–pull amplifier
- Powerful telecoil
- Gain independent of maximum power output
- Surface-mount technology
- Volume control – numbered 1 (low) to 4 (high)
- M–T–O switch – 3 positions: microphone–telecoil–OFF
- Direct audio input – MLx-compatible
- 2-tone, beige/taupe housing
- Unfiltered earhook
- Fitting is supported by NOAH-compatible Unifit or Standalone Unifit
- Extended low-frequency hearing loss and left corner audiograms (US 80 PPL BTE only)
- Suitable for fitting severe to profound hearing losses

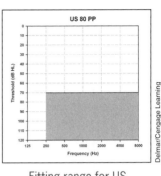

Fitting range for US 80 PP BTE

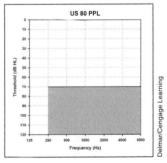

Fitting range for US 80 PPL BTE

Options of US 80 PP BTE and US 80 PPL BTE

- Tamper-resistant battery compartment/volume control cover
- CROS/BiCROS

UNITRON

- Filtered earhook
- Child-sized earhook
- Taupe, gray/taupe, brown/taupe housings

Technical data sheets not available for US 80 PP and US 80 PPL BTE Conventional.

PRODUCT 14: UE 10 AND UE 12 CONVENTIONAL

Product Application

UE 10 BTE
UE 12 PP BTE
UE 12 PPL BTE

Features of UE 10 BTE

- Powerful push–pull amplifier
- 3 controls provide full fitting flexibility:
  - C – compression
  - T – active low-cut tone
  - P – power control
- Controls continuously adjustable with end stops
- Powerful telecoil
- Frequency-dependent input compression (PDC)
- Adjustable compression threshold of 30 dB
- Low harmonic distortion
- Surface-mount technology
- Volume control numbered – 1 (low) to 4 (high)
- M–T–O switch – 3 positions: microphone–telecoil–OFF
- Unfiltered earhook
- Fitting is supported by NOAH-compatible Unifit or Standalone Unifit
- Suitable for fitting moderately severe to profound hearing losses including recruitment and discrimination problems

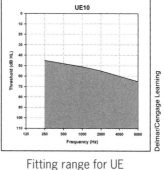

Fitting range for UE 10 BTE

Options of UE 10 BTE

- Filtered earhook
- Child-sized earhook

Features of UE 12 PP BTE

- Powerful push–pull amplifier
- 3 controls provide full fitting flexibility:
  - P – power control
  - G – gain
  - T – low-cut tone

- Controls continuously adjustable with end stops
- Powerful telecoil
- Gain independent of maximum power output
- Surface-mount technology
- Volume control numbered – 1 (low) to 4 (high)
- M–T–O switch – 3 positions: microphone–telecoil–OFF
- Unfiltered earhook
- Fitting is supported by NOAH-compatible Unifit or Standalone Unifit
- Suitable for fitting moderate to severe/ profound hearing losses including fluctuating or progressive losses

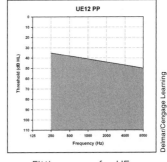

Fitting range for UE 12 PP BTE

Options of UE 12 PP BTE

- Filtered earhook
- Child-sized earhook

Features of UE 12 PPL BTE

- Powerful push–pull amplifier
- 3 controls provide full fitting flexibility:
  - P – power control
  - G – gain
  - T – low-cut tone
- Controls continuously adjustable with end stops
- Powerful telecoil
- Adjustable gain control provides moderate-to-high gain

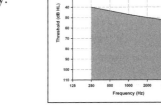

Fitting range for UE 12 PPL BTE

- Gain independent of maximum power output
- Surface-mount technology
- Volume control numbered – 1 (low) to 4 (high)
- M–T–O switch – 3 positions: microphone–telecoil–OFF
- Unfiltered earhook
- Fitting is supported by NOAH-compatible Unifit or Standalone Unifit
- Suitable for fitting moderate to severe/profound hearing losses including left corner audiograms

Options of UE 12 PPL BTE

- Direct audio input
- CROS/BiCROS
- Filtered earhook
- Child-sized earhook

Technical data sheets not available for UE 10 and UE 12 Conventional.

UNITRON

PRODUCT 15: UM60 CONVENTIONAL

Product Application

UM60 AGCo Mini-BTE
UM60 Mini-BTE
UM60 D Mini-BTE
UM60 H Mini-BTE
UM60 PP BTE

Features of UM60 AGCo Mini-BTE

- Output compression
- Powerful telecoil
- 2 controls provide fitting flexibility:
  - T – active tone control
  - P – power control
- Controls continuously adjustable with end stops
- Gain independent of maximum power output
- Surface-mount technology
- Volume control numbered – 1 (low) to 4 (high)
- M–T–O switch – 3 positions: microphone–telecoil–OFF
- Slim mini-housing
- Unfiltered earhook
- Fitting is supported by NOAH-compatible Unifit or Standalone Unifit
- Suitable for fitting mild to moderately severe hearing losses

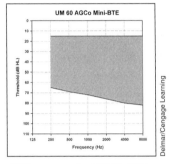

Fitting range for UM60 AGCo Mini-BTE

Options of UM60 AGCo Mini-BTE

- Filtered earhook
- Child-sized earhook
- Brown or gray housing

Features of UM60 Mini-BTE

- Powerful telecoil
- Gain tied to maximum power output
- 2 controls provide fitting flexibility:
  - T – low-cut tone
  - P –power
- Controls continuously adjustable with end stops
- Surface-mount technology
- Volume control – numbered 1 (low) to 4 (high)

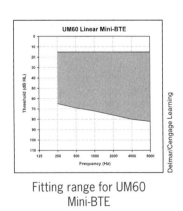

Fitting range for UM60 Mini-BTE

- M–T–O switch – 3 positions: microphone–telecoil–OFF
- Slim mini-housing
- Unfiltered earhook
- Fitting is supported by NOAH-compatible Unifit or Standalone Unifit
- Suitable for fitting mild to moderately severe hearing losses

Options of UM60 Mini-BTE

- Filtered earhook
- Child-sized earhook
- Brown or gray housing

Features of UM60 D Mini-BTE

- Frequency-dependent input compression (FDC)
- Directional microphone
- Powerful telecoil
- 2 controls provide fitting flexibility:
  - T – active tone control
  - P – power control
- Controls continuously adjustable with end stops
- Gain tied to maximum power output
- Surface-mount technology
- Volume control – numbered 1 (low) to 4 (high)
- M–T–O switch – 3 positions: microphone–telecoil–OFF
- Slim mini-housing
- Filtered earhook
- Fitting supported by NOAH-compatible Unifit or Standalone Unifit
- Suitable for fitting mild to moderate high-frequency hearing losses

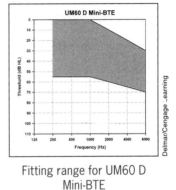

Fitting range for UM60 D
Mini-BTE

Options of UM60 D Mini-BTE

- Direct audio input
- CROS/BiCROS
- Unfiltered earhook
- Child-sized earhook
- Brown or gray housing

Features of UM60 H Mini-BTE

- Frequency-dependent input compression (FDC)
- Powerful telecoil
- 2 controls provide fitting flexibility:
  - T – active low-cut tone
  - P – power control

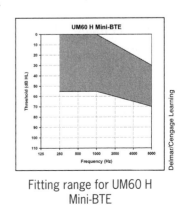

Fitting range for UM60 H
Mini-BTE

- Controls continuously adjustable with end stops
- Gain tied to maximum power output
- Volume control – numbered 1 (low) to 4 (high)
- M–T–O switch – 3 positions: microphone–telecoil–OFF
- Slim mini-housing
- Filtered earhook
- Suitable for fitting mild to moderate high-frequency hearing losses

Options of UM60 H Mini-BTE

- Unfiltered earhook
- Child-sized earhook
- Brown or gray housing

Features of UM60 PP BTE

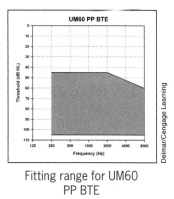

- Powerful push–pull amplifier
- Powerful telecoil
- Gain independent of maximum power output
- Surface-mount technology
- 2 controls provide fitting flexibility:
  - T – active low-cut tone
  - P – power control
- Controls continuously adjustable with end stops
- Extended-range active tone control
- Volume control numbered – 1 (low) to 4 (high)
- M–T–O switch – 3 positions: microphone–telecoil–OFF
- Slim mini-housing
- Unfiltered earhook
- Fitting is supported by NOAH-compatible Unifit or Standalone Unifit
- Suitable for fitting moderately severe to severe hearing losses

Fitting range for UM60 PP BTE

Options of UM60 PP BTE

- Direct audio input
- CROS/BiCROS
- Filtered earhook
- Child-sized earhook
- Brown or gray housing

Technical data sheets not available for UM60 series.

CHAPTER TWELVE

Tinnitus and the Hearing Instrument Marketplace

*"Only my ears whistle and buzz continuously day and night. I can say
I am living a wretched life. . . ."*

Ludwig van Beethoven, 1801

Tinnitus is one of those phenomena that is almost easier to define by exclusion. Tinnitus is *not*, for instance, voices in your head. Tinnitus is *not* that 20 seconds of ringing everyone gets in one ear once in a while. Tinnitus *is* any number of sounds that are perceived for which there is no external, physical stimulus. Clinically significant tinnitus is characterized as constant, severe, and unrelieved (Erlandsson, 2000). These sounds, while most often described as "ringing" (one or a few pure tones), can have any number of other percepts, including buzzing, humming, whooshing, rushing, roaring, whistling, and so on.

Hearing professionals vary drastically in the amount of their tinnitus training Therefore, this chapter is designed to provide a broad view of epidemiology, various types of tinnitus management techniques that use sound therapy—namely, tinnitus masking (TM) and tinnitus retraining therapy (TRT)—and the efficacy of these techniques, and to provide the reader with a list of resources that provide a comprehensive background on these topics as well as clinical implementation. As this book is related to hearing instruments, the various topics that are covered will be discussed in relation to hearing instruments. Therefore, the discussed tinnitus management techniques will be limited to those that include sound therapy, typically in the form of a wearable device.

The specific epidemiological data for tinnitus is difficult to quantify. A number of studies have been performed and report varying results. While unreliable in their absolute numbers, several trends are consistent across these studies. The overall prevalence of tinnitus ranges from 4.4 percent to over 15 percent in the adult population (see Hoffman & Reed, 2004 for a summary of the epidemiological studies). Roughly ten studies suggest that tinnitus prevalence and age are strongly correlated. Most studies are in agreement that the prevalence of tinnitus for persons under 30 is less than 10 percent (Hoffman & Reed, 2004; Davis & Refaie, 2000). This prevalence remains under 10 percent until 50-plus years of age. At that age, prevalence increases, peaks around the sixties or seventies, and then tapers off in the eighties. The peak prevalence ranges from 7.9 to 44 percent (Hoffman & Reed, 2004; Davis & Refaie, 2000). This contrasts with hearing-loss data, in which the prevalence continues to increase with age (Lockwood et al., 2002). Using these numbers and current population estimates, Henry et al. (2002) approximated there to be 40 to 50 million persons in the United States with tinnitus; 2.5 million of those are affected severely enough to be considered debilitated. Because of the vastly varying degrees of severity, it's logical to deal with tinnitus patients differently depending on how severe they report their tinnitus to be.

It is well known that noise exposure is one of the most common causes of tinnitus. Military personnel are particularly prone to tinnitus, especially during times of war. Tinnitus is the most common disability related to ongoing conflicts. In 2006, 395,000 veterans were service-connected for tinnitus, 51,360 of whom became service-connected in 2006 (Veterans Benefits Administration, 2006, 17). Similarly, tinnitus is the second most prevalent disability in the Veterans Administration, second only to hearing loss, which affects 444,583 veterans (Veterans Benefits Administration, 2006, 14). In 2007, it was reported that between March and June, 176,000 U.S. veterans of ongoing conflicts (Iraq and Afghanistan) applied for disability compensation. The most common complaint was tinnitus, for which 36,000 claims were granted, followed by back strain (33,000) and post-traumatic stress disorder (16,000) (Hoffman, 2007). Tinnitus has been extremely costly; in 2005, the Veterans Administration paid $418 million in tinnitus-related disability payments (Lite, 2007).

The common lore among hearing professionals is that the vast majority of tinnitus patients can be treated successfully with hearing aids. Some take a more nuanced approach to define the "vast majority" to include their patients with mild to moderate tinnitus. Admittedly, the proposition is attractive. It's a two-for-one deal: Treat the first complaint with hearing aids, and the added (read: free to the patient) bonus is de facto tinnitus relief. Even though the number debilitated by tinnitus is in the millions, it represents just a few percent of those who experience tinnitus. So, do hearing aids really do that well? The answer is not quite as promising as the lore suggests. The assumption, which is consistent with dispensing practice, is that the hearing aid is used without any additional tinnitus management (e.g., counseling). The following studies are consistent with this assumption. One study reports that only 7 percent of patients experience tinnitus relief with hearing aids (Vernon & Meikle,

2000). Another study, including 598 patients, reported that hearing aids were effective for only 16 percent of patients (Dobie & Sullivan, 1997). A recent survey reported a bit more success. This survey reported that 22.1 percent of tinnitus patients received major relief with the use of hearing aids, while 21.4 and 16.6 percent received moderate and minor relief, respectively. Fortunately, even though a sizeable 39 percent received no relief, only 1.7 percent of tinnitus patients' tinnitus worsened (Kochkin & Tyler, 2008). Why was this survey so much more optimistic than two studies previously discussed? Perhaps the answer is in the method employed. The two studies were follow-up studies, where the patients were the source of the data. The respondents to the survey, on the other hand, were hearing professionals, which is a less direct source of information than patient responses. In my estimation, it would be easy for this survey to be tainted by the hearing professionals' biases that hearing aids are a truly successful approach to treating tinnitus patients. Regardless, the fact remains that when tinnitus patients are surveyed about their own experiences with hearing aids, they report that hearing instruments are not effective at relieving their tinnitus.

Clearly, there are appropriate situations in which hearing aids are likely to assist in tinnitus relief. Hearing loss notwithstanding, the use of hearing aids in tinnitus management may depend on the management techniques one is employing. For instance, for TM, it has been suggested that hearing aids may be more beneficial for those with non-high-pitch tinnitus (Vernon & Meikle, 2004, 329–330). Alternatively, if one is using TRT, the use of hearing aids in sound enrichment largely depends on the "category" of patient (Jastreboff & Jastreboff, 2000, 111).

When the data addressing various questions about tinnitus are reviewed together, it is clear that tinnitus is a real problem that is not being addressed adequately. First, there are many tinnitus sufferers, and millions who are debilitated by it. Second, hearing aids have not proven themselves to be terribly helpful, at least in the eyes of the patient. The field of hearing professionals needs to take a more active approach, both in therapy and devices, in addressing their tinnitus patients' needs.

How Can I Help My Patient?

A few topics need to be addressed to understand current ways to truly help tinnitus patients. First, I will summarize two of the more common tinnitus management techniques that include sound therapy as a critical component of the management regimen (after all, this *is* a book on hearing-related devices): tinnitus masking and tinnitus retraining therapy. Second, since both therapies use sound therapy as part of the regimen, the success of these therapies will be discussed. Third, products consisting of wearable devices will be summarized. Of course, there are other tinnitus management strategies, such as cognitive—behavioral therapy (CBT), that are applied to tinnitus. The goal of CBT is to apply cognitive and behavioral therapies to help the tinnitus patient to modify

TINNITUS

negative thought patterns and behaviors. However, since this and other tinnitus management regimens do not prescribe sound therapy, it will not be described in detail. A list of excellent texts is included later in the chapter that provides detailed descriptions of available strategies, measurement tools, epidemiological data, and even guides to implement these strategies.

Certainly, many more management regimens exist besides TM and TRT; however, many are not appropriate for hearing professionals or do not include sound therapy. These two are of particular interest to hearing professionals, as some form of sound therapy is prescribed. The primary mode of sound therapy includes a wearable device (e.g., hearing aid) or personal music player (PMP) form factor. In terms of the method of treatment, there is considerable disagreement over the actual "best" formula for employing TRT. It is not my intent to pick one, or even to cover every available combination, but rather to give a broad foundation of the variety of implementations as they are described by the referenced authors. There are several books, tutorial articles, and courses on TRT available for any clinician desiring to maximize impact in helping tinnitus patients.

Tinnitus masking is a straightforward use of sound therapy. As the name suggests, TM uses sounds to obscure the perception of tinnitus. Counseling is not required for TM. In the clinical setting, certain criteria are established (e.g., pitch and loudness) for the tinnitus, allowing the hearing professional to program the device. The programming can vary greatly depending on the device, the patient profile, and the philosophy to which the hearing professional subscribes. If the device can only present one type of noise (e.g., white or pink noise), it is reasonable to expect no real programming for the noise, except to ensure that the user has control of when to activate the sound and control over the volume. Other devices are more sophisticated, having complex, programmable filters for differing selections of noise. One way to think about TM is that it is a step up from amplification through the use of hearing aids. With hearing aids, the sound therapy is the amplified sound and sometimes circuit noise (one tinnitus masker actually used a noisy hearing-aid circuit to generate the masking noise). TM increases the intervention by generating the therapeutic sound, which, depending on the sophistication of the device, can allow considerable control over the acoustic characteristics of the sound.

While TM is simply the practice of adding more sound to the phantom sounds the patient already hears, it has also been shown to be quite effective. Available products have increased in sophistication in that in addition to presenting a broadband noise, complex filtering and narrow-band noise generators have been introduced. Furthermore, so-called "combination devices" that include the tinnitus masker with the hearing aid have been available for some time. The product line has been a moving target as the tinnitus market has been largely undeveloped. Products from major hearing instrument manufacturers and start-up companies come and go rather quickly, often without a replacement. Later in this chapter, I will provide a discussion of why this is.

While there is no formal training in TM of which I am aware, it is important for any hearing professional to become well-versed in the literature before making TM a regular practice with patients. There are many misconceptions to TM. One example is the use of the term "masking." Though technically correct, it lends itself to the idea that the patients' tinnitus ought to be completely obscured by the masking noise. The confusion in this case is not making the distinction between partial and complete masking. This small error will absolutely lead to extremely poor success rates, as the masking levels can be quite bothersome and can even worsen tinnitus.

Tinnitus retraining therapy addresses tinnitus from a much more complex vantage point. TRT is based on the neurophysiological mechanisms of tinnitus (Jastreboff & Jastreboff, 2000; Kaltenbach, 2000). As a result, TRT has a much more complex philosophy incorporating not only the entire auditory pathway but also the impacts of tinnitus as a neural signal on the entire central nervous system. As graduate programs typically do not include much training in tinnitus, it behooves any audiologist who aspires to be effective in treating severe tinnitus patients to take a training course. In the following paragraphs, I will provide a description of the philosophy underlying TRT as well as its general implementation.

Tinnitus retraining therapy is based on the neurophysiological mechanisms of tinnitus (Jastreboff & Jastreboff, 2000; Kaltenbach, 2000). The essence of the model is that it accounts for cortical systems that go beyond mechanisms specific to hearing. Specifically, the model describes a relationship between the auditory system and the limbic and autonomic nervous systems. The driving force behind the model is that through the tinnitus experience, an association between the tinnitus and a strong, negative reaction (i.e. anxiety, stress, etc.) is made. It is precisely this association, rather than the actual tinnitus, that leads to the perception of severity. The goal, therefore, of TRT is to disassociate the perception of tinnitus from the reaction to tinnitus. This disassociation is the first part of the habituation process. The second part of habituation is the reduction in awareness of the tinnitus. Since the tinnitus is actually still occurring, the habituation likely manifests to modulate the patient's attention away from the tinnitus, with the patient thus becoming unaware that it is there.

Tinnitus retraining therapy places any individual patient's experience into one of five categories (Henry et al., 2002; Henry et al., 2007; Jastreboff & Hazel, 2004; Jastreboff & Jastreboff, 1999). Category 0 describes a patient with mild tinnitus from which there is little impact on his or her life. Category 1 patients experience tinnitus with high severity, and hearing loss is absent. Category 2 patients have the indicators in Category 1 as well as hearing loss. Category 3 includes patients with significant hyperacusis who may or may not have tinnitus. This category also includes patients that have tinnitus as the primary complaint, in conjunction with hyperacusis. Finally, Category 4 patients present with tinnitus and/or hyperacusis that worsen with sound exposure. Category 4 patients are considered to be the most difficult to treat (Jastreboff & Hazell, 2004).

Two critical components of TRT to achieve habituation are the enrichment of patients' auditory environment and directive counseling. Enriching one's listening experience is achieved through the use of external sound generators. These generators are typically wearable devices, but can include other devices such as desktop noise generators. Often the wearable device the so-called "tinnitus masker" can be used in TRT. Unlike TM, the sound therapy component is not used for instant relief from tinnitus. Rather, the relief experienced by patients in TRT occurs within several months of the program. The sound generator should have the following attributes: (1) should allow the listener to hear natural sounds, (2) should slowly increase the level from soft to listening level (note that the listening level should be such that the tinnitus is still perceived), (3) should have a broad frequency response, (4) should have a steady spectrum, and (5) should have acceptable aesthetics (Jastreboff & Hazell, 2004, 120; Jastreboff & Jastreboff, 2000). Of course, the chosen sound should be pleasing to the patient, so as not to cause further negative reactions (Jastreboff & Hazell, 2004, 120).

The second critical component of TRT, directive counseling, further helps the patient in the habituation process. The main goal of counseling is to help the patient remove negative thoughts related to the tinnitus (Jastreboff & Hazell, 2004). In that regard, sound therapy without counseling is not likely to result in a successful outcome (Jastreboff & Jastreboff, 2000). In the counseling sessions, tinnitus is described as an innocuous by-product of normal human function. Also, the neurophysiological model is conveyed to the patient in a manner accessible to the patient (Jastreboff & Hazell, 2004, 85).

Whichever treatment method is chosen, it is in the best interest of the patient for the hearing practitioner to be as well-informed as possible. With the availability of peer review research, instructional texts, and courses, there is no excuse to be practicing in your technical scope of practice without the proper information to practice ethically. A recent survey reported that only 44 percent of respondents (hearing care professionals who treat tinnitus) have never taken a course in tinnitus[1] (Kochkin & Tyler, 2008). Tinnitus manifests quite differently than hearing loss; the therapies for tinnitus are customized not just to the disorder, but to the individual's experience as well. It is paramount that those incorporating tinnitus treatment in their practice have the proper background to do so.

To assist in your understanding of each treatment method, including design, underlying philosophy, and clinical implementation, below is a list of excellent books on the topic. Also, there are several tutorial articles in various

---

[1] It should be added that the survey report did not include information on self-study of tinnitus treatment, for which there are excellent resources. Therefore, it is possible that 44 percent may be an overestimate of those not prepared to treat tinnitus.

journals (e.g., Journal of the American Academy of Audiology) in the reference section:

Henry, J. A., Trune, D. R., Robb, M. J. A., & Jastreboff, P. J. (2007). *Tinnitus Retraining Therapy: Clinical Guidelines.* San Diego, CA, Plural Publishing, Inc.

Jastreboff, P. J., & Hazell, J. W. (2004). *Tinnitus Retraining Therapy: Implementing the Neurophysiological Model.* Cambridge UK, Cambridge University Press.

Snow, J. B. (2004). *Tinnitus: Theory and Management.* Hamilton, Ontario, BC Becker, Inc.

Tyler, R. S. (2000). *Tinnitus Handbook.* San Diego, USA, Singular.

Tyler, R. S. (2005). *Tinnitus Treatment: Clinical Protocols.* New York, NY, Thieme.

Effectiveness

Tinnitus masking and TRT are two frequently used methods for clinical management of tinnitus. Both of these methods have a long history of development, application, and refinement, as well as a track record of clinical success (Henry et al., 2002, 560).

Tinnitus retraining therapy and tinnitus masking are the two most common therapies designed to treat tinnitus; both prescribe sound therapy in moderate and severe cases. TRT is a therapy protocol that is designed to help the sufferer habituate to the tinnitus according to a neurophysiological model. In TRT, once the assessment of the tinnitus is made, a combination of directive counseling and sound therapy is provided. The sound therapy is a critical component that allows an externally generated sound to "blend" with the sufferer's tinnitus. Generally, the therapy can persist up to 18 months. TM, on the other hand, is a protocol designed for immediate relief. In that regard, the sound therapy is presented at a level that partially masks the tinnitus, therefore providing relief to the sufferer.

Several studies have been performed assessing the efficacy of TRT and TM. The more recent studies employed more rigorous and controlled methods. Therefore, the more recent studies will be reviewed and the less controlled studies will be used as supporting evidence to the more recent, more controlled studies.

Henry et al. (2006) conducted a controlled, clinical study that included 118 patients. This 18-month study investigated the efficacy of TRT and TM. Five validated assessment tools were used to assess the severity of tinnitus before, during, and after treatment. These tools have been validated for internal consistency and reliability. In their extensive findings, TRT was found to be more effective in severe cases of tinnitus, though TM was still effective. However, in moderate cases of tinnitus, both TRT and TM were similarly effective. Specifically, the more severely afflicted patients were aware of their tinnitus 77.8 percent of the time before the TM therapy and only 33.2 percent of the time after 18 months of TM therapy. Patients treated with TRT were aware of their tinnitus 66.5 percent of the time before treatment and only 14.7 percent of the time after 18 months. In terms of how often patients were annoyed by their tinnitus, the TM-treated patients were annoyed 52.6 percent of the time before and 24.2 percent of the time after 18 months of TM therapy, while TRT-treated patients were annoyed 47.3 percent of the time before and 6.3 percent of the time after TRT treatment. Overall, 88 percent of the patients treated with TRT showed significant improvements as defined by a greater-than-or-equal-to 5-point improvement on their tinnitus severity index (Henry as cited in Jastreboff & Jastreboff, 2006).

Another interesting study investigated the effectiveness of the use of ear-level devices, which included hearing instruments and noise generators (Folmer & Carroll, 2006). One hundred fifty patients were split evenly into three groups: a hearing aid group, a noise generator group, and a control group who did not use any ear-level device. All three groups participated in other aspects of tinnitus treatment that did not include sound therapy. While all three groups showed improvement after 18 months, the two groups who used ear-level devices showed greater improvement. They concluded that ear-level devices offer benefits beyond those of other tinnitus management techniques (e.g., counseling) alone.

Herraiz et al. (2005) studied TRT in 158 tinnitus patients over a period of 12 months. According to a self-evaluation of the patients, a 78 percent and 82 percent improvement was observed after 6 and 12 months, respectively. Patients who followed through on the TRT treatment improved more than patients who discontinued the treatment.

Jastreboff (1998) reported on 152 consecutive patients who received treatment for a 6-month period. Success was defined as a minimum of 20 percent improvement in two of three outcome areas (performance of daily activities affected by tinnitus, annoyance resulting from tinnitus, and percentage of time of tinnitus awareness). Of 152 patients, 129 used sound therapy and directive counseling. Jastreboff reported that 81.4 percent of these patients met the success criteria. Similarly, Jastreboff (1999) reported data from 223 patients from his clinic, all of whom used sound therapy. Employing the same criteria for success as in his 1998 study, he reported an 81 percent improvement.

Sheldrake et al. (1999) performed a retrospective study of 483 patients from the London Tinnitus and Hyperacusis Center. Of this pool, 224 patients received full TRT. Their criteria for improvement were a 40 percent improvement in annoyance and awareness, or a 40 percent improvement in annoyance or awareness plus an improvement/facilitation of a life factor. Of the 224 TRT patients, 83.9 percent met these rather strict criteria.

McKinney et al. (1999) studied the benefit of tinnitus therapy in 182 patients. Success was met when a minimum of 40 percent improvement was made in two or more scales evaluating the effects of tinnitus. These scales included annoyance (from the tinnitus), impact of tinnitus on quality of life, tinnitus loudness, and percentage of time of awareness. Of the 182 patients, 148 received counseling and sound therapy (54 counseling only; 72 ear-level sound generators; 56 hearing aids). Of those who received counseling only, 72.2 percent improved.

Of those who used hearing aids only, 70.7 percent improved. Of those using sound generators set to a particularly low level, or "just audible level," 75 percent improved. Of those receiving the "truest" form of TRT (higher level of sound presentation), 83.3 percent improved. These various success figures give a range of what would be a reasonably expected benefit given the various treatments. However, data from this and the other studies discussed support the notion that benefit is maximized when sound therapy is used as part of TRT.

Bartnik et al. (1999) studied the benefits of TRT by randomly selecting 120 patients from a pool of 556. Next, they created five groups based on severity. Each group included 24 patients. All patients were treated for at least 12 months. Overall, 77.6 percent of the patients improved. Of patients exhibiting hyperacusis as the primary complaint, 75 percent improved. Of the patients with mild tinnitus, (Category 0) 93 percent improved. Patients with severe tinnitus (Category 1) and severe tinnitus with hearing loss (Category 2) improved at rates of 83 percent and 71 percent, respectively. Finally, 67 percent of the patients with prolonged, loud tinnitus (Category 4) improved.

Herraiz et al. (1999) reported follow-up evaluations from 84 patients after a year of tinnitus treatment. Three criteria were used to determine significant improvement: patient report of improvement (better, worse, or no change), the Tinnitus Handicap Inventory (Newman et al., 1998), and visual analog scale of tinnitus intensity. Of their patient pool, 37 percent received directive counseling, 37 percent received counseling plus sound therapy, and 46 percent received counseling plus hearing aids. Of those who received counseling only, 93.7 percent improved. For the patients who received counseling along with sound therapy, 83.3 percent improved. For those who received counseling plus hearing aids, 84.2 percent improved. Overall, an 88.1 percent success rate was noted for all three groups combined.

From the nine studies reviewed, two trends become apparent. First, there is notable variability in how TRT and TM are employed. Second, despite the variability of treatment protocol, the use of sound therapy as part of tinnitus management shows a consistent success rate that typically exceeds 80 percent. The consistency and high levels of success across all these studies supports the use of sound therapy in tinnitus therapy regimens.

What Is Out There, and What Is Needed?

There are several products available. Historically, products have come and gone due to their limited success. General Hearing Instruments (GHI) is an exception to this; they have been producing wearable sound generators for years with considerable success. There are several start-up companies developing tinnitus products; a couple will be described.

GHI is the nation's leader in tinnitus products. I believe this is due to not only their strong record of customer support but their genuine dedication to the tinnitus population. They have several tinnitus devices; refer to Chapter 3 for a complete description of each device.

TINNITUS

Beltone has introduced a product line of tinnitus devices, the Tinnitus Breaker™, which includes most form factors common to hearing aids—CIC, ITC, open-fit, and BTE. Beltone's combination device has the ability to generate white noise as well as having all of the features of their Reach™ hearing aid, making it a great solution for the vast majority of tinnitus patients, as most have concurrent hearing loss.

Neuromonics Inc. (a combination of "neural" and "harmonics"), formerly Tinnitech, Inc., is a company that produces a tinnitus sound therapy device. The hardware is similar to a PMP with high-quality earphones. Instead of simply selling the device, Neuromonics describes a complete, 6-month customized therapy (Neuromonics, 2009). Unfortunately, being a PMP-style device, there is no hearing-aid capability, hence requiring the vast majority of patients to buy two sets of products.

Sonitus Medical is a start-up company developing a line of products relating to an interesting application of bone conduction. Their patents describe some form of oral appliance that is connected to an oscillator. Apparently, they are seeking to develop a line of devices, including hearing aids and a tinnitus masker. At the time of this writing, the specifics of their application are unclear; however, this technology has the potential to challenge the status quo.

Why Isn't There More Out There?

The technology to build effective, user-friendly combination devices makes the product development a minimal exercise in engineering from a research-and-development perspective. Sufficient intellectual property exists outlining various protocols for fitting and device specifications to make reasonable products. So, why aren't these products more prevalent? The problem has been well-established: There are millions of patients in the United States, not to mention tens of millions worldwide, with tinnitus severe enough to greatly impact their quality of life and ability to thrive. These are the patients who benefit most from sound therapy. Sufficient products exist, even if not for long enough to penetrate the market. GHI has been making tinnitus products for years. Neuromonics has aggressively pursued the U.S. market, especially Veterans Affairs, where tinnitus is a particular problem. Major hearing-aid manufacturers have introduced and discontinued products due to their lack of success. Why then, aren't products "sticking," at least in the U.S. market, if (1) patient need them (which they do) and (2) the products are effective (which they generally are)?

In my view, the main obstacle involves the relationship of manufacturer expectations (or rather, their understanding of the market), and the path of the tinnitus patient. Hearing instrument manufacturers have tended to treat the tinnitus market like the hearing-aid market. In the U.S., this doesn't work. For example, a person with hearing loss makes an appointment with his or her medical practitioner (MP), often a general practitioner or otolaryngologist. Once the MP becomes aware of hearing loss, he or she will typically refer the patient for a hearing evaluation and mention the possibility of hearing aids. The MP will often provide medical clearance for hearing aids during that office visit. Alternatively, the patient is aware of his or her own hearing loss and will go directly to a hearing professional. In either case, the path of the patient is known and predictable. The end result is that the patient ends up at the hearing professional's office.

On the surface, it seems that the path of the tinnitus patient would be similar to the hearing-aid patient. To understand this, one must grapple with the experience of the severe tinnitus sufferer. First, let's consider the differences in experiences for someone who might have hearing loss versus someone who might have tinnitus with or without hearing loss. Hearing loss, in a manner of speaking, is passive. If you sit in your living room chair with no one around, it is quiet. In some ways, sleep might even be enhanced due to the reduced perception of external sounds. The problems for people with hearing losses arise when they are in communication situations, but if burdened by them, or feeling psychologically vulnerable, they can escape to a quiet place. The experience of tinnitus, however, is active. There is no escape from tinnitus, especially for the severe tinnitus patient. Sitting in your quiet house might be the most troubling. Tinnitus patients often report difficult falling and/or staying asleep. Even in my own experience as a mild/moderate tinnitus sufferer, there have been many times I have been woken up by my tinnitus. To say that this is not one of my favorite experiences in life is an understatement.

Unfortunately, as tinnitus severity increases, so does the psychological impact. Tinnitus has often been described as paralleling chronic pain (Erlandsson, 2000). Many patients report that the severity of their tinnitus fluctuates over time. Often, there is no obvious trigger to times of increased severity. So there are two characteristics that are different for the tinnitus patient than for the hearing-loss patient. One is that there is no control over the severity of the tinnitus. Second, the experience during these severe times can be quite debilitating. The psychological impact of this can be dramatic. There is an increased prevalence of depression and low self-esteem, sometimes leading the patient to grasp at straws to find ways to manage the tinnitus (Erlandsson, 2000). Numerous patients have reported that MPs tell them there is nothing they can do and they'll just have to live with it. The patient, then, is not made aware that there are professionals who are not only capable of treating tinnitus for which there is no cure, but can have great success in doing so.

The problem is worsened when manufacturers of tinnitus-therapy devices try to reach their market. Hearing professionals, especially audiologists, would appear to be the natural target for manufacturers. But with the large number of tinnitus patients being turned away at the medical practitioner level, hearing professionals don't ever get access to a large percentage of the patients seeking medical attention. Manufacturers and hearing professionals have had difficulty in getting a receptive audience from MPs for tinnitus patient referrals. It appears that many medical practitioners really don't want to deal with debilitated tinnitus patients, and so many sufferers don't get help.

TINNITUS

As a result of all these factors, the simple way to describe the U.S. tinnitus market is "undeveloped." Major hearing instrument manufacturers are unlikely to make great strides in this market, as it is expensive to do so. The eye is on start-up companies to make the efforts to penetrate this market. The challenge for start-ups is even greater, as most investors demand early success, which does not lend itself well to developing a distribution market. Start-up companies are also limited in their financial and human capital, which puts serious strain on their ability to get the product out and work on a second-generation product. Nevertheless, whoever has success in doing so will likely open the floodgates of product offering from several manufacturers.

Hearing-Related Philanthropic Organizations

Acoustical Society Foundation, Inc.

11 St. Ebbas Dr
Penfield, NY 14526
Phone: 1 (585) 275-8130
Fax: 1 (585) 271-8552
E-mail: asf@q.ent.rochester.edu
Web site: http://www.acousticalfoundation.org

The mission of the Acoustical Society Foundation (ASF) is to plan and carry out comprehensive fundraising activities and campaigns for the benefit of the Acoustical Society of America. . . . The goal is to help the Acoustical Society of America meet the challenges of furthering its position as a worldwide professional organization and enhance acoustical research and applications into the twenty-first century. (Acoustical Society Foundation, 2007)

American Academy of Audiology Foundation (AAAF)

11730 Plaza America Dr, Ste 300
Reston, VA 20190
Phone: 1 (703) 790-8466
E-mail: aaafoundation@audiology.org
Web site: http://www.audiologyfoundation.org/

The mission of the American Academy of Audiology Foundation is to raise funds and support programs of excellence in education, promising research, and public awareness in audiology and hearing science. (American Academy of Audiology Foundation, 2007)

The American Academy of Otolaryngology – Head and Neck Surgery Foundation (AAO-HNSF)

One Prince St
Alexandria, VA 22314-3357
Phone: 1 (703) 836-4444
TTY: 1 (703) 519-1585
Web site: http://www.entnet.org

The . . . [AAO-HNS] Foundation sponsor[s] continuing medical education, professional meetings, new scientific research, and practice management guidance for more than 11,000 ear, nose, and throat specialists in the United States and abroad. (AAO-HNS Foundation, 2007)

American Hearing Research Foundation (AHRF)

8 South Michigan Ave, Ste #814
Chicago, IL 60603-4539
Phone: 1 (312) 726-9670
Fax: 1 (312) 726-9695
E-mail: ahrf@american-hearing.org
Web site: http://www.american-hearing.org

The AHRF serves two vital roles: to fund significant research in hearing and balance disorders, and to help educate the public. They fund eight to ten research projects per year, with an average grant of $20,000. (AHRF, 2007)

The American Speech-Language-Hearing Foundation (ASHFoundation)

10801 Rockville Pike
Rockville, MD 20853
Phone: 1 (301) 296-8700
E-mail: foundation@asha.org
Web site: www.ashfoundation.org

[The ASHFoundation's] . . . mission is to advance knowledge about the causes and treatment of hearing, speech, and language problems. [They] . . . raise funds from individuals, corporations, and organizations to support research, graduate education, and special projects that foster discovery and innovation in the field of communication sciences.

Audiology Foundation of America

8 North Third St, Ste 406
Lafayette, IN 47901-1247

Phone: 1 (765) 743-6283
E-mail: info-afa@audfound.org
Web site: http://www.audfound.org/

The goal of the Audiology Foundation of America is to transform audiology into a healthcare profession with the Doctor of Audiology (Au.D.) as the first professional degree. The AFA is committed to fostering the education and training of these audiologists and to promote the autonomous practice of audiology for the benefit of the general public. (AFA, 2007)

Better Hearing Institute (BHI)

Better Hearing Institute
515 King St, Ste 420
Alexandria, VA 22314
Phone: 1 (703) 684-3391
E-mail: mail@betterhearing.org
Web site: http://www.betterhearing.org

BHI is a not-for-profit corporation that educates the public about the neglected problem of hearing loss and what can be done about it. They are working to erase the stigma that prevents people from seeking help for hearing loss, show the negative consequences of untreated hearing loss, [and] promote treatment for hearing loss. (Better Hearing Institute, 2007)

Deafness Research Foundation (DRF)

2801 M St NW
Washington, D.C. 20007
Phone: 1 (202) 719-8088
Toll-Free: 1 (866) 454-3924
TTY: 1 (888) 435-6104
Fax: 1 (202) 338-8182
E-mail: info@drf.org
Web site: http://www.drf.org/

DRF is the leading national source of private funding for basic and clinical research in hearing and balance science. Since its founding in 1958, DRF has awarded almost 1,900 grants, totaling over $23 million. (Deafness Research Foundation, 2007; DRF Web site)

The EAR Foundation

PO Box 330867
Nashville, TN 37203
Toll-Free (voice/TDD): 1 (800) 545-HEAR
Phone (voice/TDD): 1 (615) 627-2724
Fax: 1 (615) 627-2728
E-mail: info@earfoundation.org
Web site: http://www.earfoundation.org/index.asp

The EAR Foundation exists for three basic purposes: to provide the general public support services, to provide practicing ear specialists continuing medical education courses, [and] to educate young people and adults about hearing preservation and early detection of hearing loss. (EAR Foundation, 2007)

FLD Tinnitus Assistance Fund

PO Box 5
Portland, OR 97207-0005
Toll-Free: 1 (800) 634-8978
Phone: 1 (503) 248-9985
Fax: 1 (503) 248-0024
E-mail: tinnitus@ata.org
Web site: http://www.ata.org

The Fund will offer individual financial assistance grants up to $1,500 per person for tinnitus evaluation, treatment, devices, and travel in order to help patients who would otherwise be unable to afford or access healthcare services. (American Tinnitus Association, 2007)

Hear the World Foundation

Phonak AG
Laubisrütistr 28
CH-8712 Stäfa
Phone: +41 44 928 01 01
Fax: +41 44 928 07 07
E-mail: info@hear-the-world.com
Web site: http://www.hear-the-world.com

Hear the World is a charitable foundation that seeks to educate the public on the importance of hearing, social and emotional implications of hearing loss, and available solutions for those with hearing impairment. It provides technology and financial assistance to groups of people and research studies that work towards the improvement of the quality of life of people with hearing impairments. (Hear the World Foundation, 2007)

The Hearing and Speech Foundation

1619 East Broadway Avenue
Maryville, TN 37804
Phone: 1 (865) 977-0981
Fax: 1 (865) 980-7099
E-mail: info@handsf.org
Web site: www.hsfweb.org

The Hearing and Speech Foundation's mission is to assist low-income individuals with communication impairments, to provide training and education for professionals, and to conduct research and development to promote the best methods available for teaching the hearing- and speech-impaired. (The Hearing and Speech Foundation, 2007)

Helen Keller Foundation for Research & Education

Laura Beckwith
Executive Director
1201 11th Ave S, Ste 300
Birmingham, AL 35205
Phone: 1 (860) 306-2496
Fax: 1 (386) 424-1809
E-mail: laura_beckwith@bellsouth.net
Web site: http://www.helenkellerfoundation.org/home.asp

Based on the legacy of Helen Keller, the Foundation strives to prevent blindness and deafness by advancing research and education. The Foundation aspires to be a leader in integrating sight, speech, and hearing research with the greater biomedical research community, creating and coordinating a peer-reviewed, worldwide network of investigators and institutions. (Helen Keller Foundation, 2007)

Hope for Hearing Foundation

5855 Green Valley Cir, Ste 305
Culver City, CA 90230
Phone: 1 (310) 410-0900
Fax: 1 (310) 410-0080
Web site: http://hope4hearing.org/index.html

The mission of Hope for Hearing is to support various research projects, to educate the community, and to help hearing-impaired children and adults with a Community Outreach Program consisting of a Hearing Loss Workshop, counseling, and lip-reading. (Hope for Hearing, 2007)

International Hearing Foundation (IHF)

701 25th Ave S
Minneapolis, MN 55454
Phone: 1 (612) 339-2120
E-mail: trp-mmp@prodigy.net
Web site: http://www.internationalhearingfoundation.org/

The IHF has a threefold mission of service, education, and research. The foundation is dedicated to learning more about hearing problems, about cures, and to educate doctors around the world. IHF sponsors support groups for patients and their families to help them cope with chronic ear disease. (International Hearing Foundation, 2007)

Lions Sight & Hearing Foundation

3427 North 32nd St
Phoenix, AZ 85018-5606
Phone: 1 (602) 954-1723
Fax: 1 (602) 954-1768
E-mail: office@ls-hf.org
Web site: http://www.lions-sight-and-hearing-foundation.org

The Lions Sight & Hearing Foundation "helps people afflicted with sight and hearing impairments," regardless of their Lions Club affiliation. Their mission is "to restore these senses whenever possible through competent medical care." (Lions Sight & Hearing Foundation, 2007)

The Oticon Foundation

William Demants og Hustru Ida Emilies Fond
Kongebakken 9
DK-2765 Smørum
Denmark
Phone +45 3917 7100
Fax +45 3927 7900
E-mail: fonden@oticon.dk
Web site: www.oticonfonden.dk

As one of the world's oldest foundations, the Oticon Foundation sponsors social and educational programs, publications, conferences, cultural activities, and campaigns—both for researchers, hearing care professionals, and the general public. (Oticon, 2007d)

The Starkey Hearing Foundation

6700 Washington Ave S
Eden Prairie, MN 55344
Phone: 1 (800) 769-2799
Fax: 1 (952) 828-6946
Web site: http://www.sotheworldmayhear.org/

The Starkey Hearing Foundation delivers more than 20,000 hearing aids annually through more than 100 hearing missions a year in countries stretching from the United States to Vietnam. Besides giving the gift of hearing, the Foundation promotes hearing health awareness while supporting research and education. (Starkey Hearing Foundation, 2007)

List of Acronyms and Terms

AGC-O:	automatic gain control output compression
AZ:	audio zoom
BiCROS:	bilateral contralateral routing of signals; type of hearing instrument
BTE:	behind-the-ear hearing instrument
CAMISHA:	computer-aided manufacturing of individual shells for hearing aids
CIC:	completely-in-the-canal hearing instrument
CROS:	contralateral routing of signals; type of hearing instrument
Crossover:	a hearing-instrument form factor coined by Unitron to describe their device that sits in the ear like a CIC but includes the benefits of an open-fit device
D:	directional microphone
DAI:	direct audio input
DM:	directional microphone with microphone matching
dAZ:	digital audio zoom
dSZ:	digital surround zoom
form factor:	This refers to the style of hearing instrument, such as BTE, ITE, and the like.
FS:	full shell
HS:	half shell
ITC:	in-the-canal hearing instrument
ITE:	in-the-ear hearing instrument
MC:	mini canal
MIC:	mini in the canal

Moda:	Unitron's open-fit BTE collection
mZ:	mini zoom
open-ear:	*see* open fit
open-fit:	a fitting form factor marked by a digital BTE with feedback cancellation technology and a nonoccluding, noncustom ear mold
OTE:	on the ear
P:	power
RIC:	receiver in canal
RIE:	receiver in ear
RITE:	receiver-in-the ear
SSVC:	screw-set volume control
SP:	super power
UP:	ultra power
VC:	volume control
VC-A:	absolute analog volume control
WDRC:	wide dynamic range compression
WTC:	wireless transfer communication

References

AAO-HNS Foundation. (2007). American Academy of Otolaryngology – Head and Neck Surgery Foundation. Retrieved March 5, 2007, from http://www.entlink.net/academy/mission/history.cfm

About. (2009). Cheers for Wisconsin's cochlear implant/hearing aid bill. Retrieved June 18, 2009, from http://deafness.about.com/b/2009/05/16/cheers-for-wisconsins-cochlear-implanthearing-aid-bill.htm

Acoustical Society Foundation. (2007). Acoustical Society Foundation. Retrieved March 5, 2007, from http://www.acousticalfoundation.org

AFA. (2007). Audiology Foundation of America. Retrieved March 5, 2007, from http://www.audfound.org/index.cfm?pageID=8

American Academy of Audiology Foundation. (2007). American Academy of Audiology Foundation. Retrieved March 5, 2007, from http://www.audiologyfoundation.org

American Hearing Research Foundation (AHRF). (2007). About us. Retrieved March 5, 2007, from http://www.american-hearing.org/about.html

American Tinnitus Association. (2007). American Tinnitus Association. Retrieved March 5, 2007, from http://www.ata.org

ASHA (2009). State insurance mandates for hearing aids. Retrieved June 16, 2009, from http://www.asha.org/advocacy/state/issues/ha_reimbursement.htm#ri

ASHFoundation. (2007). American Speech-Language-Hearing Foundation. Retrieved March 5, 2007, from http://www.ashfoundation.org/foundation

Audiology Foundation of America (AFA). (2005). $10,000 Donation from GN ReSound Funds AuD Education. Retrieved February 27, 2007, from http://www.audiologyonline.com/news/news_detail.asp?news_id=1791

AudiologyOnline. (2006a). AFA/ReSound Scholarships now available. Retrieved February 27, 2007, from http://www.audiologyonline.com/news/news_detail.asp?news_id=2113

AudiologyOnline. (2006b). GN enters into agreement to sell GN ReSound to Phonak. Retrieved February 27, 2007, from http://www.audiologyonline.com/news/news_detail.asp?wc=1&news_id=2285

AudiologyOnline (2008). Colorado sends children's hearing aid insurance mandate to governor's desk. Retrieved June 16, 2009, from http://www.audiologyonline.com/news/news_detail.asp?news_id=3265

Bartnik, G., Faijanska, J., & Rogowski, M. (1999). Our experience in treatment of patients with tinnitus and/or hyperacusis using the habituation method. In J. W. P. Hazell (Ed.), *Proceedings of the Sixth International Tinnitus Seminar 1999*, 415–417. London: The Tinnitus and Hyperacusis Centre.

Beck, D. (2005). Interview with Cameron Hay, president and CEO, Unitron Hearing. Retrieved February 27, 2007, from http://www.audiologyonline.com/interview/interview_detail.asp?wc=1&interview_id=335

Bernafon. (2006a). 60 years of innovative hearing instruments from Bern. Retrieved February 20, 2007, from http://www.bernafon.com/eprise/main/_downloads/10_UK_English/Bernafon/Press/PressReleases/060901_PressReleaseEnglish.pdf

Bernafon. (2006b). The Bernafon Group at a glance. Retrieved February 20, 2007, from http://www.bernafon.com/eprise/main/_downloads/10_UK_English/Bernafon/Press/PressReleases/060901 Fact_sheet_Bernafon.pdf

Bernafon. (2007a). Company milestones. Retrieved February 20, 2007, from http://www.bernafon.com/eprise/main/com_en/Corporate/AboutBernafon/BernafonHistory/CompanyMilestones

Bernafon. (2007b). Personal communication with Shayla on February 23, 2007.

Bernafon. (2009). The World of Bernafon. Bern, Switzerland: Bernafon.

Better Hearing Institute. (2007). About BHI. Retrieved March 5, 2007, from http://www.betteringhearing.org/about

Blue Cross Blue Shield of Rhode Island. (2009). Medical Coverage Policies: Hearing Aid Mandate. Retrieved June 16, 2009, from https://www.bcbsri.com/BCBSRIWeb/plansandservices/services/medical_policies/HearingAidMandate.jsp

Christman, W. (2007). Personal communication.

Clemens, M., & Sørensen, T. W. (2003, October 2). Hearing aid industry: In best shape ever (pp. 1–28). Denmark: Carnegie Securities Research.

Davis, A., & Refaie, A. E. (2000). Chapter 1: Epidemiology of Tinnitus. In R. S. Tyler (Ed.), *Tinnitus Handbook* (pp. 1–24). San Deigo, CA, Thomson Delmar Learning.

Deafness Research Foundation. (2007). About. Retrieved March 5, 2007, from http://www.drf.org/about/about.htm

Dobie, R. A., & Sullivan, M. D. (1997). Antidepressant drugs and tinnitus. In J. A. Vernon (Ed.), *Tinnitus: Treatment and Relief* (pp. 43–51). Boston: Allyn & Bacon.

Dorich, A. (2005, June). Connecting lives: Unitron hearing of Ontario says it works to make life easier for the end user. *US Business Review*, 166–167.

EAR Foundation. (2007). About. Retrieved March 5, 2007, from http://www.earfoundation.org/about.asp

Erlandsson, S. I. (2000). Psychological profiles of tinnitus patients. In R. S. Tyler, (Ed.), *Tinnitus Handbook* (p. 37). San Diego, CA, Thompson Delmar Learning.

Feussner, J. (1998) Clinical research in the Department of Veterans Affairs: Using research to improve patient outcomes. *J Invest Med*, 46, 264–267.

Folmer, R. L., & Carroll, J. R. (2006). Long-term effectiveness of ear-level devices for tinnitus. *Otolaryngology – Head and Neck Surgery*, 134, 132–137.

GHI. (2009). General Hearing Instruments. Retrieved June 23, 2009, from http://www.generalhearing.com/explore.cfm

GHI. (2007). Personal communication with Stephanie on February 23, 2007.

Global Markets Direct. (2008a). GN ReSound A/S Company Profile. *Global Markets Direct*, 1–28.

Global Markets Direct. (2008b, August 30). Sonic Innovations, Inc. Company Profile. *Global Markets Direct*.

Gretler, C. (2004). Hearing devices: Holt Review. Credit Suisse First Boston Holt – Small & Mid-Cap Advisor, pp. 1–3.

Gretler, C. (2006). Phonak: FY 2006 results comment. Credit Suisse Equity Research Europe, June 2, 2006, pp. 1–8.

Gretler, C., Hilliker, I., & Beford, T. (2008). Hearing Device Industry. Credit Suisse Equity Research Europe, September 8, 2008, pp. 1–22.

Handelsbanken. (2006a, March 8). William Demant. Company update: Equity research, Handelsbanken. *Capital Markets*, 1–24.

Handelsbanken. (2006b, October 4). W Demant Holding: Poised to benefit from new industry order. Company update: Equity research, Handelsbanken. *Capital Markets*, 1–15.

Healthy Hearing. (2009a). Federal employee hearing aid insurance benefits take effect January 1. Retrieved June 16, 2009, from http://www.healthyhearing.com/releases/33780-federal-employee-hearing-aid

Healthy Hearing. (2009b). Senator Harkin reintroduces hearing aid tax credit and expands coverage to people of all ages. Retrieved June 16, 2009, from http://www.healthyhearing.com/releases/39208-senator-harkin-reintroduces-hearing

Hear the World Foundation. (2007). Hear the World Foundation. Retrieved March 5, 2007, from http://www.hear-the-world.com

Hearing Loss Association of America. (2009). State mandates for hearing aid insurance. Retrieved June 16, 2009, from www.hearingloss.org/advocacy/govtassistance.asp

Hearing Loss Web. (2009). Hearing aid insurance legislation update. Retrieved June 18, 2009, from http://www.hearinglossweb.com/Issues/Access/EquipmentCost/HearingAids/HAIns/rak.htm and http://www.hearinglossweb.com/Issues/Access/EquipmentCost/HearingAids/HAIns/rakb.htm

Hearing Review. (2005). GN ReSound donates $10,000 to AFA. Retrieved November 16, 2007, from http://www.hearingreview.com/issues/articles/

Hearing Review. (2008). Colorado Passes Hearing Aid Insurance Mandate for Kids. Retrieved June 16, 2009, from www.hearingreview.com/insider/2008-05-29_10.asp

Hearing Review. (2009a). Oticon's campaign nets $50k donation to AAAF. Retrieved June 24, 2009, from http://www.hearingreview.com/news/2009-05-01_04.asp

Hearing Review. (2009b). Sonic Innovations parent company renamed Otix Global. Retrieved June 16, 2009, http://www.hearingreview.com/news/2009-06-16_03.asp

Hearing and Speech Foundation. (2007). Mission. Retrieved March 5, 2007, from http://www.discoveret.org/hsf/mission.htm

Helen Keller Foundation. (2007). About the foundation. Retrieved March 5, 2007, from http://www.helenkellerfoundation.org/foundation.asp

Henry, J. A. Effectiveness of TRT judged by Tinnitus Severity Index. Personal communication.

Henry, J. A., Jastreboff, M. M., & Jastreboff, P. J. (2002). Assessment of patients for treatment with tinnitus retraining therapy. *Journal of the American Academy of Audiology, 1*, 523–544.

Henry, J. A., Schechter, M. A., Nagler, S. M., & Fausti, S. A. (2002). Comparison of tinnitus masking and tinnitus retraining therapy. *Journal of the American Academy of Audiology, 13*, 559–581.

Henry, J. A., Schechter, M. A., Zaugg, T. L., Griest, S., Jastreboff, P. J., Vernon, J. A., et al. (2006). Outcomes of clinical trial: tinnitus masking versus tinnitus retraining therapy. *Journal of the American Academy of Audiology, 17*, 104–132.

Henry, J. A., Trune, D. R., Robb, M. J. A., & Jastreboff, P. J. (2007). *Tinnitus retraining therapy: Clinical guidelines* (pp. 57–60). Abingdon, UK: Plural Publishing Inc.

Herraiz, C., Hernandez, F. J., & Machado, A. (1999). Tinnitus retraining therapy: Our experience. In J. W. P. Hazell (Ed.), *Proceedings of the Sixth International Tinnitus Seminar 1999* (pp. 483–484). London: The Tinnitus and Hyperacusis Centre.

Herraiz, C., Hernandez, F. J., Plaza, G., & de los Santos, G. (2005). Long-term clinical trial of tinnitus retraining therapy. *Otolaryngology – Head and Neck Surgery, 133*, 774–779.

HJ Report. (2003). HJ Report. *The Hearing Journal, 56*, 6–7.

Hoffman, L. (2007). Disability claims soar from Bush's wars. Capitol Hill Blue. Retrieved February 2, 2009, from http://www.capitolhillblue.com/cont/node/2689

Hoffman, H. J. & Reed, G. W. (2004). Chapter 3: Epidemiology of tinnitus. In J. B. Snow (Ed.), *Tinnitus: Theory and Management* (pp. 16–41). Hamilton, Ontario BC Becker, Inc.

Hope for Hearing. (2007). What Is Hope for Hearing? Retrieved March 5, 2007, from http://www.hope4hearing.org

International Hearing Foundation. (2007). About us. Retrieved March 5, 2007, from http://www.internationalhearingfoundation.org/aboutus.html

Jastreboff, M. M. & Jastreboff, P. J. (1999). Questionnaires for assessment of the patients and their outcomes. In J. W. P. Hazel (Ed.), *Proceedings of the Sixth International Tinnitus Seminar* (pp. 48–91). London: The Tinnitus and Hyperacusis Centre.

Jastreboff, P. J. (1998). Tinnitus: The method of Pawel J. Jastreboff. In G. Gates (Ed.), *Current Therapy in Otolaryngology – Head and Neck Surgery* (pp. 90–95). St. Louis, MO: Mosby-Year Book Inc.

Jastreboff, P. J. (1999). Categories of the patients in TRT and the treatment outcome. In J. W. P. Hazell (Ed.), *Proceedings of the Sixth International Tinnitus Seminar 1999* (pp. 394–398). London: The Tinnitus and Hyperacusis Centre.

Jastreboff, P. J., & Hazel, J. W. (2004). *Tinnitus Retraining Therapy: Implementing the Neurophysiological Model* (pp. 83–84). Cambridge, UK, Cambridge University Press.

Jastreboff, P. J., & Jastreboff, M. M. (2000). Tinnitus retraining therapy (TRT) as a method for treatment of tinnitus and hyperacusis patients. *Journal of the American Academy of Audiology, 11*, 162–177.

Jastreboff, P. J., & Jastreboff, M. M. (2006). Tinnitus retraining therapy: A different view on tinnitus. *ORL, 68*, 23–30.

Jones, D. (2006). Will wireless ALD hybrids save the hearing industry? *The Hearing Review, 13*(1), 38.

Kaltenbach, J. A. (2000). Neurophysiological mechanisms of tinnitus. *Journal of the American Academy of Audiology, 11*, 125–137.

Kirkwood, D. (2006). Phonak to buy ReSound Group. *The Hearing Journal, 59*(11), 7.

Klemme, K. (2008a). Starkey Laboratories wins Spark Design Award for Zōn™. Retrieved October 20, 2009, from http://www.starkeypro.com/public/pdfs/pr_spark_award_1008.pdf

Klemme, K. (2008b). Starkey's Zōn™ wins the Smithsonian's Cooper-Hewitt, National Design Museum's 2008 People's Design Award. Retrieved October 27, 2008, from http://www.starkeypro.com/public/pdfs/pr_cooper-hewitt_award.pdf

Kochkin, S. (2003). MarkeTrak VI: On the issue of value: Hearing aid benefit, price, satisfaction, and repurchase rates. *The Hearing Review, 10*(2), 12–26.

Kochkin, S. (2004). An open letter from Sergei Kochkin to the hearing healthcare community. *The Hearing Journal, 47*(3), 41.

Kochkin, S. (2005). MarkeTrak VII: Hearing loss population tops 31 million people. *The Hearing Review, 12*(7), 16–29.

Kochkin, S. (2009). MarkeTrak VIII: 25-year trends in the hearing-health market. *The Hearing Review, 16*(11), 12-31.

Kochkin, S., & Tyler, R. (2008). Tinnitus treatment and the effectiveness of hearing aids: Hearing care professional perceptions. *The Hearing Review, 15*(13), 14–18.

Krcmar, S. (2006, January/February). The general at General Hearing. Hearing products report.

Lane, E. (2009). Boston-Power's Battery Technology to Boost HP PCs. *Green Tech Media.* Retrieved February 2, 2009, from http://greenlight.greentechmedia.com/

2009/01/15/boston-power%E2%80%99s-battery-technology-to-boost-hp-pcs-976/

Lesiecki, W. (2006). Does the in-office electronic scanning of impressions really change everything? *The Hearing Review, 13*(1), 32–35, 94.

Life Sciences Analytics. (2008, August 14). Sonic Innovations, Inc. Company Profile Reports, Life Science Analytics Inc.

Lions Sight & Hearing Foundation. (2007). Lions Sight and Hearing Foundation. Retrieved November 28, 2007, from http://www.lions-sight-and-hearing-foundation.org

Lite, J. (2007). Iraq & Afghanistan war vets suffer from hearing loss, tinnitus. *New York Daily News.* Retrieved February 2, 2009, from http://www.nydailynews.com/lifestyle/health/2007/11/11/2007-11-11_iraq_afghanistan_war_vets_suffer_from_h.html

Lockwood, A. H., Salvi, R. J., & Burkard, R. F. (2002). Tinnitus. *New England Journal of Medicine, 347*(12), 904–910.

LSHA. (2009). ACT 816 insurance mandate for children's hearing aids legislation. Retrieved June 18, 2009, from http://www.lsha.org/2003_legislation.htm

Management Decision and Research Center, Department of Veterans Affairs. (1998). Clinical Practice Guidelines. Boston: Management Decision and Research Center; Washington, D.C.: VA Health Services Research and Development Service in collaboration with Association for Health Services Research.

McKinney, C. J., Hazell, J.W.P., & Graham, R. L. (1999). An evaluation of the TRT method. In J. W. P. Hazell (Ed.), *Proceedings of the Sixth International Tinnitus Seminar 1999* (pp. 99–105). London: The Tinnitus and Hyperacusis Centre.

Micro-Tech. (2003). Selective amplification systems. Plymouth, MN: Author.

Micro-Tech. (2006a). Micro-Tech hearing instruments. Retrieved June 23, 2006, from http://www.hearing-aid.com/Docs/AboutMicroTech.htm

Micro-Tech. (2006b). Mission. Retrieved June 23, 2006, from http://www.hearing-aid.com/Docs/Mission.htm

Mueller, H. G. (2006). Open is in. *The Hearing Journal, 59*(11), 11–13.

Myers, D. (2005). Heard around the world! Hearing aid compatibility and wireless assistive devices. *The Hearing Review, 12*(1), 22–25, 86.

National Institute on Deafness and Other Communication Disorders (NIDCD). (2009). Quick Statistics. Retrieved June 16, 2009, from http://www.nidcd.nih.gov/health/statistics/quick.htm

Neuromonics. (2009). Helping you help patients take back control over tinnitus. Retrieved January 23, 2009, from http://www.neuromonics.com/professional/treatment/index.aspx?id=138

New Mexico State Legislature. (2007). Relating to insurance; requiring insurance coverage for hearing aids for eligible children. Retrieved June 22, 2009, from http://legis.state.nm.us/Sessions/07%20Regular/final/SB0529.pdf

Newman, C. W., Sandridge, S. A., & Jacobson, G. P. (1998). Psychometric adequacy of the Tinnitus Handicap Inventory (THI) for evaluating treatment outcome. *Journal of the American Academy of Audiology, 9,* 153–160.

Nickish, C. (2008). Boston Co. gets a charge out of laptop batteries. *National Public Radio's Morning Edition.* Retrieved February 2, 2009, from http://www.npr.org/templates/story/story.php?storyId=98435455

Northern, J. L., & Beyer, C. (1999). Hearing aid returns analyzed in search for patient and fitting patterns. *The Hearing Journal, 52*(7), 46–52.

Oticon. (2007a). About Oticon. Retrieved February 20, 2007, from http://www.oticon.com/eprise/main/Oticon/com/SEC_AboutUs/AboutOticon/_Index

Oticon. (2007b). About OtoKids. Retrieved March 4, 2007, from http://www.otikids.com/eprise/main/Oticon/com/SEC_Products/SEC_OtiKids/Parents/AboutUs/_Index

Oticon. (2007c). Oticon through the years. Retrieved February 20, 2007, from http://www.oticon.com/eprise/main/Oticon/com/SEC_AboutUs/AboutOticon/OticonThroughTheYears/_Index

Oticon. (2007d). The Oticon Foundation. Retrieved February 20, 2007, from http://www.oticon.com/eprise/main/Oticon/com/SEC_AboutUs/AboutOticon/CNT01_OticonFoundation

Oticon. (2008a). Beauty & Brains by Desing! Retrieved October 30, 2009, from http://www.oticon.com/com/Information/PressReleases/downloads/oticon_dual_pressrelease.pdf

Oticon. (2008b). New Vigo Pro and Vigo offer more performance, choice and value in attractively priced hearing instruments. Retrieved October 30, 2009, from http://www.oticon.com/com/Information/PressReleases/downloads/vigo_press_release_uk.pdf

Oticon. (2009). Oticon through the years. Retrieved June 23, 2009, from http://www.oticon.com/com/AboutOticon/CorporateCulture/OticonThroughTheYears/index.htm

Parkhøi, M. (2006, October 2). *William Demant: The consolidation game is on* (pp. 1–5). London: Danske Equities.

Parkhøi, M., & Jessen, P. E. (2003, January 6). Medical technology, hearing industry: Further consolidation on the way? (pp. 1–9). London: Danske Equities.

Parkhøi, M., & Jessen, P. E. (2005, October 18). Health equipment and supplies, hearing aids: A view from three players (pp. 1–5). London: Danske Equities.

Phonak. (2006a). The world of sound: Investor presentation. Stafa: Author.

Phonak. (2006b, October 2). Phonak and ReSound join forces. Phonak Holding AG Media Release.

Phonak. (2007). Sonova information leaflet: The holding company of the Phonak Group shall be named Sonova Holding AG (p. 1). Switzerland: Phonak Group.

Phonak. (2009). Phonak history & product milestones. Retrieved June 24, 2009, from http://www.phonak.com/company/profile/product_milestones.htm

ReSound. (2003). Warranties terms services. Bloomington, MN: Author.

Rhode Island State House. (2006). Assembly approves increase in hearing aid coverage. Retrieved June 18, 2009, from http://www.rilin.state.ri.us/news/pr1.asp?prid=3412

Ricketts, T., Mueller, H. G., & Armstrong, S. (2007, April 19). Open canal fittings: It's not your father's "Tube Fit." Presented at the Annual Conference of the American Academy of Audiology. Denver, CO.

Sheldrake, J. B., Hazell, J. W. P., & Graham, R. L. (1999). Results of tinnitus retraining therapy. In J. W. P. Hazell (Ed.), *Proceedings of the Sixth International Tinnitus Seminar 1999* (pp. 292–296). London: The Tinnitus and Hyperacusis Centre.

Siemens. (2005). Products and services price guide: Effective October 1, 2005. Piscataway, NJ: Siemens Hearing Instruments.

Siemens. (2006a). Siemens. Retrieved June 23, 2006, from http://www.siemens.com

Siemens. (2006b). Siemens Hearing Instruments. Retrieved June 23, 2006, from http://www.siemens-hearing.com

Siemens. (2006c). Siemens Hearing Instruments. Retrieved June 23, 2006, from http://www.siemens-hearing.com/geninfo/aboutus_a1.aspx

Siemens. (2006d). Siemens Hearing Instruments. Retrieved June 23, 2006, from http://www.siemens-hearing.com/geninfo/history_a1.aspx

Siemens. (2006e). Siemens Hearing Instruments. Retrieved June 23, 2006, from http://www.siemens-hearing.com/geninfo/timeline_a1.aspx

Siemens. (2006f). Annual report 2006. Munich, Germany: Author.

Siemens. (2007). Personal communication, July 23, 2007.

Siemens. (2009a). Family Guide. Piscataway, NJ: Author.

Siemens. (2009b). Our Employees. Retrieved November 10, 2009 from http://w1.siemens.com/annual/08/en/glance/employees.htm

Siemens Foundation. (2005a). Siemens Foundation. Retrieved June 23, 2006, from http://www.siemens-foundation.org/about/

Siemens Foundation. (2005b). Siemens Teacher Scholarships. Retrieved June 23, 2006, from http://siemens-foundation.org/TeacherScholarhip/

Simonian, H. (2007, August 10). Sonova pulls out of ReSound deal. *The Australian Business*. Retrieved November 10, 2007, from http://www.theaustralian.news.com.au/story/0,25197,22216884-36375,00.html

Sonic. (2008a). Sonic Innovations: About. Retrieved September 23, 2008, from http://www.sonici.com/consumer/aboutsonic/default.aspx

Sonic. (2008b, May 22). Sonic Innovations established donation fund for the armed forces foundation. Sonic Innovations: Company Press Release.

Sonic. (2008c). Mission, Vision and Values. Retrieved September 23, 2008, from http://www.sonici.com/corporate/mission/default.aspx

Sonic. (2008d, June 12). Sonic Innovations teams up with hearing clinics across the country to provide free hearing screenings. Sonic Innovations: Company Press Release.

Starkey. (2006a). Starkey Laboratories. Retrieved June 23, 2006, from http://www.starkey.com

Starkey. (2006b). Starkey Laboratories. Retrieved June 23, 2006, from http://www.starkey.com/pages/yhi/yhiWarrantyTypes.html

Starkey. (2006c). About Starkey. Retrieved June 23, 2006, from http://www.starkey.com/pages/about/index.html

Starkey. (2006d). Starkey innovations. Retrieved June 23, 2006, from http://www.starkey.com/pages/about/aboutInnovations.html

Starkey. (2009a). Starkey Audiology Series presents Paul Pessis, Au.D., Alan Freint, M. D., and Gyl Kasewurm, Au.D. Retrieved June 17, 2009, from http://www.starkeypro.com/public/corporate/news/news/200906_sas_class.jsp

Starkey. (2009b). Starkey introduces the next generation of hearing aids: S Series with drive architecture. Retrieved April 2, 2009, from http://www.starkeypro.com/public/corporate/news/news/200904_s_series.jsp

Starkey. (2007). Starkey Laboratories. Personal communication.

Starkey Hearing Foundation. (2009, April). So the world may hear. Retrieved from http://www.sotheworldmayhear.org/uploads/newsletters/q2newsletter.pdf

Starkey Hearing Foundation. (2006a). The Starkey Hearing Foundation. Retrieved March 5, 2007, from http://www.sotheworldmayhear.org/aboutus/

Starkey Hearing Foundation. (2006b). About us. Retrieved June 23, 2006, from http://www.sotheworldmayhear.org/forms/hearnow.php

Starkey Hearing Foundation. (2006c). World Focus. Retrieved June 23, 2006, from http://www.sotheworldmayhear.org/worldfocus/index.php

Starkey Marketing Services. (2005a, August 20). Starkey Hearing Foundation's gala raises record $4 million-plus. Starkey Marketing Services.

Starkey Marketing Services. (2005b, September 7). Starkey Laboratories offers $40 million for Katrina relief efforts. Starkey Marketing Services.

State of Illinois. (2009). Bill status of SB0068: 96th General Assembly. Retrieved June 18, 2009, from http://www.ilga.gov/legislation/BillStatus.asp?DocNum=68&GAID=10&DocTypeID=SB&SessionID=76

State of Virginia. (2009). HB 237 Health Insurance; mandated coverage for hearing aids for minors. Retrieved June 18, 2009, from http://leg1.state.va.us/cgi-bin/legp504.exe?081+sum+HB237

State of Wisconsin. (2009). 2009 Senate Bill 27. Retrieved June 18, 2009, from http://www.legis.state.wi.us/2009/data/SB-27.pdf

Strom, K. E. (2001). *The Hearing Review* 2000 Dispenser Survey. *The Hearing Review, 8*(6), 20–42.

Strom, K. E. (2006). Hal-Hen & Widex USA celebrate landmarks. *The Hearing Review, 13*(11), 40–48.

Strom, K. (2007). Happier returns? Retrieved June 19, 2009, from http://www.hearingreview.com/issues/articles/2007-05_09.asp

Stursberg, S. (2005, December 15). Phonak: Initiation of coverage with a buy rating. Equity Note, Sarasin.

Stursberg, S. (2006, October 26). Phonak in the fast lane. Auerbach Grayson, Western European Large Cap Research.

Unitron. (2009a). About Unitron. Retrieved June 24, 2009, from http://www.unitron.com/us/ccus/about_us.htm

Unitron. (2009b). New Passport premium hearing instrument exemplifies Unitron's commitment to purpose-driven innovation. Retrieved June 24, 2009, from http://www.unitron.com/us/ccus/about_us/news_us/news_passport_us.htm

Unitron. (2009c). Unitron unveils new company brand identity and two new products at Audiology NOW! 2009. Retrieved June 24, 2009, from http://www.unitron.com/us/ccus/about_us/news_us/news_brand_us.htm

Vernon, J. A. & Meikle, M. B. (2000). Tinnitus masking. In R. S. Tyler (Ed.), *Tinnitus Handbook*. San Diego, CA, Thomson Delmar Learning.

Veterans Benefits Administration. (2006). Annual Benefits Report: Fiscal Year 2006.

Wayner, D. S. (2005). Aural rehabilitation adds value, lifts satisfaction, cuts returns. *The Hearing Journal, 58*(12), 30–38.

Yanz, J. (2006). The future of wireless devices in hearing care. *The Hearing Review, 13*(1), 18–20, 93.

Zable, J., & Anand, A. (2008, August 6). Sonic Innovations: First call note. Natixis Bleichroeder, Medical Devices.

Index

631